D1567943

Veterinary Hematology

and Clinical Chemistry

Veterinary Hematology

and Clinical Chemistry

Mary Anna Thrall, D.V.M., M.S., D.A.C.V.P.

Professor, Department of Microbiology, Immunology,
and Pathology
College of Veterinary Medicine and Biomedical Sciences
Colorado State University
Fort Collins, Colorado

Dale C. Baker, D.V.M., Ph.D., D.A.C.V.P.

Pathologist, Genentech, Inc.
South San Francisco, California

Terry W. Campbell, D.V.M., Ph.D.

Professor, Department of Clinical Sciences
College of Veterinary Medicine and Biomedical Sciences
Fort Collins, Colorado

Dennis DeNicola, D.V.M., Ph.D., D.A.C.V.P.

Chief Veterinary Educator
IDEXX Laboratories
North Grafton, Massachusetts

Martin J. Fettman, D.V.M., M.S., Ph.D., D.A.C.V.P.

Associate Dean, College of Veterinary Medicine and
Biomedical Sciences
Colorado State University
Fort Collins, Colorado

E. Duane Lassen, D.V.M., Ph.D., D.A.C.V.P.

Professor, Department of Microbiology, Immunology,
and Pathology
College of Veterinary Medicine and Biomedical Sciences
Colorado State University
Fort Collins, Colorado

Alan Rebar, D.V.M., Ph.D., D.A.C.V.P.

Dean, School of Veterinary Medicine
Purdue University
West Lafayette, Indiana

Glade Weiser, D.V.M., D.A.C.V.P.

Vice President, Diagnostics/Clinical Pathologist
Heska Corporation
Fort Collins, Colorado

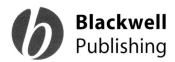

Blackwell
Publishing

Blackwell Publishing Professional
2121 State Avenue, Ames, Iowa 50014, USA

Orders: 1-800-862-6657
Office: 1-515-292-0140
Fax: 1-515-292-3348
Web site: www.blackwellprofessional.com

Blackwell Publishing Ltd
9600 Garsington Road, Oxford OX4 2DQ, UK
Tel.: +44 (0)1865 776868

Blackwell Publishing Asia
550 Swanston Street, Carlton, Victoria 3053, Australia
Tel.: +61 (0)3 8359 1011

Library of Congress Cataloging-in-Publication Data
Veterinary hematology and clinical chemistry / Mary Anna Thrall; co-authors, Dale C.
   Baker ... [et al.].
      p. ; cm.
   Includes bibliographical references and index.
   ISBN-13: 978-0-7817-6850-4

   1. Veterinary hematology. 2. Veterinary clinical chemistry. I. Thrall, Mary Anna.
[DNLM: 1. Hematologic Diseases—veterinary. 2. Clinical Chemistry Tests—methods. 3.
Hematologic Diseases—diagnosis. 4. Laboratory Techniques and Procedures. SF 769.5
V586 2001]
SF769.5.V48 2001
636.0899615—dc21   00-061850

The last digit is the print number: 9 8 7 6 5

The authors wish to dedicate this book to their mentors, the pioneers in veterinary clinical pathology. In particular, the book is dedicated to Drs. Maxine Benjamin, Oscar Schalm, and J. J. Kaneko for their respective first-generation textbooks addressing veterinary clinical pathology, hematology, and clinical chemistry, and their inspiration to many subsequent careers in veterinary clinical pathology. Mary Anna Thrall also wishes to thank Dr. Maxine Benjamin for her generosity, patience, and friendship.

PREFACE

There will be a supplemental book available that contains over 50 detailed case studies, grouped by primary system abnormality, to help you to recognize patterns of disease and boost your diagnostic accuracy. This free supplement will be available to all who purchase this main text. Please contact Lippincott Williams & Wilkins at (800) 638-3030 and a copy will be forwarded to you.

The publication of Veterinary Hematology and Clinical Chemistry marks a new and unique contribution to veterinary clinical pathology. The product of a collaborative effort by a team of experts in the field, this text combines critical information about performing diagnostic tests, viewing pertinent clinical pathology, and interpreting laboratory data with an innovative approach to incorporating color visual content.

AUDIENCE

A current trend in the field is the movement of laboratory diagnostics into the veterinary facility, enabled by technological advancements in point-of-care diagnostic capability. This movement to in-house testing increases the need for education in veterinary clinical pathology. Although this book was written primarily for veterinary students and practitioners, it has applications for a much broader audience, serving as a useful adjunct for the educational and reference needs of a variety of other users. The following audiences will benefit from this resource:

- Students in professional veterinary medical education programs
- Veterinary health professional teams in veterinary care facilities
- Veterinary clinical pathologists and clinical pathologists in training
- Research and product development groups utilizing veterinary clinical pathology

ORGANIZATION

Veterinary Hematology and Clinical Chemistry is organized into six parts, arranged as follows:

- Part I presents principles of laboratory technology and test procedures used in veterinary labs to generate laboratory results.
- Part II presents hematology and hemopathology of common domestic species. This includes all aspects of the hemogram or complete blood count, bone marrow, hemostasis, and transfusion medicine.
- Part III presents hematology of common nondomestic species encountered in veterinary practice.
- Part IV presents clinical chemistry of common domestic species and is organized primarily by organ system.
- Part V presents clinical chemistry of common nondomestic species.

UNIQUE ART PROGRAM

Many aspects of veterinary clinical pathology are highly visual. The most unique feature of this book is the quantity and quality of color artwork. This was facilitated by digital image acquisition and processing performed by the authors. Optimization and standardization of images was performed by digital image engineering techniques to achieve an improvement in imagery over what is possible with conventional photomicrography. Our goal was to bring a new level of realism to the visual communication of concepts pertaining to microscopy. In some instances, visual content has been amplified by combining images from multiple microscopic fields into a single figure or showing different levels of magnification within the same figure. Digital image engineering also allows for image manipulation; an example is arrangement of cells that are randomized on a microscope field into a specific order to convey a concept such as cell maturation. We believe that the fidelity of visual imagery, as well as its liberal integration with text content, makes this work the first of its kind.

AUTHOR TEAM

Contributing content and expertise to this project are a number of recognized authorities in the field of veterinary clinical pathology. These individuals have helped shape the existing curriculum, train the existing faculty, and create the disciplines of comparative laboratory medicine and diagnostic cytology as we know them today. It is through the combined efforts of so many experts in the field that this book was made possible.

We hope you find this publication to be an excellent resource in the clinical laboratory and for laboratory data interpretation.

M. G. Weiser and M. A. Thrall
Fort Collins, Colorado

CONTENTS

SECTION THREE
HEMATOLOGY OF COMMON NONDOMESTIC MAMMALS, BIRDS, REPTILES, FISH, AND AMPHIBIANS

SECTION FOUR
CLINICAL CHEMISTRY OF COMMON DOMESTIC SPECIES

SECTION FIVE

CLINICAL CHEMISTRY OF COMMON NONDOMESTIC MAMMALS, BIRDS, REPTILES, FISH, AND AMPHIBIANS

O N E

GENERAL PRINCIPLES

OF LABORATORY TESTING

AND DIAGNOSIS

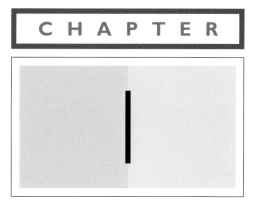

CHAPTER

1

LABORATORY TECHNOLOGY
FOR VETERINARY MEDICINE

This chapter presents an overview of the laboratory technology used to generate data for hematology and clinical biochemistry. For the procedures and technologies likely to be employed within veterinary hospitals, general instructions and descriptions provide a review of the principles previously learned in laboratory courses. This, in conjunction with the instructions accompanying different devices and consumables, should enable users to reproduce the procedures to a satisfactory performance standard. For technologies more likely to be used only in large commercial or research laboratories, the overview provides familiarity with the basic principles.

HEMATOLOGIC TECHNIQUES

Basic Techniques Applicable for any Veterinary Hospital

The procedures outlined here are most appropriate for the in-house veterinary laboratory in most practice settings. These procedures require minimal investment in equipment and technical training. These basic hematologic procedures include:

▪ Blood mixing
▪ Packed cell volume or hematocrit by centrifugation
▪ Plasma protein estimation by refractometry

▪ Leukocyte concentration by Unopette (Becton Dickinson, East Rutherford, NJ) dilution and hemocytometer microscopy
▪ Preparation of blood films
▪ Differential leukocyte count and blood film examination

Blood Mixing

The blood sample generally is assumed to have been freshly and properly collected into an ethylenediaminetetraacetic acid (EDTA) tube (as described in Chapter 2). When performing any hematologic procedure, it is important that the blood is thoroughly mixed. Cellular components may settle rapidly while the tube sits on a counter or in a tube rack *(Fig. 1.1)*. As a result, failure to mix the sample before removing an aliquot for hematologic measurement may result in a serious error. Mixing can be performed by manually tipping the tube back and forth a minimum of 10 to 15 times (Fig. 1.1). Alternatively, the tube may be placed on a rotating wheel or tilting rack designed specifically to mix blood *(Fig. 1.2)*.

Packed Cell Volume

The packed cell volume value is the percentage of whole blood composed of erythrocytes. It is measured in a

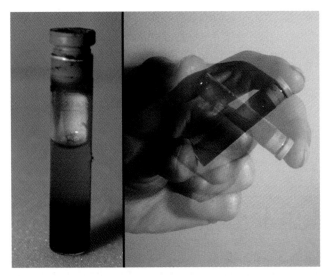

Figure 1.1 **Left.** Gravity sedimentation of whole blood. **Right.** A gentle, repetitive, back-and-forth tube inversion technique used to manually mix blood before removing aliquots for hematologic procedures.

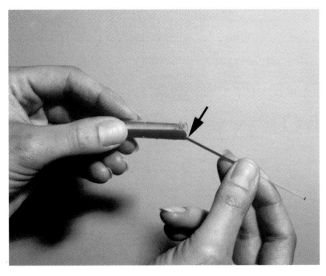

Figure 1.3 Proper technique for filling a microhematocrit tube. The tube should be positioned horizontally or tilted slightly downward to facilitate filling by capillary action. Capillary action is established by touching the upper end of the tube to the blood (arrow).

column of blood after centrifugation that results in maximal packing of the erythrocytes. Tools for performing the packed cell volume include 75- × 1.5-mm tubes (i.e., microhematocrit tubes), tube sealant, a microhematocrit centrifuge, and a tube-reading device.

The procedure is performed using the following steps. First, the microhematocrit tube is filled via capillary action by holding it horizontally or slightly downward and then touching the upper end to the blood of the opened EDTA tube *(Fig. 1.3)*.

Next, allow the tube to fill to approximately 70% to 90% of its length. Hold the tube horizontally to prevent blood from dripping out of the tube, and seal one end by pressing the tube into the tube sealant once or twice *(Fig. 1.4)*. Note that air may be present between the sealant and the blood (Fig. 1.4). This is not a problem, however, because the trapped air is removed during centrifugation.

The tube is then loaded into the microhematocrit centrifuge according to the manufacturer's instructions

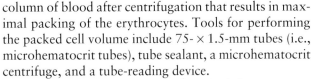

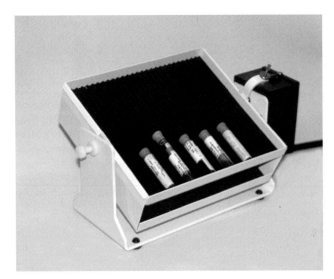

Figure 1.2 Representative mechanical blood-mixing table. The surface holds several tubes on a ribbed rubber surface and tilts back and forth at the rate of 20 to 30 oscillations per minute.

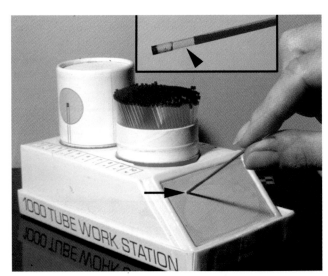

Figure 1.4 A microhematocrit tube is sealed by pressing two to three times into the clay sealant (arrow). Note that a small amount of air trapped between the blood and white clay is not a problem (arrowhead in the inset).

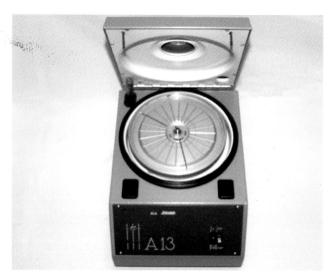

Figure 1.5 Representative microhematocrit centrifuge. The head and motor are designed to spin the tubes at very high speeds to achieve maximal erythrocyte packing.

(Figs. 1.5 and 1.6). The microhematocrit centrifuge is designed to spin the lightweight tube at very high speeds to generate sufficient centrifugal force to completely pack the red cells within 2 to 3 minutes. With such centrifugal force, most (or all) of the plasma is removed from the layer of packed red cells.

Three distinct layers that may be observed in the tube after removal from the centrifuge: the plasma column at the top, the packed erythrocytes at the bottom, and a small, middle white band known as the buffy coat

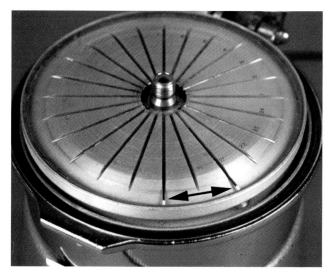

Figure 1.6 Placement of microhematocrit tubes on a micro-hematocrit centrifuge head. Note the proper orientation of two microhematocrit tubes, with the clay-sealed end positioned at the outer ring of the centrifuge head (double arrow).

(Fig. 1.7). The buffy coat consists of nucleated cells (predominantly leukocytes) and platelets, and it may be discolored red when the nucleated erythrocyte concentration is prominently increased. Observations of any abnormalities in the plasma column above the red cells should be recorded. Common abnormalities such as icterus, lipemia, and hemolysis are shown in Fig. 1.7. Icterus is excessively yellow pigmentation of the plasma column that suggests hyperbilirubinemia; the magnitude of this hyperbilirubinemia should be confirmed by a biochemical determination of serum bilirubin concentration (see Chapter 23). The observation of an icteric coloration to the plasma is diagnostically useful in small animals. It is not reliable in large animal species, however, because their serum usually has a yellow coloration from the normal carotene pigments associated with their herbivorous diet. Lipemia is a white, opaque coloration of the plasma column because of the presence of chylomicrons. Lipemia most commonly is associated with the postprandial collection of blood, but it also may be associated with disorders in-

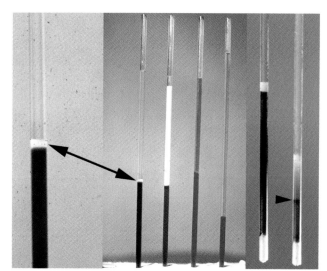

Figure 1.7 Normal and abnormal spun microhematocrit tubes (4 tubes in middle panel). The tube on the left is normal. Note the packed erythrocytes at the bottom, plasma layer at the top, and buffy coat in the middle (arrow; enlarged at left). The second tube illustrates lipemia, the third hemolysis, and the fourth icterus. Note also that the hematocrit is considerably decreased in the fourth tube. Two additional tubes illustrate buffy-coat abnormalities (enlarged at right). The first of these tubes has an increased buffy coat that correlates with an increased leukocyte concentration. The second (right) is from a sheep with leukemia and has a dramatically increased buffy coat. The leukocyte concentration was greater than 400,000 cells/μL. There is also severe anemia. With such major abnormalities in cell concentration, separation of erythrocytes and leukocytes is not complete, and division may be blurred. What is interpreted as being the "top" of the erythrocyte column is indicated by the arrowhead. The red discoloration of the buffy coat may be caused by a prominent increase in nucleated erythrocytes.

volving lipid metabolism (see Chapter 28). Hemolysis is a red discoloration of the plasma column, which usually results from artifactual lysis of red cells induced during the collection of blood. A small quantity of lysed erythrocytes is sufficient to impart visual hemolysis. Therefore, if the hematocrit is normal, one may assume it is an artifact. Less commonly, causes of anemia that result in intravascular hemolysis give rise to observable hemolysis in the plasma fraction, which also is known as hemoglobinemia (see Chapter 8).

The packed cell volume is measured on a reading device, such as a microhematocrit card reader *(Fig. 1.8)*. The procedure is performed by positioning the erythrocyte—clay interface on the 0 line and the top of the plasma column on the 100 line. The position of the top of the erythrocyte column then is read on the scale as the packed cell volume.

Plasma Proteins by Refractometry

After measurement and observation of the microhematocrit tube, the plasma column may be used to measure the plasma protein concentration on the refractometer *(Fig. 1.9)*. This instrument may be used to estimate the concentration of any solute in fluid according to the principle that the solute refracts (or bends) light passing through the fluid to a degree that is proportional to the solute concentration. The principle or property being measured is

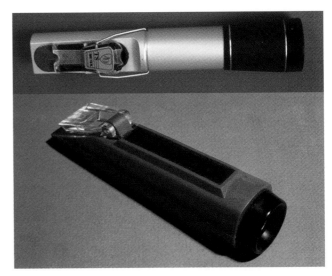

Figure 1.9 Refractometers. The lower refractometer is more rugged, because it is encased in rubber. It is known as a veterinary refractometer, and it has a canine and feline urine specific gravity scale that calibrates for minor differences between species during this determination.

the refractive index relative to distilled water. The scale for a particular solute can be developed from refractive index measurements calibrated to solutions with known solute concentrations. In clinical diagnostics, refractometry is used to estimate the plasma protein concentration and urine specific gravity.

Plasma protein is measured using the plasma column in the microhematocrit tube. The tube is broken above the buffy coat layer *(Fig. 1.10)*, and the portion of the tube containing the plasma is used to load the refractometer

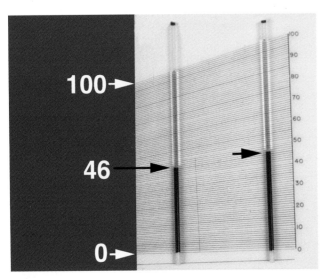

Figure 1.8 Determination of packed cell volume on a microhematocrit tube card reader using two tubes of blood from the same patient sample. Note that the scale allows the tube to be read over a considerable range of filling levels. The steps are to line up the erythrocyte–clay interface with the 0 line, line up the top of the plasma column with the 100 line, and then read the top of the erythrocyte column on the scale. The positions of these steps are indicated by the arrows. Note in this example that the packed cell volume is 46%.

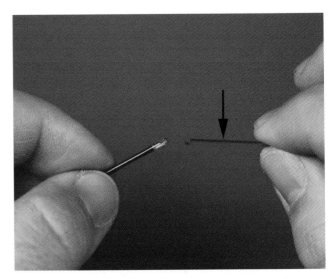

Figure 1.10 Preparation of the microhematocrit tube for measuring plasma protein concentration. The tube is broken just above the buffy coat to yield a column of plasma (arrow).

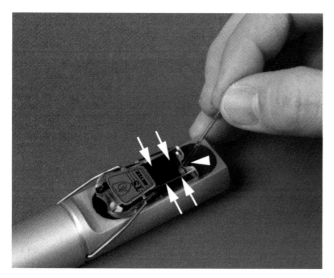

Figure 1.11 Loading plasma from the microhematocrit tube to the refractometer. To wick plasma onto the refractometer, capillary action is established by touching the end of the plasma tube at the notch of the prism cover (arrowhead). Flow should establish a thin layer of plasma under the plastic cover to fill the area delineated by arrows. After reading, the plastic cover is flipped back and wiped clean with a laboratory tissue.

(Fig. 1.11). The instrument then is held so that an ambient light source can pass through the prism wetted with plasma, and the light refraction is read on a scale through an eyepiece *(Fig. 1.12)*.

The protein measurement is regarded as being an estimate based on calibration, assuming that other solutes in the serum are present in normal concentrations. The measurement may be influenced by alterations in other solutes.

Most notably, lipemia may artificially increase the protein estimate by as much as 2 g/dL. Other alterations of solutes such as urea and glucose influence the protein estimate to a much lesser, and usually negligible, degree.

Determination of Total Leukocyte Concentration

Two general approaches are available to determine the leukocyte concentration: the Unopette dilution, which is done in conjunction with hemocytometer microscopy; and instruments designed to employ either particle counting or expanded buffy coat analysis technology. The total leukocyte count is the concentration of nucleated cells, because the techniques detect all the nuclei in solutions from which erythrocytes have been removed by lysis or centrifugation. Therefore, nucleated erythrocytes usually are included in this count.

The Unopette system consists of a commercial kit for preparing blood dilutions; it comes with detailed user instructions. The Unopette (#5853) with acetic acid diluent is recommended. In addition, a hemocytometer counting chamber and a microscope are required for enumerating cells *(Fig. 1.13)*. The Unopette capillary is used to transfer 20 μL of blood into 1.98 mL of acetic acid diluent *(Fig. 1.14)*. This results in a 1:100 dilution. The acid lyses cytoplasmic membranes, thereby eliminating erythrocytes and platelets and leaving behind nucleated particles. After appropriate incubation and mixing, an aliquot is transferred onto the hemocytometer counting chamber *(Fig. 1.15)*. The chamber then is covered by a planar coverglass, thereby creating a three-dimensional space.

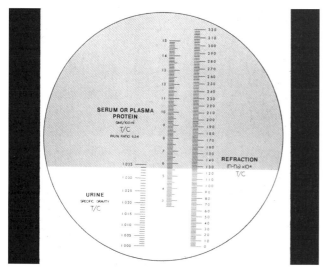

Figure 1.12 Representative refractometer scale as seen through the eyepiece. Light refraction creates a shadow–bright area interface that is read on the appropriate scale.

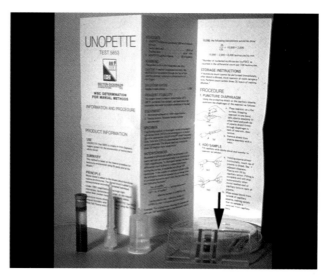

Figure 1.13 Components of the Unopette leukocyte counting system. Note the glass hemocytometer resting on a Petri dish (arrow). Other components include the blood tube, dilution capillary, reservoir of diluent, and an instruction sheet. A microscope also is required.

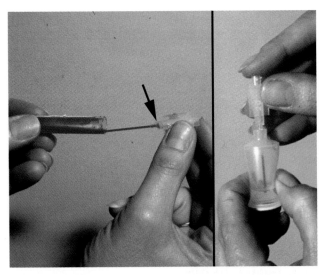

Figure 1.14 Manipulations of the Unopette capillary system. **Left.** The capillary tube is filled with blood by surface tension action and is designed to fill to the hub (arrow). Blood flows into the tube and abruptly stops at the hub. Blood on the outside of the capillary is wiped off with a laboratory tissue. **Right.** The contents of the capillary are transferred to the reservoir of diluent fluid. Squeezing gently on the reservoir moves the diluent up and down in the capillary, resulting in the complete transfer of blood, which completes the dilution step.

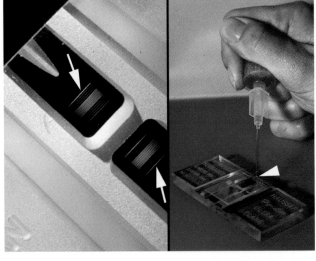

Figure 1.15 Hemocytometer. **Left.** Middle portion of the hemocytometer, where the grids are located (arrows). These grids ordinarily are not visible; they have been photographed here with polarized light to facilitate their visualization. **Right.** Technique for loading fluid from the Unopette system to the hemocytometer. Fluid is allowed to flow from the capillary under the coverglass to cover the area of the grid. (See product inserts for details.)

An etched grid marking the boundaries for the counting procedure delineate a specific volume within the space. The hemocytometer is examined using the ×10 objective. Particles are counted within all nine major squares of the counting grid *(Fig. 1.16)*, and the total volume of the area covered by the counting procedure is 0.9 μL. The leukocyte concentration of blood is calculated by taking the total number of cells counted in the grid, adding 10% (to yield the number of cells in 1.0 μL, and then multiplying this result by the dilution factor of 100. An example of such a count and its calculations is presented in Fig. 1.16. The microscopic appearance of the hemocytometer grid lines and leukocyte particles is illustrated in *Figures 1.17* and *1.18*.

More convenient instrument systems also may be used—if the user is willing to make the necessary investments in equipment. A variety of electronic cell counters operate by enumerating nuclear particles in an isotonic dilution in which a detergent is used to lyse the erythrocytes. These systems must be engineered for animal blood, however, to generate accurate measurements of cell concentrations. (For principles of operation, see the discussion of advanced hematologic procedures later in this chapter.) The quantitative buffy coat analysis system (QBC, Becton Dickinson) estimates the leukocyte concentration by measurement of the buffy coat layer in a specialized

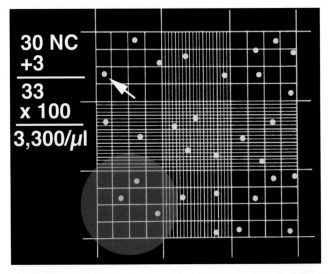

Figure 1.16 Example of a count on a hemocytometer grid and the necessary calculations. The complete grid delineating a volume of 0.9 μL is made of nine primary squares. One primary square is counted at a time using the ×10 objective. The approximate field of view with a microscope is indicated by the blue-shaded area covering the lower left primary square. Leukocyte particles (arrow) are counted while systematically moving across all nine primary squares. In this example, 30 cells are counted. Ten percent (3 cells) are added to yield the number of cells in 1.0 μL. The number of cells then is multiplied by the dilution factor (100) to give the total concentration of cells per microliter of blood.

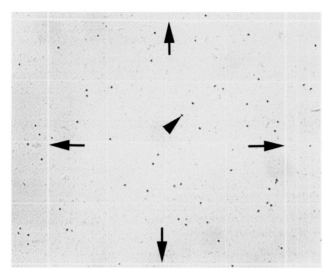

Figure 1.17   Appearance of one primary square on a hemocytometer using the ×10 objective. Note the boundaries of the square (arrows), the leukocyte particles dispersed throughout the grid, and the representative leukocyte (arrowhead).

microhematocrit tube, in which a float is present to expand the buffy coat region for optical scanning.

In isolation, the total leukocyte count is not particularly useful for interpretive purposes; this value is used to determine the concentration of various leukocyte types that make up the differential count. The concentration of individual leukocytes is the most useful value for the interpre-

tation of disease processes. This information is determined by evaluating the stained blood film (discussed later).

Preparation of Blood Films

The stained blood film is an essential tool for determining the concentrations of individual leukocyte types (i.e., differential count) and for evaluating important pathologic abnormalities involving leukocytes, erythrocytes, and platelets. Successful derivation of information from the blood film requires a proper technique, which both creates a monolayer of individually dispersed cells and a minimal disturbance of relative cell distributions that reflect the cell concentrations in mixed blood. A poorly prepared film presents confusing artifacts and may result in cell distributions on the slide that lead to serious errors in the differential count.

Preparation of a good-quality blood film requires mastery of a specific technique (*Figs. 1.19* through *1.21*). The most common procedure is known as the wedge or push technique and uses two glass microscope slides. A drop of blood is placed near one end of the first slide supported on the counter. The second slide is placed on the first in a way that forms a "wedge" consisting of a 30° to 45° angle in front of the drop of blood. The second slide, which is known as the pusher slide, then is backed into the drop of blood and advanced forward to the end. This should be accomplished in one rapid motion that involves a flip of the wrist holding the pusher slide. Downward pressure on the pusher slide should be minimal. Learning this technique in the presence of someone experienced

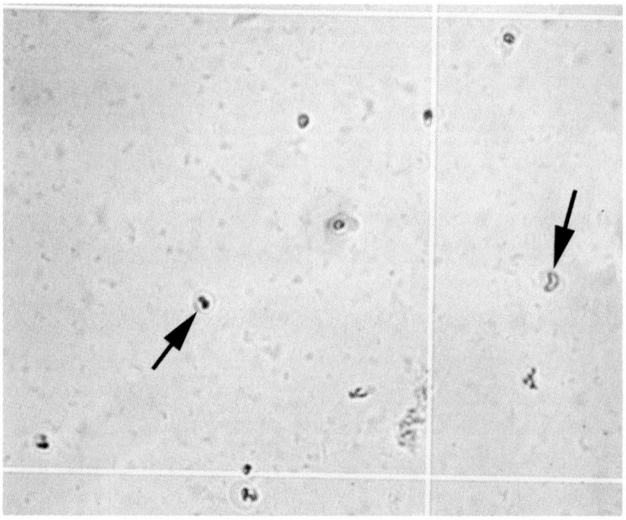

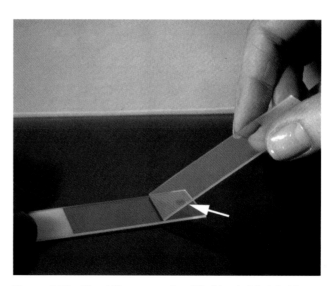

Figure 1.18   Higher-magnification view of a hemocytometer chamber. Note representative leukocytes (arrows). By focusing upward and downward, a nuclear particle surrounded by a faint halo may be visualized. Fine granular debris in the background represents erythrocyte membrane debris.

Figure 1.19   Blood film preparation. The blood slide is held on a firm surface, and a drop of blood is placed near the end (arrow). The pusher slide then is placed on the blood slide in front of the drop of blood to form an angle of approximately 30°.

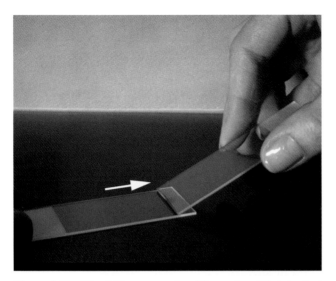

Figure 1.20 Blood film preparation. The pusher slide is backed into the drop of blood with a directional movement (arrow).

Staining

After preparation, the blood film usually is stained within minutes. However, it may be stained within hours to days if being sent to a diagnostic laboratory. The staining system used for microscopic evaluation of cellular elements is the Wright stain, or a Wright stain modified by the addition of Giemsa. This is a relatively complex procedure that requires care and maintenance, thus often being limited to larger laboratory facilities. Quick-stain procedures that mimic the classical Wright stain are available, however, and for convenience, these are the most commonly used stains in the veterinary practice setting. The best-known stain kit is Diff-Quick (Dade Diagnostics, Aguada, Peurto Rico). Quick stains may result in nuclear overstaining and blurring of chromatin detail, but they provide sufficient quality for differential leukocyte counting and screening for morphologic abnormalities. Examples of simple to complex staining systems are shown in *Figure 1.22.*

with making good films is helpful, and considerable practice is advised. A common poor technique is to push the pusher slide too slowly, thereby creating a film that is too thin. This results in very poor distribution of leukocytes at the end of the film and artifacts in the evaluation of erythrocytes. In blood with reduced viscosity, such as that from patients with severe anemia, increasing the angle to avoid a slide that is too thin is useful.

Expertise for Examination of Blood Films

Once stained, the anatomy of a blood film must be known to properly orient the slide for microscopic viewing *(Fig. 1.23)*. The largest part of the film is the thick area or

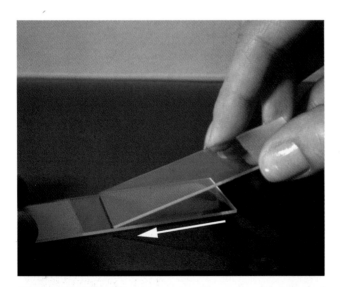

Figure 1.21 Blood film preparation. The pusher slide is pushed forward with a rapid directional movement (arrow). It is important that the movements shown in Figures 1.19 through 1.21 are a single, rapid procedure involving a flip of the wrist. Considerable practice is required to develop this skill. The result should be a uniform film of blood that gets progressively thinner (see Fig. 1.23).

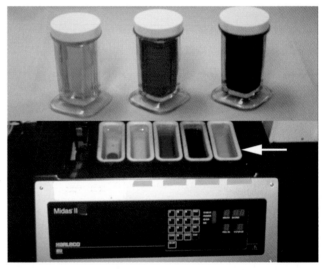

Figure 1.22 Blood film and cytology staining apparatus. **Top.** Manual staining jars containing Diff-Quick stain. Slides are manually moved from one jar to the next according to the manufacturer's instructions. **Bottom.** An automated stainer used for higher-throughput situations. Note the mechanical arm that moves a rack of slides (not shown) through the sequence of staining procedure baths (arrow). The stainer may be programmed to control the timing in each bath. Most such machines provide the ability to stain as many as 20 to 25 slides per cycle.

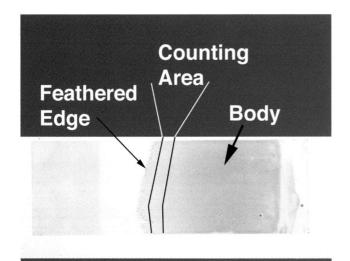

Figure 1.23 Anatomy of a stained blood film. Note the feathered edge (thin arrow) and the thick area or body of the slide (thick arrow). The counting area containing a monolayer of cells is present in a relatively small area, which is delineated approximately by the lines across the slide. This gross examination of the slide is very helpful in orienting the observer before placing the slide on the microscope stage. This facilitates alignment of the optics over the proper area of the slide, making it easier and faster to perform low-magnification observations and to find the counting area.

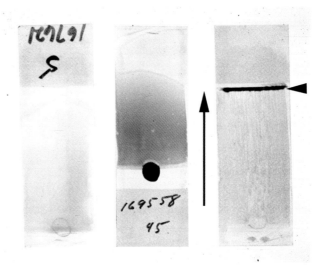

Figure 1.24 Gross appearance of blood films. All three of these films are oriented the same way. The drop of blood was placed near the bottom of the picture, and the film was made by pushing in the direction of the arrow. The middle film has a normal appearance and intensity of color. The appearance is homogeneous but gets progressively thinner as one approaches the feathered edge. The film on the left is very pale; this is the appearance when severe anemia is present. With severe anemia, blood viscosity is reduced, resulting in a much thinner film. The film on the right is made improperly and does not yield accurate information. The pusher slide was pushed too slowly, making a thin film with streaks. Note the streaking and irregularity over most of the slide. Blood was still present at the end of the slide as well, resulting in a line of densely concentrated cells (arrowhead). It is not possible to find a good monolayer for evaluation of erythrocyte morphology on this slide. In addition, the leukocytes are disproportionately concentrated at the end of the slide, which ordinarily has a feathered edge. Performing a differential count will be difficult in this case—and likely not accurate. A thin slide as a result of pushing too slowly is the most common problem in technique found at veterinary facilities.

body, in which cells are superimposed and leukocytes are rounded up, thereby making microscopic evaluation of all components difficult. The feathered edge occurs at the end of the film. Artifacts in this area include broken leukocytes and the inability to evaluate the erythrocyte central pallor. The counting area is a small area between the thick portion and the feathered edge, and it consists of a monolayer of cells in which microscopy is optimal. Leukocytes are flattened out so that the internal detail is most evident.

The amount of interpretive disease relevance that can be gained from examination of the blood film is proportional to the expertise available for the examination. Success in dealing with all components of such examination depends on the quality of film making, ability to look in the correct place, ability to differentiate preparation artifacts from morphologic abnormalities, and experience with interpretive blood film pathology. To the extent the user cannot make these distinctions, abnormal blood films should be referred to a specialist for examination and/or second opinions.

It is important to examine the gross appearance of blood films as a correlate to artifact recognition. Improper preparation can be recognized, thereby alerting the observer to artifacts that can be avoided and preventing any associated, errant interpretations. Common abnormalities

that may be recognized grossly are presented in *Fig. 1.24*. The most common and important abnormality is a slide that is too thin, which can be recognized by streaks progressing toward the feathered edge. This results in a leukocyte distribution that presents major errors in the differential count. In addition, there is not an area adequate for the evaluation of erythrocyte abnormalities.

The observer should locate the counting area using the 10× objective. The feathered edge is recognized by a loss of erythrocyte central pallor and a reticulated pattern of erythrocyte distribution on the film *(Fig. 1.25)*. Quick, low-power examination of the feathered edge is useful for the detection and identification of abnormalities such as microfilaria, platelet clumps, and unusual, large cells that are preferentially deposited here *(Fig. 1.26)*. The thick area is recognized by a progressive superimposition

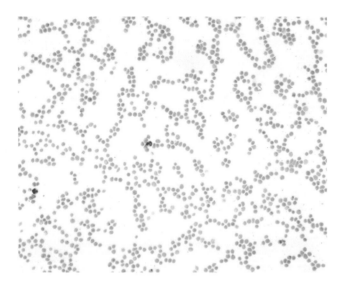

Figure 1.25 Low-magnification appearance of the feathered edge. Note the reticulated pattern of erythrocyte distribution. Artifactual loss of central pallor makes evaluation of erythrocyte morphology difficult, and false interpretation of pathologic abnormalities is likely to occur in this area.

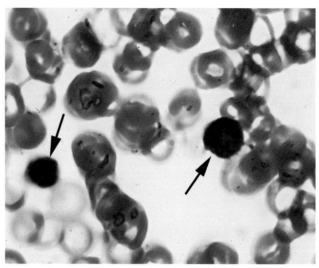

Figure 1.27 High-magnification appearance of cells in the thick area or body of slide. Note the superimposition of erythrocytes, thus making evaluation of erythrocyte morphology difficult. In addition, specifically identifying leukocytes (arrows) is difficult to impossible. In this area, leukocytes are spherical or rounded-up rather than flattened. It is not possible to see intracellular detail or even the delineation between the cytoplasm and the nucleus.

of cells as the observer moves further into the thick area of the slide. In very thick areas, the evaluation of cells is severely compromised *(Fig. 1.27)*. The counting area is recognized by a monolayer of evenly dispersed cells *(Fig. 1.28)*.

Once the counting area is located, the experienced observer can estimate the leukocyte concentration on a well-prepared blood film. This is useful as a quality-control measure, and it is recommended that the observer gain

experience at this by repetitive comparison of leukocyte density on well-prepared blood films with total leukocyte counts from a reliable procedure. The low-power appearances of a leukocyte count in the normal range, marked leukopenia, and marked leukocytosis are shown in *Figures 1.29, 1.30,* and *1.31*, respectively.

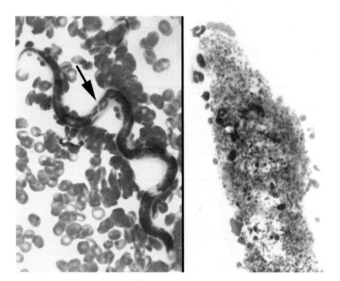

Figure 1.26 Large items pushed to the feathered edge. **Left.** Microfilaria (arrow) in an animal with heartworm disease. **Right.** A large clump of platelets with trapped leukocytes. Several hundred platelets are contained in this microclot.

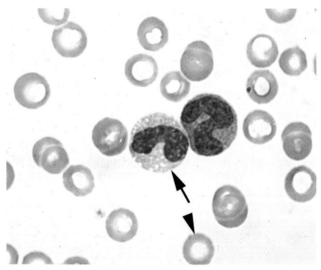

Figure 1.28 High-magnification appearance of cells in the counting area or monolayer. Note the minimal superimposition of erythrocytes, which facilitates evaluation of erythrocyte morphology (arrowhead). Leukocytes (arrow) are flattened on the slide, which makes it possible to see details of the cytoplasm and nucleus. Note that the nuclear borders are sharply delineated from the surrounding cytoplasm.

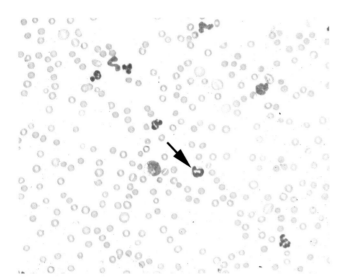

Figure 1.29 Low-magnification appearance of the counting area. Note the evenly dispersed cells and the ability to visualize the erythrocyte central pallor. The density of leukocytes (arrow) is that expected with a leukocyte concentration in the normal range.

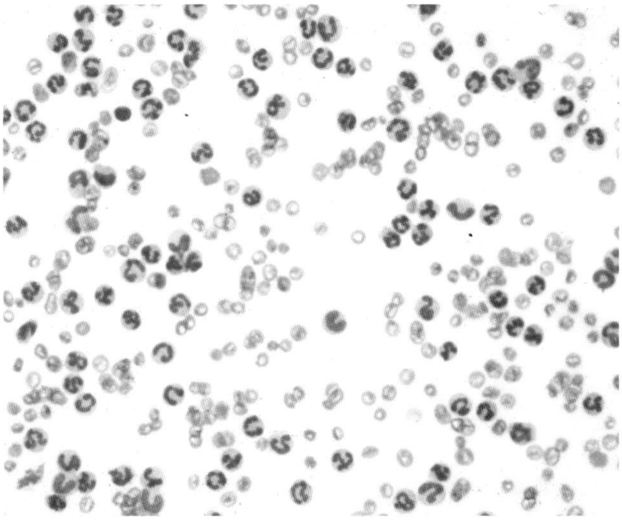

Figure 1.31 Low-magnification appearance of the counting area with a marked increase in leukocyte concentration. The density of leukocytes is considerably greater than that seen in Figure 1.29.

Procedures Using the 100×, Oil-Immersion Objective

Once the counting area is located, these assessments are completed and the microscope adjusted for high-power observation, and the observer should perform a systematic evaluation of the three major cell lines. This includes a differential count for leukocytes, evaluation of erythrocyte morphology, and evaluation of platelet numbers.

The differential leukocyte count is performed by counting a minimum of 100 consecutively encountered cells as the observer moves across fields within the counting area. Cells are classified into a minimum of five to six categories, with the presence of abnormal cells being recorded into a category of "other," in which a specification is made for the individual sample. The common six categories of cells—neutrophil, band neutrophil, lymphocyte, monocyte, eosinophil, and basophil—are shown in *Figure 1.32*. (See Chapter 10 for additional visual details regarding leukocyte identification that may be helpful in differential counts.)

The result of counting 100 cells is that the number of each leukocyte type is a fraction of 100, or a percentage of the leukocyte population. Once cells are categorized into percentages, they must be converted to absolute numbers for interpretation purposes. This is done by multiplying the total leukocyte concentration by the percentage of each leukocyte type, which yields the absolute number or concentration of each leukocyte in the blood sample. The following example illustrates the conversion of percentages to absolute numbers:

Example 1.1. Conversion of Percentage Counts to Absolute Concentrations

Total white-blood-cell count = 10,000

Differential white-blood-cell count:

	Percentages	Absolute Numbers/μL
Neutrophils	60%	(6000)
Lymphocytes	30%	(3000)
Monocytes	5%	(500)
Eosinophils	5%	(500)

Any abnormalities in leukocyte morphology also should be noted. Important morphologic abnormalities are detailed in Chapter 12.

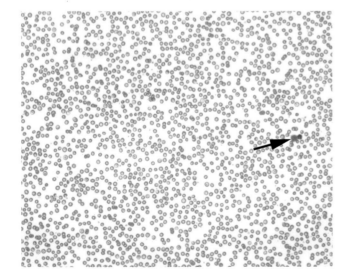

Figure 1.30 Low-magnification appearance of the counting area with a marked decrease in the leukocyte concentration. A rare leukocyte per field is present (arrow).

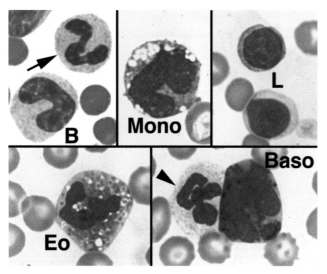

Figure 1.32 Basic leukocytes encountered in the differential count. **Upper left.** Neutrophils. Note the asegmented neutrophil (arrow) and the constrictions in the nuclear contour. The band neutrophil (B) has smooth, parallel nuclear contours. **Upper middle.** Monocyte (Mono). The nucleus may have any shape, from round to bean-shaped to ameboid and band-shaped, as in this example. The cytoplasm is blue-gray and may variably contain vacuoles. **Upper right.** Two lymphocytes (L). **Lower left.** An eosinophil (Eo). Note that granules stain similar to the surrounding erythrocytes. Occasionally, granules may wash out in the staining procedure, leaving vacuoles. **Lower right.** Basophil (B) with dark granules that stain similar to nuclear chromatin. Note the adjacent neutrophil (arrowhead) and that neutrophils may have small, poorly staining granules that are much smaller than those of eosinophils or basophils.

Erythrocyte morphology then is systematically evaluated. The observer should note any important erythrocyte shape or color abnormalities; this is particularly important for evaluating anemias. (See Chapter 5 for a review of morphologic erythrocyte abnormalities.)

The presence of platelet adequacy may be interpreted from a properly prepared blood film. A minimum of 6 to 10 platelets per high-power (×1000) field may be interpreted as adequate. The number seen may be considerably greater than this, however, because of the wide range of normal platelet concentrations. This number is only a guideline for most microscopes with a wide field of view. It should be adjusted downward when using a microscope with a narrow field of view and upward if using one with a superwide field of view. If the platelets appear to be decreased, a search for platelet clumps on a low-power setting at the feathered edge should be performed. Morphology of platelets also may be noted. Platelets that approach the diameter of erythrocytes or larger are referred to as macroplatelets. In dogs, these suggest accelerated platelet regeneration, but this interpretation usually is not applied to macroplatelets in cats.

Advanced Hematologic Techniques Usually Performed in Commercial Laboratories

Hemograms performed in commercial laboratories provide some additional measurements that are obtained using automated instrumentation. Some of this capability now also exists in some hematology analyzers available for use in veterinary practices. A trend during the past 10 to 15 years has been a decreasing cost of producing basic automated hematology equipment, thereby making such instrumentation affordable for use in many veterinary clinics. The predominant differences of the larger, more expensive systems used by commercial laboratories are throughput rate, automated tube handling, and sophisticated differential counting technology. (See Chapter 2 for additional discussion of equipment and laboratories.)

Values or measurements provided by more advanced techniques include:

Items determined by spectrophotometry or calculation:
   Hemoglobin concentration of blood, g/dL
   Mean cell hemoglobin content, pg/dL
   Mean cell hemoglobin concentration (MCHC), g/dL

Items determined by cell (particle) counting and sizing:
   Erythrocyte concentration of blood, $\times 10^6$ cells/μL
   Mean cell volume (the average size of erythrocytes; MCV), fL
   Hematocrit (equivalent to the packed cell volume), %
   Platelet concentration of blood, cells/μL
   Total and differential leukocyte concentrations, cells/μL

The method and applicability for each of these measurements are now described.

Items Determined by Spectrophotometry or Calculation

Hemoglobin Concentration. This measurement of the quantity of hemoglobin per unit volume, expressed as g/dL, is performed in conjunction with the total leukocyte count. Briefly, a blood sample is diluted, and a chemical agent is added to rapidly lyse cells, thereby liberating hemoglobin into the fluid phase. Nucleated cells remain present in the form of a nucleus with organelles collapsed around it. A chemical such as potassium cyanide may be present in the lytic agent to rapidly convert the hemoglobin to a stable pigment, such as cyanmethemoglobin. The absorbance of light at a specific wavelength then may be measured by spectrophotometry in a small flow cell known as a hemoglobinometer. The absorbance of light is proportional to the concentration of hemoglobin. The system is calibrated with material of known hemoglobin concentration using reference techniques.

Interpretation of the hemoglobin concentration is the same as that of the packed cell volume. It is an index of the red cell mass per unit volume of blood in the patient. Because it is roughly equivalent to the packed cell volume, however, it is not particularly useful for clinical interpretations. Most clinicians are more familiar or experienced with interpreting packed cell volumes. Still, a nuance is that the hemoglobin value may serve as a quality-control adjunct for laboratory personnel when used to calculate the MCHC.

Mean Cell Hemoglobin. The mean cell hemoglobin is calculated from the hemoglobin concentration and erythrocyte concentration. It is regarded as being redundant to other measurements and, therefore, is not useful.

Mean Cell Hemoglobin Concentration. The MCHC is calculated from the hemoglobin concentration and the hematocrit. It provides an index for the quantity of hemoglobin (HGB) relative to the volume of packed erythrocytes (expressed as g/dL):

$$\frac{\text{HGB (g/dL)}}{\text{PCV (\%)}} \times 100 = \text{MCHC (g/dL)}$$

where PCV is the packed cell volume. An example calculation is

$$\frac{10 \text{ g/dL}}{30\%} \times 100 = 33.3 \text{ g/dL}$$

A universal relationship among mammalian species, other than the camel family, is that the hemoglobin value normally is approximately one-third of the hematocrit value. Thus, from the relationship described, the MCHC for all mammalian species ranges from approximately 32 to 36 g/dL. Because members of the camel family (camel, llama, alpaca, vicuna) have relatively more hemoglobin within their cells, their MCHCs are expected to range from 41 to 45 g/dL.

The MCHC is not particularly useful for clinical interpretations; however, it is useful to laboratorians for monitoring instrument performance. The rationale is that the packed cell volume and hemoglobin are determined on different blood aliquots, which are diluted in two different subsystems of the instrument. A malfunction in either of these subsystems may result in a mismatch between the hemoglobin and the packed cell volume, which is reflected by a deviation from range of the 32 to 36 g/dL. In addition, some abnormalities of blood can result in an artifactually increased MCHC, and these can include any factor that causes a false increase in the spectrophotometric determination of hemoglobin relative to the packed cell volume. Hemolysis in the sample is a common cause of an increased MCHC. Alternatively, common examples of increased turbidity that interfere with light transmittance are lipemia and a very large number of Heinz bodies (see Chapter 8) in cats.

Two erythrocyte responses related to anemia may be associated with a slightly decreased MCHC. The first is marked regenerative anemia. Reticulocytes or polychromatophilic cells are still synthesizing hemoglobin and, therefore, have not yet attained the cellular hemoglobin concentration of a mature erythrocyte. A very high fraction of reticulocytes is required, however, such as greater than 20%, to develop a detectable decrease in MCHC. The second is severe iron deficiency, in which cells have a reduction in hemoglobin content because they are smaller (i.e., microcytic) but also may have a minor reduction in cellular hemoglobin concentration. There are no causes of a dramatically decreased MCHC (<28 g/dL) other than an analytic instrument error.

Items Determined by Cell (Particle) Counting and Sizing

Cell Counting and Sizing Technologies. A brief overview of cell counting and sizing technology common to all of these measurements is now appropriate. One of two technologies are used by most hematology instrument systems.

The first is light-scatter measurement of cells passing through a light source. Cells are passed through a flow cell that is intersected by a focused laser beam. The physical properties of the cell scatter light to different degrees and at different angles relative to the light source. Cell passages eliciting scatter events may be counted to derive the cell concentration. The degree of scatter in the direction of the light beam, which is known as forward-angle scatter, is proportional to the size of the cell. In addition, measurement of light scattered to different angles may be correlated with cellular properties, which leads to the ability to differentiate cell types. Light-scatter technology currently is limited to more expensive instrumentation used only in large laboratories.

The second is more common and incorporated into a wider range of instrument designs, some of which are affordable in veterinary hospital settings. This is electronic cell counting, which is also known as impedance technology or Coulter technology (after the original inventor). It is based on the principle that cells are suspended in an electrolyte medium, such as saline, that is a good conductor of electricity. The suspended cells, however, are relatively poor conductors of electricity. Thus, these cells impede the ability of the medium to conduct current in this sensing zone. By simultaneously passing current and cells through a small space or aperture, deflections in current can be measured (*Fig. 1.33*). In addition, the size of the cell is proportional to the resultant deflection in current.

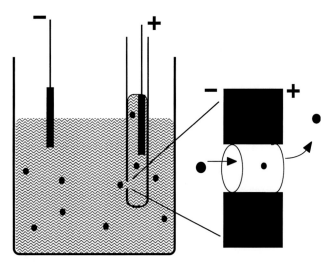

Figure 1.33 Principle of electronic impedance cell counting. **Left.** Overview of the fluidic chamber. Cells (dots) are diluted in an isotonic fluid (wavy lines). Two electrodes (+ and –) are separated by a glass tube containing a small opening or aperture. Electric current is conducted by the isotonic fluid across the electrodes via the aperture. Vacuum is applied to move the fluid and cells through the aperture. **Right.** Magnified, diagrammatic view of the aperture. Cells flow through the aperture (arrows). The aperture is a cylindric shape with a volume called the sensing zone. Although occupying space within the aperture, cells transiently impede the flow of current. Cell passages are counted as deflections in the current voltage. In addition, the magnitude of voltage deflection is proportional to the volume of the cell.

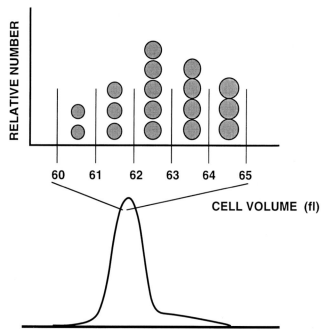

Figure 1.34 Cell volumes assigned to size bins. In the case of erythrocytes, a cell volume scale of approximately 30 to 250 fL is divided into a large number of discrete size bins (e.g., 60–61 fL, 61–62 fL). As the cells are counted, they are assigned to size bins (circles). Accumulation of many cells allows the construction of a size distribution histogram on the cell-volume scale (curve tracing at bottom). The drawing of bins at the top would represent a small area of the total curve.

The principle of size discrimination may be used to measure the size distribution of erythrocytes, to discriminate platelets from erythrocytes, and to differentiate leukocytes. Cells within a given population are counted and assigned to a size distribution by particle-size analyzer circuitry *(Fig. 1.34)*. The particle-size analyzer assigns each cell to a size scale that is divided into a large number of discrete size "bins" of equal size. The size scale is calibrated with particles of known size. By rapidly accumulating several thousand cells, a frequency distribution of the sizes of the cell population may be constructed *(Fig. 1.35)*.

The size distribution curve is most useful for the evaluation of erythrocytes in the laboratory. It also may be used analytically, however, by the instrument to derive leukocyte differential and platelet information.

The following measurements derive from the described cell counting and sizing technology. Because of the considerable differences in erythrocyte and platelet sizes between species, instrument systems require careful design and/or adjustment to accurately obtain the various measurements. For example, instruments manufactured for the analysis of human blood do not perform accurately for most animal species without modification.

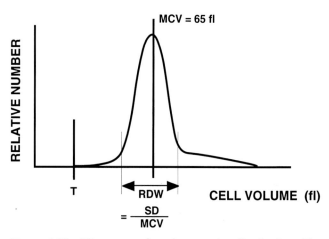

Figure 1.35 Histogram of erythrocyte size distribution. The *x*-axis is the cell volume, and the *y*-axis is the relative number of cells at each volume. Only cells above a specified volume or threshold are included in the analysis; this is indicated by the vertical bar (T). The mean cell volume (MCV) is indicated by the large vertical bar. The RDW (red-cell distribution width) value, an index of volume heterogeneity, is the standard deviation (SD) divided by the MCV, with the SD being that of the volumes of erythrocytes within the region indicated by the fine lines marked by the double arrow.

Erythrocyte Concentration. The erythrocyte concentration is derived by counting the erythrocyte particles in an isotonic dilution of blood. This value is not useful for purposes of clinical interpretation. It generally parallels the packed cell volume and hemoglobin concentration, but again, the packed cell volume is the preferred value for the interpretation of erythrocyte mass. The erythrocyte concentration is used by the instrument to calculate the packed cell volume (described later).

Mean Cell Volume, Erythrocyte Histogram, and Red Cell Distribution Width. As the erythrocytes are counted, their size distribution is simultaneously constructed (Fig. 1.35), and from this size distribution, the MCV is easily calculated. The red cell distribution width (RDW) is a mathematic index describing the relative width of the size distribution curve. It is the standard deviation of most the erythrocytes divided by the MCV. The tails of the erythrocyte distribution usually are excluded from this mathematic treatment.

These values are useful for the evaluation of anemia. Iron deficiency results in the production of microcytic erythrocytes, and accelerated erythrocyte regeneration results in the production of macrocytic erythrocytes. Early in these responses, a widening of the erythrocyte size distribution and RDW value may be observed (Fig. 1.35). As a larger proportion of these cells accumulate during the response, the curve shifts in the respective direction, and eventually, the MCV falls out of the reference range. The RDW is more useful in the laboratory, in conjunction with the examination of blood films, whereas interpretation of the MCV is used by the laboratorian and the clinician. Examples of interspecies variation and representative reference ranges for MCV are

Humans	80–100 fL
Dogs	60–72 fL
Cats, Horses, and Cows	39–50 fL
Sheep	25–35 fL
Llama	21–29 fL
Goat	15–25 fL

For additional detail on microcytic and macrocytic anemias and other breed-specific information regarding erythrocyte size, see Chapter 6.

Hematocrit. One of the advantages of hematology instrumentation is that the hematocrit may be determined by calculation, thereby avoiding the need for microhematocrit centrifugation. The hematocrit (HCT) is calculated by the instrument using the erythrocyte concentration (RBC) and the MCV:

$$\text{MCV } 10^{-15} \text{ L} \times \text{RBC} \times 10^{12} \text{ L} = \text{HCT}$$

Or, simplified:

$$\frac{\text{MCV} \times \text{RBC}}{10} = \text{HCT}$$

Thus, for example:

$$\frac{\text{MCV 70 fL} \times 7.00 \text{ RBC}}{10} = \text{HCT } 49\%$$

Platelet Concentration. Platelets may be counted simultaneously with erythrocytes. Because platelets are considerably smaller than erythrocytes, however, they may be analyzed in a separate particle-size analyzer from the erythrocytes. Most species have little or no overlap between platelet and erythrocyte volume, thereby making such analysis both simple and accurate. Cats are an exception, in that their platelets are approximately twice the volume of those in other domestic species. In addition, macroplatelet production is a frequent response during most hematologic disturbances in cats. This response is not specific for any specific disease pattern, but it results in considerable overlap between erythrocyte and platelet size distributions, thus making determination of accurate counts difficult. Therefore, feline platelet counts should be regarded as being estimates only. Because large platelets tend to get counted as erythrocytes, the platelet concentration frequently may be artifactually low. In general, if the platelet concentration falls in the reference range, it may be regarded as being adequate. If the platelet concentration is decreased, however, the blood film should be examined by a laboratorian to confirm this finding.

Platelets also may be enumerated by microscopy using a hemocytometer and Unopette kit. This procedure requires considerable experience, however, and should be performed by laboratorians familiar with the technique.

White Blood Cell and Differential Leukocyte Concentrations. To analyze leukocytes, a lytic agent is first added to a dilution of blood. This agent rapidly lyses or dissolves cytoplasmic membranes, thereby making the erythrocytes and platelets "invisible" to the detection technologies. Only nuclear particles of nucleated cells remain, around which is found a "collapse" or condensation of cytoskeleton and any attached organelles. These particles are measured by one of the detection technologies previously described to obtain the leukocyte concentration. Using specially formulated lytic reagents, the degree of collapse may be controlled to different degrees in different leukocyte types. The result is a differential size that can be measured by a particle-size analyzer or light-scatter technology. Automated differential leukocyte counting is not as perfected in domestic animals as in humans; however, the procedure is reasonably accurate for normal blood and, therefore, is very useful in situations such as safety assessment trials, in which most (or all) of the blood samples to be analyzed are normal. When blood is abnormal, however, the frequency of analytic error in the differential count increases considerably. Analytic errors are handled by using the blood film for comparison and the visual differential count whenever an instrument analytic error is either present or suspected. It is essential to monitor instrument performance by visual inspection of the histogram or cytogram display for each sample to know when analytic failure occurs. It is very difficult, if not impossible, to determine this simply by monitoring numeric data from the instrument. Therefore, use of this technology requires considerable training and expertise by the operator to monitor the instrument performance and appropriately intervene with visual inspection of the blood film.

Summary of Blood Analysis by Automated or Semiautomated Instrumentation

The flow of dilutions, analysis, and calculations within an automated hematology instrument is summarized in *Figure 1.36*. This flow has two main pathways. In one, an isotonic dilution of blood is made for erythrocyte and platelet analysis. In the other, a dilution is made, into which a lytic agent is added; in this pathway, leukocytes and hemoglobin are measured.

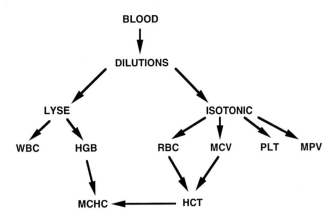

Figure 1.36 Summary of blood analysis pathways in an automated instrument. Two major dilutions are made (see text). In the left pathway, a lytic agent is added, and leukocytes are counted and the hemoglobin concentration measured. In the right pathway, erythrocytes and platelets are counted and sized. From the direct measurements, the hematocrit is calculated. A cross-check between the two pathways is provided by calculation of the mean cell hemoglobin concentration (MCHC).

Hemograms obtained with automated instrumentation have several advantages. First, with the exception of automated differential counts, the results generated in this way are more highly controlled and very reproducible. Second, a more complete hematologic assessment is obtained compared with that using manual techniques. In particular, information regarding erythrocyte size is helpful in characterizing anemias. Third, these instruments generate results much more rapidly, and the cost of consumable reagents is minimal. Therefore, use of this instrumentation is very cost-effective in large laboratories and may be moderately cost-effective in veterinary hospital settings in which laboratory testing forms an integral component of the medical practice activities.

Reticulocyte Concentration

Reticulocyte Enumeration. The reticulocyte concentration is very useful in the evaluation of anemias. The rate of release of reticulocytes from the bone marrow is the best assessment regarding the function of the erythroid component of bone marrow. (See Chapters 6–8 for a more detailed discussion of the anemias.)

The basis for the reticulocyte count involves the events in the maturation of erythroid cells. The developing erythroid cell is heavily involved in aerobic metabolism and protein (i.e., hemoglobin) synthesis. As it nears the final stages of maturity, the nucleus undergoes degeneration and is extruded from the cell, and the organelles supporting the synthetic and metabolic events are removed. After denucleation of the metarubricyte, the remaining erythrocyte undergoes its final maturation, which involves the loss of ribosomes and mitochondria during a 1- to 2-day period. To enumerate reticulocytes, a stain is applied to erythrocytes, thereby causing aggregation of these residual organelles. This results in visible, clumped granular material that can be seen microscopically *(Fig. 1.37)*. The aggregation is referred to as reticulum, hence the name reticulocyte. Reticulocytes are equivalent to the polychromatophilic cells observed on the Wright-stained blood films (Fig. 1.37). Evaluation of polychromatophilic cells on the Wright-stained blood film can provide an assessment of the bone marrow response to anemia. The appearance of these cells, however, is more subjective, and they are more difficult to quantitate than counting the corresponding cells on the reticulocyte stain.

Stains that can be used are new methylene blue (liquid) and brilliant cresyl blue, which is available in disposable tubes that facilitate the procedure *(Fig. 1.38)*. First, several drops of blood are added to the stain in a tube. The tube then is mixed and incubated for 10 minutes. From this mixture, a conventional blood film is made and air-dried. A total of 1000 erythrocytes are counted and categorized as either reticulocytes or normal cells. From this, the percentage of reticulocytes is derived. Interpretation

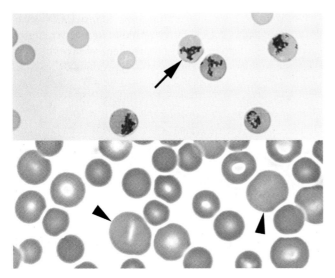

Figure 1.37 Reticulocytes. **Top.** Representative reticulocyte (arrow) using new methylene blue stain. Note the dark-staining, aggregated organelles in several reticulocytes. **Bottom.** Blood film stained with Wright-Giemsa stain. Polychromatophilic cells (arrowheads) are roughly equivalent to reticulocytes on the counterpart stain.

of the percentage reticulocytes is somewhat misleading, however, because it does not account for the degree of anemia. Thus, for purposes of interpretation, the absolute reticulocyte concentration should be calculated by multiplying the erythrocyte concentration (RBC) by the percentage of erythrocytes that are reticulocytes:

$$RBC/\mu L \times \% \text{ Reticulocyte} = \text{Reticulocytes}/\mu L$$

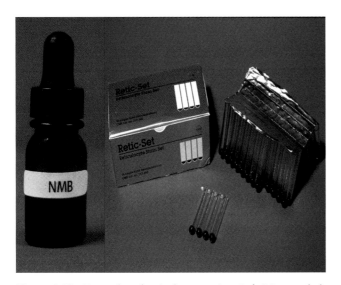

Figure 1.38 Examples of reticulocyte stains. **Left.** New methylene blue in a liquid dropper bottle. **Right.** Commercial preparation of brilliant cresyl blue. The stain is coated on the bottom of disposable tubes.

Interpretation of the Reticulocyte Concentration. The reticulocyte concentration is most useful in dogs and cats, and it also has some application in cows. It is not used in horses, however. Reticulocyte maturation is confined to the marrow space in the horse, and reticulocytes almost never are released into their circulation. Reference ranges for domestic mammals are the concentrations to be expected when the hematocrit is normal:

Dogs and Cats	0–60,000 cells/μL
Cows	0 cells/μL
Horses	Do not release reticulocytes

When anemia is present, a greater degree of release from the marrow is to be expected if the marrow can respond to the anemia. This gives rise to the following guidelines for the interpretation of reticulocyte concentrations with respect to the type of anemia present:

Nonregenerative anemia to very poor regeneration	0–10,000 cells/μL
Nonregenerative to poorly regenerative anemia	10,000–60,000 cells/μL
Regenerative anemia with mild to moderate output	60,000–200,000 cells/μL
Maximal regeneration	200,000–500,000 cells/μL

Reticulocyte Maturation. In dogs, reticulocyte maturation occurs in 24 to 48 hours. Maturation involves a continuum of progressive loss of the visible organelles *(Fig. 1.39)*.

Cats are unique in that more than one kind of reticulocyte may be present. These reticulocytes are of the aggregate and the punctate forms *(Fig. 1.40)*. The aggregate reticulocyte has a clumped reticulum that appears to be identical to that of other species. In the punctate reticulocyte, discrete dots are seen without any clumping; other species do not have this reticulocyte counterpart. Only aggregate reticulocytes appear to be polychromatophilic with Wright stain. Punctate reticulocytes are indistinguishable from normal, mature erythrocytes with Wright stain.

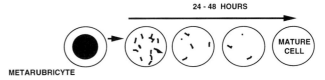

Figure 1.39 Sequential erythroid maturation as related to the reticulocyte stain and interpreted in dogs. The metarubricyte denucleates on leaving the reticulocyte. Reticulum is progressively lost during a 24- to 48-hour period, resulting in a mature erythrocyte.

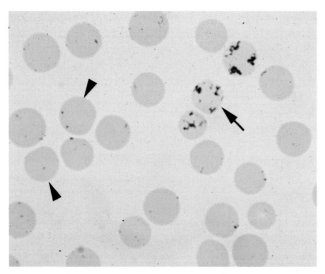

Figure 1.40   Feline reticulocyte morphology with new methylene blue stain. Three aggregate reticulocytes are in the field; note the representative one (arrow). The remainder of the cells are punctate reticulocytes; note the representative cells (arrowheads).

Reticulocyte maturation in cats also may be viewed as a continuum *(Fig. 1.41)*. Aggregate reticulocytes mature to the punctate form in approximately 12 hours; the punctate cells may continue to mature for another 10 to 12 days. Because of the short maturation time of aggregate reticulocytes, these cells are the best indicator of ac-

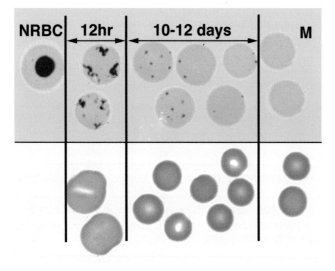

Figure 1.41   Feline reticulocyte maturation, progressing from left to right. **Top.** Cells stained with new methylene blue. After denucleation of the metarubricyte (NRBC), an aggregate reticulocyte is formed. This cell matures to the punctate form in approximately 12 hours. The punctate forms continue to mature by slow loss of punctate granules during a 10- to 12-day period. Mature cells (M) on the right have no granularity. **Bottom.** Corresponding cells stained with Wright-Giemsa stain. Note that polychromatophilic cells correspond to aggregate reticulocytes. Punctate and mature cells are indistinguishable with Wright-Giemsa stain.

tive marrow release. Therefore, only aggregate cells are counted in cats, and interpretive guidelines apply to this cell type only. Experience is required to exclude punctate cells when performing the reticulocyte count.

Organization of the Complete Blood Count (Hemogram)

It is useful to summarize the described basic and advanced determinations in a way that shows the organization of how they are performed and interpreted. This provides a mental framework for simplifying the complexity of this information into an everyday, intuitive tool: the hemogram. The techniques for generating data may be organized conceptually as direct measurements, microscopic procedures, and calculations. The complete blood count may include:

Direct Measurements
Packed cell volume
Hemoglobin
Red count
Mean corpuscular volume (MCV)
White cell count
Plasma proteins (by refractometer)
Platelet count
Mean platelet volume

Microscopic Procedures
Differential white cell count
Red cell morphology
Platelet morphology and assessment of adequacy
Reticulocyte enumeration in patients with anemia

Calculations
Erythrocyte indices (e.g., MCHC, mean cell hemoglobin content, and RDW)
Absolute white blood cell differential values
Absolute reticulocyte count

These determinations are organized into a report form that aids the clinician in efficiently interpreting the information. The best way for this information to be organized is into banks of data that relate to the three major cell lines (i.e., erythrocytes, leukocytes, and platelets). For each cell line, all pieces of relevant information are organized in one place on the form.

Laboratory Tests Useful in the Diagnosis of Immune-Mediated Hemolytic Anemia

Coombs' or Antiglobulin Test.   The Coombs of antiglobulin test is used as an aid in establishing the diagnosis of immune-mediated hemolytic anemia by detecting species-specific immunoglobulin that is adsorbed or attached to the surface of erythrocytes. The test uses the Coombs reagent, which is a polyclonal serum (usually prepared in rabbits) to the immunoglobulins of the species of interest. Some reagent manufacturers claim their reagent also detects complement. The procedure involves washing the erythrocytes in saline to remove plasma proteins and immunoglobulin that is nonspecifically associated with erythrocytes. An aliquot of washed cells then is incubated with Coombs' serum. If appreciable patient immunoglobulin is attached to the erythrocytes, the Coombs' serum induces erythrocyte agglutination. By means of two binding sites per molecule, the Coombs reagent immunoglobulin binds the patient immunoglobulin attached to the erythrocytes. The two binding sites result in progressive bridging of erythrocytes, which is visualized as agglutination. The absence of agglutination is interpreted as being a negative result, whereas the presence of agglutination is interpreted as being a positive result. Appropriate controls are performed as well.

False-negative reactions are a common problem with the Coombs' test, likely because of the elution of pathologically adsorbed immunoglobulin or immune complexes during washing of the erythrocytes in preparation for the test. The best evidence for this is that prominent autoagglutination may disappear with washing. Autoagglutination, if confirmed microscopically, may be interpreted as being equivalent to a positive Coombs test. False-positive reactions also may occur but are less well documented, because the test is only performed when one suspects the disease.

Saline Fragility Test. Resistance of patient erythrocytes to hemolysis is measured in decreasing concentrations of saline. This test is not commonly used because of its complexity and labor intensity. It remains a useful diagnostic aid, however, in occasional cases of immune-mediated hemolytic anemia in which other hallmark pieces of information are not clearly interpretable. An equal aliquot of erythrocytes is added to a series of tubes containing decreasing concentrations of saline. After incubation, the tubes undergo centrifugation, and the hemoglobin concentration then is measured on the supernatant. A tube with distilled water serves as an index for 100% hemolysis. Interpretation is facilitated by plotting the percentage hemolysis and the concentration of saline, as shown in *Figure 1.42*.

These tests must not be used or interpreted in isolation. They are to be used in conjunction with analysis of other hematologic data and morphologic evaluation of the blood film by the laboratorian. Because of the frequency of false-negative and -positive results with the Coombs' test, interpreting the results of this test in the light of the other available hematologic information is important.

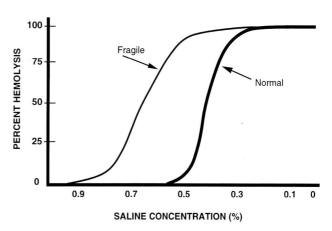

Figure 1.42 Erythrocyte fragility curve. Percentage hemolysis is plotted against decreasing saline concentration. Note the normal curve (arrow marked Normal). Increased erythrocyte fragility is recognized by a shift of the curve to the left (arrow marked Fragile).

(See Chapter 8 for a detailed discussion of the strategy for diagnosing immune-mediated hemolytic anemia.)

CHEMISTRY TECHNIQUES

A wide variety of techniques, which have been incorporated into many different instrument designs, are used in veterinary clinical chemistry. No attempt is made here to discuss all of these techniques and instruments, but the basic information on a variety of chemistry techniques used in analyzing samples from animals is provided. A complete understanding of these techniques is not necessary for veterinarians who send clinical chemistry samples to a reference laboratory; however, an increasing number of chemistry instruments are being marketed to veterinarians for in-practice use. Therefore, an understanding of how these instruments work is important for understanding the advantages and disadvantages of the various instruments, the laboratory techniques necessary for their use, the problems that might arise during their use, and the basic principles underlying their variations in design.

The chemistry techniques discussed in this chapter and the substances that may be measured with them are listed in *Table 1.1*. Absorbance or reflectance photometry is used to measure most of the substances in clinical chemistry profiles. Fluorometry also is used to measure certain analytes in some clinical chemistry analyzers. Blood pH, partial pressures of carbon dioxide and oxygen, and concentrations of electrolytes such as sodium, potassium, and chloride most commonly are measured by electrochemical methods. Sodium and potassium concentrations less frequently are measured by flame photometry. Atomic absorption spectrophotometers are not commonly used in clinical chemistry laboratories; rather, they are more

> **TABLE 1.1   TECHNIQUES IN VETERINARY CLINICAL CHEMISTRY AND SUBSTANCES MEASURED WITH THOSE TECHNIQUES**

Technique	Substances Measured
Photometry	
Absorbance photometry	Glucose, BUN, creatine, calcium, phosphorus, magnesium, protein, albumin, bilirubin, bile acids, ammonia, cholesterol, bicarbonate, total CO_2, enzymes
Reflectance photometry	Similar to those measured by absorbance photometry
Flame photometry	Sodium and potassium[a]
Atomic absorption spectrophotometry	Many elements including nutrients and toxicants (e.g., calcium,[b] magnesium,[b] lead, arsenic)
Fluorometry	Glucose, bilirubin, bile acids, calcium, magnesium, enzymes, antithrombin III, heparin, plasminogen, hormones, drugs
Light-scatter techniques	
Turbidimetry	Immunoglobulins, antigen–antibody complexes, other large proteins, drugs
Nephalometry	Immunoglobulins, antigen–antibody complexes, other large proteins, drugs
Electrochemical methods	
Potentiometry	Blood pH, P_{CO_2}, sodium,[c] potassium,[c] chloride[c]
Amperometry	P_{O_2}
Coulometry and conductometry[d]	BUN
Osmometry	Osmolality or osmolarity
Protein electrophoresis	Albumin, α-globulin, β-globulin, Υ-globulin

BUN, blood urea nitrogen.

[a] This technique has been replaced by potentiometric methods (ion-selective electrodes) for measuring serum sodium and potassium concentrations in most laboratories.

[b] May be used to measure the concentration of these substances in solid tissues that have been ashed or digested. Absorbance photometry is more commonly used to measure concentrations of these substances in serum or plasma.

[c] Electrodes used to measure concentrations of these electrolytes are called ion-selective electrodes.

[d] Conductometry also is used to perform cell counts in some hematology analyzers.

common in laboratories testing for elements considered to be nutrients and/or toxicants. Osmometers are common in clinical chemistry laboratories and are used to measure blood osmolality or osmolarity. Protein electrophoresis is used to measure concentrations of the various protein fractions comprising the total serum protein, especially in samples with either decreased or increased protein concentrations. Light-scatter techniques are used less commonly to measure the concentrations of substances such as large protein molecules.

Photometry

Photometry is a general term used to describe an analytic chemistry technique in which the concentrations of substances and the activities of enzymes are determined by measuring the intensity of light passing through or emitted from a test chamber. This test chamber contains the substance to be detected and, in many cases, chemicals that are reacting with that substance. Strictly speaking, the term *spectrophotometry* should be applied when the

instrument being used has the ability to produce light of a variety of wavelengths through some type of light-fractionating device, such as filters, prisms, or diffraction gratings.

Absorbance Spectrophotometry

Absorbance spectrophotometry is an analytic technique in which concentrations of substances are determined by directing a beam of light through a solution containing the substance to be detected (or a product of that substance) and then measuring the amount of light that either of these absorb.

To understand absorbance spectrophotometry, some basic knowledge regarding light is necessary. Typically, light is classified by its wavelength, which is measured in nanometers (nm). Light with the shortest wavelengths (<380 nm) is termed ultraviolet (UV) light *(Table 1.2)*. Light in the visible spectrum has wavelengths of 380 to 750 nm. Light with the longest wavelengths (>750–2000 nm) is termed infrared (IR) light. The energy of light

TABLE 1.2 WAVELENGTHS RESULTING IN ULTRAVIOLET LIGHT, VARIOUS COLORS OF VISIBLE LIGHT, AND INFRARED LIGHT

Wavelength (nm)	Color
<380	None (ultraviolet)
380–440	Violet
440–500	Blue
500–580	Green
580–600	Yellow
600–620	Orange
620–750	Red
750–2000	None (infrared)

is inversely proportional to its wavelength; therefore, UV light has the highest energy and IR light the lowest.

The visible spectrum includes a variety of wavelengths that represent the colors with which we are familiar. It is important to remember that color results from the transmittance or reflectance of light. In other words, a green object is that color because it reflects the green area of the visible spectrum and has absorbed the other wavelengths of light in that spectrum. Likewise, a green solution is green because it allows light in the green area of the visible spectrum to be transmitted through it and has absorbed the visible light of other wavelengths. These same principles also apply to light outside the visible spectrum. Different substances absorb and reflect different wavelengths of UV or IR light in a pattern that is typical for that substance. The pattern in which a substance absorbs light at various wavelengths is known as its absorption spectrum, and each substance has its own unique absorption spectrum.

A basic absorbance spectrophotometer is diagrammed in *Figure 1.43*. Various sources of light can be used, with the choice being based on the portion of the spectrum desired plus issues such as longevity of the bulb and the basic

instrument design. In the application of absorbance spectrophotometry for measuring the concentration of a substance, a wavelength of light that is absorbed by that substance (or by a product of that substance) is used. This wavelength is determined by examining the absorption spectrum of the substance of interest. Usually, the wavelength chosen is the one at which the maximum absorbance occurs. Occasionally, however, some other wavelength is chosen to avoid interference with substances such as hemoglobin and bilirubin, which may be present in serum samples secondary to hemolysis (in vitro or in vivo) or disease leading to high bilirubin concentration. Hemoglobin and bilirubin have their own absorption spectrums, and one should avoid using the wavelengths that these substances strongly absorb.

Monochromators narrow the spectrum of light that passes through the cuvette. Monochromators can be filters, prisms, or diffraction gratings. When attempting to produce light of a specific wavelength, the actual range of wavelengths produced by a monochromator is called the spectral bandwidth. Each type of monochromator can produce rays of light at certain spectral bandwidths. Monochromators capable of producing light of a narrow spectral bandwidth have more spectral purity. The importance of spectral purity varies with the type of spectrophotometry, however, and with the substance being analyzed. Filters may be a thin layer of colored glass that transmits light at wavelengths corresponding to the filter's color, or they may be more complex structures, with a layer of dielectric material sandwiched between two pieces of glass coated with a thin layer of silver. The latter type of filter transmits light at wavelengths equal to or at multiples of the thickness of the dielectric layer. In some cases, multiple filters may be placed in series to produce light of greater spectral purity. Prisms separate the wavelengths of white light by refracting this light. As light passes through a prism, shorter wavelengths are bent more than longer wavelengths, thus separating them. The desired wavelength then can be selected from this spectrum for transmission. Diffraction gratings are a metal or glass plate covered with a layer of metal alloy into which multiple parallel grooves have been etched. When the grating is illuminated, each groove separates the light into a spectrum, and light of specific wavelengths is produced as wavelengths that are in phase are reinforced and those that are not in phase are cancelled.

The focusing devices usually are lenses or slits that are inserted before and/or after the monochromator. This placement varies with the instrument. Focusing devices are used to narrow the light beam, to produce parallel light rays, and/or to regulate the intensity of the light reaching the photodetector. In some modern instruments, application of fiber optics has eliminated some of the lens and slits used for narrowing and directing the light beams.

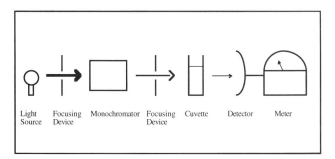

Figure 1.43 Components of a simple absorbance spectrophotometer. Arrows represent light.

Cuvettes are also known as absorption cells. They have constant dimensions for a given instrument, and they can be made of various materials (e.g., glass, quartz or plastic) and be of various shapes (e.g., round, square, or rectangular). The materials or shapes used depend on the instrument design and on the portion of the light spectrum being used. During analysis, a solution containing the absorbing substance is placed in the cuvette, and the light rays that have been produced pass through the cuvette walls and the solution. If the correct wavelength has been chosen, the substance absorbs this light in direct proportion to its concentration. In addition to the absorbing substance, the cuvette walls and the solution in which the substance is suspended also absorb small amounts of light. It is, therefore, necessary to "zero" spectrophotometers in order to eliminate the effect of these other factors, and this typically is accomplished by taking an absorbance reading on a cuvette containing only the solution in which the substance is suspended (i.e., the solution contains none of the absorbing substance). The absorbance reading of the instrument typically is set to zero while reading the absorbance of this "blank." Some spectrophotometers are designed to read the absorbance of the test solution and the blank solution simultaneously, which requires splitting the light beam and then shining each beam through either the test or the blank cuvette.

Photodetectors collect the light that has passed through the cuvette (i.e., the light that has not been absorbed). Several different technologies can be used in photodetectors. Factors such as cost, sensitivity, speed of response to changes in light intensity, propensity to fatigue (i.e., decreased response over time despite constant light intensity), and heat sensitivity help to determine which technology is used in a given application. Regardless of the type of photodetector, the underlying mechanism involves the production of electrons and, therefore, an electrical current in response to light striking the detector. This electrical current then is transmitted to a readout device or meter.

Readout devices or meters measure the electrical current produced by the photodetector. This current can be read out directly, but more commonly, this information is converted to a readout that gives either the absorbance or the actual concentration of the substance being measured. This conversion usually requires some type of microprocessor, which can store and use calibration information (discussed later) and also automatically adjust for the reading of the blank sample. The actual readout might be presented as some type of digital display, but it more commonly is printed.

Modern readout devices also incorporate recorders for obtaining multiple absorbance readings on the same sample over time. This is most useful in kinetic assays. In such

assays (discussed later), a reaction is allowed to occur over a period of time, and the production or disappearance of the absorbing substance is evaluated at several time points by measuring the absorbance of light normally absorbed by that substance. The change in absorbance over the time period is proportional to the activity of an enzyme or to the concentration of a substance, depending on which is being assayed. Such an assay obviously requires a device that can record and use data produced over time.

In addition to the basic instrumentation of absorbance spectrophotometry, the basic physical chemistry principles used in obtaining measurements via this technology also should be understood. When a light beam of a certain wavelength is projected through a solution containing a substance that absorbs light at that wavelength, the light is absorbed in direct proportion to the concentration of that substance. The intensity of the light leaving the solution, therefore, is less than the intensity of the light entering the solution. If these two intensities are known, the percentage transmittance of light (%T) can be calculated. For instance, if the intensity of light entering the cuvette is designated as I_1 and the intensity of light leaving the cuvette as I_2, then %T is calculated as

$$\%T = \frac{I_2}{I_1}$$

The intensity of light entering the cuvette is measured by projecting light of the appropriate wavelength through a cuvette containing the solution in which the substance to be measured is suspended. In this case, however, the solution contains none of the substance. Therefore, %T is set at 100% for this "blank" solution. The solution containing the substance to be measured is then placed in a similar cuvette, and the light is intensity measured, after which the %T can be assessed.

In the described situation, transmittance varies inversely and logarithmically with the concentration of the substance being measured. If %T versus the concentration of such a substance is plotted, a curved line results (Fig. 1.44). Light that is not transmitted is absorbed; therefore, transmittance and absorbance are inversely related, as described by the formula

$$\text{Absorbance} = 2 - \log \%T$$

Because of this relationship, absorbance of light increases linearly with increasing concentration of the substance being measured (Fig. 1.44). This linear relationship between absorbance and concentration makes it more convenient to deal with absorbance than with transmittance during spectrophotometric analysis. Modern spectrophotometers measure transmittance but then convert transmittance to absorbance. In addition, micro-

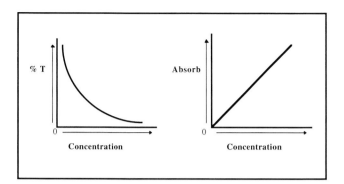

Figure 1.44   The relationships between percentage transmittance (%T), absorbance (Absorb), and concentration of a substance being measured. Note that as the concentration increases, %T decreases geometrically and absorbance increases linearly.

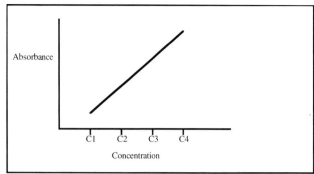

Figure 1.45   Use of calibrators to establish a calibration curve. In this case, four calibrators (C1, C2, C3, C4) were used. Note the linear relationship between concentration of the substance being measured and resulting absorbance.

processors in most spectrophotometers convert absorbance results to concentrations or activities and then report these.

The concentration of a substance can be calculated from the absorbance by use of Beer's law:

$$A = a\,bc$$

where A is the absorbance measured, a is the molar absorptivity (also known as the proportionality constant), b is the light path in centimeters (the diameter or width of the cuvette through which the light passes), and c is the concentration of the substance in question. The concentration (c) then can be calculated as

$$\text{Concentration} = \frac{A}{ab}$$

For Beer's law to apply, a linear relationship must exist between concentration and absorbance. In some cases, this might be true only up to certain concentrations or absorbance levels. To assure that Beer's law applies to a given assay, calibration solutions (also known as calibrators), which contain known concentrations of the substance to be measured, are used. The ranges of concentrations used as calibrators should include those that might be measured in samples from patients. Absorbance results for each calibrator are plotted against the concentrations of these calibrators to establish a calibration curve. Ideally, this curve is a straight line rather than an actual curve, showing that a linear relationship exists between absorbance and concentration *(Fig. 1.45)*. In most applications, one or more calibrators are included with each series of sample measurements. It is best, however, to re-establish the calibration curve at frequent intervals (at least daily), because many slight day-to-day changes in the conditions

of the test can affect this curve. These changes (e.g., light intensity, temperature, condition of reagents) can occur even in situations when instruments and reagents have been designed to minimize such variation. If a linear relationship does exist between the concentrations of the calibrators and the resulting absorbances, the solutions are said to obey Beer's law, and the calibrators can be used to establish a calibration constant (K):

$$K = \frac{\text{Concentration of the calibration solution}}{\text{Absorbance of the calibration solution}}$$

If K is known, then the concentration of an unknown solution can be calculated as

$$\text{Concentration of unknown} = (\text{Absorbance of unknown}) \times K$$

Microprocessors in instruments can plot absorbance results from calibrators, assure that a linear relationship exists, and calculate the calibration constant. These results are stored, and the concentrations of unknowns then can be calculated by measuring their absorbances and using the calibration constant as previously derived.

A linear relationship between concentration and absorbance over the possible range of unknown concentrations is highly desirable, but a nonlinear calibration curve also can be used to derive unknown concentrations. In such a case, enough calibrators must be used to define the shape of the calibration curve, and as with a linear calibration curve, the range of calibrator concentrations should include the possible range of concentrations that might be found in samples from patients.

In absorbance spectrophotometry, two types of assay methods—end point or kinetic—may be used. In both types, the same principles of spectrophotometry described earlier apply. End-point assays usually are applied when measuring the concentration of some pre-existing substance in serum or plasma. In such an assay, some type of reagent is added to a quantity of serum, and a chemical reaction occurs. The product resulting from this reaction then is measured by spectrophotometry. In other words, the solution in which the reaction has occurred is placed in a cuvette (or the reaction itself might have occurred in the cuvette), a light beam of a wavelength absorbed by the product is projected through a cuvette, and the absorbance is measured. By using a calibration curve and/or a calibration constant, the concentration of the substance being measured then is calculated. An example of an end-point assay is a method for measuring the concentration of calcium:

$$\text{calcium} + o\text{-cresolphthalein complexone} \rightarrow$$
$$\text{calcium–cresolphthalein complexone}$$

In this assay, the substance of interest (i.e., calcium) is complexed with cresolphthalein complexone, which has a purple color and absorbs light at a wavelength of 570 nm. This reaction is allowed to occur long enough to allow nearly all of the calcium in the sample to be complexed. More calcium–cresolphthalein complexone produced results in more light being absorbed and a higher concentration of calcium reported by the instrument. After the absorbance is determined, it is compared with the absorbance of a calibration solution, and the absorbance of the unknown then is calculated as:

$$\begin{array}{l}\text{Concentration of} \\ \text{the unknown}\end{array} = \begin{array}{l}\text{Absorbance of} \\ \text{the unknown}\end{array} \times \dfrac{\begin{array}{l}\text{Concentration of the} \\ \text{calibration solution}\end{array}}{\begin{array}{l}\text{Absorbance of the} \\ \text{calibration solution}\end{array}}$$

Note that the second portion of this formula is the calibration constant (K).

Kinetic assays typically have been used to measure enzyme activities but also have been adapted to measure the concentrations of many pre-existing substances in the blood. As noted in Chapter 23, enzyme concentrations are not measured directly in clinical chemistry. Rather, the amount of enzyme in the serum usually is gauged indirectly, by the activity of that enzyme. Enzymes are proteins that catalyze (i.e., speed-up) chemical reactions, with the result that substrate is converted to product more quickly:

$$\text{Substrate} \xrightarrow{\text{Enzyme}} \text{Product}$$

To measure an enzyme's activity, the rate at which it converts a substrate to a product must be assessed. The more quickly conversion occurs, the higher the enzyme activity is assumed to be. To measure the rate of conversion from substrate to product, the rate at which the product is being produced must be assessed, and this requires multiple measurements of the product concentration over time. Because this type of assay is a dynamic process, it is termed a *kinetic assay*. In a kinetic assay of enzyme activity, a solution containing the substrate of the enzyme of interest is added to the sample serum in a cuvette that already is in a spectrophotometer. When enzyme in this serum begins to convert substrate to product, absorbance is measured periodically by the same methods and using the same principles of spectrophotometry described previously (i.e., using a light beam of a wavelength absorbed by the product). In this process, the conversion rate of substrate to product is monitored. This rate can be converted to enzyme activity by using a formula involving the rate of absorbance change and several constants related to the absorptivity of the product as well as to test characteristics such as sample volume, total sample volume, and light path.

An example of a kinetic enzyme assay is an assay of alanine aminotransferase (ALT) activity:

$$\alpha\text{-Ketoglutarate} + \text{L-Alanine} \xrightarrow{\text{ALT}} \text{L-Glutamate} + \text{Pyruvate}$$

$$\text{Pyruvate} + \text{NADH} + \text{H}^+ \xrightarrow{\text{LDH}} \text{L-Lactate} + \text{NAD}^+$$

where LDH is lactate dehydrogenase. In this assay, NADH is converted to NAD^+ at a rate proportional to the activity of ALT in the sample. The NADH absorbs light at 340 nm, and its rate of disappearance is measured by periodically assessing the absorbance of the reaction mixture. The rate of absorbance change in this mixture can be converted to units of ALT activity.

As previously noted, kinetic assays also are used for measuring the concentrations of pre-existing substances in the blood. In these assays, the rate of appearance or disappearance of an absorbing substance is monitored by periodically measuring the absorbance of the reaction mixture. An example of a kinetic assay for measuring the concentration of a pre-existing substance is an assay of the blood urea nitrogen (BUN) concentration, which uses the chemical reaction

$$\text{Urea} + \text{H}_2\text{O} + 2\text{H}^+ \xrightarrow{\text{Urease}} \text{CO}_2 + 2\,\text{NH}_4^+$$

$$\text{NH}_4^+ + \alpha\text{-Ketoglutarate} + \text{NADH} \xrightarrow{\text{GLDH}} \text{L-Glutamate} + \text{NAD}^+ + \text{H}_2\text{O}$$

where GLDH is glutamate dehydrogenase. In this reaction, the disappearance rate of NADH is monitored by periodically assessing the absorbance of the reaction mixture at a wavelength of 340 nm. The disappearance rate is proportional to the urea nitrogen concentration in the serum being tested. The BUN concentration is calculated by relating the rate of change in the absorbance of the sample with that of a calibrator.

Enzyme activity also can be measured by end-point methods, which involve mixing serum with reagent containing substrate for the enzyme and then allowing the conversion of substrate to product to proceed for a specific period of time. At the end of that period, the concentration of substrate or product is measured. The more substrate used or product produced during the time period, the higher the enzyme activity is assumed to be.

Reflectance Photometry

The principle of reflectance photometry is used in a few large, automated clinical chemistry analyzers and in several of the smaller clinical chemistry analyzers marketed for in-practice use. Most of these instruments use "dry chemistry" systems, in which the fluid to be analyzed is placed on a carrier that contains the reagents for the assay. This carrier can take different forms, including a dry fiber pad or a multilayer of film. After the fluid is applied, the chemical reaction occurs in this carrier, and a product is formed in a concentration proportional to that of the substance being measured. The carrier then is illuminated with diffused light, and the intensity of the light reflected from the carrier is measured and compared with that of either the original illuminating light or the intensity of light reflected off a reference surface. Reflectance photometry, therefore, is analogous to absorbance photometry in that the chemical reaction occurring in the carrier results in a product that absorbs a portion of the illuminating light. The remaining light is reflected, analogous to transmittance in absorbance spectrophotometry, to a photodetector that measures its intensity. The intensity of the reflected light is not related linearly to the concentration of the substance being produced. As a result, formulas are required to convert the reflectance results to concentrations. These formulas vary with the type of instrument being used.

Flame Photometry

Flame photometry, which also is known as flame emission photometry, most commonly is used for measurement of serum sodium and potassium concentrations and less commonly for measurement of lithium concentrations. The basic principle of flame photometry is that when atoms of many metallic elements are heated to a very high temperature (e.g., in a hot flame), they emit light at characteristic wavelengths. When heat is applied to a metallic atom, this energy is absorbed by orbital electrons, and this absorption of energy causes those electrons to "jump" to a different orbital level. These electrons are unstable in their excited state and, as a result, jump back to their original, lower-energy or ground state, which in turn results in a loss of energy that is emitted as a photon of light. The light released is of specific wavelengths that are typical for that element. Each element has a characteristic emission spectrum. One wavelength from this emission spectrum is isolated and measured, and the intensity of the light measured is proportional to the number of atoms emitting light and, therefore, to the concentration of the element in the solution.

A typical flame photometer is diagrammed in *Figure 1.46*. The sample first is aspirated and then converted to fine droplets by an atomizer. These fine droplets enter the flame, and a small percentage of the metal ions are converted to atoms. Electrons of these atoms can absorb energy from the flame, jump to a higher-energy state, and then return to the ground state, thereby emitting light. Only a very small percentage of the ions entering the flame actually participate in this process (e.g., only 1%–5% of sodium atoms in the flame reach the excited state). Some elements, such as sodium, potassium, and lithium, are excited more easily by this technique, whereas elements such as calcium, are not easily excited. Thus, only certain analytes can be accurately analyzed using flame photometry. The flame is produced by compressed gas and also emits light. It is very important that a proper temperature be produced for the excitation of electrons to occur.

As previously stated, each element maximally emits light at specific wavelengths (e.g., sodium emits light at 330, 589, and 819 nm). One wavelength from the element's emission spectrum is chosen to be measured. The chosen wavelength should be different from those in the emission spectrum of the flame itself and from those in the emission spectrums of any potentially interfering substances. This wavelength also must be of an adequate intensity to allow the needed sensitivity in the measurement.

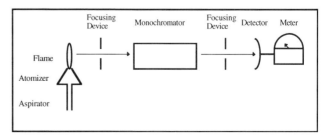

Figure 1.46 Basic components of a flame photometer. Arrows represent light.

The monochromator is used to isolate the chosen, emitted wavelength of light. The monochromator, therefore, excludes those wavelengths of light emitted from other nonionic materials in the flame as well as the light from the flame itself. Because of the variety of wavelengths being produced by other nonionic materials and the flame, the bandwidth of light isolated by the monochromator should be as narrow as possible. Therefore, monochromators used in flame photometry usually must be of higher quality than those used in absorbance spectrophotometry. Detectors, meters, and other readout devices used in flame photometry are similar in principle to those used in absorbance spectrophotometry. To convert the measured emissions to concentrations of sodium and potassium, a calibration curve must be established, just as in absorbance spectrophotometry. This involves use of calibrators with known sodium and potassium concentrations, which are analyzed just as the unknown samples are. The results from these calibrators are used to establish a calibration curve, and the concentrations of the unknowns then can be determined from this curve, as discussed earlier.

In flame photometry, several variations in test conditions that might affect the results can occur from one sample aspiration to the next. These involve fluctuations in air pressure (affecting atomization) as well as solution viscosity and gas pressure (possibly affecting the flame). To minimize the effect of these fluctuations, most flame photometers use an internal lithium or cesium standard. Both lithium and cesium have high emission intensity at wavelengths different from those of sodium and potassium. A standard concentration of lithium or cesium is added to all calibrators, blanks, and unknowns, and the emission of these elements is measured along with those of sodium and potassium. In each case, the emission readout for sodium and potassium is adjusted for any variations from what would be expected in the lithium or cesium emission, thereby minimizing the effects of the variables mentioned earlier. An additional benefit from the addition of lithium to the assay is its effect as a radiation buffer. Without lithium in the aspirated solution, the emission by potassium is enhanced by sodium. This results from a transfer of energy from an excited sodium atom to a potassium atom. When lithium is present, however, lithium rather than potassium atoms absorb this energy.

The presence of substances in the serum that displace water volume can alter both sodium and potassium concentrations as measured by flame photometry. This is most important in the case of lipemia. In lipemic serum samples, lipids displace a portion of the aqueous fluid in the blood, and little sodium or potassium is present in the lipid portion. The concentrations of these electrolytes, therefore, are decreased when measured with a flame photometer. In other words, the instrument atomizes all components of the lipemic serum sample, and the emissions from sodium and potassium ions are decreased because of the relative dilution by lipids. This problem is eliminated when electrochemical methods of measuring serum sodium and potassium concentrations are used (see the discussion of potentiometry).

Atomic Absorption Spectrophotometry

Atomic absorption spectrophotometry (AA) is used for measuring the concentrations of many elements in fluids as well as tissues. Advantages of AA compared with flame photometry include its superior sensitivity (i.e., it can detect smaller concentrations) and its ability to measure the concentrations of elements whose electrons do not easily jump to the excited state in a flame. As the name implies, AA differs from flame photometry in that it involves measuring absorption rather than emission of energy by atoms. This technique involves heating a sample in a flame that is hot enough to cause the element in question to dissociate from its chemical bonds and form neutral atoms—but not hot enough to cause large numbers of electrons to jump to the excited state. These atoms then are in a low-energy (i.e., ground) state and can absorb light of a narrow wavelength that is specific for that element. If a light of this wavelength is projected through the flame, the amount of light absorbed is proportional to the concentration of the element in the sample. Measurement of the amount of light absorbed, therefore, allows the concentration of that element in the sample to be calculated.

The components of an atomic absorption spectrophotometer are diagrammed in *Figure 1.47*. The hollow cathode tube is the source of light and is made of the same element as that which is to be measured. A different cathode usually is needed for each element to be analyzed. Alloy cathodes, which are made from more than one element and which, therefore, can analyze more than one element, are available for some applications. Heating of the hollow cathode produces light at wavelengths specific

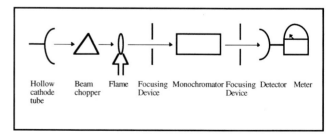

Figure 1.47 Basic components of an atomic absorption spectrophotometer. Arrows represent light.

to that element. These wavelengths typically are very narrow (i.e., of high spectral purity).

The light from the hollow cathode tube is projected through a beam chopper and then the flame. The beam chopper helps to eliminate interfering effects by pulsating the flow of light through the flame. Sources of light leaving the flame include projected light that was not absorbed (i.e., the light that one wants to measure), light emitted by the flame itself, and light emitted from atoms in the sample. By analyzing the emissions from the flame during the period when the pulsed light is off, the latter two sources of light can be measured and then subtracted from the total light leaving the flame. This process leaves only the unabsorbed portion of the projected light, which then is used to calculate the concentration of the element in question.

Production of a flame in which the sample is burned involves use of an aspirator, atomizer, and source of compressed gas for fuel. Unlike flame photometry, in which a very small percentage of atoms are excited by the flame, most atoms in the flame of an atomic absorption spectrophotometer absorb light. This makes AA a much more sensitive technique than flame photometry.

So-called "flameless" AA instruments also are available. In these instruments, the sample is placed in a depression in a carbon rod and then heated in a chamber to the point where it dries, chars, and eventually, atomizes. Light from the hollow cathode tube then is projected through the atomized material. This variation of AA is more sensitive and allows the analysis of trace elements.

Focusing devices, photodetectors, meters, and readout devices serve the same purposes in AA as in other types of spectrophotometry.

Fluorometry

Fluorometric techniques can be used in a wide variety of applications, ranging from measurement of the concentrations of substances to assessment of the numbers and other characteristics of larger particles, including cells. This section discusses use of these techniques in measuring concentrations of various substances in body fluids.

Among the substances that can be measured by these techniques are some that commonly are measured in clinical chemistry analysis (e.g., bilirubin, bile acids, glucose, calcium, magnesium, and various enzymes), substances related to coagulation (e.g., antithrombin III, heparin, and plasminogen), drugs, and hormones. Some of these substances are fluorescent; in other cases, measurement of these substances is possible by linking other fluorescent substances to the analyte of interest, either directly or indirectly, as the result of a series of chemical reactions.

The basic principle underlying use of fluorometry is that certain substances, when exposed to light of the

proper wavelength, will fluoresce. Fluorescence results when a substance absorbs light at one wavelength and then emits light at a longer (i.e., lower energy) wavelength. The basic mechanism by which this occurs is diagrammed in *Figure 1.48*. When a substance capable of fluorescence is exposed to light, some electrons at ground state jump to a higher-energy state known as the first excited state. Both the ground and first excited states have various energy levels within them, which are known as vibrational energy levels. An electron excited by light can jump to any of the vibrational energy levels in the first excited state. After this jump, electrons in the higher vibrational energy levels of the first excited state drop to the lowest vibration energy level in this state, which then is followed by a jump to one of the vibrational energy levels of the ground state. This latter jump produces light energy, which is seen as fluorescence. Electrons also can jump directly from a higher vibrational level of the excited state to the ground state, but this jump produces more energy, which is expressed as heat rather than fluorescence. Fluorescence occurs more readily in some compounds than in others. The ability to fluoresce varies with a compound's chemical structure; therefore, not all compounds can be readily measured by fluorometry.

The basic design of a fluorometer is shown in *Figure 1.49*. A variety of light sources, including various types of bulbs and lasers, can be used. Most fluorescent compounds absorb light at 300 to 550 nm; therefore, light sources must produce light at these wavelengths. The primary monochromator isolates light at the proper wavelength to produce fluorescence in the substance being analyzed. Each compound can best be caused to fluoresce at specific wavelengths, and these wavelengths are known

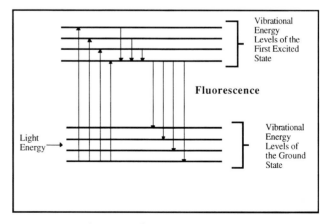

Figure 1.48 Changes in electron energy states resulting in fluorescence. Light energy causes electrons to jump from the ground state to one of the vibrational energy levels of the first excited state. After returning to the lowest vibrational energy level of the first excited state, electrons jump back to the ground state, thereby producing fluorescence.

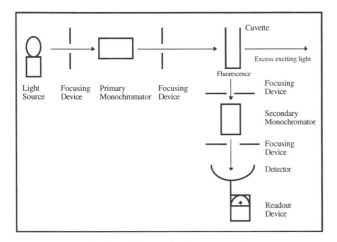

Figure 1.49   The basic design of a fluorometer. Arrows represent light.

as the apparent excitation spectrum of the compound. Of these wavelengths, a narrow band at which peak fluorescence is caused usually is chosen to be isolated by the primary monochromator and, from there, transmitted to the cuvette. When light strikes the solution in the cuvette, it sets off the mechanisms previously described and produces fluorescence in the substance being measured. The detector of this fluorescent energy usually is placed at a 90° angle from the projected (i.e., the exciting) light beam. This placement means that light from the exciting light beam continues straight through the cuvette and does not need to be dealt with by the secondary monochromator or the detector. Because fluorescent energy is projected in all directions, this energy can be measured at 90° without measuring the energy from the exciting light beam. Some fluorometers incorporated into absorbance spectrophotometers measure fluorescence directly in the path of exciting light (i.e., an end-on design), because this is the typical light path for absorbance spectrophotometers. In such cases, mechanisms must be incorporated to exclude excitation light that has passed through the cuvette.

The secondary monochromator excludes light from sources other than the fluorescence itself and allows only a narrow band of wavelengths to pass to the photodetector. Just as each fluorescent compound has an apparent excitation spectrum of light in which optimum fluorescence occurs, each compound also has an emission spectrum, which is the spectrum of wavelengths in which most of the emitted fluorescent energy from that compound is found. To develop a fluorescent assay, the emission spectrum of the compound of interest must be determined. Then, the narrow band of wavelengths in which maximum emission occurs is isolated by the secondary monochromator. Light passing from the monochromator is collected by a photodetector, measured, and processed in

a manner similar to that described for spectrophotometry. Various lenses, slits and in some cases, polarizing devices are included in fluorometers to help direct and/or polarize light as well as to reduce stray light in the system.

A wide variety of fluorometer designs are available. Strictly speaking, fluorometers are instruments that can produce light at only a few wavelengths, because their primary monochromator is a filter. Many instruments that use fluorometry have primary monochromators that are diffraction gratings or prisms. These instruments can produce a spectrum of excitation wavelengths and are known as spectrofluorometers. Some fluorometers are designed to compensate for variations in the intensity of the light source and, therefore, decrease the frequency with which calibration is required (i.e., ratio referencing). Fluorometers also might use a pulsed light source and measure fluorescence only during those periods of time when the source is off. This technique, which is known as time-resolved fluorometry, eliminates the effects of light scatter.

Several variables affect fluorescence, including pH, temperature, light scatter, the inner-filter effect, and interference by other molecules. The pH has a marked effect on the ability of molecules to fluoresce and, therefore, must be carefully controlled. At higher temperatures, molecules in solutions move more rapidly, which causes these molecules to collide. Such collisions dissipate energy that otherwise would produce fluorescence. Therefore, increased temperature reduces fluorescence, whereas decreased temperature increases fluorescence.

Although most of the exciting light passes straight through the cuvette and is not measured by the photodetector placed at a 90° angle, some of the exciting light rays do collide with particles in solution and then scatter in all directions, including that of the photodetector. In some cases, some of the energy from the exciting light is absorbed by molecules other than those of interest, and the resulting scattered light has a longer wavelength than that of the exciting light. The resulting light falls into the emission spectrum of the substance being measured and can interfere with its analysis. These "light-scattering" factors are controlled by adjusting the wavelengths of the exciting light and/or the emitted light to avoid the wavelengths of the scattered light. Narrowing the slit width of light passing to the secondary monochromator also controls light-scatter effects.

The inner-filter effect occurs in solutions with very high concentrations of fluorescing substances. In these solutions, exciting light is absorbed in significant quantities as it progresses through the contents of the cuvette; therefore, it causes less fluorescence as it travels. In the fluorometer diagrammed in Figure 1.49, fluorescence is measured primarily from the center of the cuvette. If the inner-filter effect is occurring, fluorescence from the center of the cuvette is considerably less than that from the front of the cuvette. Some fluorometers are designed to read only fluorescence emitted from the front surface of the cuvette, thus eliminating problems with the inner-filter effect.

Interference by other molecules is a potential problem when biologic fluids are being analyzed by fluorometry. Some of these molecules fluoresce (e.g., bilirubin and some proteins), whereas others scatter light (e.g., proteins and lipids). When developing assays on biologic fluids, adjustments must be made to minimize the effects of these molecules.

Although the mechanism of measuring concentrations is different, the basic procedure for performing fluorometry is similar to that for absorbance spectrophotometry. Calibrators are used to establish a calibration curve, and blanks are used to negate any effects other than those attributable to the substance of interest. At low concentrations of fluorescing substances (e.g., resulting in an absorbance of <2% of the exciting light), a direct, linear relationship usually exists between fluorescence and concentration. If the concentration of the fluorescing substance is high (e.g., >2% of the exciting light is absorbed), the relationship between fluorescence and concentration might be nonlinear. The inner-filter effect plays a part in this phenomenon.

Light-Scatter Techniques

Light-scatter techniques can be used to measure the concentrations of larger molecules in fluids. When light is projected through solutions containing large molecules such as immunoglobulins and other large proteins, antigen–antibody complexes, and some drugs, these molecules cause light to scatter in all directions. These techniques, therefore, are potentially useful in measuring the concentrations of these substances. With light scattering, the wavelength of the light being scattered is the same as that of the light being projected into the solution. By assessing the degree of light scattering, the concentration of the substance of interest can be measured. Two techniques, turbidimetry and nephalometry, use the principles of light scattering to make such measurements.

In turbidimetry, the decreased intensity of a light beam passing through a turbid solution is measured. The intensity of light decreases, because a portion of it has been scattered by the large molecules of interest. A basic turbidimeter is diagrammed in *Figure 1.50*. In a turbidimeter, light rays are projected through a cuvette containing the analyte in solution, and the intensity of light leaving the solution (i.e., the transmitted light) is measured in a straight line from the transmitted light. The decrease in transmitted light intensity is proportional to the concentration of the analyte. A turbidimeter, therefore, is similar in principle to an absorbance spectrophotometer.

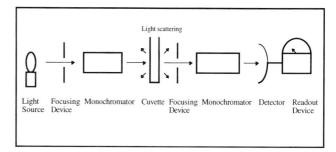

Figure 1.50   A basic turbidimeter. Arrows represent light.

In nephalometry, a beam of light also is projected through a solution containing the analyte, but the photodetector is placed at a 90° angle to the cuvette *(Fig. 1.51)*. In addition, scattered rather than transmitted light is measured. The intensity of the scattered light is proportional to the concentration of the analyte. Nephalometry, therefore, is analogous to fluorometry in terms of configuration of the light path. If a solution is not visibly turbid, nephalometry is a somewhat better technique than turbidimetry.

A direct relationship exists between the concentrations of light-scattering molecules and the degree of light scattering. A direct relationship also exists between the sizes of the light-scattering molecules and the degree of light scattering. When developing light-scatter techniques, the size of the particles being measured must be considered, because larger particles (e.g., immunoglobulin M, chylomicrons, and antigen–antibody complexes) cause an asymmetric distribution of scattered light. In some cases, the position of the photodetector must be altered to adjust for this. Large molecules or particles other than

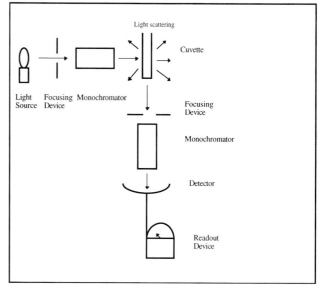

Figure 1.51   A basic nephalometer. Arrows represent light.

those of interest can interfere with light-scatter techniques as well.

With light-scatter techniques, the analytic procedures are similar to those of absorbance spectrophotometry. Calibrators are used to establish a calibration curve, and blanks are used to negate the effects of reagents and other light-scattering molecules.

Electrochemical Techniques

A variety of electrochemical techniques are used in clinical chemistry and most often are applied in measurements of various ions as well as partial pressures of oxygen and carbon dioxide in blood. These techniques also can be used to measure other substances if the chemical reactions used in the assay system result in production of an ion. Basic information on electrochemical techniques and examples of some of their applications are described in this section. Note, however, that in-depth understanding of electrochemical techniques requires detailed understanding regarding the physical chemistry principles underlying these techniques. Instilling such an understanding is not the goal of this section, and only those physical chemistry principles necessary for understanding the basic theory of these techniques are described. Electrochemical methods are applied through a wide variety of electrode and instrument configurations; this section does not attempt to be an all-inclusive summary of these variations.

Potentiometry

Potentiometry is commonly used for measurements of pH (i.e., hydrogen ion concentration), partial pressure of carbon dioxide in the blood, and concentrations of certain electrolytes in the blood or serum. In potentiometry, the electrical potential between two electrodes is measured, thereby giving a value that can be used to calculate the concentrations of various electrolytes.

Electrical potential is illustrated in *Figure 1.52*, which diagrams a small plate composed of a metal (M) that has been placed in a solution composed of a cationic form of that metal (M^{+1}) and an anionic substance (Cl^{-1}). As the metal plate lies in the solution, a small amount of the metal leaves the plate and becomes ionic metal (M^{+1}). The degree to which metal cations (M^{+1}) leave the plate relates directly to the activity (and concentration) of the metal cations originally in the solution. The higher the original activity (and concentration) of these cations, the fewer cations leave the plate to enter the solution. The process diagrammed in Figure 1.52 results in the metal plate gaining one electron as each molecule of metal is ionized and leaves the plate (i.e., the electron is left behind on the plate). Because the cations (M^{+1}) and the anions (Cl^{-1}) in the original solution were equal in number, the addition

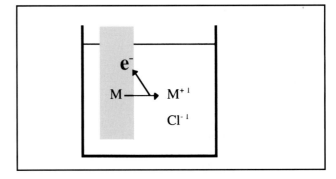

Figure 1.52 A simple electrode. A plate composed of a metal (M) has been placed in a solution of metal cations (M^{+1}) and an ion (Cl^{-1}). As a metal ion leaves the plate, an electron is left on the plate, which gives the plate a net negative charge.

of more cations to the solution makes it more positively charged (i.e., no extra Cl^{-1} ions are available to neutralize the M^{+1} ions leaving the plate). Addition of free electrons to the plate makes it more negatively charged. The net effect is that the plate becomes more negatively charged than the solution.

In the situation just described, work is required to add another electron to the plate, because it already is negatively charged. The amount of work required depends on the magnitude of the charge on the metal plate: the more negatively charged the plate, the more work required to add another electron. As noted earlier, the magnitude of this charge relates directly to the activity (and concentration) of metal cations in the original solution. The work needed to neutralize this charge relates to the electrical potential according to the equation

$$\text{Electrical potential} = \frac{\text{Work}}{\text{Valence of the ion}}$$

In this equation, work is defined as described earlier (e.g., the energy needed to add an electron to the metal plate). The valence of the ion is the net negative or positive charge of that ion (e.g., chloride = Cl^{-1} = valence of 1, sulfate = SO_4^{-2} = valence of 2). Because the valence is constant for a given ion in a specific electrode, the only variable in the electrical potential of that electrode is the work required to transfer an electron to the metal plate. As noted, this work depends on the charge of the metal plate, which in turn relates directly to the activity of metal ions in the solution. The activity of the metal ions relates directly to the concentration of these ions. In other words, the concentration of metal ions in the solution directly influences the electrical potential developed in an electrode. Therefore, the electrical potential can be assessed on the metal plate in this example and then used to determine the concentration of metal ions originally in the solution.

In this example, note that the metal in the plate and the metal ions in the solution that are being measured are the same element. This is the basic feature of many electrodes used with electrochemical techniques. In addition, note that measuring the potential produced by the electrode described here is not possible. To measure potential, two electrodes are needed that are electrically connected in two ways: through an instrument designed to measure electrical potential (i.e., a potentiometer), and through some type of membrane or bridge that completes the electrical circuit. An example of two electrodes connected to produce an electrical potential is diagrammed in *Figure 1.53*. The electrode on the left in this figure is a silver plate coated with silver chloride (i.e., a silver/silver chloride electrode) and immersed in a solution of potassium chloride of both known and consistent concentration. In this electrode, potential develops because of the addition of a small amount of silver to the electrode through the reaction

$$2 \text{ AgCl (from the coating)} + 2 \text{ electrons} \rightarrow 2 \text{ Ag (metal added to plate)} + 2 \text{ Cl}^-$$

This plate, therefore, becomes slightly positively charged, because it loses electrons that combine with Ag^+ to form metallic Ag. At the hydrogen electrode, hydrogen gas is lost from the electrode through the reaction

$$H_2 \rightarrow 2H^+ + 2 \text{ electrons}$$

This electrode, therefore, gains electrons and becomes negatively charged. The total potential in this system is the sum of the potentials of the two electrodes. The net effect, however, is an electrical potential between these electrodes that is proportional to the only variable in the system: the hydrogen ion concentration. In this case, the higher the concentration of hydrogen ions in the solu-

tion, the less likely that the hydrogen gas in the hydrogen electrode will become ionized. Therefore, the electrode will develop less of a charge, and the potential between the hydrogen and Ag/AgCl will be less. In other words, the potential measured relates inversely to the hydrogen ion concentration in the tested fluid. The salt bridge in this example allows electrical contact between the two electrodes without changing the potential. This is a very simplified version of a pH meter.

In summary, electrochemical techniques such as potentiometry require two electrodes. One is the reference electrode (i.e., the Ag/AgCl electrode in the example), and the other is the measuring electrode (i.e., the hydrogen electrode in the example). Because the conditions in the reference electrode are defined by the instrumentation, the potential of this electrode is both known and consistent. Any difference in potential, therefore, results from the measuring electrode and relates to differences in the activity of the ion of interest in the solution. Because the basic measurement in potentiometry is electrical potential, the activity rather than the concentration of ions is being measured. Thus, it is possible to calculate the concentration from the activity. In practice, these instruments are calibrated with solutions of known concentrations; therefore, the results are reported directly as concentrations rather than as activities. That activity rather than concentration is being measured might seem like an esoteric point, but this difference helps to explain why the measurement of ions such as sodium and potassium in markedly lipemic serum is more valid by potentiometric techniques than by flame photometry. (This difference is discussed later, along with ion specific membrane electrodes.)

As noted earlier, the electrochemical cell in Figure 1.53 is a very basic form of pH meter. In clinical chemistry laboratories, pH meters can be stand-alone instruments but also can be incorporated into blood-gas analyzers. Modern pH meters are available in a variety of designs, but the basic components as diagrammed in Figure 1.53 are still included. These designs arrange these components in more compact configurations. A pH-sensitive glass commonly is incorporated into the design of these electrodes, and pH-measuring electrodes also have been designed for use with continuously flowing fluid.

Potentiometry also has been adapted to measure a number of other ions. The electrodes used in these measurements commonly are designated as ion-selective membrane electrodes, or simply as ion-specific electrodes. The design and materials used to manufacture these electrodes are variable. The basic components of and theory behind the operation of these electrodes are the same as those described earlier. An important component of each electrode is a membrane that is sensitive to the ion that electrode measures. This membrane might be a special type

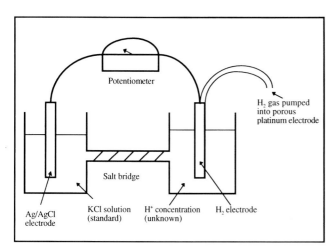

Figure 1.53 An electrochemical cell designed to measure hydrogen ion concentration.

of glass (i.e., glass electrode), a single crystal of some ion-selective material or this same material imbedded in an inert matrix (i.e., solid-state electrode), or an ion-sensitive material dissolved in an inert solvent (i.e., ion-exchange electrode). Regardless of the type of membrane chosen, the basic principle is that contact of the ion-sensitive membrane with the test solution causes a membrane potential to develop. This membrane potential is proportional to the activity of the ion of interest in that solution, and it can be measured with use of a reference electrode and a potentiometer and then converted to readout the concentration of the ion.

As noted, the electrical potential that is measured when using ion-specific electrodes relates directly to the activity of the ion of interest. The concentration of that ion then is calculated using certain assumptions and the formula

$$\text{Concentration of ion} = (\text{Activity of ion}) \times (\text{Appropriate factor for that ion } [F])$$

The activity of the ion is, of course, measured by the potentiometer, but the appropriate factor (F) for that ion must be calculated. This is a constant for a given ion and is calculated using the formula

$$F = \frac{\text{Mass concentration of water in serum or plasma}}{\text{Activity coefficient of the ion} \times \text{Degree of ion dissociation}}$$

In potentiometry, all of these factors are constant for each ion; therefore, the value of F is constant for each ion. The activity coefficient relates to the ionic strength of a solution and has been estimated for each ion in a biologic solution. The degree of dissociation is the proportion of the total ions which is free in the serum or plasma. This varies with different ions. The mass concentration of water is the mass of water found in 1 L of serum or plasma. In other words, if 0.90 kg of water are present in 1 L of serum, this serum has a mass concentration of 0.90 kg/L.

The mass concentration of water can change depending on whether other constituents of plasma or serum displace water. This can happen when extremely high concentrations of lipids or protein are present. In such cases, the mass concentration of water in serum or plasma decreases. The assumed value for the mass concentration of water used in the previous equation, which is used to convert ion activity to ion concentration, does not change. As a result, high lipid or protein concentrations in serum or plasma do not alter the concentration as reported by potentiometric applications. In other words, in lipemic samples, potentiometric assays measure the ion activity in

the water component of the serum or plasma and report ion concentrations with the assumption that the proportion of water in the blood is normal. Flame photometry, however, measures and reports the ion concentrations of the water and lipid components combined. Because the concentration of ions in the lipid component are low and the ion concentrations in the water compartment are the physiologically important ones, the concentrations as reported by potentiometry are considered to be more physiologically valid than those reported by flame photometry.

The partial pressure of carbon dioxide (PCO_2) in the blood also is measured by potentiometry. This method is used in sophisticated blood-gas analyzers and in patient-side analyzers. Whereas CO_2 is not an ion, the CO_2 electrode is designed to produce an ion in proportion to the PCO_2 in the blood. The design of such an electrode is shown in *Figure 1.54* as a modified pH electrode. In this electrode, a chamber containing sodium bicarbonate solution is separated from the blood sample by a thin membrane. The CO_2 passes through the membrane into the sodium bicarbonate solution, and the following chemical reaction occurs:

$$CO_2 + H_2O \rightarrow H_2CO_3$$
$$H_2CO_3 \rightarrow H^+ + HCO_3^-$$

The amount of CO_2 that diffuses through the membrane affects the H^+ concentration in the sodium bicarbonate solution in direct proportion to the PCO_2. The remainder of this electrode is a pH electrode that senses the change in H^+ concentration of the sodium bicarbonate solution.

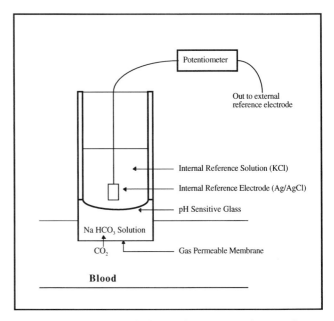

Figure 1.54   An electrode designed to measure the partial pressure of carbon dioxide in the blood.

These changes alter the electrical potential of this electrode, and the instrument then calculates the P_{CO_2} from these changes.

Amperometry

Amperometry is a technique that measures the electrical current passing between two electrodes in a chemical cell while a constant voltage is applied. This differentiates the technique from potentiometry, in which no electrical current flows and no voltage is applied. The most common application of amperometry in clinical chemistry is electrochemical measurement of the partial pressure of oxygen (P_{O_2}) in blood.

The technique is most easily understood by considering how this electrochemical cell operates. A typical P_{O_2} electrode is diagrammed in *Figure 1.55*. An electrical potential of –0.65 V is applied to this electrode, and almost no current passes through this electrode if no oxygen is present. When this electrode is submersed in blood, O_2 from the blood diffuses through the O_2-permeable membrane and comes into contact with the tip of the platinum electrode. The O_2 then is reduced by the reaction

$$O_2 + 2H_2O + 4 \text{ electrons} \rightarrow 4 \text{ OH}^-$$

This process consumes electrons and, therefore, produces an electrical current under these conditions. This current can be measured by an ammeter as amperage. The amount of current produced is proportional to the P_{O_2} of the blood. Calibration solutions are used to relate the amperage to the P_{O_2} of the unknown.

Coulometry and Conductometry

Coulometry and conductometry are two other electrochemical methods that occasionally are used to measure the concentrations of substances. Coulometry involves measurement of the amount of electrical energy passing between two electrodes in an electrochemical cell. This electrical current is produced by chemical reactions occurring at the surfaces of each of two electrodes, resulting in the loss or gain of electrons by these electrodes. The amount of electrical current produced is directly proportional to the concentration of the substance being measured. This substance is consumed in an electron-using or electron-producing process. Unlike potentiometry, the actual current rather than the potential between two electrodes is measured, and unlike amperometry, no outside voltage is applied to the system. This method has been applied to the measurement of serum chloride concentrations.

Conductometry involves measurement of a fluid's ability to conduct an electrical current between two electrodes when a voltage is applied to the system. This property, which is known as electrolytic conductance, occurs via movement of ions in the fluid. The conductivity of an aqueous fluid depends on the concentration and ionic strength of the electrolytes in that fluid: the higher the electrolyte concentration, the higher the conductivity. Conductometry can be used to measure the production of ions by chemical reactions. Therefore, it is possible to measure the concentration of a substance in a fluid if it is used in a chemical reaction producing ions in numbers proportional to the substance of interest. The increased conductivity resulting from the production of these ions would then be proportional to the original concentration of the substance being measured.

Osmometry

Osmometry involves measurement of the concentrations of particles in a fluid. The clinical significance of these concentrations, which are reported as osmolality (particles per kilogram of solvent [osmol/kg]) or osmolarity (particles per liter of solvent [osmol/L]), is discussed in Chapter 22. To understand osmometry, the changes that occur in a solution when concentrations of particles (i.e., solute) dissolved in a fluid (i.e., solvent) increase must be understood. These changes, which are known as colligative properties, are increased osmotic pressure, decreased vapor pressure, increased boiling point (because of decreased vapor pressure), and decreased freezing point. Any of these colligative properties could be used to measure osmolality or osmolarity. Among those properties that actually are used to make these measurements are freezing point depression and decreased vapor pressure.

The freezing-point depression technique is the most commonly used. As the name implies, this type of osmometer measures the freezing point of a solution through a number of steps involving freezing, thawing, and freezing

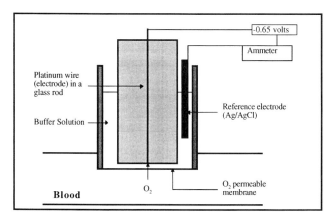

Figure 1.55 An electrochemical cell designed to measure the partial pressure of oxygen in the blood.

again. This process is monitored by a thermistor, which measures temperature, and it determines the freezing point by determining the temperature at an equilibrium between freezing and thawing. The osmolality or osmolarity of the fluid then is determined by comparing this temperature with those of various calibration fluids with known osmolality or osmolarity.

Vapor pressure osmometers are less commonly used. These instruments measure the osmolality or osmolarity of a fluid by determining the dew point (i.e., the temperature at the point of equilibrium between vaporization and condensation) of that fluid. The dew point is a gauge of vapor pressure: the higher the osmolality or osmolarity of a fluid, the lower its dew point. In general, vapor pressure osmometers are not considered to be as precise as freezing-point osmometers. In addition, volatile substances such as ethanol are not detected by vapor pressure osmometers, whereas they are detected by the freezing-point depression technique.

Protein Electrophoresis

Electrophoresis is an analytic technique based on the movement of charged particles through a solution under the influence of an electrical field. In clinical chemistry, electrophoretic techniques most commonly are used to separate and analyze serum proteins. When serum is placed on or in a supporting substance that allows migration of these proteins and can carry an electrical charge, these proteins move through this material just as other charged particles do. The movement of proteins through such a substance depends on the net charge on the protein molecule, the size and shape of the protein molecule, the strength of the electrical field applied, the type of supporting medium, and the temperature. In a given electrophoresis application, the latter three items are held constant. Therefore, the migration of protein molecules depends on the net charge and on the size and shape of the molecules. As a result, different serum proteins migrate at different rates and, possibly, in different directions in the supporting substance.

A simple electrophoresis chamber is demonstrated in *Figure 1.56*. Small amounts of serum are placed in specific areas on the surface of the supporting substance or in small depressions cut at one end. Supporting substances commonly used include agarose gel and cellulose acetate. Starch gel is less commonly used in clinical applications. Polyacrylamide gel also can be used for protein electrophoresis and separates more serum protein fractions than the other supporting substances. Polyacrylamide electrophoresis does produce interesting information, but the clinical applications of this information in veterinary medicine are not yet widely understood. The common supporting substances usually are in the

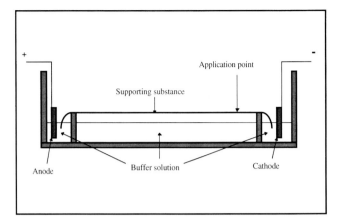

Figure 1.56   A simple electrophoresis chamber.

form of a sheet, and they either have buffer incorporated into them when they are produced or are soaked in buffer before use. The buffer determines the pH at which the process occurs, and the pH determines the type of charge as well as the net charge on each type of protein molecule. Both ends of the supporting substance are in contact with buffer solution in an adjacent well. These buffer solutions are not in contact with each other, however, or with the buffer solution in the center well. The electrical current is applied to the system by electrodes placed into each of these wells. A negatively charged cathode is placed in the well at one end, and a positively charged anode is placed in the well at the other end. The serum sample typically is applied at the end near the cathode, because most proteins are negatively charged and migrate toward the anode. When an electrical current is applied to this system, proteins migrate toward either the anode or the cathode, depending on whether they are negatively charged (i.e., toward the anode) or positively charged (i.e., toward the cathode). As noted, the rate of this migration depends on both the net charge of the molecule and its size and shape, and because these vary with the different types of proteins, different proteins migrate at different rates. If this migration is allowed to occur for a fixed period of time, various protein fractions are isolated along a straight line in the supporting substance.

A typical distribution of serum protein fractions in a sheet of supporting substance after electrophoretic separation is shown in *Figure 1.57*. Albumin is the smallest of the serum proteins and has the highest net negative charge relative to its size. Albumin, therefore, migrates faster than the other proteins, and it advances further toward the anode during the time allowed for separation. The globulins are larger than albumin and, because of this, do not migrate as far toward the anode. The relative migration distances of the globulins depend on the relationship of their size to their net negative charge. The

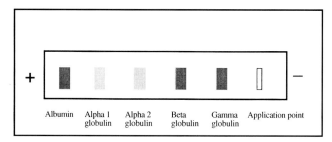

Figure 1.57 Typical electrophoretic separation of serum proteins in a sheet of supporting substance. The type and number of fractions actually separated depends on the type of electrophoresis application and on the species from which the serum was sampled.

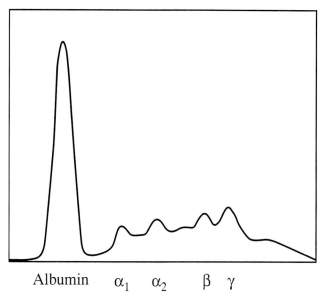

Figure 1.58 A densitometer scan (electrophoretic scan) of a serum protein electrophoresis separation.

gamma globulins have the smallest net negative charge relative to their size and, therefore, migrate the shortest distance toward the anode. In some techniques, the application point actually might lie in the gamma-globulin region, with some gamma globulins migrating to the cathode side of this point. The number of fractions separated depends on the electrophoretic technique used and the species being analyzed. (These separations are discussed in more detail in Chapter 26.)

Once electrophoretic separation is completed, the protein fractions usually are identified and quantitated. Staining these fractions aids in this process. Various types of dye that stain protein can be used, including amido black, bromphenol blue, Coomassie brilliant blue, nigrosin, and ponceau s. After staining, it is possible, with experience, to visually identify the various proteins fractions based on their order of migration. Visual examination also sometimes reveals apparently increased quantities of some protein fractions. This quantitation is more easily accomplished using a densitometer to scan the protein pattern and calculate the percentages and absolute quantities of protein in each fraction. A densitometer measures the amount of protein in each fraction by projecting light through these fractions as these are mechanically passed over the light source. A photodetector determines the width and density of each fraction. Results are reported as a densitometer scan, which more commonly is known as an electrophoretic pattern or electrophoretogram, as shown in *Figure 1.58* and as both a percentage and an absolute value for each protein fraction. The absolute value for each fraction is calculated by the microprocessor in the instrument using the total protein concentration, which is entered by the operator, and the percentage of each fraction as determined by the densitometer:

$$\text{Absolute quantity of each fraction} = \frac{\text{Percentage of each fraction} \times \text{Total serum protein}}{100}$$

Most densitometers automatically identify each fraction as well as the boundaries between these fractions. The operator can and should change these in some cases.

Once the absolute quantities in the various fractions are determined, they can be compared with known reference ranges for that species, and any abnormalities can be identified. Use of such data in clinical chemistry of proteins is discussed in Chapter 26.

SUGGESTED READINGS

Hematology
Beutler E, Lichtman MA, Coller BS. William's hematology. 5th ed. New York: McGraw-Hill, 1994.
Jain NC. Schalm's veterinary hematology. 4th ed. Philadelphia: Lea & Febiger, 1986.

Chemistry
Durst RA, Siggaard-Andersen O. Electrochemistry. In: Burtis CA, Ashwood ER, eds. Tietz textbook of clinical chemistry. 2nd ed. Philadelphia: WB Saunders, 1994:159–183.
Epstein E, Karcher RE. Electrophoresis. In: Burtis CA, Ashwood ER, eds. Tietz textbook of clinical chemistry. 2nd ed. Philadelphia: WB Saunders, 1994:191–205.
Evenson MA. Photometry. In: Burtis CA, Ashwood ER, eds. Tietz textbook of clinical chemistry. 2nd ed. Philadelphia: WB Saunders, 1994:103–131.
Freier EF. Osmometry. In: Burtis CA, Ashwood ER, eds. Tietz textbook of clinical chemistry. 2nd ed. Philadelphia: WB Saunders, 1994:184–190.
Tiffany TO. Fluorometry, nephelometry, and turbidimetry. In: Burtis CA, Ashwood ER, eds. Tietz textbook of clinical chemistry. 2nd ed. Philadelphia: WB Saunders, 1994:132–158.
Vap LM, Mitzner B. An update on chemistry analyzers. Vet Clin North Am Small Anim Pract 1996;26:1129–1154.

CHAPTER

2

SAMPLE COLLECTION, PROCESSING, AND ANALYSIS OF LABORATORY SERVICE OPTIONS

In the previous chapter, laboratory technology was reviewed. To take advantage of this technology and its medical diagnostic capability, however, samples for the respective procedures must be properly collected and prepared. From this rather vast array of diagnostic options, the veterinarian must also make decisions regarding implementation of these procedures, which will be influenced by several factors. The important factors include the type of practice (e.g., general, outpatient clinic, emergency facility, specialty referral center), geographic location, and practice style of the individuals involved. This chapter presents rules for proper sample processing and guidelines for selecting the appropriate laboratory diagnostic options.

SAMPLE COLLECTION AND PROCESSING

Regardless of the technique or laboratory used for any diagnostic test, obtaining reliable results starts with

proper collection and handling of the sample. Sample collection, processing, testing, and interpretation all must be properly performed as a complete, sequential chain of events for a diagnostic result to have its intended value. For example, even the most reliable test, performed in the most reliable facility and interpreted by the most skilled diagnostician, cannot overcome the error introduced by an inappropriate technique used in sample collection or handling. This section provides guidelines for sample collection and handling that will ensure the initial sequence of events are properly performed.

Containers for Sample Collection

A variety of commercially available tubes are used for blood collection. These tubes contain the appropriate anticoagulant for the various diagnostic procedures and a vacuum for drawing in the appropriate volume of blood. These tubes are commonly known as vacutainer tubes (after the trademark of Becton-Dickinson). The following commonly used vacuum tubes are described in the approximate order of their frequency of use. Tubes are commonly referred to by their stopper color, which is used to identify the type of anticoagulation system the tube contains *(Fig. 2.1)*.

Red-Top or Serum Collection Tube

The red-top of serum collection tube contains no anticoagulant. Blood that is placed in this tube is expected to clot so that serum may be harvested. This tube is used to collect serum for common biochemical determinations, such as those tests used in creating biochemical profiles.

Lavender-Top Tube

The lavender-top tube contains the anticoagulant ethylenediaminetetraacetic acid (EDTA) salt. This tube is used to collect blood for hematologic determinations. The EDTA anticoagulant results in the most consistent preservation of cell volume and morphologic features on stained films. The liquid tripotassium salt is the most commonly used form of EDTA, and this form is preferred for use in preservation of cell volumes as measured on automated hematology analyzers. Powdered forms are not recommended because of slower, inconsistent mixing with blood that is added to the tube.

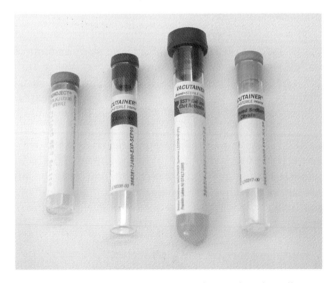

Figure 2.1 Representative vacuum tubes used in the collection of blood samples for diagnostic tests. The tubes are, from left to right, a lavender-top EDTA tube, a red-top tube without anticoagulant, a serum-separation tube, and a blue-top citrate tube. Note that the serum-separation tube contains a yellow gel at the bottom.

Green-Top or Heparin Tube

The green-top tube contains heparin. This anticoagulant is used for certain special biochemistry tests, particularly those that require a whole-blood aliquot for determination and that might be influenced by the presence of other chemical anticoagulation systems.

Blue-Top or Citrate Tube

The blue-top tube contains sodium citrate. It is used for coagulation biochemistry determinations.

Sure-Sep Tube

The Sure-Sep tube is a variation of the red-top tube containing no anticoagulant. The stopper is red with black mottling, and the tube contains a gel that separates packed cell fractions from serum when it undergoes centrifugation. It is convenient for use in situations when centrifugation at the site of collection and transport to the laboratory without the transfer of serum to a separate tube are desirable. The gel physically separates cells from the serum fluid, thus preventing analyte metabolism from occurring at the cell/fluid interface.

Gray-Top or Fluoride Tube

The gray-top tube contains sodium fluoride. Fluoride is not an anticoagulant, however. Rather, it inhibits enzymes in the glycolytic pathway and prevents erythrocytes from metabolizing glucose while whole blood is transported to the laboratory. It is not commonly used.

Tips for Filling Vacuum Tubes

A few simple habits must be developed for appropriately filling tubes:

1. The ratio of blood to anticoagulant volume is designed to be fixed. This is particularly important for hematology and blood coagulation biochemistry tests; therefore, a tube with anticoagulant should be filled to the volume specified for that tube. The amount of vacuum in the tube facilitates this, but the user should watch to ensure that this consistently occurs.
2. When collecting blood for several diagnostic procedures, fill the tube(s) containing anticoagulant first and the tube containing no anticoagulant last. The most commonly used combination of tubes is an EDTA and clot/serum tube. The EDTA tube should be filled first so that any clot formation is minimized. This is unimportant in the tube without anticoagulant, however, because the blood is expected to clot in that tube.

3. Vacuum tubes should be filled using minimal positive force, because forceful passage of blood through the needle may cause hemolysis, which in turn may cause an error in the biochemical measurements. Smaller-gauge needles are more likely to cause hemolysis. An 18- to 20-G needle is best for most collection procedures.

4. Clean venipunctures with no tissue contamination are important. Tissue contamination may result in unwanted platelet aggregation and clotting in samples collected using anticoagulants. As a result, select venipuncture sites (e.g., the jugular vein) that likely will yield the appropriate volume of blood needed for the diagnostic tests being ordered for a given patient.

5. Select a venipuncture site that will yield the desired amount of blood easily. This means being able to draw the blood with little or no collapse of the vein so that blood may be transferred to the anticoagulant tubes as rapidly as possible. Recommended venipuncture sites for diagnostic screening procedures such as a hemogram and biochemical profile include: the jugular vein for small dogs, cats, horses, and cows; and the cephalic or jugular vein in medium to large dogs. These procedures generally require 5 to 12 mL of blood depending on the laboratory and the complexity of the screening procedures.

General Sample Handling Procedures

Hematologic Procedures

Blood collected for a complete blood count (CBC) should be analyzed within 1 hour or be prepared in the proper way for analysis at a later time. If the blood is not analyzed within 1 hour, a blood film should be prepared and the tube refrigerated. Morphologic features of cells may deteriorate rapidly on storage of blood in an EDTA tube; an air-dried blood film preserves the morphology of such cells for later examination. Refrigeration of the blood tube also helps to preserve the cell components that are measured by automated cell-counting systems. For example, cell swelling that could produce artifactual increases in mean cell volume (MCV) and hematocrit occurs as blood is stored in a tube at room or higher temperature. For some analytical systems with differential capability, it is recommended by the laboratory that blood be held at room temperature. Blood should never be frozen, however, because this will result in lysis of the cells. In addition, blood films should not be refrigerated, because water condensation on the glass may damage the cellular morphology.

For hematologic measurements, the EDTA tube should be filled to the specified volume, and tissue contamination during venipuncture should be avoided. Underfilling the EDTA tube results in excess EDTA, which osmotically shrinks erythrocytes. In turn, this results in falsely decreased packed cell volume and MCV when the microhematocrit procedure is used. Tissue contamination during venipuncture results in platelet aggregation *(Fig. 2.2)*, and this artifactually decreases the platelet concentration as determined by cell-counting systems and may contribute to fluidic obstruction on some hematology instruments.

Clinical Biochemistry Procedures

Blood collected in the red-top tube is allowed to clot for 15 to 30 minutes and then centrifuged to separate the cellular components from the resultant serum. The fluid phase of the blood should be separated from the cellular elements, because cells metabolize certain chemical components in the serum. The most notable example is glucose. If left in contact with cellular elements, glucose is metabolized at a rate of approximately 10% per hour. After centrifugation, serum is harvested by a transfer pipette to a second tube or is dispensed directly to devices for biochemical determinations *(Fig. 2.3)*. Harvested serum should be analyzed quickly; otherwise, it can be refrigerated for as long as 24 to 48 hours. If serum is to be held for longer than 24 to 48 hours, it should be frozen, and serum that is to be held frozen indefinitely (e.g., for archival purposes) should be stored at −70°. Most chemical constituents are stable under these conditions. If serum is frozen and then thawed for analysis, the thawed aliquot should be thoroughly mixed before testing.

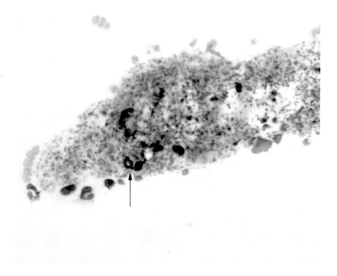

Figure 2.2 Platelet aggregation observed on a stained blood film. Tissue contamination may result in microclots that consist of hundreds of platelets, which falsely decrease the platelet concentration. Microclots also may trap leukocytes. Note the representative leukocyte (arrow); low magnification.

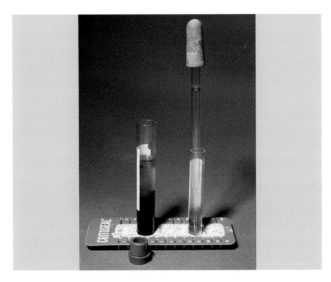

Figure 2.3 Serum preparation for biochemical tests. The tube on the left was allowed to clot and then centrifuged to pack the cells below the serum layer. A transfer pipette is used to transfer serum from the centrifuged sample to the tube on the right.

Serum enzymes require separate consideration regarding storage. A general rule is that for best reliability, serum enzyme activities should be determined within 24 hours of collection. Long-term archival storage of samples for determination of serum enzyme activity is not advised. Data on the exact stability of serum enzyme activity under various storage conditions is difficult to interpret. Knowledge regarding this subject has not been updated in any systematic way during recent years, and historical data were not collected in any consistent manner. Thus, our current understanding of enzyme stability during storage may be summarized as follows: Commonly measured enzymes, including alanine aminotransferase (ALT), aspartate aminotransferase, and alkaline phosphatase, and amylase activities are satisfactorily stable (>70% activity) when stored at 4°C. Freezing, however, may result in considerably accelerated loss of ALT activity. Creatine kinase activity should be measured as soon as possible, because considerable activity is lost after 24 hours regardless of the storage conditions.

Special Procedures

Special laboratory diagnostic procedures are usually performed by centralized or commercial laboratories because of the complexity or specialized instrumentation involved. These procedures are performed less frequently, and they are more dependent on unique requirements of the technology employed by the laboratory undertaking the procedure. As a result, the laboratory protocol materials for sample collection and handling should be consulted rather than committing these requirements to memory.

ANALYSIS OF DIAGNOSTIC SERVICE IMPLEMENTATION OPTIONS

The veterinarian has several options for obtaining laboratory diagnostic data. These may be generally considered as falling into three categories:

1. In-house (performed on the premises).
2. Commercial veterinary laboratory.
3. Human laboratory or community hospital.

Several factors should be considered when formulating a strategy for using one (or more) of these options. The veterinary facility should self-assess the following:

1. Type of practice (e.g., general practice, outpatient clinic, emergency facility, specialty referral center).
2. Geographic location (proximity to reliable service options).
3. Practice style of the individuals involved.
4. Willingness to implement and evaluate quality-assurance programs.
5. Willingness to invest the time to evaluate and troubleshoot diagnostics with varying degrees of complexity.
6. Willingness to invest in a good microscope and training of personnel regarding basic clinical microscopy.
7. Desired turnaround times.
8. Ability to invest in instrumentation and training for the operators.

Advantages and Disadvantages of In-House Laboratory Testing

Advantages of in-house laboratory testing include rapid turnaround time and control over when testing is performed relative to when samples are drawn in a particular practice setting. In-house testing may also have economic advantages in certain situations.

Disadvantages of in-house laboratory testing include the issue of technical operator expertise for basic laboratory technology, which may not be available or affordable in many veterinary facilities. Attention to detail and quality assurance also must be managed by someone on site, and an investment in equipment is required. In addition, access to a clinical pathologist to help with the characterization of abnormal screening tests, particularly blood film analysis for hematology, must be cultivated, and arrangements for specialized testing to supplement in-clinic diagnostic tests must be procured.

Advantages and Disadvantages of Commercial Veterinary Laboratories

The major advantages of commercial veterinary laboratories are the cost leveraging of automated instrumentation and centralized testing volume, a complete menu of testing services, professional oversight of technical performance, and pathology support. Because the automated instrumentation is dedicated to animal-specific diagnostics, it is usually already adapted for the proper analysis of animal samples. Quality-control programs are usually implemented as well, but these are variable.

The major disadvantages of commercial veterinary laboratories include relatively fixed turnaround times, which are dictated by sample transportation logistics. In addition, sample transportation is a major part of the cost of the service. Pathology support and consultation may be variable as well.

Advantages and Disadvantages of Human Laboratory Facilities

The advantage of human laboratory facilities is that they may be the only available option in less-populated areas. The disadvantages, however, are considerable. The instrumentation, particularly for hematology, is usually not modified for animal-specific diagnostics, and knowledge about the consequences is often lacking. Animal-specific pathology support is usually nonexistent or minimal. The technologists do not have training in veterinary hematology, and nobody on site can provide that training. In addition, turnaround times for animal testing may not receive the appropriate priority relative to the primary purpose of the laboratory.

FACTORS TO CONSIDER WHEN COMMITTING TO IN-HOUSE TESTING

Investment in Instrumentation

Acquiring a diagnostic capability in chemistry and hematology requires an investment of approximately $10,000 to $25,000—or more. The cost of equipment has somewhat stabilized in this range, but the technical capability for this investment continues to improve. For example, a diagnostic capability in hematology that cost in excess of $80,000 during the 1980s may now be obtained for $10,000 to $15,000. The useful technical life span of most instrumentation should be viewed as being from 5

to 7 years. Lease plans may facilitate the acquisition of instrumentation in ways that involve planned replacement at 3- to 7-year intervals.

Commitment to Personnel

Commitment to personnel requires hiring—and retaining—a technologist who is capable of reliable performance in diagnostics. Essential elements include an understanding of the basic laboratory technology, an ability to perform these procedures, a willingness to implement quality control, and a mindset that allows the technologist to seek consultation when he or she is confronted with uncertainty.

Commitment to Quality Assurance

A commitment to quality assurance involves a willingness to invest in periodic training regarding diagnostic technology for the personnel who perform these procedures as well as in the oversight of a regular quality assurance program. The latter involves regular monitoring of equipment accuracy and precision using commercial control materials with known target values. This may cost from $100 to $300 per month for materials.

Establishing a Pathology Consultation Relationship

A working relationship with a veterinary clinical pathologist to provide help with data interpretations and morphologic assessments in difficult cases, as well as cytopathology support, is highly desirable. A relationship with an anatomic pathologist is also required for interpretations of surgical biopsy specimens.

The Business Plan

Veterinarians who are considering in-house testing must have a mind-set that allows them to use diagnostics liberally as part of their practice style. Instrument salespersons may make a compelling case for how one or two CBCs per day will pay for the cost of an instrument system. The same occurs in chemistry as well. First and foremost, these schemes are profitable for the seller, but this may or may not be true for the buyer. One should not make this investment without first analyzing the costs of various alternatives, such as the use of external laboratories. Veterinarians who perform only occasional diagnostic workups likely are better off using an external laboratory. Alternatively, diagnostics may be viewed as a source of revenue if the practice style calls for a combination of frequent diagnostic workups, preanesthetic testing, and wellness testing programs. Thus, a business plan should be created that projects the number of diagnostic tests to be performed across the practice caseload. Multiplying these numbers by the projected internal charge for laboratory tests will yield the gross revenue of the proposed in-house testing effort. Recommended target values are the charges for similar tests imposed by a veterinary commercial laboratory in the region. The projected gross revenue then should be compared with the projected costs, including instrumentation amortization, consumable supplies, personnel, training, quality assurance, and time for supervision.

For chemistry, one must also consider the style of use. Most of the currently available systems are not economically favorable for performing biochemical profiles in-house. For example, the cost of consumables per test with an in-house system may easily exceed $1 to $3 per test, whereas a complete biochemical profile may be obtained from a laboratory for approximately $16. With these circumstances, it makes sense to use in-house chemistry testing for single tests or mini-panels, but not for profiling (unless other laboratory options are not available).

FACTORS TO CONSIDER WHEN SELECTING EXTERNAL LABORATORY SERVICES

Instrument Adaptation

Instrumentation must be suitably adjusted for animal blood testing. This is particularly important regarding hematologic analyses. Such adaptation is likely to occur in veterinary commercial laboratories, and it is much less likely to be found in human hospital laboratories that analyze animal samples as a secondary priority.

Sample Pick-Up Service

Many veterinary laboratories offer once or twice daily sample pick-up service to facilitate the shortest possible time from sample collection to the return of results. The trade-off is that courier services represent a considerable fraction of the cost of the laboratory service. Human laboratory facilities usually rely on users to transport samples to the facility.

Appropriate Turnaround Time

In general, the rate-limiting step is transporting the sample to the laboratory. The trend toward consolidation of laboratory services, however, often results in very large transportation distances, thus extending the turnaround time. Once a sample arrives at the laboratory, most facilities perform the analyses as rapidly as possible and then return the results by fax or electronic transmission. Laboratories that prioritize animal samples behind a busy human diagnostics schedule may not provide convenient timing for the delivery of results.

Species-Specific Ability

The laboratory should have the ability to recognize and interpret species-specific morphologic and pathologic abnormalities. In addition, the laboratory should be able to provide knowledgeable evaluation of abnormalities in data and morphology on blood films and cytology.

Telephone Consultation

The veterinary user must be able to consult with laboratory staff and pathologists regarding abnormal or unusual data generated by the laboratory.

Decision Process

The analysis of one's diagnostic options may be summarized as follows: The decision process for implementing diagnostic support is complex, and this complexity is enhanced by rapidly changing technologies and services. It is advisable to run some experiments to facilitate this analysis. To maintain flexibility when uncertainty exists, it is advisable to avoid entering long-term purchase or service agreements.

SUGGESTED READINGS

Jain NC, ed: Schalm's veterinary hematology. 4th ed. Philadelphia: Lea & Febiger, 1986.
Kaneko JJ, Harvey JH, Bruss ML, eds: Clinical biochemistry of domestic animals. 5th ed. New York: Academic Press, 1997.

CHAPTER
3

PERSPECTIVES IN DATA
INTERPRETATION

The ability to interpret laboratory data is based on knowledge regarding the normal physiologic mechanisms underlying each laboratory test and recognition of the effects of diseases on these normal physiologic mechanisms and, therefore, on the test results themselves. With these perspectives, one can assess all possible explanations for an alteration in a laboratory test result, and one can sort through these possibilities to identify the most likely explanations. If performed properly, laboratory testing and interpretation of laboratory data can provide significant insights regarding diseases and therapeutic approaches. Most chapters in this book discuss normal physiologic mechanisms and the effects of disease processes on these mechanisms as well as on laboratory test results; this chapter provides basic information that applies to the interpretation of all types of laboratory data.

REFERENCE RANGES

To recognize laboratory results as being abnormal, the ranges of the values from healthy animals must be known. These ranges are commonly referred to as *reference ranges* or *normal values*. Different methods can be used to establish reference ranges, but all of them begin with the sampling of animals from a healthy population. In most cases,

healthy animals are those that have no apparent illness and that exhibit behavior considered to be normal for that species.

Reference ranges must be established for each species being tested, but such ranges should also be established for the subdivisions within that species when some characteristic of a subgroup results in significantly different reference ranges compared with those for the species as a whole. These subdivisions might occur on the basis of age, breed, gender, pregnancy status, or type of husbandry. Because establishing reference ranges is an expensive, time-consuming task, ranges for such subdivisions are usually not established, and veterinarians generally use a single reference range for all animals of a given species. When this is the case, it is important to consider variations in those test results that could relate to the previously mentioned characteristics (e.g., age, breed, gender) and to consider these characteristics when evaluating the possible causes of values falling outside the reference range (especially mildly abnormal values).

Adequate numbers of normal animals also must be sampled to develop ranges that are valid for healthy animals from the population in question. In general, the more animals that are sampled, the more likely the reference range will truly reflect the range of values to be expected from healthy animals. Sampling large numbers of animals to make the results most reflective of the healthy overall population is desirable, but practical constraints (e.g., availability of apparently healthy animals, costs of obtaining samples and of performing large numbers of tests) dictate limits on the number of animals that can actually be tested. For acceptable precision, at least 120 samples should be analyzed when establishing reference ranges. The minimum number of samples to establish reference ranges is generally considered to be 40.

Several statistical methods exist for establishing reference ranges. The choice of method to be used partially depends on the distribution of values obtained from the sampled population. If these values are plotted by their frequency of occurrence, they may form a normal, Gaussian or bell-shaped distribution *(Fig. 3.1A)*. With such a distribution, parametric tests are appropriate for determining the reference range. Conversely, if the plotted frequencies do not form a normal, Gaussian or bell-shaped distribution *(Fig. 3.1B)*, parametric statistical tests are not appropriate. In these cases, the data are either analyzed by nonparametric statistical methods or transformed to produce a more normal distribution, which can then be analyzed by parametric methods. Visual inspection of the distribution of values is usually not sufficient to indicate whether the sampled values have a normal distribution; statistical tests should be applied to determine whether the distribution is, in fact, normal. An alternate and practical approach is to assume the distribution is not normal and to apply nonparametric methods for determining reference ranges. If the data are normally distributed, these nonparametric methods will result in a reference range similar to that which would have been determined by using parametric methods.

Regardless of the method used to establish reference ranges, a few values from the apparently healthy population that was sampled to establish these ranges might be markedly higher or lower than most of the other values. These extreme values are known as *outliers*. If outliers are included in the sampled values when the ranges are calculated, they will widen the reference ranges, thus making the test less sensitive for the detection of unhealthy animals. If these outliers are deleted when the ranges are calculated, the reference ranges will be narrower; however, this could exclude more values from the healthy animals than is desirable. One relatively simple and statistically robust rule-of-thumb for dealing with this dilemma is to determine the distance between the highest (or lowest) value and the second highest (or lowest) value. If this distance exceeds one-third of the range of all values, then consider the highest (or lowest) value to be an outlier, and eliminate it when calculating the reference ranges. Once this value has been eliminated, the same test can be applied to the next highest (or lowest) value. For example, *Figure 3.2* presents the blood glucose

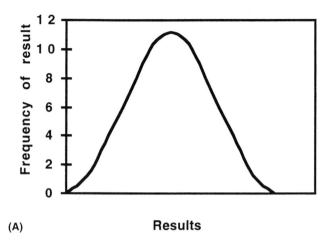

(A)   **Results**

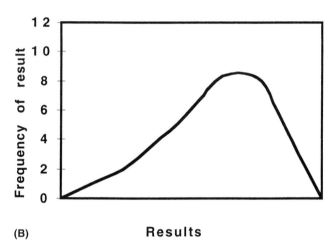

(B)   **Results**

Figure 3.1 Two distributions of values resulting from sampling a large number of apparently healthy animals. **A.** Plotted by their frequency of occurrence, these values form a symmetric, bell-shaped curve. This is known as a normal or Gaussian distribution. **B.** Plotted by their frequency of occurrence, these values form an asymmetric distribution that is skewed toward the higher values. This is not a normal distribution (a non-Gaussian distribution).

values obtained from a population of 120 apparently healthy animals plotted in a frequency distribution histogram. One value (30 mg/dL) is obviously much lower than the others. The difference between this value and the next lowest value is 25 mg/dL, and the range of all values is 70 mg/dL (30–100 mg/dL). Because 25 mg/dL is greater than one-third of the range of all values ($70 \div 3 = 23.3$), the lowest value (30 mg/dL) should be considered for elimination as an outlier. If this value is eliminated, the difference between the remaining lowest value (55 mg/dL) and the next lowest value is then 10 mg/dL. This is less than one-third of the range of all remaining values ($45 \div 3 = 15$) and, therefore, should not be eliminated as an outlier. This method is useful for identifying outliers, but

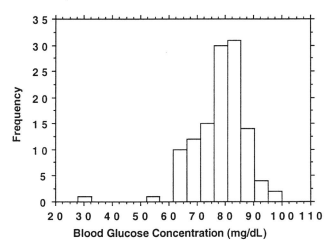

Figure 3.2 Blood glucose values obtained from a population of 120 apparently healthy animals and plotted in a frequency distribution histogram. Frequency represents the total number of samples with that blood glucose concentration.

the values identified as such should not be eliminated automatically. Possible circumstances that justify classification of the value as an outlier should be considered, and lacking those circumstances, inclusion of the value in the calculation of reference ranges may be justified.

If the values obtained from a sample population of apparently healthy animals are determined to be normally distributed, then parametric statistics may be applied. In such a case, the mean and standard deviation (SD) are calculated, and the central 95% of values (the mean ± 2 SD *[Fig. 3.3])* are considered to be the reference range.

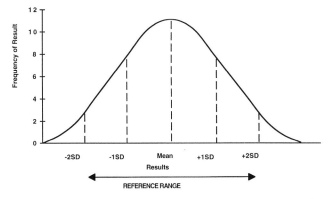

Figure 3.3 The frequencies with which various values were derived when applying a laboratory test to a number of apparently healthy animals in a theoretic case. The distribution of these frequencies has formed a bell-shaped curve (a normal or Gaussian distribution). The mean and SD have been calculated for these results. Because the data have a normal distribution, the reference range for this test is arbitrarily determined as being the mean ± 2 SD. If adequate numbers of truly healthy animals were sampled, then 95% of the values derived from healthy animals should fall within this reference range.

If the values obtained from a sample population of apparently healthy animals do not form a bell-shaped curve (e.g., the distribution is not normal or Gaussian) when graphed by their frequency of occurrence, or if statistical tests to determine whether the distribution is normal are not applied, then nonparametric statistical methods are appropriate. Like parametric methods, nonparametric methods also attempt to identify the central 95% of values in establishing reference ranges, and these ranges are usually derived by ranking the values and then applying statistical methods to determine the most likely values for defining the upper and lower limits of the 95% range. An example of establishing a reference range by a nonparametric method is presented in *Table 3.1*, which uses the data as presented in Figure 3.2. As noted earlier, one value (30 mg/dL) has been eliminated as an outlier; therefore, the range of the remaining 119 values is 55 to 100 mg/dL. These values are given a numeric rank from the lowest to the highest. Usually, however, it is only necessary to determine the ranks of the lowest and highest 5 to 10 values. The central 95% of these ranked values are then determined by identifying and eliminating those values in the lowest 2.5% and in the highest 2.5%. The rank of highest value in the lower 2.5% of ranked values is determined by the calculation 0.025 × (number of observations + 1). The rank of lowest value in the upper 2.5% of ranked values is determined by the calculation 0.975 × (number of observations + 1). Values with ranks equal to or lower than that determined for the lower 2.5%, and values with ranks equal to or higher than that determined for the upper 2.5%, are eliminated from the reference range. Thus, in Table 3.1, the third ranked value and those values with lower rankings (rank 1 and rank 2) are eliminated from the lower end of the reference range, and the 117th ranked value as well as those with higher rankings (rank 118 and rank 119) are eliminated from the upper end of the reference range. Therefore, the reference range is defined by the fourth through the 116th ranked values, which corresponds to the range from 65 to 95 mg/dL. If the rank value as calculated to determine the lower or upper 2.5% is not a whole number, however, the value corresponding to that rank may need to be extrapolated. For instance, if the lower rank value is 10.4, the tenth ranked value is 66, and eleventh ranked value is 67, then the appropriate reference limit is 66.4. In some cases, 90% confidence intervals for the lower and upper limits also may be calculated, but this requires use of a sophisticated formula or a table designed for this purpose.

The statistical methods described here are applicable when the sampled population includes 40 or more animals. If fewer than 40 animals are sampled, the lower and upper 2.5% of values cannot be reliably determined. In such a case, the reference range is then considered to be the observed range of values that remains after the outliers

TABLE 3.1   AN EXAMPLE OF NONPARAMETRIC DETERMINATION OF A REFERENCE RANGE[a]

Lowest 10 Values and Their Ranks

Value	30	55	65	65	65	65	65	65	65	65
Rank	1	2	3	4	5	6	7	8	9	10

Highest 10 Values and Their Ranks

Value	90	90	90	90	95	95	95	95	100	100
Rank	110	111	112	113	114	115	116	117	118	119

Highest value of the lower 2.5% = 0.025 × (number of values + 1)
Highest value of the lower 2.5% = 0.025 × (119 + 1) = **3**

Lowest value of the upper 2.5% = 0.975 × (number of values + 1)
Lowest value of the upper 2.5% = 0.975 × (119 + 1) = **117**

Lower Values Eliminated from Reference Range

Value	30	55	65
Rank	1	2	3

Upper Values Eliminated from Reference Range

Value	95	100	100
Rank	117	118	119

Resulting reference range = 65–95

[a] Blood glucose concentrations were obtained from 120 apparently healthy animals, and one of these values was eliminated as an outlier (see Fig. 3.2). The method involves ranking values from lowest to highest, calculation of ranks representing the highest rank of the lower 2.5% of values and the lowest rank of the upper 2.5% of values, and eliminating values corresponding to these ranks as well as values corresponding to lower and higher ranks, respectively. The remaining values are the central 95% and are used as the reference range.

have been eliminated. Such a reference range is less reliable than those determined from a larger population using the statistical methods described.

Regardless of which statistical methods are used, the resulting reference ranges include the central 95% of values obtained from the sampled population. Theoretically, this excludes 5% of the values obtained from the healthy population (2.5% below the lower limit, and 2.5% above the upper limit). In other words, as defined by such reference ranges, approximately 5% of healthy animals would have values that were considered to be abnormal for any given test. Including all values that could possibly be obtained from healthy animals in the reference ranges might seem to be desirable. Use of only the central 95% of values for these ranges is practical, however, because the values from healthy and unhealthy animals overlap at each end of the reference range (Fig. 3.4). If 100% of values obtained from healthy animals were included in the reference ranges, then these values in unhealthy animals would be considered to be normal, thus resulting in failure to identify a certain number of unhealthy animals. Limiting reference ranges to 95% of values obtained from healthy animals is a compromise that makes a test more sensitive for detecting unhealthy animals.

One practical implication of using the central 95% of values obtained from the healthy animals sampled to establish reference ranges is that a few healthy animals can have test results that fall slightly above or below the reference range for that test, because 5% of their values have been excluded from the reference range. If many tests are performed for one animal, the likelihood of finding an abnormal test result—even if the animal is healthy—increases with the number of tests performed. For instance, in a 10-test profile, approximately 40% of healthy animals will have at least one abnormal value, and in a 20-test profile, approximately 64% of healthy animals will have at least one abnormal value. If the animal is indeed healthy, then such values will be only slightly above or below the reference range. When such test results do not correlate with the patient history, clinical signs, or other laboratory data, they may represent a normal result for that animal. Test results that are markedly above or below the reference range, however, must be considered more seriously, regardless of their correlation with history, clinical signs, or other laboratory data, because these values are unlikely to represent normal results that have been excluded because of the method used to establish the reference ranges.

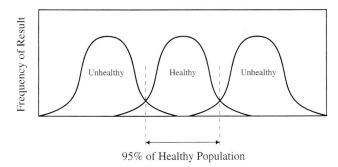

Figure 3.4 The overlap of laboratory values that can be expected from healthy and unhealthy populations (populations with diseases that cause either decreases or increases in the values for a given test). Note that defining the reference range at 95% of the healthy population excludes the values from some healthy animals, but it also excludes the values from some unhealthy ones (i.e., it allows one to recognize these animals as being potentially unhealthy). If the reference range was broadened to include more of the potential values from healthy animals, it would also recognize these values from unhealthy animals as being normal (i.e., the unhealthy animal might not be detected). Using a reference range that includes 95% of the healthy population is a compromise that increases the sensitivity of the test for recognizing unhealthy animals while causing only a few healthy animals to be recognized as being potentially unhealthy.

INTERPRETING LABORATORY DATA

General Approach

Laboratory data typically are analyzed after obtaining a thorough patient history and performing a physical examination, and they should not be interpreted without considering this information. Most laboratory abnormalities have multiple potential causes, and the history and physical examination results should be used to determine which of these potential causes is most likely. Using a combination of history, physical examination results, and pattern of laboratory abnormalities, the veterinarian should attempt to recognize the pathogenesis of the disease process. If such a pathogenesis can be logically discerned, a correct diagnosis is more likely to result. Similar history, physical examination results, and pattern of laboratory abnormalities can result from more than one disease process, however, so keeping an open mind when interpreting these abnormalities is important.

The results of laboratory tests can be used to rule in or out previously established differential diagnoses established on the basis of history or physical examination findings, can suggest additional differential diagnoses, and in some cases, can even confirm a specific diagnosis. When reporting test results, most laboratories also designate which of the tests are abnormal. A good first step when interpreting laboratory data is to quickly review these

abnormal results. Those that are most markedly outside the reference ranges are usually the best indicators of the primary disease process. Those that are slightly outside the reference ranges also may be significant, but they could be normal for that particular animal as well.

Recognizing patterns of abnormal results often suggests which tissue or organ systems are affected, which pathologic processes are occurring, or both. For instance, a combination of an increased concentration of blood urea nitrogen (BUN; a test of kidney function) with a urine specific gravity indicative of inadequate urine concentration is very suggestive of renal failure, whereas an increased BUN with concentrated urine (high specific gravity) is more suggestive of conditions such as dehydration or shock.

Analyzing changes in laboratory values for the same animal over time also can be helpful in establishing a diagnosis and assessing progress of the disease. For instance, periodic determinations of BUN in an animal with renal failure may indicate whether treatment to reestablish renal function is succeeding (i.e., BUN should be decreasing).

Of course, not every abnormality will fit neatly into one disease process, nor will every laboratory profile result in a specific diagnosis. In some cases, more than one disease process may be occurring, thereby producing a confusing combination of abnormalities. Sometimes profiles simply eliminate previously established differential diagnoses, and sometimes they offer no useful information at all.

Sensitivity, Specificity, and Predictive Values

When interpreting laboratory abnormalities, the concepts of sensitivity, specificity, and predictive values must be considered.

Sensitivity is a measure of the frequency with which the test result will be positive or abnormal in animals with the disease. The following formula is used to determine sensitivity:

$$\text{Sensitivity (\%)} = \frac{TP}{TP + FN} \times 100$$

where TP (true positive) is the total number of animals that tested positive and actually have the disease and FN (false negative) is the total number of animals that tested negative but actually have the disease. For instance, if the sensitivity of a test for a disease is 99%, then 99 of 100 animals with that disease will have a positive (i.e., abnormal) result. One percent of the animals with the disease will have a negative (i.e., normal) result; that is, 1% of the tests would have false-negative results.

Specificity is a measure of the frequency with which the test result will be negative or normal in animals without the disease one wishes to detect. The following formula is used to determine specificity:

$$\text{Specificity } (\%) = \frac{TN}{TN + FP} \times 100$$

where *TN* (true negative) is the total number of animals that tested negative and actually do not have the disease and *FP* (false positive) is the total number of animals that tested positive but actually do not have the disease. For instance, if the specificity of a test for a disease is 99%, then 99 of 100 nonaffected animals will have negative (i.e., normal) results. One percent of nonaffected animals will have a positive (i.e., abnormal) result; that is, 1% of the tests would have false-positives results.

Sensitivity and specificity are established by applying the test in question to animals with known disease status (i.e., animals known to have or not have the disease in question). Another diagnostic procedure, often termed the "gold standard," is used to establish which animals do or do not have the disease. This gold standard is often another laboratory test known to be reliable for detecting the disease. Sensitivity and specificity, therefore, do not apply directly to animals of unknown disease status, but they do provide information regarding the reliability of the test in question for detecting that disease.

In practice, one needs to know the reliability of a test for detecting a certain disease in animals with unknown disease status. In other words, how reliable is an abnormal or a normal test result for predicting whether the animal does or does not have the disease in question? In this situation, predictive values define the chances that abnormal or normal test results are reliable indicators of disease status. Predictive values depend on the sensitivity and specificity of a test, but the prevalence or likelihood of the disease in the population being tested affects predictive values as well. Such prevalence or likelihood of disease is established based on the judgement of the veterinarian, before performing the test, of the chance (expressed as a percentage) that the animal has the disease in question. This judgement can be based on several other observations, including patient history, clinical signs, other test results, and epidemiologic data.

Both positive (i.e., abnormal) and negative (i.e., normal) test results have predictive values. The predictive value of a positive test is the percentage of animals with a positive (abnormal) value that actually have the disease:

$$\text{Predictive value of a positive test } = \frac{TP}{TP + FP} \times 100$$

where, again, *TP* is the total number of animals that tested positive and actually have the disease and *FP* is the total number of animals that tested positive but actually do not have the disease. The higher the predictive value of a positive test result, the more likely that an animal with a positive (i.e., abnormal) test actually has the disease in question.

The predictive value of a negative test result is the percentage of animals with a negative (i.e., normal) value that do not have the disease:

$$\text{Predictive value of a negative test } = \frac{TN}{TN + FN} \times 100$$

where, again, *TN* is the total number of animals that tested negative and actually do not have the disease and *FN* is the total number of animals that tested negative but actually do have the disease. The higher the predictive value of a negative test result, the more likely that an animal with a negative or a normal test does *not* have the disease in question.

As stated previously, predictive values are determined from a combination of the sensitivity and specificity of the test and the veterinarian's pretest judgement regarding the likelihood of the disease in that animal. A rather complex formula to estimate predictive values based on these factors does exist, but the roles of sensitivity, specificity, and disease prevalence or likelihood in the interpretation of diagnostic test results can be understood without it. The roles of these three factors are best understood by considering a hypothetic situation in which an excellent diagnostic test is used to detect a specific disease. This test has a previously determined sensitivity of 99% (i.e., it will be positive or abnormal in 99 of 100 animals with the disease) and a previously determined specificity of 99% (i.e., it will be negative or normal in 99 of 100 animals without the disease). If this test is used for screening a population of animals in which you, as the veterinarian, judge there is a 1% chance of the disease being present, the following predictive values result:

Predictive value of a positive test = 50%
Predictive value of a negative test = 100%

In other words, a positive or abnormal test is correct 50% of the time and incorrect 50% of the time. This result is equivalent in reliability to flipping a coin, and it might lead one to question the wisdom of performing such a test in a population with a low likelihood of disease. In this situation, however, a negative or normal test result is almost 100% reliable in ruling out the possibility that an animal has the disease (i.e., the predictive value of a negative test is approximately 100%). In addition, the described combination of excellent test sensitivity and specificity with low prevalence or likelihood of disease is quite common when using serologic tests to screen for various infectious diseases.

Because most diagnostic tests have an inherent sensitivity and specificity, the most easily altered factor that affects the predictive value is the pretest likelihood of the disease. Veterinarians can use this to enhance the predictive values. For instance, in the previous example, a test with excellent sensitivity and specificity was used to screen for a disease in a population with a low prevalence of that disease. This resulted in a low positive predictive value. If, however, a veterinarian were presented with an animal that had a history, clinical signs, and other features suggesting that disease, such an animal would represent a different population, and the veterinarian would establish a different, higher pretest likelihood for that disease. In such a case, the veterinarian would, perhaps, be 75% certain that the animal had the disease in question. Therefore, the predictive value of a positive test result would be nearly 100%, and the predictive value of a negative test result would be approximately 97%. The test result in this scenario would, in fact, be very reliable for predicting the presence or absence of the disease in question.

In summary, the more likely before performing the test that an animal has a certain disease, the more reliable a positive or abnormal test result suggesting the presence of that disease will be. The effect of the pretest likelihood of disease on the positive and negative predictive values of a test are demonstrated in *Figures 3.5* and *3.6*. In practice, most veterinarians incorporate this ap-

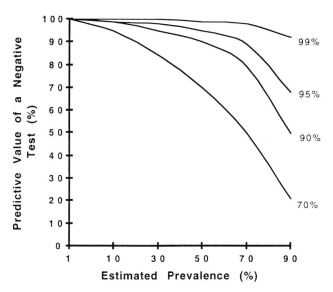

Figure 3.6 The effect of various pretest estimates of disease likelihood on the predictive value of a negative test. Each line represents a different level of sensitivity and specificity (99% = 99% sensitivity and specificity, 95% = 95% sensitivity and specificity, and so on). The predictive value of a negative test increases as the pretest estimate of disease likelihood decreases.

proach to diagnostic testing instinctively. If the test result is compatible with the disease the veterinarian suspected before conducting the test, this result is considered to be supportive evidence that the animal has the disease; if the result is not compatible with the suspected disease, the veterinarian does not completely rule out that disease but does begin to consider other options more seriously. Biochemical abnormalities that suggest a disease that was not strongly suspected before the profile was completed will occasionally be detected, and in this situation, these abnormalities are *not* as reliable in predicting that disease as they would be had the disease been previously suspected.

Most routine clinical pathology tests (i.e., hematology, biochemistry, and urinalysis) have sensitivities and specificities for detecting any given disease that are considerably less than the 99% in the previous example. This makes the pretest likelihood of disease an even more important factor in this type of testing. For instance, both the sensitivity and specificity of the pancreatic enzyme amylase for detecting pancreatitis are controversial, but most agree they are quite low. Serum amylase activity is routinely measured on some biochemical profiles. Thus, an increased serum amylase activity on a biochemical screen from a dog in which pancreatitis was not previously suspected would have a very low positive predictive value, because the sensitivity, specificity, and pretest likelihood of pancreatitis are all low. On the other hand, an increased serum amylase activity on a biochemical

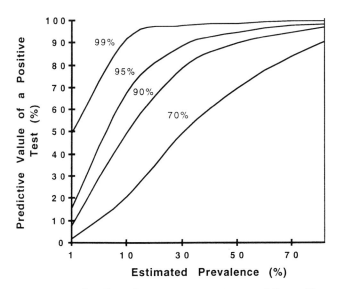

Figure 3.5 The effect of various pretest estimates of disease likelihood on the predictive value of a positive test. Each line represents a different level of sensitivity and specificity (99% = 99% sensitivity and specificity, 95% = 95% sensitivity and specificity, and so on). The predictive value of a positive test decreases as the pretest estimate of disease likelihood decreases.

profile from a dog with clinical signs that suggest pancreatitis would have a much higher positive predictive value. This concept is important to remember whenever unexpected abnormalities are detected on any routine clinical pathology test.

QUALITY CONTROL

To obtain reliable laboratory test results, the quality of the results being produced must be monitored so that they are both accurate and precise. Accuracy is a gauge of how close the result is to the true value for that test, and precision is a gauge of how repeatable the result is when assaying the same sample. A single result might be accurate, for instance, but if a similar result cannot be obtained repeatedly using the same sample (i.e., if the test is not precise), then the results for that assay are not reliable. It also is possible to obtain the same result repeatedly using the same sample, but if that result does not reflect the true value for the substance being measured (i.e., if the test is not accurate), then the results again are not reliable.

Reputable laboratories maintain quality-control programs to ensure the accuracy and precision of their results. This is accomplished by assaying control samples at previously determined intervals (often during each run of a test) along with the samples from patients. These intervals might be daily or several times per day, depending on the workload of the laboratory. The control samples are similar to those from patients (e.g., blood or serum) and usually are obtained from a commercial source. Control samples can be either assayed (i.e., the probable accurate value for the test in that control sample has been previously determined) or unassayed (i.e., the probable accurate value for the test in that control sample has not been previously determined). If unassayed control samples are obtained, the laboratory then establishes the probable accurate value for that sample using methods similar to those summarized earlier (see the discussion of reference ranges). Because establishing such probable accurate values is both time-consuming and expensive, most laboratories use assayed rather than unassayed control samples.

During routine laboratory operation, the result from each control sample is compared with what is considered to be the accurate result for that sample (as previously established). This tests the accuracy of the assay. In addition, results obtained from the control sample over time are analyzed to determine if the value obtained changes over time, thus establishing the precision of the test. Both accuracy and precision usually are assessed by graphing the values obtained from the control sample on a quality-control chart *(Fig. 3.7)*. If the results obtained from the control sample are outside the previously established ac-

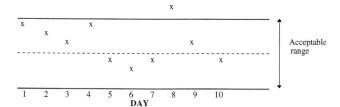

Figure 3.7   An example of a quality-control chart used to assure the accuracy and precision of an assay. To produce this chart, a control sample was assayed each day along with the patient samples. Daily results from the control sample are plotted (×), and the dashed line (---) represents the expected value from this sample. Solid lines (—) delineate acceptable variations from this value. Note that the result on Day 8 was outside this acceptable range, which should have triggered the rejection of all results for this test on this day and an assessment of the instrument, reagents, and operator's methodology to identify the problem. This problem was solved by Day 9, and the test was back in "control."

ceptable range, which is also known as the control limit (usually ±2–3 SD from the mean), or if the results drift either up or down over time, then a problem with the analytic instrument, reagents, or operator may exist. Results obtained from patient samples during these "out-of-control" periods are rejected, and the analytic methods used are carefully evaluated.

Quality-control programs are common in large reference laboratories, but they are also important for clinic laboratories. Manufacturers may supply quality-control materials with laboratory instruments. These programs should be followed in detail to have some assurance that the results produced by the in-clinic laboratory are both accurate and precise.

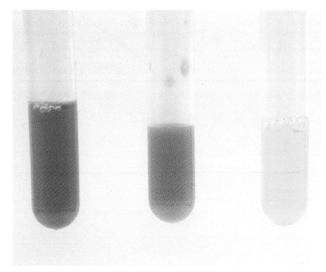

Figure 3.8   Hemolysis, lipemia, and hyperbilirubinemia (left to right) in serum samples. Lipemic serum is often pink because of in vitro hemolysis.

EFFECTS OF LIPEMIA, HEMOLYSIS, AND HYPERBILIRUBINEMIA

Hemolysis, lipemia, and increased serum bilirubin *(Fig. 3.8)* can potentially affect the results of biochemical assays. Hemolysis refers to the breakdown of erythrocytes, either in the circulating blood (in vivo) or, more commonly, during or after blood collection (in vitro). Hemolysis can interfere with assay results by spillage from erythrocytes into serum of increased amounts of the substance being measured, resulting in falsely increased concentrations; by dilution of normal substances in the serum, resulting in falsely decreased concentrations; or by interference with spectrophotometric assays. For instance, horses have high concentrations of potassium within erythrocytes, whereas dogs (except Akitas) and cats do not. Hemolysis may result in a falsely increased serum potassium concentration in horses and cattle, but not in most dogs or in cats.

Lipemia causes visible clouding of the serum. It can result in dilution of normal substances in the aqueous component of serum, resulting in falsely decreased concentrations, or it can interfere with the results of spectrophotometric assays.

Increased serum bilirubin concentrations result in a serum with a darker-yellow color than normal for that species. This increased color can interfere with the results of spectrophotometric assays.

The potential alterations in biochemistry results caused by hemolysis, lipemia, and hyperbilirubinemia vary with the substance being assayed and with the method being used for the assay itself. Reference laboratories usually can provide specific information regarding the effects of hemolysis, lipemia, or hyperbilirubinemia on test results.

SUGGESTED READINGS

Gerstman BB, Cappucci DT. Evaluating the reliability of diagnostic test results. J Am Vet Med Assoc 1986;188:248–251.
Muray W, Peter AT, Teclaw RF. The clinical relevance of assay validation. Comp Cont Educ 1993;15:1665–1676.
Solberg HE. Establishment and use of reference values. In: Burtis CA, Ashwood ER, eds. Tietz textbook of clinical chemistry. 2nd ed. Philadelphia: WB Saunders, 1994:454–484.
Solberg HE. Statistical treatment of collected reference values and determination of reference limits. In: Gräsbeck R, Alström T, eds. Reference values in laboratory medicine. London: John Wiley and Sons, Ltd., 1981.

CHAPTER

4

IMMUNODIAGNOSTICS AND OTHER EMERGING DIAGNOSTIC TECHNOLOGIES

ROY R. MONDESIRE

Historically, the diagnosis of infectious disease has required demonstration of the presence of an organism through morphologic identification or microbial culture. For many organisms, however, these procedures were not useful because of technical difficulty, the time required to achieve results, or both. The advent of immunodiagnostics provided an additional set of tools for establishing the diagnosis of infectious disease, either indirectly by detection of antibodies or directly by detection of antigen associated with the presence of the organism. The advantages of immunodiagnostics are simplicity and rapid results, and an increasing number of these diagnostics are now available as in-clinic tools. In addition, new tools from molecular biology are being developed. The detection of nucleic acid targets that are specific for an infectious agent also provides a sensitive, alternative technique.

The invasive presence of a foreign organism results in antibody responses to antigens that are recognized by and appropriately presented to the body's immune system. Detection of antibody responses is accomplished by measurement of blood or serum reactivity to a known antigen reagent system. Alternatively, antigens may be released continually by the invading organism in selected infectious diseases in such a way that allows for diagnostic detection. Antigen in patient serum is detected by reactivity to a fabricated antibody system. This involves production of polyclonal (in an experimental animal) or monoclonal antibodies to the antigen of interest, and these antibodies are used as the reagent detection system. Detection of either antibody or antigen in patient blood or serum is the basis for immunodiagnostic tests. These types of immunodiagnostic technologies have been employed for many years, and they remain the most important diagnostic tools for infectious disease.

One limitation of this technology is that detection of an antibody does not necessarily equate to detection of an active infection. This interpretation of an antibody response depends on the biology of the specific disease or host-agent interaction. In many infectious diseases, an antibody response clears the body of infection. In these instances, the interpretation of positive antibody tests is that the animal has been infected by the organism, but the status of an active infection is not certain.

For infectious agents that are not effectively eliminated by antibody responses, detection of antibody responses may correlate better with an interpretation of active infection. Detection of antigen is a more direct determination for the presence of active infection. The limitation, however, is that antigen detection technology currently is limited to a few diseases; a good working example is canine heartworm disease. A more recent innovation is the ability to detect foreign organisms directly by detection of nucleic acid sequences or targets. This technology is still in its infancy regarding our understanding of the biology of specific diseases and its application in a widely available, reliable format. It is beyond the scope of this chapter to do justice to the enormous and rapidly evolving field of immunodiagnostics. An attempt is made, however, to provide an overview regarding the essential components of this technology, with a projection into the future.

In the late 1950s, Yalow and Berson (1) were the first to describe the principles of immunoassay technology. By the 1970s and 1980s, this technology had evolved from research and development and been incorporated in many large central and local hospital laboratories. Immunoassays have been applied to both qualitative and quantitative analyses, and they have probably been the most significant contributions to in vitro diagnostics in this century. Immunoassays have been applied to virtually all aspects of biomedical research, enabling investigators to study numerous molecules of importance. This injection of impressive scientific and technologic innovations into the in vitro medical device industry has resulted in dramatically increased use of immunodiagnostic products.

ANTIBODIES IN IMMUNOASSAYS

Antibodies are glycoproteins secreted by B lymphocytes, and they comprise the primary arm of the humoral immune response. The development of B lymphocytes occurs in specific inductive microenvironments and includes both antigen-independent and -dependent processes. Antigen-specific, naive B lymphocytes are retained in secondary lymphoid organs on recognition of receptor-specific antigen. Secondary lymphoid organs contain B lymphocyte–rich follicles, in which these naïve, antigen-specific B lymphocytes undergo clonal expansion. In turn, clonal expansion results in the generation of memory B lymphocytes or of antibody-secreting plasma cells.

Vertebrate immune systems have evolved a variety of strategies with which to diversify antigen-receptor molecules. DNA recombination events result in mature antigen-receptor genes from separate gene segments. Three gene segments are involved in this event and are designated as variable (V), diversity (D), and joining (J). As the

B cell matures, it rearranges (or shuffles) these gene segments and selects among hundreds of DNA segments. Specific sequences of DNA are then cut, and selected pieces are spliced together *(Fig. 4.1)*.

For antibody, the V gene segment encodes most of the variable domain, including complementarity-determining regions 1 and 2 (CDR1 and CDR2). The D segments and the DJ junctions encode CDR3. In the mouse, an extensive immunoglobulin (Ig) repertoire is achieved by a large group of genes encoding the variable regions of the heavy (H) and light (L) chains (V_H and V_L). In humans, however, the lesser numbers of V_H and V_L are compensated for by the relatively longer CDR3.

For the heavy chain of antibody, the variable regions derive from gene rearrangement and recombinations of the V_H, D_H, and J_H. For the light chain, the variable regions derive from the V_L and J_L gene segments. Humans have approximately 10^5 V(D)J germline exons and 10^3 V_L exons. Thus, the germline has 10^8 different possibilities. Maturation and selection of B-cell clones in the germinal center results in the production of high-affinity antibodies, and during this time, antigen-specific B-cell clones undergo isotype switches and somatic hypermutation. In the T cell–dependent regions of the peripheral lymphoid organs, B cells react with specific antigen and proliferate with the assistance of T and accessory cells.

Structure and Function of Antibodies

Our knowledge regarding antibodies has been derived primarily from studies on human and murine immunology. Antibodies are glycoproteins that belong to the Ig supergene family. Five major isotypes occur within this family and are present in most species of higher mammals. These isotypes have been designated IgG, IgM, IgA, IgD, and IgE. Size, charge, amino acid composition. and carbohydrate content distinguish the isotypes.

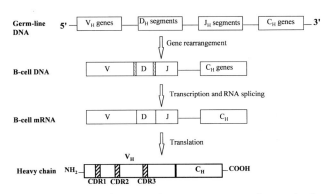

Figure 4.1 General pattern for rearrangement of genes in the production of an antibody heavy chain.

IgG

Usually depicted as the basic Ig molecule (H_2L_2), IgG is a monomeric glycoprotein composed of two identical heavy chains (H) and two identical light chains (L). It is the predominant antibody in normal serum, and it accounts for 70% to 75% of the total Ig content. Human IgG has a sedimentation coefficient of 7S and a molecular mass (MM) of approximately 160 kDa. Four subclasses are recognized for human IgG and are designated IgG1, IgG2, IgG3, and IgG4. *Figure 4.2* illustrates the general structure of IgG.

IgM

The first Ig isotype detected early in a primary immune response, IgM accounts for approximately 10% of the total antibody pool. It is pentameric, with each unit having a MM of 180 kDa. Thus, the relative MM is approximately 900 kDa. Monomers of IgM are linked by disulfide bonds in a circular array. A cysteine-rich "J chain" joins two of the monomers to complete the circle *(Fig. 4.3)*.

IgA

The second most abundant Ig in humans, IgA is rich in carbohydrates. In most other mammals, IgA forms a rel-

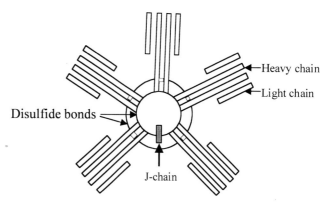

Figure 4.3   General schematic of IgM showing its pentameric configuration, interchain disulfide bonds, and J chain.

atively small part of the plasma pool. Dimeric IgA predominates in mammals and consists of two IgA molecules in association with a secretory component. A J-chain links the dimeric form via the Fc. At the mucosae, IgA is the predominant Ig, and it plays an important role in protection at these surfaces.

IgD

With a MM of 170 kDa, IgD accounts for only a small fraction of circulating Ig. The structure of IgD confers a high susceptibility to proteolysis and heat. It is present primarily on the surface of circulating B lymphocytes in association with IgM, and although its function has not been established, it may play a role in B-cell differentiation.

IgE

With a MM of 200 kDa, IgE is primarily found in association with the high-affinity IgE receptor (Fc[RI]) on the membranes of mast cells and basophils. It mediates type I hypersensitivity reactions, and it may play a role in immunity to some parasitic diseases. IgE has a relatively short half life and is easily denatured by heat.

Two distinct functions, antigen binding and effector functions, are associated with antibodies. The binding site on an antibody is located on the hypervariable domain of the Fab region of the Ig, and this binding site (or "paratope") is located in the N-terminal portion of the molecule. This paratope can recognize and bind to an epitope on a corresponding antigen.

The effector functions reside in the C-terminal portion of the molecule in the Fc constant domain region. Examples of effector functions include complement fixation and cell surface binding via Fc receptors expressed on phagocytic or other effector cells.

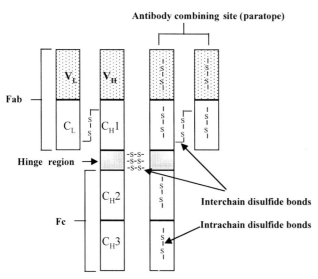

Figure 4.2   Schematic of an antibody molecule showing the domains that make up the heavy (H) and light (L) chains. The variable region of the molecule is designated V. Note that the V_L and V_H regions together form the antibody combining site. In IgG, there are three constant (C_H) domains designated C_H1, C_H2, and C_H3. The domains C_H2 and C_H3 constitute the Fc region of the molecule. In addition, there are intra- and interchain disulfide bonds (-s-s-). The hinge region, which imparts segmental flexibility to the molecule, is shaded.

Immunodiagnostic technology has focused on antigen and antibody recognition. The binding of antigenic epitopes to antibody paratopes involves multiple noncovalent bonds. The attractive forces involved in binding include the hydrogen bond, electrostatic, van der Waals, and hydrophobic interactions. Hydrophobic interactions account for approximately 50% of the total strength of bonding, and they result primarily from the interaction of nonpolar hydrophobic residues where contact with water molecules is greatly reduced. These noncovalent interactions depend greatly on the distance between the interacting residues.

Anti-Idiotypic Antibodies

As described earlier, distinct regions within the V_H and V_L Ig chains constitute the paratope, which can react with a specific antigenic epitope. The functional specificity for a unique antigenic epitope generally is used to define a particular antibody; however, an antibody also can be defined in terms of its idiotype (Id). The Id is a collection of idiotopes (i.e., unique antigenic regions) associated with V_H and V_L regions on an Ig molecule. By virtue of their uniqueness, idiotypes have the potential to stimulate anti-idiotypic (anti-Id) antibodies, which in some cases can mimic antigenic determinants recognized by the original antibody and, thus, can act as antigens. Interactions between idiotypes and anti-idiotypes may constitute a mechanism whereby the immune system regulates itself. Idiotypy has found practical use in the development of immunodiagnostic tests (2).

Hybridoma Technology

In 1976, immunology was revolutionized by Köhler and Milstein (3), who showed that individual antibody-producing cells could be immortalized when fused with a myeloma cell line, thus making it possible to produce a virtually unlimited supply of antibodies with the same specificity. These are called monoclonal antibodies (MAbs). Large quantities of specific antibodies can now be produced, purified, and adapted as tools for in vitro diagnostics, in vivo diagnostics, or therapeutics.

Antibody Purification

Antibody destined for use in an immunoassay must first undergo purification, for which several techniques are available. Salt fractionation with ammonium sulfate, followed by exhaustive dialysis to remove all the ammonium sulfate, is commonly used; this technique exploits differences in the solubility of various proteins at different ionic strengths. Gel filtration chromatographic methods exploit the differences in the molecular sizes of molecules in

a mixture. A suitable solid phase of known exclusion limits allows for separation of molecular mixtures at different retention times. Anion- and cation-exchange chromatography also are powerful techniques that are based on the interaction of various ionic species of molecules for the chromatographic matrix. Salt or pH gradients are used to elute fractions. Affinity chromatography is a chromatographic technique in which the affinity of the molecules to be purified is exploited.

ELEMENTS OF IMMUNOASSAYS

Heterogeneous Enzyme Immunoassays

Heterogeneous EIAs are those with at least one separation step to distinguish reacted from unreacted reagents.

Certain features characterize antigen–antibody interactions at solid–liquid interfaces. Some of these include:

1. The binding of antibody to immobilized antigen is diffusion rate limited.
2. Steric interactions occur at certain levels of immobilized ligand.
3. Solid-phase antigen–antibody reactions have a lower intrinsic and reverse reaction rate than solution-phase reactions.
4. Antigen–antibody reactions at the solid-liquid interface are virtually irreversible.

Figures 4.4 to *4.7* illustrate some of the principles of heterogeneous EIAs.

The enzyme-linked immunosorbent assay (ELISA) is a heterogeneous EIA. First described by Engvall and Perlmann (4), this technique applies to all immunoassays in which one or more of the reactants is immobilized onto a solid phase. This solid phase typically is used to immobilize specific antibody or antigen, depending on the assay configuration. Other components of immunoassays

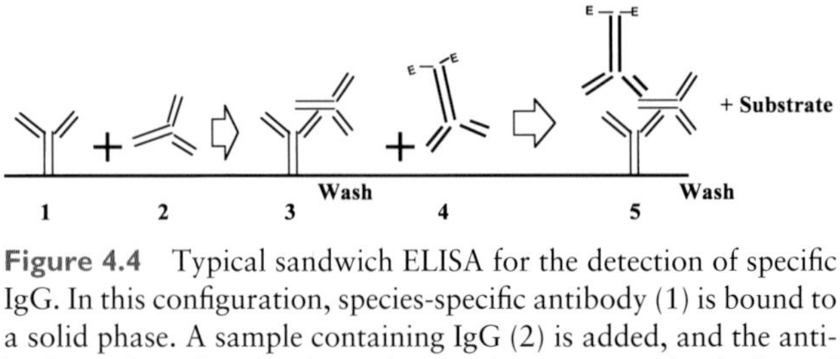

Figure 4.4 Typical sandwich ELISA for the detection of specific IgG. In this configuration, species-specific antibody (1) is bound to a solid phase. A sample containing IgG (2) is added, and the antibody (Y-shaped molecule) in the sample is captured by the bound antibody (3). After a wash step, anti–species IgG enzyme (E) conjugate is added (4). The conjugate binds to the captured IgG, thereby forming a "sandwich" (5). After a second wash step, addition of the appropriate chromogenic substrate results in a color change, thus revealing binding of the specific antibody of interest.

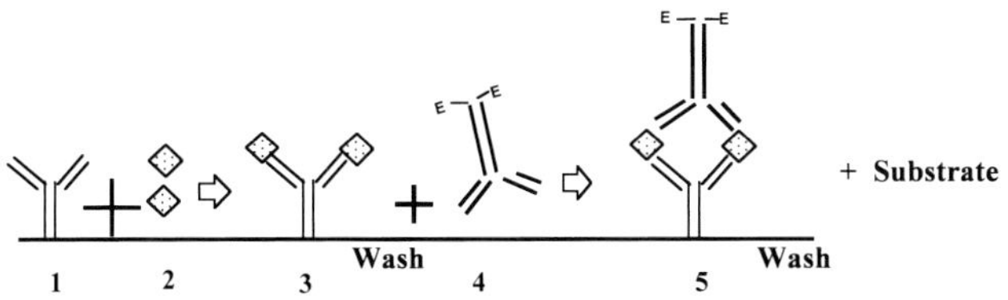

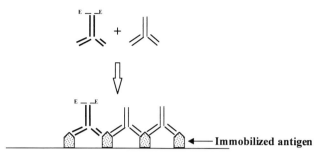

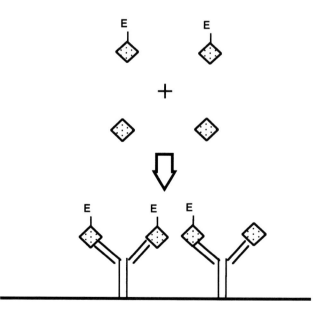

Figure 4.5 Noncompetitive ELISA for the detection of antigen. In this configuration, specific antibody (1) is bound to a solid phase. A sample containing antigen (2) is added, and the antigen in the sample is then captured by the bound antibody (3). After a wash step, an antibody enzyme conjugate is added (4). The conjugate binds to a site on the captured antigen, thereby forming a "sandwich" (5). After another wash, addition of the appropriate chromogenic substrate results in a color change, thus revealing binding of specific analyte of interest.

Figure 4.7 Principle of competitive ELISA for the detection of antibody. Both enzyme-labeled antibody and antibody in the patient's sample compete for bound antigen. The activity associated with the bound, labeled antibody is inversely proportional to the quantity of that antibody in the sample.

are the enzyme-labeled antibody or antigen. These conjugated reagents are used to probe any molecules that have reacted with the surface-bound antibody or antigen. Verification of the reaction sequence in the case of a colorimetric assay is achieved with a chromogenic substrate. Other types of detection systems are discussed later.

Homogeneous Enzyme Immunoassays

In homogeneous EIAs, the immunologic reactions and detection of changes in enzymatic activity are performed in the same solution; there is no need to separate bound and free labels. As with heterogeneous EIAs, the substrates that use homogeneous EIAs can be chromogenic, fluorogenic,

or chemiluminescent. Enzymes used for homogeneous EIAs include α-D-galactosidase, glucose-6-phosphate dehydrogenase, hexokinase, and glucose oxidase. The substrates for these labels are the fluorogenic substrate 4-methylumbelliferyl-β-D-galactopyranoside, D-glucose 6-phosphate plus NAD^+, D-hexose plus adenosine triphosphate, and glucose, respectively.

Homogeneous EIAs can be competitive or noncompetitive binding assays. Competitive assays are based on the modulation of enzyme activity because of the competitive reaction of antibody with both labeled and free antigen. Here, the enzyme activity is either activated or inhibited as a result of immune complex formation. Noncompetitive assays, however, use enzyme-labeled antibody conjugates. One approach involves a proximal linkage assay based on substrate channeling resulting from the close proximity of one enzyme with a corresponding coupling enzyme. In another method, changes in enzyme activity occur because of the binding of antigen with the corresponding antibody–enzyme conjugate.

Several competitive homogeneous EIAs have been reported. These include the enzyme-multiplied immunoassay technique, substrate-labeled fluorescein immunoassay, apoenzyme reactivation immunoassay, and cloned enzyme donor immunoassay. Noncompetitive EIAs include the associated enzyme-sensitive technique and enzyme inhibitory homogeneous immunoassay.

Soluble Labels and Detection

Enzymes are more widely used than any other label for immunoassays. The various enzymes used generate colored, fluorescent, or luminescent compounds from neutral substrates. Those used in ELISA include horseradish peroxidase (HRP), alkaline phosphatase (AP), glucose oxidase, β-galactosidase, glucoamylase, carbonic anhydrase, and acetylcholinesterase. Several covalent conjugation methods are available for coupling enzymes to antigens or anti-

Figure 4.6 Principle of competitive ELISA for the detection of antigen. Both enzyme-labeled and unlabeled antigen (derived from the patient sample) compete for antigen-binding sites on the immobilized IgG. The activity measured for the labeled antigen is inversely proportional to the concentration of that antigen in the sample.

bodies. The enzymes HRP (44 kDa) and AP (140 kDa) are the most commonly used in heterogeneous immunoassays. First, HRP catalyzes conversion of the substrate H_2O_2 to H_2O and O_2. Then, it oxidizes another substrate, thereby resulting in a colored, fluorescent, or luminescent derivative (depending on the nature of the substrate). The enzyme AP catalyzes the hydrolysis of the phosphate esters of primary alcohols, phenols, and amines.

Another commonly used approach employs biotin-avidin–binding reactions with one of the components complexed with a chromogenic enzyme. Avidin (67 kDa) can be isolated from purified egg white. This molecule has a very high affinity (association constant = 10^{15} LM^{-1}) for the small, water-soluble vitamin biotin (0.244 kDa). Four biotin molecules can bind to one avidin molecule. In a typical ELISA, biotinylated antibody and avidin-labeled enzyme are used instead of the enzyme-labeled antibody, because this combination offers a significantly enhanced signal.

SIGNAL MEASUREMENT

Colorimetry

The most common—and the simplest—detection system is colorimetry, which can be determined either visually or with the aid of a spectrophotometer. Some of the common chromogenic substrates for peroxidase are o-phenylene-diamine (OPD), 3,3′,5,5′-tetramethylbenzidine (TMB), and 2,2′-azino-bis(3-ethylbenzothiazoline-6-sulfonate). The most widely used is TMB, because it generates the highest absorbance values and low backgrounds. Furthermore, unlike OPD, it is not mutagenic. Immunoassays based on HRP offer greater sensitivity than those based on AP; the most frequently used substrate for AP is p-nitrophenyl phosphate.

Fluorometry

Fluorescence begins with the absorption of photons by fluorophores. At the appropriate wavelength, electrons are energized from a ground energy state to an excited, singlet state. Then, as the molecule returns to the ground state, it emits a photon of light at a lower energy (i.e., a longer wavelength). The difference between the excitation maximum and the emission maximum is known as the Stokes' shift *(Fig. 4.8)*.

The standard label, fluorescein isothiocyanate, has an absorption-emission time interval of only 1 nanosecond (ns). Many other compounds, however, exhibit delayed fluorescence, with much higher time intervals.

Use of fluorescence techniques in immunoassays has been reviewed elsewhere (5). Fluorometric EIAs (FIAs) are more sensitive than colorimetric immunoassays and, there-

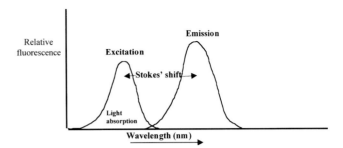

Figure 4.8 Principle of fluorescent measurement. Stokes' shift represents the difference between the maximum excitation and the maximum emission.

fore, may be used to detect or measure small concentrations of analyte. Two disadvantages, however, are the increased complexity of the procedure and the need for instrumentation. A common substrate for AP in fluorometric EIAs is 4-methylumbelliferyl phosphate (4-MUP); AP dephosphorylates 4-MUP to the form the fluorophore 4-methylumbelliferone.

Time-Resolved Fluorescence

Background interference by light scattering and the intrinsic fluorescence of sample components are two limitations of traditional fluorescent compounds. Time-resolved fluorescence is based on the principle that some lanthanides, such as europium (Eu^{3+}), form fluorescent chelates with certain organic ligands. These fluorophores have very large Stokes' shifts and decay times (200 nm and >500 ns, respectively). Time-resolved fluorescence takes advantage of these long decay times and large Stokes' shifts; thus, any short-lived fluorescence background signal or scattered excitation radiation is eliminated. In fact, signals are measured under conditions of virtually no background. Several homogeneous and heterogeneous FIAs for the detection and quantitation of various diseases markers have been developed, and many of them have been automated. Use of time-resolved fluorescence techniques in immunoassays has been reviewed elsewhere (5).

Luminescence

In chemiluminescent immunoassays, luminescent compounds emit light during a chemical reaction. Luminol derivatives or acridinium esters have been used as labels. Chemiluminescence kinetics are very fast, and light is emitted within seconds of substrate oxidation. These assays generally are very sensitive, with high dynamic ranges.

A bioluminescent immunoassay based on SeaLight Sciences' AquaLite, which is a recombinant form of the calcium-activated photoprotein aequorin, is adaptable to commercial luminometers. Attomole levels of AquaLite have been detected in some assays. This photoprotein is easily coupled to MAbs and polyclonal antibodies. Luminescent and bioluminescent immunoassays have been reviewed elsewhere (6).

In an electrochemiluminescence technique (7,8), a ruthenium metal chelate and tripropylamine are used. Both molecules become oxidized at the surface of an electrode, where they react to form an excited state of ruthenium that decays and releases a photon at 620 nm. This technology is easily adapted to immunoassays and molecular diagnostics.

PRINCIPLES OF ASSAY DESIGN AND OPTIMIZATION

Immobilization of Molecules on Solid Phases

Two types of plastics commonly are used for solid phase attachment in EIAs: polystyrene, and polyvinyl chloride. Typically, these are used in 8-, 12-, or 96-well configurations. Many factors affect the rate, extent, and quality of attachment to the solid phase. The most obvious of these are:

1. Characteristics of the solid phase used.
2. Quality of the solid phase.
3. Purity of the molecule to be attached.
4. Physicochemical characteristics of the molecule (e.g., hydrophobicity).
5. Diffusion coefficient of the molecule.
6. Concentration of the molecule in coating solution.
7. Characteristics of the coupling solution (e.g., pH, ionic strength, and temperature).
8. Time allowed for attachment of the molecule.
9. Subsequent processing and storage of the coated solid phase.

Principles of Binding

Biologic macromolecules can bind to plastic surfaces in various ways, and determining the proportion of bound molecules that are biologically active is important. The adsorption of molecules to polystyrene primarily results from intermolecular attraction forces. These forces are of two types: alternating polarities, which are known as hydrophobic interaction; and stationary polarities. Alternating polarities occur when molecules in close proximity create disturbances in their electron clouds. Molecules with stationary polarities can bind to each other through dipoles, and hydrogen bonding can result between two dipoles. Chemical groups that mediate H bonding include –OH, =O, –NH₂, =NH, and N. Knowledge regarding the properties of both the solid phase and of the molecule to be

bound is useful before immobilization of a molecule to a surface. For example, some plastics are available in either hydrophobic or hydrophilic forms, and others have both properties.

For cases in which molecules do not bind optimally to the solid phase by passive adsorption, it may be necessary to mediate binding by other means. Glutaraldehyde, succinimidyl esters, carbodiimides and poly-L-lysine have been used to enhance binding of some molecules. Irradiated wells also enhance the binding of some molecules. Furthermore, in the case of antibody, having the antibody vertically oriented with the Fc on the solid phase is desirable, because in this configuration, the Fab is free to recognize and bind to the corresponding antigenic epitope. This also allows for uninhibited segmental flexibility of the antibody molecule, which facilitates this process. For this purpose, chemistries that exploit the carbohydrate on the Fc may be used to immobilize antibody. In addition, attachment of protein A or protein G to the solid phase before addition of the capture antibody may facilitate better-oriented and more-reactive capture antibody molecules.

The geometry of a globular molecule dictates the maximum number of molecules that can be packed in the densest monolayer on a surface. The density of packing is a function of the orientation of the molecule after binding. For an elongated molecule such as IgG (150 Å × 3 Å), vertical packing results in more molecules being bound per unit area compared with horizontal packing of the molecules.

Nonspecific Interactions in Immunoassays

Nonspecific interactions can have an adverse effect on immunoassays. This effect manifests primarily as reduced specificity. Many factors can contribute to this effect. The elimination of nonspecificity is central to the performance of a reliable test, and several approaches to reduce this effect are discussed later.

Fc Interactions

Complement, rheumatoid factor, and noncovalent interaction between the Fc portions of whole-antibody molecules can contribute to nonspecific interactions in immunoassays. To circumvent this effect, F(ab')₂ and Fab IgG fragments may be used. Both F(ab')₂ and Fab Ig fragments are produced by the enzymatic actions of pepsin and papain, respectively *(Fig. 4.9)*.

The Fab' fragments may be prepared by the reduction of F(ab')₂ with 2-mercaptoethylamine. These abbreviated Ig components may confer increased rates of diffusion in immunoassays, but use of these fragments does have potential disadvantages. First, fewer residues are available for conjugation with labeling reagent, thereby making the

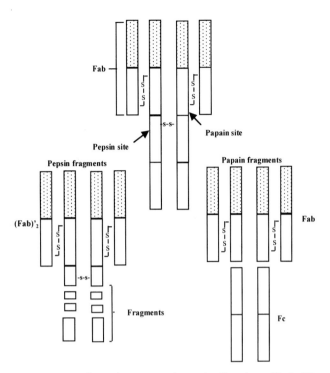

Figure 4.9 Effect of pepsin and papain digestion of IgG. The F(ab)$'_2$ fragment is used more frequently than the Fab fragment for immunoassays.

fragment less reactive than intact IgG on a molar basis. Second, IgG fragments are less stable after immobilization to solid phases. Third, elimination of the Fc portion of the Ig, in addition to shortening the molecule, affects the segmental flexibility of the molecule, thus making it more rigid and less able to access more remote antigenic epitopes.

General Approaches to Eliminate Nonspecific Interactions

General approaches to eliminate nonspecific interactions include:

1. Change the solid phase.
2. Replace reagents with more purified ones.
3. Use pure recombinant antigens and MAbs.
4. Increase the protein content in sample, label diluent, or both.
5. Optimize the detergent concentration in the assay.
6. Modify the test parameters (e.g., incubation time and temperature, sample concentration, and conjugate concentration).
7. Use blocking reagents after immobilization of ligand onto solid phase.

In the development of ELISAs, "blocking" has always been a concern. Any substance that aids in the prevention of nonspecific binding of reagents is considered to be a blocking agent. Several such agents have been used, including Tween 20, gelatin, bovine serum albumin, casein, fetal bovine serum, and sera from various other normal animals. In some instances, further treatment of the wells containing immobilized ligand is not necessary, because the presence of selected protein sources in the sample and label buffers suffices.

The processes of immunoassay optimization can be complex. The classic "one variable at a time" approach to identifying confounding elements in assay optimization is very time-consuming. Therefore, to develop products with rigorous specifications more quickly, statistical experimental designs may be employed (9,10). This process, which is known as design of experiments (DoE), uses design tools that drastically reduce the amount of experimental data needed to reach conclusions regarding a process. By minimizing the resource requirements, workers can get the most information about immunoassay parameters with less effort than would otherwise be needed. Many manufacturers of in vitro medical devices use DoE to identify the optimum combination of factors required to generate products that meet exacting specifications at minimum cost. In addition to shortening product development times, this approach results in better product performance.

PARTICLE IMMUNOASSAYS

Particles are employed as a solid phase in many important immunodiagnostic procedures. This section presents a brief overview of such particles; a comprehensive approach to understanding the history and role of particles in immunodiagnostics has been published elsewhere (11).

Agglutination Without Separation

Particle immunoassays are those using antigen or antibody immobilized onto a particle as a form of solid phase. Several particles can be used, including erythrocytes, bacteria, liposomes, microcapsules, metal sols (e.g., colloidal gold), gelatin, and latexes. For agglutination reactions, particle sizes range from 0.05 to 7 μm, and polystyrene microspheres (i.e., "uniform latex particles") are most commonly used. Latex agglutination tests are easy to perform and serve as useful point-of-care tests.

Hemagglutination reactions are conducted in round-bottom or V-shaped microtitration wells. When coated red blood cells are agglutinated, they fall to the well surface as an expanded network of particles. Unagglutinated particles are clearly differentiated as they condense and roll to the center of the well *(Fig. 4.10)*. Particles coated with antigen can be used to detect antibody through formation of cross-linked structures and subsequent agglu-

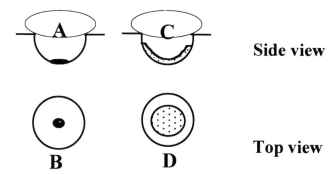

Figure 4.10 A and B. Unagglutinated erythrocytes. C and D. Hemagglutination pattern observed during an antigen–antibody reaction.

tination. Antibody-coated particles agglutinate in the presence of specific antigen. On a slide, agglutinated reactions appear as clumps, whereas unreacted particles maintain their smooth-suspension appearance *(Fig. 4.11)*.

Spectrophotometers and nephelometers have been used to measure agglutination by turbidimetry and forward light scattering, respectively. These instruments have contributed to the enhanced sensitivity of microsphere agglutination assays. Today, sensitivities of 100 pg/mL for proteins have been achieved.

Fluorochrome-dyed microspheres have become more widely used in diagnostics, and many unique applications now incorporate this technology. For example, flow cytometry capable of discriminating microspheres by size and fluorescent color has been used to perform simultaneous, real-time analyses of several assays on the surfaces of the microspheres. This assay system can simultaneously perform several different assays in a single tube with a single specimen as well.

Particle-counting immunoassay (PACIA) (12) may offer sensitivities 10- to 15-fold greater than that of turbidimetry. Using a particle counter, PACIA measures the reduction of single (unagglutinated) particles or clumps of particles during a reaction. One example of this technology is Copalis (Sienna Biotech), which is a laser-based particle sizer/counter using "optical sizing flow particle analysis."

Quasielastic light scattering (i.e., "dynamic light scattering" or "photon correlation spectroscopy") measures changes in the responses of particles according to their size distribution. Measurements of changes in the angular anisotropy (i.e., "two-angle light scattering") of scattered light intensity resulting from changes in average particle size has been used to determine the extent of particle agglutination.

Scanning laser microscopy also has been applied to the quantification of agglutination. This method, however, is more suitable for larger particles (>1 μm).

Agglutination with Separation

Particle Capture

After agglutination, colored agglutinated microspheres can be applied to a membrane. The complexes will be caught on the filter because of their larger size, and the unreacted single microspheres will pass through *(Fig. 4.12)*. The results may be visually assessed, or reflectometry or densitometry may be used for a more objective assessment. Particle capture may be followed by an ELISA procedure. In this approach, uncolored microspheres labeled with antibody are attached to a membrane. Then, sample containing antigen is added, followed by the appropriate conjugate and precipitable substrate *(Fig. 4.13)*. The extent of color formation is proportional to the amount of antigen in the sample. This approach works equally well for antibody detection when microspheres are coated with antigen.

Lateral Flow Immunoassays

Lateral or tangential flow immunoassays are conducted in single-use test devices. Such devices typically contain dyed

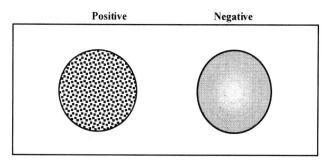

Figure 4.11 Agglutination pattern of latex microspheres.

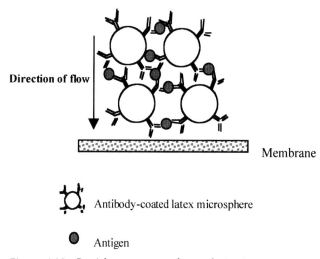

Figure 4.12 Particle entrapment after agglutination.

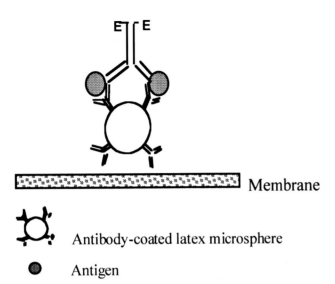

Figure 4.13   Particle entrapment with ELISA.

latex microspheres, liposomes, metallic particles, or colloids containing immobilized antigen or antibody. These mobile solid phases can migrate through a membrane support. On addition of a test sample, the analyte binds to the solid phase, and the complex migrates through the membrane until being captured at a detection zone *(Fig. 4.14)*. Aggregation of particles in the detection zone results in a distinct, visible area of color.

Paramagnetic Particles and Latexes

In another modification, paramagnetic particles containing antibody can be mixed with colored latex particles having bound analyte and transferred to a capillary tube. Application of a magnet separates the magnetic particle–latex particle complexes. The degree of change in turbidity depends on the quantity of analyte present in the complex.

BIOSENSORS

Biosensors are analytic devices in which a molecule of biologic origin (e.g., an antibody or enzyme), which serves as

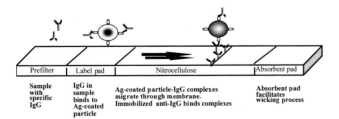

Figure 4.14   General principle of solid-phase chromatographic (lateral flow) immunoassays. (Components are not drawn to scale.)

the chemical recognition element, is in close contact with a physical transducer or detector (13). Biosensors are of various types, including biocatalytic, electrochemical, optical, mass-detection, amperometric, pharmacologic, and immunochemical (14,15). A nonseparation, sandwich-type electrochemical EIA for detecting specific molecules in undiluted whole blood has also been described (16). The principle is based on the preferential electrochemical measurement of surface-bound antibody–enzyme conjugate relative to an excess of this reagent in the sample solution. Immunologic biosensors have gained great impetus in immunodiagnostics, with a rapid influx of new applications. More recently, DNA biosensors have used single-stranded DNA immobilized on quartz optical fibers, piezoelectric crystals, and amperometric electrodes.

DIAGNOSTIC MOLECULAR PATHOLOGY

Testing with nucleic acid probes in the clinical laboratory was initiated more than 12 years ago, when Gen-Probe (San Diego, CA) introduced the first U.S. Food and Drug Administration–approved test kit for *Legionella* sp. Molecular diagnostic methods continue to play an important role in the diagnosis of a variety of diseases (17,18). The market is dominated by infectious disease diagnostics, but use of molecular tests for cancer and genetic disease is increasing. Several factors have contributed to this rapid expansion of diagnostic molecular pathology. The primary factors involve improvements in nucleic acid extraction techniques, more efficient DNA sequencing methods, diversity of nucleic acid amplification techniques, availability of several commercially available molecular detection methods, and introduction of semiautomated instrumentation for probe testing.

Procedures for molecular diagnostics may be performed with or without amplification; however, direct reaction with nucleic acid probes in which no amplification is used is less sensitive. Chiron Diagnostics (Emeryville, CA) developed a branched DNA signal amplification technique that uses multiple probes and reporter molecules. This approach is more sensitive than traditional direct probing methods, with a sensitivity of 50 nucleic acid targets.

Molecular diagnostic approaches that use target amplification offer greater sensitivity. Some of these techniques include the widely used polymerase chain reaction (PCR) of Cetus, which is based on the ability of DNA polymerase to copy a strand of DNA by the elongation of complementary strands initiated from a pair of oligonucleotide primers. Reverse transcriptase (RT)–PCR is used to amplify RNA targets, and in this process, RT converts RNA to complementary DNA, which is followed by amplification with PCR. This has been a useful test in the detection

RNA viruses. Nested PCR uses two sets of amplification primers, and this dual amplification process results in very high sensitivity. In multiplex PCR, two or more pairs of primers for different targets are introduced in the same reaction mixture; here, simultaneous amplification of more than one unique DNA sequence in a sample occurs.

Isothermal nucleic acid amplification systems include the transcription-based amplification system and its derivatives, such as nucleic acid sequence–based amplification or transcription-mediated amplification. Another non-PCR isothermal system is strand displacement amplification. The Q? replicase system for RNA amplification and the ligase chain reaction, which is a probe amplification technique, are examples of other powerful tools in molecular diagnostics.

Diagnostic molecular pathology is easily adapted to make use of the currently available detection methods, such as colorimetry, fluorescence, and chemiluminescence. Automation for nucleic acid probe tests continues to be a major factor driving the market penetration of these tests. Roche Molecular Systems was the first to launch an automated instrument for performing amplified probe assays in the clinical laboratory. This was followed by the commercialization of several diagnostic platforms and unique proprietary chemical approaches by a number of diagnostics companies. As a result, worldwide sales of nucleic acid probe tests are expected to grow to US$964 million by 2002 (19).

VETERINARY DIAGNOSTIC PRODUCTS

The worldwide potential for veterinary diagnostics is considerable, and this potential is also rapidly expanding as new and more inexpensive technologies become available. *Table 4.1* presents a small selection of the commercially available immunodiagnostic tests for cats and dogs.

Governmental regulation is an important consideration in the manufacture and sale of diagnostic products. In the United States, production and marketing of some diagnostic products is governed by the regulations within the Code of Federal Regulations. For veterinary diagnostics, implementation of these regulations is the responsibility of the U.S. Animal and Plant Health Inspection Services; similar agencies oversee diagnostic manufacturers in many other countries worldwide. A voluntary certification standard of excellence that may be achieved by manufacturers is the ISO 9000, which was initiated by the British Standards Institution. This standard is implemented by several thousand companies in more than 85 countries.

Veterinary diagnostics is a growing business. The world veterinary diagnostics market is estimated to be US$600 million. This market includes blood biochemistry, hematology, electrolyte analysis, and infectious disease diagnostics. In 1997, the worldwide diagnostics market was estimated at US$400 million, with the companion animal market (i.e., dogs, cats, and horses) being the predominant sector.

THE FUTURE OF IMMUNODIAGNOSTICS

Immunodiagnostic technology in the twenty-first century will be characterized by innovations in chemistry, molecular biology, immunology, automation, and data management. Smaller, inexpensive instrumentation will play a major role in providing more accurate and objective results for point-of-care diagnostic tests. Traditional immunoassays have focused on humoral aspects of the immune response, but immunodiagnostic technology is expected to continue expanding into the study of other immune system components in disease. For example, immunodiagnostic technology has been applied to products of the major histocompatibility complex (MHC). On the cell surface, MHC molecules provide a critical context for the recognition of antigens by the T-cell receptor.

TABLE 4.1 SELECTED VETERINARY IMMUNODIAGNOSTIC PRODUCTS AND THEIR CONFIGURATIONS

Company	Product Name	Test Use	Analyte Measured	Test Configuration
Agen	VetRed FIV	Cat	FIV antibody	Hemagglutination
Heska	Solo Step FH	Cat	Heartworm antibody	Lateral flow
Heska	Solo Step CH	Dog	Heartworm antigen	Lateral flow
IDEXX	LymeCHEK	Dog	*Borrelia burgdorferi* antibody	Indirect ELISA
IDEXX	Snap Canine Heartworm PF	Dog	Heartworm antigen	Sandwich ELISA
Synbiotics	Assure/FH	Cat	Heartworm antibody	Indirect ELISA
Synbiotics	ICT-Gold HW	Dog and cat	Heartworm antigen	Lateral flow

The World Health Organization reports that emerging infectious diseases are a serious global threat, and that a disease can emerge and spread swiftly to anywhere on the Earth. Many factors influence this category of infections, including travel, changes in social customs, changes in climate, and our ability to detect new diseases through more sophisticated diagnosis. Some of the new—and re-emerging—diseases of both animals and humans include bovine spongioform encephalopathy, equine morbillivirus infection, ehrlichioses, coccidioidomycosis, visceral leishmaniasis, Lyme disease, *Chlamydia pneumoniae* infection, dengue hemorrhagic fever, human immunodeficiency virus (acquired immunodeficiency syndrome), ebola virus, and hantavirus. Many of these diseases have been identified using classical immunodiagnostic technologies for specific IgG, IgM, or antigens associated with the respective pathogens. The global health threat posed by new and re-emerging diseases requires continual development of improved diagnostic methods.

REFERENCES

1. Yalow RS, Berson SA. Assay of plasma insulin in human subjects by immunological methods. Nature (London) 1959;184:1648–1649.
2. Skaletsky E. Antiidiotypic antibodies as diagnostic antigens. IVD Technol 1997;3:24–35.
3. Köhler G, Milstein C. Continuous culture of fused cells secreting antibodies of predefined specificity. Nature (London) 1976;256: 495–497.
4. Engvall E, Perlmann P. Enzyme linked immunosorbent assay (ELISA). Quantitative assay of immunoglobulin G. Immunochemistry 1971;8:871–875.
5. Hemmilä IL. Applications of fluorescence in immunoassays. In: Winefordner JD, ed. Chemical analysis. London: John Wiley & Sons, 1991:117.
6. Bronstein I, Sparks A. Sensitive enzyme immunoassays with chemiluminescent detection. In: Nakamura RM, Kasahara Y, Rechnitz GA, eds. Immunochemical assays and biosensor technology for the 1990s. Washington, DC: ASM Press, 1992:229–250.
7. Yang H, Leland JK, Yost D, Massey RJ. Electrochemiluminescence: a new diagnostic and research tool. Biotechnology 1994;12: 193–194.
8. Jameison F, Sanchez RI, Dong L, Leland JK, Yost D, Martin MT. Electrochemiluminescence-based quantitation of classical clinical chemistry analytes. Anal Chem 1996;68:1298–1302.
9. Atkinson AC, Donev AN. Optimum experimental designs. Oxford: Clarendon Press, 1992.
10. Montgomery DC. Design and analysis of experiments. 3rd ed. New York: John Wiley & Sons, 1991.
11. Bangs L. The latex course. Meeting Proceedings. Princeton, NJ, 1996.
12. Masson PL, Holy HW. Immunoassay by particle counting. In: Rose NR, Friedman H, Fahey JL, eds. Manual of clinical laboratory immunology. 3rd ed. Washington, DC: ASM Press, 1986:43–86.
13. Turner APF, Karube I, Wilson GS, eds. Biosensors. Fundamentals and application. Oxford: Oxford University Press, 1987.
14. Ho MYK. An introduction to biosensors. In: Nakamura RM, Kasahara Y, Rechnitz GA, eds. Immunochemical assays and biosensor technology for the 1990s. Washington, DC: ASM Press, 1992:275–290.
15. Malan PG. Immunological biosensors. In: Wild E, ed. The immunoassay handbook. New York: Stockton Press, 1994:125–134.
16. Meyerhoff ME, Daun C, Meusel M. Novel nonseparation sandwich-type electrochemical enzyme immunoassay for detecting marker proteins in undiluted blood. Clin Chem 1995;41: 1378–1384.
17. Hill CS. Molecular diagnostics for infectious diseases. J Clin Ligand Assay 1996;19:43–52.
18. Tang YW, Procop C, Persing D. Molecular diagnosis of infectious diseases. Clin Chem 1997;43:2021–2038.
19. Simonsen M. Infectious disease testing leads the way in nucleic acid diagnostics. Diagn Update 1998;1.1–7.

TWO

HEMATOLOGY OF COMMON

DOMESTIC SPECIES

CHAPTER

5

ERYTHROCYTE MORPHOLOGY

The primary function of the erythrocyte is to transport hemoglobin, which carries oxygen to the tissues. The deformable, permeable membrane that encloses the red-cell components is made of lipids, proteins, and carbohydrates. Alterations in the lipid composition (primarily phospholipids and cholesterol) of the membrane may result in abnormal red-cell shapes. Membrane proteins form the cytoskeleton of the membrane, and these proteins also play key roles in maintaining both cell shape and integrity. These membrane proteins have been named according to their relative location from the place of migration when solubilized and subjected to electrophoresis. Bands 1 and 2 (i.e., spectrin) and band 5 (i.e., actin) are the major cytoskeletal proteins. Abnormalities in membrane proteins have also been associated with abnormal red-cell shapes.

Normal erythrocyte morphology varies among different species (*Fig. 5.1*). Mammalian erythrocytes are anucleate, unlike those of all other vertebrates, which have nuclei. Erythrocytes are round and somewhat biconcave in most mammalian species, except in members of the family Camellidae (e.g., llamas, camels, and alpacas), which have oval erythrocytes. The biconcavity causes stained red blood cells to appear to have a central, pale area, because the observer is looking through less hemoglobin in this area of the cell. This central pallor is most apparent in canine erythrocytes. Species with smaller erythrocytes, such as the cat, horse, cow, sheep,

and goat, have less concavity and, thus, little to no central pallor. The biconcave disc shape is efficient for oxygen exchange, and it allows the cell to be deformable as it moves through vasculature with a smaller diameter than that of the erythrocyte itself. Briefly, the significant differences between species are size, shape, amount of central pallor, tendency to form rouleaux, presence of basophilic stippling in regenerative response to anemia, and the presence of reticulocytes in response to anemia (*Table 5.1*).

Erythrocyte morphology often is an important aid in establishing a diagnosis regarding the cause of anemia, and it sometimes is helpful in establishing the diagnosis of other disorders as well. Critical to blood-cell evaluation is adequate preparation of a blood film (see Chapter 1). The observer should examine the leukocyte counting area to evaluate erythrocyte morphology, because the red blood cells are neither too dense nor too flattened in this area. The interpretation of red-blood-cell morphology should be made in conjunction with other quantitative data from the complete blood count. For example, the degree of polychromasia in erythrocytes usually is more significant when the red-cell mass is decreased.

This chapter concentrates primarily on those morphologic characteristics that are most diagnostically useful. Morphology of erythrocytes is categorized here according to color, size, shape, structures in or on the erythrocytes, and the arrangement of cells on blood films.

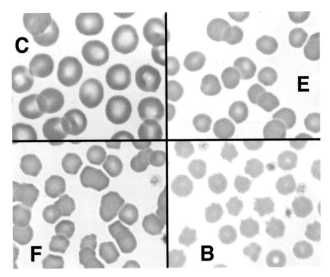

Figure 5.1 Normal canine (C), equine (E), feline (F), and bovine (B) erythrocytes. Note the larger size and marked central pallor of the canine erythrocytes compared to those of the other species. Wright stain.

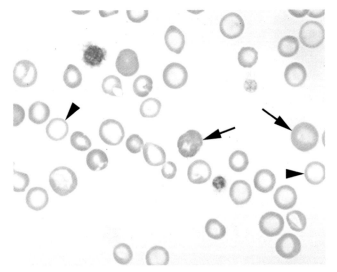

Figure 5.2 Blood film from a dog with iron-deficiency anemia. Note the lack of density of the blood film, suggesting marked anemia. Most of the erythrocytes are small and hypochromic (arrowheads). The anemia is regenerative, and numerous polychromatophilic erythrocytes are present (arrows). Wright stain.

ERYTHROCYTE COLOR

Polychromasia

Polychromatophilic cells are young erythrocytes that have been released early. Usually, they are large and more blue in color than mature erythrocytes (*Fig. 5.2*). The blue color results from organelles (i.e., ribosomes, mitochondria) that are still present in the immature cells. The presence or absence of polychromatophilic erythrocytes is very important when determining the cause of anemia. If immature cells are released, the likely cause of the anemia is blood loss or blood destruction, with the bone marrow attempting to compensate by the early release of cells (see

Chapter 8). If the anemia is caused by erythroid hypoplasia or aplasia within the marrow, then the level of polychromatophilic cells will not be increased (see Chapter 7). Horses are unique, however, in that they do not release polychromatophilic cells in the face of anemia.

The degree of polychromasia correlates well with the reticulocyte concentration, but it is more objective to quantitate the regenerative response by counting reticulocytes (see Chapter 1). The reticulocyte is analogous to the polychromatophilic erythrocyte, but it is stained with a vital stain (e.g., new methylene blue or brilliant cresyl blue), which causes the ribosomes and other organelles to clump into visible granules (see Fig. 1.37).

TABLE 5.1. SIGNIFICANT DIFFERENCES IN ERYTHROCYTES BETWEEN SPECIES

Species	Diameter (μm)	Rouleaux	Central Pallor	Basophilic Stippling	Reticulocytes (%)[a]	MCV (fL)
Dog	7.0	+	++++	−	1	60–72
Pig	6.0	++	±	−	1	50–68
Cat	5.8	++	+	±	0.5	39–50
Horse	5.7	++++	−	−	0[b]	36–52
Cow	5.5	−	+	+++	0	37–53
Sheep	4.5	±	+	+++	0	23–48
Goat	3.2	−	−	++	0	15–30

[a]With normal packed cell volume.
[b]Does not increase in response to anemia.

Hypochromasia

Hypochromic red blood cells are pale and have increased central pallor as a result of decreased hemoglobin concentration from iron deficiency (Fig. 5.2). Erythrocytes of iron-deficient dogs have more obvious hypochromasia than erythrocytes of other species with iron deficiency; erythrocytes of iron-deficient cats usually are not hypochromic at all. One needs to distinguish hypochromic cells from bowl-shaped (i.e., torocytes) or "punched-out" cells, which are insignificant (*Fig. 5.3*). Bowl-shaped cells have a sharply defined, central clear area, and they also have a thicker rim of hemoglobin than is seen in true hypochromic cells. Immature polychromatophilic erythrocytes also may appear to be hypochromic, because their hemoglobin concentration is less than normal due to their increased volume. Although hyperchromic states are not thought to exist, spherocytes appear to have increased color intensity because of their lack of concavity.

ERYTHROCYTE SIZE

Variation in erythrocyte size is termed *anisocytosis*. This variation may result from the presence of large cells (i.e., macrocytes), small cells (i.e., microcytes), or both. In itself, the term does not provide any meaningful information. Red blood cells may appear to be small on the blood film because of decreased diameter, but the cell volume is the true measurement of red-cell size and is determined electronically (see Chapter 1). The best example of this is the spherocyte, which appears to be small because of its spheric shape and subsequent decreased diameter; however, the red-cell volume of spherocytes is almost always within the reference range. Conversely, hypochromic microcytic iron-deficient red blood cells with an electronically determined decreased volume may have a normal diameter and, thus, not appear to be small on the blood film.

Microcytic Erythrocytes

Cells must be markedly small before their decreased diameter can be visually detected (Fig. 5.2). Mean corpuscular volume (MCV) is more valuable than blood film examination in assessing the true size of erythrocytes. Using automated cell-counting systems, a histogram or volume–distribution curve of the erythrocyte population can be generated. Mean cell volume is determined by analysis of the volume–distribution curve, and the hematocrit is then calculated by multiplying the MCV by the erythrocyte concentration (see Chapter 1). The most common cause of microcytosis is iron-deficiency anemia; a decreased MCV is the hallmark of such anemia. In some iron-deficient patients, the MCV may be normal even though the animal has a microcytic population of cells. In these cases, examination of the volume–distribution curve is helpful (see Chapter 1). The pathophysiology of the microcytosis is theorized to involve erythroid precursors continuing to divide until a near-normal complement of hemoglobin concentration is reached, resulting in small erythrocytes. Cells can not obtain a normal hemoglobin concentration because iron is required to make hemoglobin. If the iron deficiency is severe, microcytosis and hypochromia may be observed on the blood film. In addition, membrane defects are present, which often lead to specific abnormalities in shape and fragmentation (discussed later). Dogs with portocaval shunts may have microcytic anemia that usually is related to abnormal iron metabolism and low serum iron concentration. Some breeds of dogs (i.e., Akitas and Shiba Inus) normally have smaller erythrocytes.

Macrocytic Erythrocytes

Macrocytic erythrocytes are large and have an increased MCV (see Fig. 1.37). The most common cause of macrocytosis is increased numbers of immature erythrocytes that are polychromatophilic on Wright-stained blood films. Unlike other domestic species, horses release macrocytes that are not polychromatophilic. The associated increase in MCV usually is the only evidence of erythroid regeneration in horses. During regeneration, species other than dogs tend to produce regenerative macrocytes that are approximately twice the size of normal erythrocytes, resulting in a marked change in the MCV. Dogs, however, release macrocytes that usually are only slightly

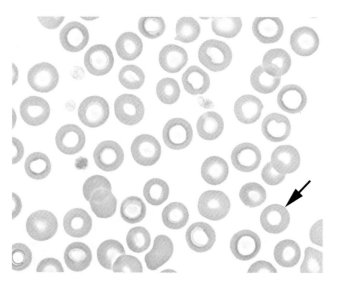

Figure 5.3   Blood film from a dog showing numerous torocytes ("punched-out" erythrocytes). Note the wide rim of hemoglobin and lack of hemoglobinization in the center of the cells (arrow). Torocytes can be mistaken for true hypochromasia. Wright stain.

larger than normal erythrocytes. Macrocytosis without polychromasia or other evidence of an appropriate regenerative response is a common finding in anemic cats with myelodysplasia and myeloproliferative disease (see Chapter 13). This macrocytosis is associated with feline leukemia virus (FeLV) infection, and it also may be seen in FeLV-infected cats that are not anemic.

Other, more infrequent causes of macrocytosis include macrocytosis of poodles and hereditary stomatocytosis. Macrocytosis of miniature or toy poodles is rare, is thought to be hereditary, and is usually an incidental finding. Affected dogs are not anemic, but their erythrocyte count may be decreased. The MCV is usually 90 to 100 fL. Other findings include increased nucleated erythrocytes, increased Howell-Jolly bodies (often multiple), and hypersegmented neutrophils. Numerous abnormalities are seen in erythroid precursors on bone marrow film examination, including megaloblasts with nuclear and cytoplasmic asynchrony of maturation. The cause of the defect is unknown, and no clinical signs are associated with the disorder. Finally, stomatocytes in Alaskan malamutes and miniature schnauzers with hereditary stomatocytosis are macrocytic (discussed later).

Some anticonvulsant drugs, such as phenobarbital, phenytoin, and primidone, have been thought to induce macrocytosis, but macrocytosis was not experimentally reproduced in dogs receiving long-term anticonvulsant drugs. Vitamin B$_{12}$ (i.e., cobalamin) and folate deficiency do not cause macrocytosis in domestic animals, but these deficiencies are a common cause of macrocytosis in humans. Giant schnauzers with hereditary cobalamin malabsorption are anemic, but this anemia is normocytic rather than macrocytic.

ERYTHROCYTE SHAPE

Abnormally shaped erythrocytes are termed *poikilocytes*. This terminology is not helpful, however, because it does not suggest a specific change in shape. Thus, no specific interpretation is possible. The most important shape changes include various types of spiculated erythrocytes, spherocytes, and eccentrocytes. Spiculated erythrocytes have one or more surface spicules and include echinocytes, acanthocytes, keratocytes, and schistocytes. One should be as specific as possible when describing shape changes, because certain types of abnormal red-cell shapes are associated with certain diseases. Less significant abnormally shaped red blood cells include leptocytes (i.e., folded or target cells), codocytes (i.e., target cells), dacryocytes (i.e., teardrop-shaped erythrocytes), and torocytes (i.e., bowl-shaped erythrocytes).

A few inherited abnormalities associated with red-cell shape change have been described in animals and include

hereditary stomatocytosis in dogs, hereditary elliptocytosis resulting from band 4.1 deficiency in dogs, and hereditary spherocytosis in Japanese black cattle resulting from band 3 deficiency. Hereditary spherocytosis has also been reported in mice. Most inherited abnormalities of red-blood-cell shape are associated with abnormalities of cytoskeletal protein, or plasma or red-cell membrane cholesterol or phospholipid concentration.

Schistocytes and Keratocytes

Erythrocyte fragments, also termed *schistocytes*, usually result from shearing of the red cell by intravascular trauma. This may be observed in animals with disseminated intravascular coagulopathy (DIC) as a result of erythrocytes being broken by fibrin strands, with vascular neoplasms (e.g., hemangiosarcoma), and with iron deficiency. Animals with DIC also may have a concurrent thrombocytopenia (*Fig. 5.4*). When erythrocyte fragments are observed in blood films from dogs with hemangiosarcoma, acanthocytes usually are present as well. Fragmentation in iron-deficient erythrocytes apparently results from oxidative injury, leading to membrane lesions or increased susceptibility to intravascular trauma. Iron-deficient erythrocytes initially develop an apparent blister or vacuole, which is thought to represent an oxidative injury and in which inner membrane surfaces are cross-linked across the cell. Exclusion of hemoglobin may account for the colorless area. These lesions subsequently enlarge and break open to form cells with one or more spicules. When one spicule is present, these cells are commonly termed *apple-stem cells*; when two or more spicules are present, they are termed *keratocytes* (*Figure 5.5*). The projections from the

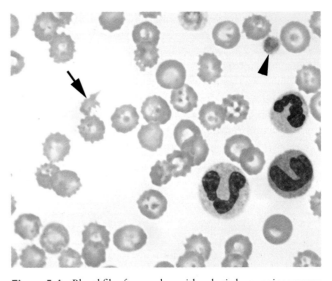

Figure 5.4 Blood film from a dog with splenic hemangiosarcoma and disseminated intravascular coagulopathy. Note the schistocyte (arrow) and single platelet in the field (arrowhead). Wright stain.

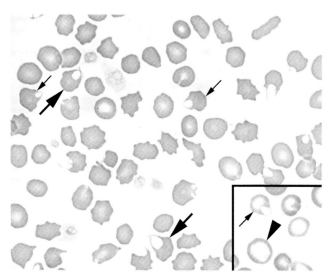

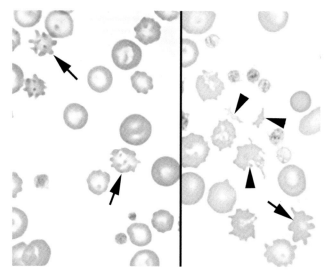

Figure 5.5   Blood film from a cat with iron-deficiency anemia. Note the erythrocyte membrane abnormalities. Lack of hypochromasia is typical for feline iron-deficient erythrocytes. Blister cells (small arrows) and keratocytes (large arrows) also are present. **Inset.** Blood film from an iron-deficient dog. Note the blister cell (small arrow) and hypochromic erythrocyte (arrowhead). Wright stain.

Figure 5.6   Blood film from an anemic dog with a ruptured hemangiosarcoma of the spleen. **Left.** Numerous acanthocytes are present (arrows). Note the large polychromatophilic cells in the same field, indicating that the anemia is regenerative. **Right.** Acanthocytes (arrow) and schistocytes (arrowheads) are typical findings in dogs with hemangiosarcoma. Wright stain.

keratocytes probably then fragment from the erythrocytes, thereby forming schistocytes.

Acanthocytes

Acanthocytes, or spur cells, are irregular, spiculated erythrocytes with few, unevenly distributed surface projections of variable length and diameter (*Fig. 5.6*). Acanthocytes are thought to result from changes in cholesterol or phospholipid concentrations in the red-cell membrane. They commonly are seen on blood films from humans with altered lipid metabolism, such as may occur with liver disease, but they rarely are observed on blood films from dogs with liver disease. Acanthocytes, however, are generally observed on blood films from cats with hepatic lipidosis and are seen quite consistently on those from dogs with hemangiosarcoma. The pathogenesis of this shape change in dogs with hemangiosarcoma is not known, but the presence of acanthocytes in middle-aged to old large-breed dogs with a concurrent regenerative anemia is very suggestive of hemangiosarcoma.

Echinocytes

Echinocytes (i.e., burr cells) are spiculated cells with numerous short, evenly spaced, blunt to sharp surface projections that are quite uniform in size and shape (*Fig. 5.7*). Echinocyte formation can be an artifactual result (i.e., crenation) of a change in pH from slow drying of blood

films, but it also has been associated with renal disease, lymphoma, rattlesnake envenomation, and chemotherapy in dogs and after exercise in horses. The echinocytes seen with rattlesnake envenomation are termed *type 3 echinocytes*, and they are quite characteristic, with numerous very fine spicules on all erythrocytes, except those that are polychromatophilic (*Fig. 5.8*). In some instances of rattlesnake envenomation, spheroechinocytes are formed. These erythrocytes appear to be spherocytes with fine

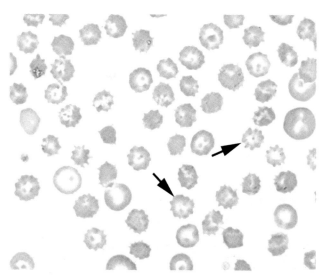

Figure 5.7   Blood film from a dog with lymphoma. Numerous echinocytes are present (arrows). Wright stain.

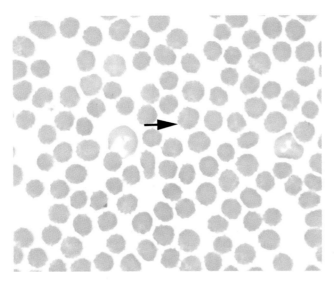

Figure 5.8   Blood film from a dog that was bitten by a rattlesnake approximately 24 hours previously. Almost all the erythrocytes are echinospherocytes (arrow). Note that the polychromatophilic erythrocytes are not affected. Wright stain.

spicules, usually present from 24 to 48 hours after envenomation, and are a reliable indication that envenomation has occurred.

Spherocytes

Spherocytes are darkly staining erythrocytes that lack central pallor (*Fig. 5.9*). They appear to be small, but their volume is normal. Spherocytes are not easily detected in species other than dogs because of the small size and lack of central pallor in the normal erythrocytes of most other domestic animals. Spherocytes have a reduced amount of membrane as a result of partial phagocytosis, which occurs because antibody or complement is on the surface of the erythrocyte. Spherocytes are very significant, in that their presence suggests immune-mediated hemolytic anemia (see Chapter 8). They also, however, may be seen after blood transfusion with mismatched blood. Spherocyte formation has been reported in dogs with bee stings and zinc toxicosis, but zinc toxicosis also may cause Heinz-body anemia. Sometimes, a small amount of central pallor will remain in a spherocyte, and it then is termed an *incomplete spherocyte* (*Fig. 5.10*). These spherocytes likely represent a continuum of membrane removal that finally results in a complete sphere.

Eccentrocytes

Features of eccentrocytes include shifting of hemoglobin toward one side of the cell, loss of normal central pallor, and a clear zone outlined by a membrane (*Fig. 5.11*). They are associated with oxidative damage, especially in dogs, and may be found in conjunction with Heinz bodies (discussed later). Animals with an inherited erythrocyte enzyme deficiency, glucose-6-phosphate dehydrogenase deficiency, may show increased susceptibility to oxidant-induced erythrocyte injury, resulting in eccentrocyte formation or increased incidence of Heinz bodies.

Leptocytes and Codocytes

Leptocytes are erythrocytes that have undergone a surface-to-volume ratio change in which there is excess membrane

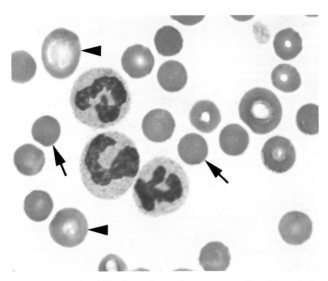

Figure 5.9   Blood film from dog with immune-mediated hemolytic anemia. Note the numerous spherocytes (arrows). The anemia is regenerative, as indicated by the polychromatophilic erythrocytes (arrowheads). Wright stain.

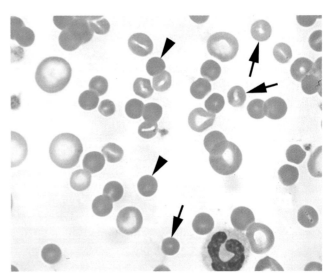

Figure 5.10   Blood film from a dog with immune-mediated hemolytic anemia. Many of the erythrocytes are spherocytes (arrowheads), and several incomplete spheres are present (arrows). Wright stain.

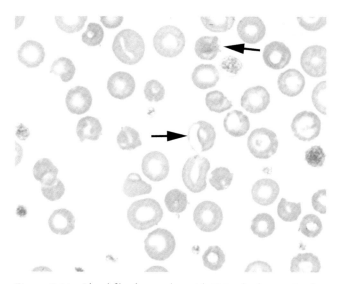

Figure 5.11 Blood film from a dog with Heinz-body anemia after ingestion of onions. Eccentrocytes are present (arrows). Wright stain.

relative to the internal contents, resulting in membrane folding and target-cell formation (*Fig. 5.12*). They have little diagnostic significance, however, and may form in vitro secondary to contact with excess ethylenediamine-tetraacetic acid (EDTA) as a result of improperly filling the blood-collection tubes. Target cells also are referred to as codocytes and are thin, bowl-shaped erythrocytes with a dense, central area of hemoglobin that is separated from the peripheral hemoglobinized region by a pale zone. Target cells may be seen in dogs with increased serum cholesterol concentration, but they also are seen in a variety of other conditions and have little significance.

Stomatocytes

Stomatocytes are uniconcave erythrocytes with a mouth-like, clear area near the cell center (*Fig. 5.13*). A few stomatocytes on the blood film usually are insignificant. Hereditary stomatocytosis has been reported in several dog breeds, including Alaskan malamutes, miniature schnauzers, and the Drentse partrijshond. All the disorders are inherited in an autosomal-recessive manner, but stomatocyte formation is caused by different defects in different breeds, involving either cell membranes or regulation of cell volume. Alaskan malamutes with hereditary stomatocytosis also have chondrodysplasia, and only a small percentage of the erythrocytes are stomatocytes. These stomatocytes are thought to form secondary to a membrane defect that allows increased sodium and water content of erythrocytes. Drentse partrijshond dogs with stomatocytosis also have hypertrophic gastritis, retarded growth, diarrhea, renal cysts, and polyneuropathy, and in this breed, the erythrocyte defect is thought to result from an abnormal concentration of phospholipids in the erythrocyte membrane. Miniature schnauzers with stomatocytosis are asymptomatic; the cause of the erythrocyte defect in this breed has not been described.

STRUCTURES IN OR ON ERYTHROCYTES

Heinz bodies

Oxidative denaturation of hemoglobin results in Heinz-body formation. Approximately 1% to 2% of erythrocytes from normal cats contain Heinz bodies, presumably

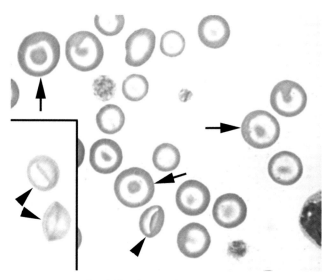

Figure 5.12 Blood film from a dog with numerous leptocytes. Note the numerous target cells (arrows) and folded cells (arrowheads). Wright stain.

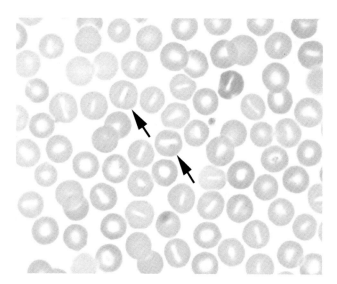

Figure 5.13 Blood film from a miniature schnauzer mix breed dog with hereditary spherocytosis. Note the numerous slit or mouth-shaped clear areas in the stomatocytes (arrows). Wright stain.

because of an unusual propensity for hemoglobin denaturation due to feline hemoglobin molecules containing twice the number of reactive sulfhydryl groups as are in hemoglobin molecules of other species. Heinz bodies appear as small, eccentric, pale structures within the red cell, and they commonly seem to protrude slightly from the red-cell margin on Wright-stained blood films (*Fig. 5.14*). Heinz bodies usually are 0.5 to 1.0 μm in diameter but may be larger. They usually occur as single, large structures in feline erythrocytes, but in canine erythrocytes, they more commonly are small and multiple. Heinz bodies are difficult to see on Wright-stained blood films, particularly with canine erythrocytes, in which eccentrocyte formation may be more apparent. When stained with vital stains (e.g., new methylene blue or brilliant cresyl blue), Heinz bodies appear as blue structures (Fig. 5.14). The presence of Heinz bodies reduces the deformability of the cell, making it more susceptible to both intravascular and extravascular hemolysis. If large numbers of erythrocytes are affected, severe hemolytic anemia may result. Oxidative drugs and compounds known to induce Heinz-body formation include onions, garlic, *Brassica* species of plants, wilted or dried leaves from red maple (*Acer rubrum*), benzocaine, zinc, copper, acetaminophen, propofol, phenazopyridine, phenothiazine, phenylhydrazine, naphthalene, vitamin K, methylene blue, and propylene glycol. Ill cats may develop a high concentration of Heinz bodies without being exposed to oxidant chemicals or drugs. The most common disorders associated with an increased concentration of Heinz bodies in cats are diabetes mellitus, lymphoma, and hyperthyroidism, but in-

creased concentrations also may be seen in association with a wide variety of other diseases (see Chapter 8).

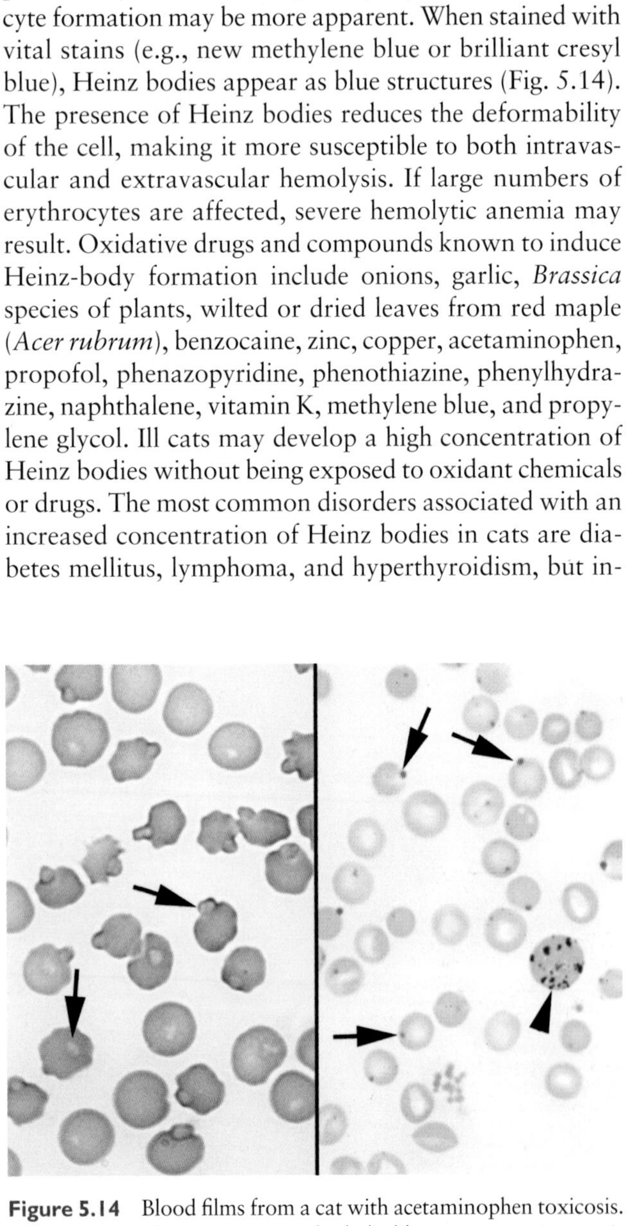

Basophilic Stippling

In vivo aggregation of ribosomes into small basophilic granules is termed *basophilic stippling* (*Fig. 5.15*). Normally, basophilic stippling is associated with immature erythrocytes in ruminants, and it may be seen to a lesser extent in cats and dogs with intensely regenerative anemia. Basophilic stippling not associated with severe anemia is suggestive of lead poisoning, but not all animals with lead poisoning have basophilic stippling. The enzyme pyrimidine 5′-nucleotidase, which is present in reticulocytes, normally catabolizes ribosomes; the activity of this enzyme is reduced in lead toxicosis and normally is low in ruminants.

Nucleated Erythrocytes

Increased numbers of erythrocytes in which the nucleus remains (Fig. 5.15) are associated with regenerative anemias and early release of these cells in response to hypoxia. Increased concentrations of nucleated erythrocytes also may be seen in animals with a nonfunctioning spleen and with increased levels of endogenous or exogenous corticosteroids. An increase in nucleated erythrocytes out

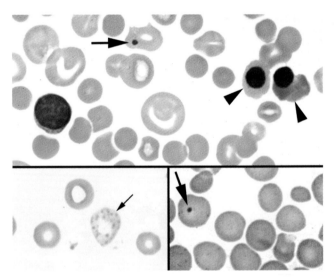

Figure 5.15 Top. Blood film from dog with immune-mediated hemolytic anemia. The anemia is very regenerative, and polychromatophilic erythrocytes, nucleated erythrocytes (arrowheads), and a Howell-Jolly body (arrow) are present. Note that the nucleated erythrocytes (metarubricytes) have variably colored cytoplasm. The one on the left has mature cytoplasm, whereas the one on the right has polychromatophilic cytoplasm. **Lower Right.** A nuclear remnant, or Howell-Jolly body, is indicated by the arrow. **Lower Left.** Basophilic stippling (small arrow) in a blood film from a dog with lead poisoning. Wright stain.

Figure 5.14 Blood films from a cat with acetaminophen toxicosis. **Left.** Heinz bodies appear as pale, light-blue structures (arrows). Wright stain. **Right.** Heinz bodies appear as blue structures (arrows). Note the reticulocyte (arrowhead). Brilliant cresyl blue stain.

of proportion to the degree of anemia frequently is associated with lead poisoning, but not all animals with lead poisoning have increased nucleated erythrocytes. In cats, the presence of nucleated erythrocytes in the absence of significant polychromasia is usually an indication of myelodysplasia or myeloproliferative disease.

Howell-Jolly Bodies

Nuclear remnants in erythrocytes are termed *Howell-Jolly bodies*. An increased concentration of Howell-Jolly bodies is associated with regenerative anemia, splenectomy, and suppressed splenic function. These bodies are small, round, dark-blue inclusions of variable size (Fig. 5.15).

Siderotic Granules

Siderotic granules are stainable iron granules within mitochondria and lysosomes. These siderotic inclusions are also referred to as Pappenheimer bodies, and their presence is thought to be associated with impaired heme synthesis. Erythrocytes containing these inclusions are termed *siderocytes* (*Fig. 5.16*). Siderocytes in domestic animals are rare, but they have been associated with chloramphenicol therapy, myelodysplasia, and ineffective erythropoiesis of unknown cause.

Parasites

Erythrocyte parasites are discussed in more detail in Chapter 8. Spherocyte formation and agglutination may be observed on blood films from animals with erythrocyte parasites, because the organisms induce an immune-mediated anemia.

The primary parasitic disease of feline erythrocytes is infection with *Hemobartonella felis* (Fig. 5.17), which is a mycoplasmal organism that is the causative agent of feline infectious anemia. These organisms are attached to the external erythrocyte membrane and appear as rod-shaped organisms on the periphery of the erythrocyte or as a delicate, basophilic ring on the cell. A less common erythrocyte parasite in cats is the protozoan *Cytauxzoon felis*, which appears as a ring (diameter, 0.5–1.5 μm) and contains a small, basophilic nucleus (*Fig. 5.18*).

In dogs, erythrocyte parasites are rare. *Hemobartonella canis* usually only occurs in dogs that have been splenectomized or that have nonfunctional spleens. The organisms appear as small dots that chain across the surface of the erythrocyte (*Fig. 5.19*). *Babesia canis* and *B. gibsoni* are protozoal red-cell parasites in the dog that produce severe hemolytic anemia. Usually, *B. canis* appears as a teardrop–shaped structure (*Fig. 5.20*), but *B. gibsoni* is smaller and varies considerably in both size and shape (Fig. 5.20). Other erythrocyte parasites include *B. bigemina*, *Eperythrozoon* sp. (*Fig. 5.21*) and *Anaplasma* sp. (*Fig. 5.22*).

Viral Inclusions

Viral inclusions are rarely seen in erythrocytes from dogs with distemper. When found, however, distemper inclusions are variable in size (~1.0–2.0 μm), number, and color (faint blue to magenta) and are more frequently seen in polychromatophilic erythrocytes (*Fig. 5.23*).

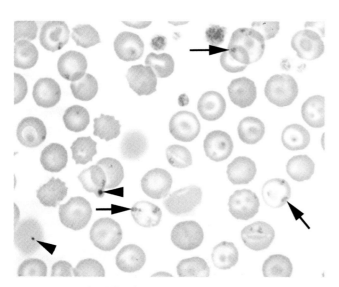

Figure 5.16 Blood film from a dog. Numerous erythrocytes (siderocytes) containing siderotic granules are present (arrows). Note the Howell-Jolly bodies (arrowheads). Wright stain.

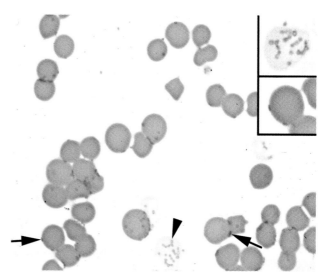

Figure 5.17 Blood film from an anemic cat. Note the numerous *Hemobartonella felis* organisms. Some of these appear as small, ring-shaped organisms on the surface of a "ghost" erythrocyte that has lysed (arrowhead). Others appear as rod-shaped structures on the edge of erythrocytes (arrows). **Insets.** Higher magnification of both the ring and the rod-shaped forms. Wright stain.

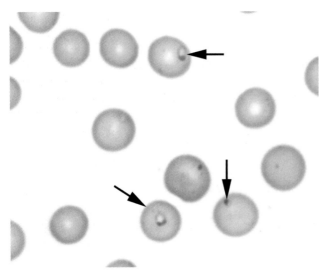

Figure 5.18   Blood film from a cat with *Cytauxzoon* organisms (arrows). Wright stain.

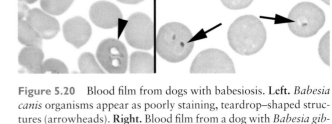

Figure 5.20   Blood film from dogs with babesiosis. **Left.** *Babesia canis* organisms appear as poorly staining, teardrop–shaped structures (arrowheads). **Right.** Blood film from a dog with *Babesia gibsoni* (arrows). Wright stain.

ERYTHROCYTE ARRANGEMENT ON BLOOD FILMS

Rouleaux Formation

Rouleaux formation is the spontaneous association of erythrocytes in linear stacks, and its appearance is similar to a stack of coins (*Fig. 5.24*). Marked rouleaux formation is normal in horses, and a slight amount also is normal in dogs and cats. Rouleaux formation is enhanced, however, when the concentration of plasma proteins such as fibrinogen or immunoglobulins is increased. Increased rouleaux formation often is suggestive of a gammopathy; animals with multiple myeloma almost always have increased rouleaux formation.

Agglutination

Agglutination of erythrocytes results in irregular, spheric clumps of cells because of antibody-related bridging (*Fig. 5.25*). Agglutination is very suggestive of immune-mediated hemolytic anemia, but it also may be seen after

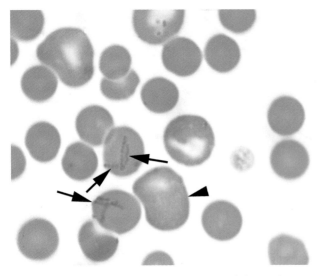

Figure 5.19   Blood film from a splenectomized dog with *Hemobartonella canis*. Note the dot-like organisms that chain across the surface of the erythrocyte (arrows). The anemia is regenerative, as indicated by the polychromatophilic cell (arrowhead). Wright stain.

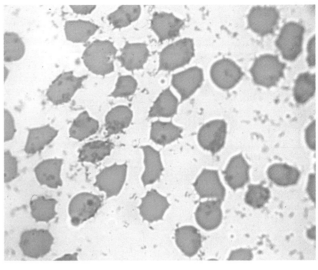

Figure 5.21   Blood film from a cow with *Eperythrozoon wenyoni*. Note the many free organisms in the plasma. Wright stain.

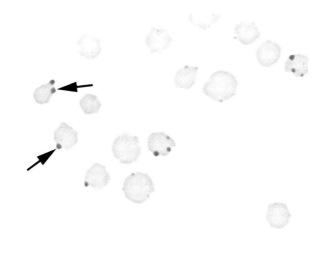

Figure 5.22 Blood film from an anemic cow with anaplasmosis. Note the numerous *Anaplasma marginale* organisms on the periphery of the erythrocytes (arrows). Wright stain.

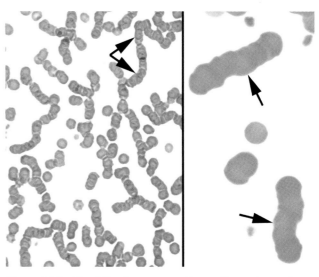

Figure 5.24 Blood film from a normal horse, illustrating rouleaux formation (arrows). Wright stain.

a mismatched blood transfusion. To confirm that agglutination is present, mix a small quantity of blood with a drop of isotonic saline. Agglutination will persist in the presence of saline (*Fig. 5.26*), whereas rouleaux formation will disperse. Agglutination may be so marked that it can be seen grossly on blood films and on the side of EDTA tubes (Fig. 5.26). Agglutination may result in a falsely increased MCV and a falsely decreased red-blood-cell count, because agglutinated red cells (i.e., doublets and triplets) may be counted as large cells (see Chapter 1).

ERYTHROID DYSPLASIA AND NEOPLASIA IN PERIPHERAL BLOOD

Dysplasia and leukemia of red blood cells is covered in more detail in Chapter 13. Briefly, erythroid dysplasia, which is commonly seen in cats associated with FeLV, is characterized by a nonregenerative anemia in conjunction with macrocytosis and megaloblastic erythroid precursors, in which there is advanced cell hemoglobinization with incomplete nuclear maturation. Red-cell leukemia

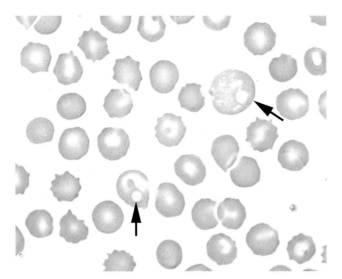

Figure 5.23 Blood film from a dog with distemper. Note the pale-blue viral inclusions of distemper with the erythrocytes (arrows). These inclusions may stain pale blue to dark magenta in color. Wright stain.

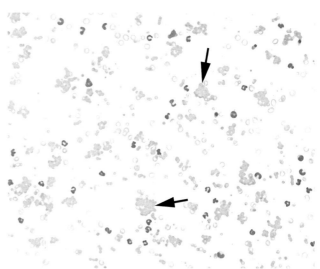

Figure 5.25 Blood film from an anemic dog with immune-mediated hemolytic anemia and marked agglutination. Note the large aggregates of spherocytes (arrows). Wright stain, low magnification.

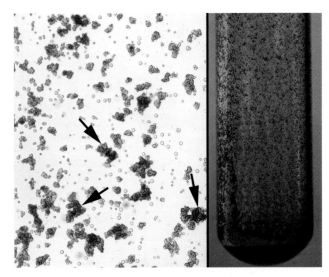

Figure 5.26   Blood from a dog with immune-mediated hemolytic anemia. **Left.** Blood has been mixed with isotonic saline, and agglutination persists (arrows). **Right.** Agglutination is so severe that it can be visualized grossly on the side of the EDTA blood-collection tube.

(i.e., erythremic myelosis, M6) is relatively rare in dogs, but in cats, it usually is associated with FeLV. In these patients, an increased concentration of quite immature nucleated erythrocytes typically is present in the face of a severe, nonregenerative anemia (see Chapter 13).

SUGGESTED READINGS

Erythrocyte Size
Bunch SE, Easley JR, Cullen JM. Hematologic values and plasma and tissue concentrations in dogs given phenytoin on a long-term basis. Am J Vet Res 1990;51:1865–1868.

Bunch SE, Jordan HL, Sellon RK, et al. Characterization of iron status in young dogs with portosystemic shunt. Am J Vet Res 1995;56:853–858.

Degen M. Pseudohyperkalemia in Akitas. J Am Vet Med Assoc 1987;190:541–543.

Gookin JL, Bunch SE, Rush LJ, et al. Evaluation of microcytosis in 18 Shiba Inus. J Am Vet Med Assoc 1998;212:1258–1259.

Fulton R, Weiser MG, Freshman JL, et al. Electronic and morphologic characterization of erythrocytes of an adult cat with iron deficiency anemia. Vet Pathol 1988;25:521–523.

Fyfe JC, Jezyk PK, Giger U, et al. Inherited selective malabsorption of Vitamin B_{12} in giant schnauzers. J Am Anim Hosp Assoc 1989;25:533–539.

Harvey JW, Asquith RL, Sussman WA, et al. Serum ferritin, serum iron, and erythrocyte values in foals. Am J Vet Res 1987;48:1348–1352.

Laflamme DP, Mahaffey EA, Allen SW, et al. Microcytosis and iron status in dogs with surgically induced portosystemic shunts. J Vet Intern Med 1994;8:212–216.

Meyer DJ, Harvey JW. Hematologic changes associated with serum and hepatic iron alterations in dogs with congenital portosystemic vascular anomalies. J Vet Intern Med 1994;8:55–56.

Schalm OJ. Erythrocyte macrocytosis in miniature poodles. California Vet 1976;3:55–57.

Simpson KW, Meyer DJ, Boswood A, et al. Iron status and erythrocyte volume in dogs with congenital portosystemic vascular anomalies. J Vet Intern Med 1997;11:14–19.

Weiser MG, Kociba GJ. Erythrocyte macrocytosis in feline leukemia virus associated anemia. Vet Pathol 1983;20:687–697.

Weiser MG, Kociba GJ. Sequential changes in erythrocyte volume distribution and microcytosis associated with iron deficiency in kittens. Vet Pathol 1983;20:1–12.

Weiser G, O'Grady M. Erythrocyte volume distribution analysis and hematologic changes in dogs with iron deficiency anemia. Vet Pathol 1983;20:230–241.

Inherited Erythrocyte Shape Abnormalities
Stomatocytes
Brown DE, Weiser MG, Thrall MA, et al. Erythrocyte indices and volume distribution in a dog with stomatocytosis. Vet Pathol 1994;31:247–250.

Fletch SM, Pinkerton PH, Brueckner PJ. The Alaskan malamute chondrodysplasia (dwarfism-anemia) syndrome—in review. J Am Anim Hosp Assoc 1975;11:353–361.

Pinkerton PH, Fletch SM, Brueckner PJ, et al. Hereditary stomatocytosis with hemolytic anemia in the dog. Blood 1974;44:557–567.

Slappendel RJ, Renooij W, de Bruijne JJ. Normal cations and abnormal membrane lipids in the red blood cells of dogs with familial stomatocytosis-hypertrophic gastritis. Blood 1994;84:904–909.

Slappendel RJ, van der Gaag I, van Nes JJ, et al. Familial stomatocytosis—hypertrophic gastritis (FSHG), a newly recognized disease in the dog (Drentse partrijshond). Vet Q 1991;13:30–40.

Elliptocytes
Conboy JG, Shitamoto R, Parra M, et al. Hereditary elliptocytosis due to both qualitative and quantitative defects in membrane skeletal protein 4.1. Blood 1991;78:2438–2443.

Mills JN, Marsden CA. Presumed hereditary elliptocytosis in a dog. Aust Vet J 1999;77:651–652.

Smith JE, Moore K, Arens M, et al. Hereditary elliptocytosis with protein band 4.1 deficiency in the dog. Blood 1983;61:373–377.

Eccentrocytes
Stockham SL, Harvey JW, Kinden DA. Equine glucose-6-phosphate dehydrogenase deficiency. Vet Pathol 1994;31:518–527.

Acquired Erythrocyte Shape Abnormalities
Spiculated Red Blood Cells (General)
Rebar AH, Lewis HB, DeNicola DB, et al. Red cell fragmentation in the dog: an editorial review. Vet Pathol 1981;18:415–426.

Weiss DJ, Kristensen A, Papenfuss N. Quantitative evaluation of irregularly spiculated red blood cells in the dog. Vet Clin Pathol 1993;22:117–121.

Acanthocytes
Biemer JJ. Acanthocytosis—biochemical and physiological considerations. Ann Clin Lab Sci 1980;10:238–249.

Christopher MM, Lee SE. Red cell morphologic alterations in cats with hepatic disease. Vet Clin Pathol 1994;23:7–12.

Gelberg H, Stackhouse LL. Three cases of canine acanthocytosis associated with splenic neoplasia. Vet Med Small Anim Clin 1977;72:1183–1184.

Hirsch VM, Jacobsen J, Mills JH. A retrospective study of canine hemangiosarcoma and its association with acanthocytosis. Can Vet J 1981;22:152–155.

Ng CY, Mills JN. Clinical and haematological features of haemangiosarcoma in dogs. Aust Vet J 1985;62:1–4.

Rebar AH, Hahn FF, Halliwell WH, et al. Microangiopathic hemolytic anemia associated with radiation-induced hemangiosarcomas. Vet Pathol 1980;17:443–454.

Schistocytes

Hammer AS, Couto CG, Swardson C, et al. Hemostatic abnormalities in dogs with hemangiosarcoma. J Vet Intern Med 1991;5:11–14.

Heyes H, Kohle W, Slijepcevic B. The appearance of schistocytes in the peripheral blood in correlation to the degree of disseminated intravascular coagulation. An experimental study in rats. Haemostasis 1976;5:66–73.

Rebar AH, Hahn FF, Halliwell WH, et al. Microangiopathic hemolytic anemia associated with radiation-induced hemangiosarcomas. Vet Pathol 1980;17:443–454.

Echinocytes

Brown DE, Meyer DJ, Wingfield WE, et al. Echinocytosis associated with rattlesnake envenomation in dogs. Vet Pathol 1994;31:654–657.

Geor RJ, Lund EM, Weiss DJ. Echinocytosis in horses: 54 cases (1990). J Am Vet Med Assoc 1993;202:976–980.

Walton RM, Brown DE, Hamar DW, et al. Mechanisms of echinocytosis induced by *Crotalus atrox* venom. Vet Pathol 1997;34:442–449.

Weiss DJ, Geor RJ, Smith CM II. Effects of echinocytosis on hemorrheologic values and exercise performance in horses. Am J Vet Res 1994;55:204–210.

Weiss DJ, Geor R, Smith CM II, et al. Furosemide-induced electrolyte depletion associated with echinocytosis in horses. Am J Vet Res 1992;53:1769–1772.

Weiss DJ, Kristensen A, Papenfuss N, et al. Quantitative evaluation of echinocytes in the dog. Vet Clin Pathol 1990;19:114–118.

Wong P. A basis of echinocytosis and stomatocytosis in the disc-sphere transformations of the erythrocyte. J Theor Biol 1999;196:343–361.

Spherocytes

Breitschwerdt EB, Armstrong PJ, Robinette CL, et al. Three cases of acute zinc toxicosis in dogs. Vet Hum Toxicol 1986;28:109–117.

Inaba M, Yawata A, Koshino I, et al. Defective anion transport and marked spherocytosis with membrane instability caused by hereditary total deficiency of red cell band 3 in cattle due to a nonsense mutation. J Clin Invest 1996;97:1804–1807.

Klag AR, Giger U, Shofer FS. Idiopathic immune-mediated hemolytic anemia in dogs: 42 cases (1986–1990). J Am Vet Med Assoc 1993;202:783–788.

Latimer KS, Jain A, Inglesby HB, et al. Zinc-induced hemolytic anemia caused by ingestion of pennies by a pup. J Am Vet Med Assoc 1989;195:77–80.

Messer NT IV, Arnold K. Immune-mediated hemolytic anemia in a horse. J Am Vet Med Assoc 1991;198:1415–1416.

Mills JN, Day MJ, Shaw SE, et al. Autoimmune haemolytic anaemia in dogs. Aust Vet J 1985;62:121–123.

Noble SJ, Armstrong PJ. Bee sting envenomation resulting in secondary immune-mediated hemolytic anemia in two dogs. J Am Vet Med Assoc 1999;214:1026–1027.

Swenson C, Jacobs R. Spherocytosis associated with anaplasmosis in two cows. J Am Vet Med Assoc 1986;188:1061–1063.

Weiser MG, Thrall MA. Immune-mediated hemolytic anemia in dogs (letter). J Am Vet Med Assoc 1993;202:1786–1788.

Wysoke JM, Bland van-den Berg P, Marshall C. Bee sting-induced haemolysis, spherocytosis and neural dysfunction in three dogs. J S Afr Vet Assoc 1990;61:29–32.

Eccentrocytes

Ham TH, Grauel JA, Dunn RF, et al. Physical properties of red cells as related to effects in vivo. IV. Oxidant drugs producing abnormal intracellular concentration of hemoglobin (eccentrocytes) with a rigid-red-cell hemolytic syndrome. J Lab Clin Med 1973;82:898–910.

Lee K-W, Yamato O, Tajima M, et al. Hematologic changes associated with the appearance of eccentrocytes after intragastric administration of garlic extract to dogs. Am J Vet Res 2000;61:1446–1450.

Reagan WJ, Carter C, Turek J. Eccentrocytosis in equine red maple leaf toxicosis. Vet Clin Pathol 1994;23:123–127.

Ward PC, Schwartz BS, White JG. Heinz-body anemia: "bite cell" variant—a light and electron microscopic study. Am J Hematol 1983;15:135–146.

Erythrocyte Inclusions

Heinz Bodies

Christopher MM. Relation of endogenous Heinz bodies to disease and anemia in cats: 120 cases (1978–1987). J Am Vet Med Assoc 1989;194:1089–1095.

Christopher MM, Broussard JD, Peterson ME. Heinz body formation associated with ketoacidosis in diabetic cats. J Vet Intern Med 1995;9:24–31.

Christopher MM, Perman V, Eaton JW. Contribution of propylene glycol-induced Heinz body formation to anemia in cats. J Am Vet Med Assoc 1989;194:1045–1056.

Christopher MM, White JG, Eaton JW. Erythrocyte pathology and mechanisms of Heinz body–mediated hemolysis in cats. Vet Pathol 1990;27:299–310.

George LW, Divers TJ, Mahaffey EA, et al. Heinz body anemia and methemoglobinemia in ponies given red maple (*Acer rubrum* L.) leaves. Vet Pathol 1982;19:521–533.

Harvey JW, Rackear D. Experimental onion-induced hemolytic anemia in dogs. Vet Pathol 1985;22:387–392.

Hickman MA, Rogers QR, Morris JG. Effect of diet on Heinz body formation in kittens. Am J Vet Res 1990;51:475–478.

Houston DM, Myers SL. A review of Heinz-body anemia in the dog induced by toxins. Vet Hum Toxicol 1993;35:158–161.

Lincoln SD, Howell ME, Combs JJ, et al. Hematologic effects and feeding performance in cattle fed cull domestic onions (*Allium cepa*). J Am Vet Med Assoc 1992;200:1090–1094.

Luttgen PJ, Whitney MS, Wolf AM, et al. Heinz body hemolytic anemia associated with high plasma zinc concentration in a dog. J Am Vet Med Assoc 1990;197:1347–1350.

Robertson JE, Christopher MM, Rogers QR. Heinz body formation in cats fed baby food containing onion powder. J Am Vet Med Assoc 1998;212:1260–1266.

Soli NE, Froslie A. Chronic copper poisoning in sheep. I. The relationship of methaemoglobinemia to Heinz body formation and haemolysis during the terminal crisis. Acta Pharm Toxicol 1977;40:169–177.

Tennant B, Dill SG, Glickman LT, et al. Acute hemolytic anemia, methemoglobinemia, and Heinz body formation associated with ingestion of red maple leaves by horses. J Am Vet Med Assoc 1981;179:143–150.

Weiss DJ, McClay CB, Christopher MM, et al. Effects of propylene glycol-containing diets on acetaminophen-induced methemoglobinemia in cats. J Am Vet Med Assoc 1990;196:1816–1819.

Torrance AG, Fulton RB Jr. Zinc-induced hemolytic anemia in a dog. J Am Vet Med Assoc 1987;191:443–444.

Basophilic Stippling, Nucleated Red Blood Cells, and Howell-Jolly Bodies

Burrows GE, Borchard RE. Experimental lead toxicosis in ponies: comparison of the effects of smelter effluent-contaminated hay and lead acetate. Am J Vet Res 1982;43:2129–2133.

George JW. Duncan JR. Pyrimidine-specific 5′-nucleotidase activity in bovine erythrocytes: effect of phlebotomy and lead poisoning. Am J Vet Res 1982;43:17–20.

Johnson KA, Powers BE, Withrow SJ, et al. Splenomegaly in dogs. Predictors of neoplasia and survival after splenectomy. J Vet Int Med 1989;3:160–166.

Knecht CD, Crabtree J, Katherman A. Clinical, clinicopathologic, and electroencephalographic features of lead poisoning in dogs. J Am Vet Med Assoc 1979;175:196–201.

Velcek FT, Kugaczewski JT, Jongco B, et al. Function of the replanted spleen in dogs. J Trauma Injury Crit Care1982;22:502–506.

Zook BC, McConnell G, Gilmore CE. Basophilic stippling of erythrocytes in dogs with special reference to lead poisoning. J Am Vet Med Assoc 1970;157:2092–2099.

Siderocytes

Canfield PJ, Watson ADJ, Ratcliffe RCC. Dyserythropoiesis, sideroblasts/siderocytes and hemoglobin crystallization in a dog. Vet Clin Pathol 1987;16:21–27.

Harvey JW, Wolfsheimer KJ, Simpson CF, et al. Pathologic sideroblasts and siderocytes associated with chloramphenicol therapy in a dog. Vet Clin Pathol 1985;14:36–42.

Weiss DJ, Lulich J. Myelodysplastic syndrome with sideroblastic differentiation in a dog. Vet Clin Pathol 1999;28:59–63.

Erythrocyte Arrangement

Agglutination

Porter RE, Weiser MG. Effect of immune-mediated erythrocyte agglutination on analysis of canine blood using a multichannel blood cell counting system. Vet Clin Pathol 1990;19:45–50.

Rouleaux

Allen BV. Relationships between the erythrocyte sedimentation rate, plasma proteins and viscosity, and leukocyte counts in thoroughbred racehorses. Vet Rec 1988;122:329–332.

Baumler H, Neu B, Donath E, et al. Basic phenomena of red blood cell rouleaux formation. Biorheology 1999;36:439–442.

Talstad I, Scheie P, Dalen H, et al. Influence of plasma proteins on erythrocyte morphology and sedimentation. Scand J Haematol 1983;31:478–484.

6

CLASSIFICATION OF AND DIAGNOSTIC APPROACH TO ANEMIA

Anemia is a decrease in the red blood cell (RBC) mass that results in decreased oxygenation of tissues. The RBC mass is determined by measuring the packed cell volume (PCV; i.e., hematocrit), the amount of hemoglobin in the blood, and the erythrocyte count (see Chapter 1). Of these three, PCV is used most commonly as the primary value for interpretation in North America.

Anemia is a manifestation of an underlying disease that has produced increased erythrocyte destruction, increased erythrocyte loss through hemorrhage, decreased production of erythrocytes, or some combination of these events. Clinical signs usually relate to decreased oxygenation or associated compensatory mechanisms and may include pale mucous membranes, lethargy, reduced exercise tolerance, increased respiratory rate or dyspnea, increased heart rate, and murmurs caused by increased blood turbulence. Nonspecific clinical signs, such as weight loss, anorexia, fever, or lymphadenopathy, may be present if the animal has an underlying systemic illness. Specific clinical signs that are associated with blood destruction may include splenomegaly, icterus, and darkly pigmented urine resulting from hemoglobinuria or bilirubinuria.

The severity of clinical signs usually relates to the duration of onset, because animals with a slow onset, resulting from chronic blood loss or bone marrow dysfunction, usually compensate to some extent for the hypoxemia. Compensatory mechanisms include increased concentration of erythrocyte 2,3-diphosphoglycerate, which decreases the oxygen–hemoglobin affinity and, thus, enhances the delivery of oxygen to tissues, increases cardiac output, and aids in the redistribution of blood flow to vital organs. Death may occur in animals that experience severe acute blood loss or blood destruction. Appropriate therapy and prognosis is facilitated by determining whether the anemia is a result of erythrocyte destruction, blood loss, or lack of erythrocyte production, followed by establishing the diagnosis of the underlying disease. This chapter addresses the classification of and diagnostic approach to anemia.

CLASSIFICATION OF ANEMIA

Three general schemes are used to classify anemia: erythrocyte size and hemoglobin concentration, bone marrow response, and classification by pathophysiologic mechanism. The classification by erythrocyte size and bone marrow response are the most useful for clinical purposes, because they are tools that allow veterinarians to follow a mental pathway to a differential diagnosis. The pathophysiologic classification merely provides a conceptual framework for a diagnostic library of disorders that cause anemia.

Erythrocyte Size and Hemoglobin Concentration

Traditionally, anemia has been classified by erythrocyte volume (i.e., mean cell volume [MCV]) and the amount of hemoglobin within erythrocytes (i.e., mean corpuscular hemoglobin concentration [MCHC]). An anemia is referred to as being microcytic when the erythrocytes are small, normocytic when they are of normal volume, and macrocytic when they are larger than the reference interval. Moreover, anemia is referred to as being hypochromic when the cells contain a less-than-normal hemoglobin concentration and as normochromic when they contain a normal hemoglobin concentration. Hyperchromic anemias do not occur, but the MCHC is falsely increased when the hemoglobin determination is falsely increased because of intravascular hemolysis, lipemia, or the presence of Heinz bodies. The MCHC is also falsely increased if the erythrocyte size falls below the threshold of RBC detection in the hematology analyzer. This will effectively reduce the PCV and increase the MCHC. Although spherocytes appear to be hyperchromic on blood films because of their shape, the hemoglobin concentration is normal in these erythrocytes. The MCHC, however, may be falsely increased in patients with immune-mediated hemolytic anemia because of intravascular hemolysis or agglutination, which causes errors in measurement of the RBC mass.

This classification system is useful, particularly as it relates to cell volume, in that microcytic anemias almost always result from iron deficiency. Other causes of microcytosis include hepatic portocaval vascular shunts in dogs, and normal canine breed variations in Akitas and Shiba Inus. A macrocytic anemia usually indicates that the marrow is functional and is releasing immature cells that are larger than normal in size. Macrocytosis without polychromasia or reticulocytosis should be evaluated further, because a regenerative response likely is not the cause in these patients. The MCV is of particular value in horses, because reticulocytes are almost never released into the circulation. Other causes of macrocytosis include feline leukemia virus, myelodysplasia, poodle macrocytosis, and hereditary stomatocytosis (see Chapter 5). Animals with a normocytic anemia usually have a nonregenerative or a preregenerative anemia. (Preregenerative refers to anemia in animals with blood loss or blood destruction, but in which evidence of regeneration in the peripheral blood is not yet evident.) Animals with a regenerative anemia, however, may have an MCV within the reference interval and, thus, be classified as having a normocytic anemia. The generated histogram or computer graphic is valuable in these patients, in that the subpopulation of macrocytic cells can be observed even though the MCV is normal (discussed later).

The MCHC is less useful in the classification of anemia, in that hypochromia usually is simply associated with an increased concentration of large, immature cells (i.e., regenerative anemia). Reticulocytes are still synthesizing hemoglobin; therefore, their hemoglobin concentration is less than that of mature erythrocytes. Occasionally, animals with iron deficiency may have a hypochromic as well as a microcytic anemia, but in most iron-deficient animals, the MCHC is within the reference interval.

Historically, MCV and MCHC were derived by calculations based on the PCV, hemoglobin concentration, and erythrocyte count. The MCV was calculated by dividing the PCV by the erythrocyte (RBC) count. For example, if the patient's PCV is 42% and its RBC count is 6.0×10^6, then the PCV divided by the RBC count is 70 fL (i.e., 42/6 = 7). In terms of mathematical logic, 1 μL = 10^9 fL, and 42% of 10^9 fL is 420,000,000 fL. Therefore, the MCV = 70 fL (i.e., 420,000,000 ÷ 6,000,000). The MCHC, which is the ratio of the weight of hemoglobin to the volume of erythrocytes in grams per deciliter, can be calculated by the following equation:

$$\text{Hemoglobin} \left(\text{g/dL}\right) \div \text{PCV} \left(\text{mL/100mL}\right) \times 100$$
$$= \text{MCHC} \left(\text{g/dL}\right)$$

For example, if the hemoglobin is 14 g/dL and the PCV is 42%, then the MCHC is 33.3 g/dL.

Electronic cell counters have made calculation of the MCV obsolete, because the cell volume can be measured electronically. Thus, the MCV and RBC are used to calculate the PCV (see Chapter 1). This technology has improved the usefulness of this classification of anemia, because subpopulations of microcytic or macrocytic erythrocytes can be observed in histograms or computer graphics, even when the MCV is within the reference interval (*Fig. 6.1*). The RBC distribution width, which describes the width of the RBC size distribution, increases when subpopulations of either microcytic or macrocytic erythrocytes are present and often is increased before the MCV value falls out of the reference interval. The MCHC is still derived using the hemoglobin and PCV determinations; however, laser-detection technology using light scatter now allows for direct determination of the amount of hemoglobin within cells. Hemoglobin concentration using this type of technology is reported as corpuscular hemoglobin concentration mean (CHCM). Using this detection system, lipemia or hemolysis will not falsely increase the CHCM. Heinz bodies, however, may, because erythrocytes containing Heinz bodies are more optically dense.

Bone Marrow Response

Classification of anemia based on responsiveness of the bone marrow is very useful diagnostically. An anemia is classified as either regenerative or nonregenerative based on the number of immature erythrocytes that are circulating. Early release of immature erythrocytes is a normal marrow response to increased erythropoietin production, primarily by renal tissue, secondary to hypoxia. Increased numbers of immature erythrocytes are released into the circulation after blood loss or blood destruction, and they are indicative of a regenerative anemia. An increased concentration of immature erythrocytes usually is seen within 2 to 4 days after blood loss or destruction. A lack of circulating immature erythrocytes in the face of anemia indicates a nonregenerative anemia and should be considered as evidence of marrow dysfunction.

Immature erythrocytes observed using a Wright-stained blood film are polychromatophilic, and they have a blue-staining reticulum (i.e., reticulocyte) when new methylene blue or brilliant cresyl blue stains are used (see Chapters 1 and 5). In general, an anemia is considered to be regenerative if the reticulocyte concentration is greater than 60,000 cells/μL (see Chapter 1). Horses, however, almost never release reticulocytes into the circulation.

Pathophysiologic Classification

The pathophysiologic classification of anemia essentially is a categorization based on the underlying disorder. Nonregenerative anemia results from defective or decreased erythropoiesis (see Chapter 7). Decreased erythropoiesis usually is classified according to whether neutrophil and platelet production are also decreased (i.e., aplastic anemia) and whether RBC production is simply decreased (i.e., hypoplasia) or is completely absent (i.e., aplasia). Moreover, impaired erythrocyte production may be caused by an intrinsic (i.e., primary) marrow disorder, such as myelofibrosis, myelodysplasia, or myeloproliferative disorder, or it may be caused by an extrinsic (i.e., secondary) disorder. Secondary disorders include chronic renal disease; some endocrine disorders; inflammatory diseases; infectious agents, such as *Ehrlichia* sp., equine infectious anemia virus, and feline leukemia virus; immune-mediated destruction of erythrocyte precursors; and drug- or chemical-induced damage (see Chapter 13).

Regenerative anemia is caused by blood loss or erythrocyte destruction (see Chapter 8). Blood loss may be external or internal, and it may be acute or chronic. Causes of acute blood loss include trauma, bleeding lesions (e.g., tumors or large ulcers), and hemostatic disorders (e.g., thrombocytopenia or an inherited or acquired coagulopathy such as warfarin toxicosis or disseminated vascular coagulopathy). Common causes of chronic blood loss include bleeding lesions, particularly within the gastrointestinal tract, and gastrointestinal or external parasites. Erythrocyte destruction (i.e., hemolysis) may be either intravascular or extravascular, and it may result from intrinsic (i.e., primary) defects, such as hereditary membrane defects or enzyme deficiencies, or from extrinsic (i.e., secondary) causes, such as erythrocyte parasites or immune-mediated destruction. Intravascular hemolysis is the actual lysis of erythrocytes within the vascular system. Extravascular hemolysis occurs when abnormal erythrocytes are phagocytized by macrophages, usually within the spleen or liver. Common causes of erythrocyte destruction include immune mediated mechanisms, erythrocyte parasites, and drugs and chemicals that produce oxidative damage, resulting in Heinz body formation. Less common causes of hemolysis include hypophosphatemia, water intoxication in young ruminants, bacteria (e.g., *Leptospira* and *Clostridium* sp.), heparin overdose, and hereditary erythrocyte enzyme deficiencies and membrane defects.

DIAGNOSTIC APPROACH

When presented with an anemic patient, the ultimate goal is to establish a definitive diagnosis of the underlying disorder so that appropriate therapy can be initiated and a prognosis established. Information can be obtained from the laboratory evaluation, the patient history, and the physical examination. The most clinically useful approach to anemia is based on the classification schemes involving a combination of bone marrow response and erythrocyte size and hemoglobin concentration.

Laboratory Evaluation

The classification of an anemia based on erythrocyte size and marrow response (discussed earlier) is very important. Essential laboratory data include PCV, MCV, and reticulocyte count. Either blood loss or destruction will result in a regenerative anemia, and marrow dysfunction will result in a nonregenerative anemia. Furthermore, microcytosis usually is evidence of iron-deficiency anemia, and macrocytosis usually is evidence of regeneration. Additional information may be obtained from examination of the blood film; erythrocyte morphology may even reveal a definitive diagnosis (see Chapter 5).

Other laboratory procedures that may provide helpful information include plasma protein estimation by refractometry (see Chapter 1). Blood loss usually results not only in a loss of erythrocytes but also in a loss of other blood components, including protein. Thus, patients with blood loss may be hypoproteinemic. Other causes of hypoproteinemia, however, still must be considered (see Chapter 26). If blood is lost internally, such as within a body cavity, the protein usually is reabsorbed within hours.

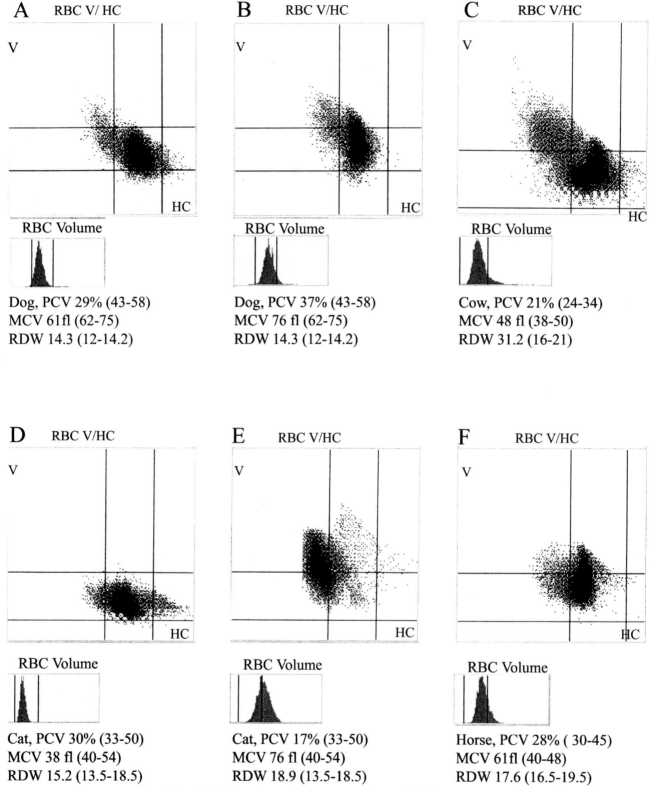

A RBC V/ HC

RBC Volume

Dog, PCV 29% (43-58)
MCV 61fl (62-75)
RDW 14.3 (12-14.2)

B RBC V/HC

RBC Volume

Dog, PCV 37% (43-58)
MCV 76 fl (62-75)
RDW 14.3 (12-14.2)

C RBC V/HC

RBC Volume

Cow, PCV 21% (24-34)
MCV 48 fl (38-50)
RDW 31.2 (16-21)

D RBC V/HC

RBC Volume

Cat, PCV 30% (33-50)
MCV 38 fl (40-54)
RDW 15.2 (13.5-18.5)

E RBC V/HC

RBC Volume

Cat, PCV 17% (33-50)
MCV 76 fl (40-54)
RDW 18.9 (13.5-18.5)

F RBC V/HC

RBC Volume

Horse, PCV 28% (30-45)
MCV 61fl (40-48)
RDW 17.6 (16.5-19.5)

Figure 6.1 Red-blood-cell volume/hemoglobin concentration (RBC V/HC) cytograms and RBC Volume histograms from six anemic animals generated by a Bayer Advia 120 (Bayer Corporation, Tarrytown, NY). On the RBC V/HC cytogram, hemoglobin (Hgb) concentration is plotted along the x (i.e., horizontal) axis, and cell volume is plotted along the y (i.e., vertical) axis. Each RBC is displayed based on volume and Hgb concentration, and normocytic normochromic cells are in the center box of each nine-box

Other components of the complete blood count (CBC) also may provide useful information. For example, if a patient is severely thrombocytopenic, anemia may be caused by blood loss secondary to impaired clot formation. On the other hand, if the leukocyte concentration, platelet concentration, and PCV are all decreased and the anemia is nonregenerative, then complete bone marrow failure is the likely cause of the anemia. An animal with a mild, nonregenerative anemia and increased immature neutrophils likely has an anemia of inflammatory disease (see Chapter 7).

Specific laboratory tests can be performed to help confirm or exclude a suspected diagnosis. If spherocytes are observed on the blood film of an anemic patient, then a Coombs' or a saline fragility test (see Chapter 1) can help

to confirm immune-mediated hemolytic anemia. In patients with microcytic anemia, serum iron should be measured to determine if the microcytosis is caused by iron deficiency. In addition, the feces should be examined for blood, because chronic blood loss from the gastrointestinal tract is a common cause of iron-deficiency anemia (see Chapter 8). Anemic dogs, particularly those with a concurrent thrombocytopenia and hyperglobulinemia, should be tested for ehrlichiosis, and anemic cats should be tested for feline leukemia virus and feline immunodeficiency virus. Anemic horses should be tested for equine infectious anemia.

The biochemical profile also may provide essential information. Patients with mild to moderate, nonregenerative anemia may have disorders that are extrinsic to the

Figure 6.1 (continued) cytogram. Larger cells are displayed toward the top of the cytogram and hypochromic cells toward the left; thus, macrocytic hypochromic cells are displayed to the upper left of the cluster of normal erythrocytes. The RBC Volume histogram represents the distribution of the RBCs by cell volume; normal samples have a bell-shaped curve. The mean corpuscular volume (MCV) and RBC distribution width (RDW) are determined from this histogram. The MCV is the mean of the RBC Volume histogram, and the RDW is the coefficient of variation of the population. Each animal's species, packed cell volume (PCV), MCV, and RDW are provided beneath the RBC V/HC cytogram and RBC Volume histogram. Reference ranges are in parentheses. A. A 12-year-old, mixed-breed dog with a mild anemia, mildly decreased MCV, and mildly increased RDW. The RBC V/HC cytogram shows that many of the erythrocytes are toward the bottom of the middle square, indicating they are microcytic. In addition, a population of hypochromic cells is present, some of which are normocytic and some of which are macrocytic. The RBC Volume histogram is shifted toward the left, also indicating that many of the erythrocytes are slightly small. Iron-deficiency anemia was suspected in this patient and was confirmed by decreased serum iron concentration. The dog had a 3-month history of epistaxis associated with a nasal passage chondrosarcoma. B. A 12-year-old, miniature schnauzer with a very mild anemia, mildly increased MCV, and mildly increased RDW. The RBC V/HC cytogram shows a population of cells above the middle square that represents large cells. A population of macrocytic hypochromic cells is present as well. The RBC Volume histogram is shifted slightly toward the right, and a population of macrocytic cells is evident. This is indicative of a regenerative anemia. C. A 1-week-old anemic calf. Note the population of macrocytic hypochromic cells, even though the MCV is within the reference interval. The RDW is markedly increased. The reticulocyte count is 90,000 cells/μL (2%). The presence of macrocytic cells and reticulocytes indicates that the anemia is regenerative. The calf's umbilical stump had been bleeding since birth, and it also had blood in the feces for 3 days. The PCV on the previous day was 9%, and the calf received a blood transfusion at that time. Many of the normocytic cells probably are donor erythrocytes. The calf responded well to supportive therapy and 1 week later, the PCV was 27%. D. A 13-year-old cat with a mildly decreased MCV. The RBC V/HC cytogram and RBC Volume histogram are similar to those of the dog in *panel A*, suggesting iron-deficiency anemia. The cat had blood in the feces, as a result of intestinal (primarily colonic) lymphoma, for several weeks before this CBC was performed. The reticulocyte count is 108,000 cells/μL, indicating that the anemia is regenerative, but the immature erythrocytes are also small because of iron deficiency. E. A 6-year-old cat with a slightly increased RDW. Note that most of the cells are macrocytic and hypochromic. The RBC Volume histogram is shifted far toward the right because of numerous large erythrocytes, and the reticulocyte count is 233,260 cells/μL (10.7%), indicating a very regenerative anemia. The cat was Coombs' positive, and a diagnosis of immune-mediated hemolytic anemia was made. No *Haemobartonella* organisms were observed on blood films taken during various days, but polymerase chain reaction for *Haemobartonella felis* was not performed. The cat was negative for feline leukemia virus. F. A 12-year-old horse with a macrocytic anemia. Note the population of large cells, some of which are hypochromic. The RBC Volume histogram is shifted toward the right, indicating a subpopulation of large cells. Reticulocytes are not released in horses, but the presence of macrocytic erythrocytes suggests that the anemia is regenerative. The horse was dehydrated, so it likely was more anemic than would be indicated by the PCV. Blood loss or blood destruction should be suspected in this case.

marrow but that affect the marrow function. For example, animals with a nonregenerative anemia that are also azotemic because of kidney dysfunction likely have decreased erythropoietin production. All patients with an unexplained nonregenerative anemia should undergo bone marrow aspiration and examination (see Chapter 13).

Signalment and History

A complete and accurate patient history from the owner may provide valuable information. In some cases, the signalment is also helpful, because certain disorders are more common in certain breeds. For example, immune-mediated hemolytic anemia is relatively common in cocker spaniels. Acute blood loss results in acute onset of clinical signs, whereas both chronic blood loss and marrow dysfunction result in chronic onset of clinical signs. Therefore, determining if the onset of clinical signs was acute or chronic may be helpful. Asking the owner if other clinical signs are present may be useful as well. For example, a dog that is also experiencing polyuria and polydipsia may be anemic as a consequence of renal dysfunction. Alternatively, a dog that is experiencing periodic episodes of weakness may have recurring, intermittent, intra-abdominal hemorrhage secondary to a bleeding lesion (e.g., hemangiosarcoma). One should also determine any history of trauma or recent surgery and if the owner has observed any evidence of blood loss, such as hematuria or epistaxis. (Melena, on the other hand, must be very severe to be obvious by visual examination of feces.) Finally, one should inquire if the patient has had any possible exposure to plants, drugs, or chemicals that might induce blood destruction, marrow dysfunction, or gastrointestinal ulceration and associated blood loss.

Physical Examination

A careful, routine physical examination may reveal additional information. For example, if bruising, petechia, or ecchymoses are present in an anemic patient, the anemia may be secondary to decreased or dysfunctional platelets or to a coagulation disorder (see Chapter 14). If abdominal distension is present, intra-abdominal hemorrhage should be suspected, and an abdominal paracentesis and fluid evaluation should be performed. If the mucous membranes are icteric as well as pale, erythrocyte destruction should be suspected. If the mucous membranes are cyanotic or brown as well as pale, methemoglobinemia, which may accompany Heinz-body anemia, may be present.

SUMMARY

In summary, the clinical signs, laboratory evaluation, signalment, history, and physical examination are all important in establishing a diagnosis for the underlying cause of anemia. Chronic external blood loss usually results in iron-deficiency anemia, which can be diagnosed on the basis of decreased MCV and serum iron. Acute external blood loss usually can be diagnosed during the physical examination; however, internal blood loss may initially be difficult to differentiate from blood destruction. Significant internal blood loss usually occurs within a body cavity, so careful physical examination, body-cavity aspiration, or other methods of visualization usually are diagnostic. Furthermore, many causes of blood destruction, such as immune-mediated destruction, Heinz bodies, or erythrocyte parasites, can be detected based on examination of blood films and erythrocyte morphology. (Diagnostic procedures for specific causes of anemia are discussed in more detail in Chapters 7 and 8.)

SUGGESTED READINGS

Schalm OW. Morphologic classification of the anemias. Vet Clin Pathol 1978;7:6–8.
Tvedten HW. Morphologic classification of anemia. Vet Clin Pathol 1999;28:80–82.

CHAPTER

7

NONREGENERATIVE ANEMIA

Anemia is classified as either regenerative or nonregenerative based on the number of circulating immature erythrocytes (polychromatophilic erythrocytes or reticulocytes). A lack of circulating immature erythrocytes indicates a nonregenerative anemia and provides evidence of marrow dysfunction. Most nonregenerative anemias are normocytic.

Nonregenerative anemia is further subclassified based on whether granulopoiesis (neutrophil production) and thrombopoiesis (platelet production) are also affected. Animals with nonregenerative anemia in conjunction with neutropenia and thrombocytopenia (pancytopenia) have either reversible or irreversible stem cell injury. Irreversible stem cell injuries are discussed in Chapter 13 and represent an intrinsic defect in proliferative behavior and/or regulation of stem cell entry into differentiated hematopoiesis. Some irreversible injuries may be induced by drugs, chemicals, viruses (e.g., feline leukemia virus [FeLV]), radiation, and immune-mediated stem cell injury, but the cause often is never discovered. Manifestations of stem cell injury range from dysplasia to lack of cell production (aplastic anemia) to uncontrolled neoplastic proliferation. Reversible stem cell injury is transient but also may be caused by drugs, chemicals, viruses, radiation, and immune-mediated destruction of stem cells. Reversible stem cell injury does not progress to neoplasia; however, both reversible and irreversible stem cell damage may be associated with myelofibrosis in response to the injury.

Pancytopenia also may result from myelophthisic disorders in which nonhematopoietic neoplasms, such as

lymphoma and malignant histiocytosis, either metastasize to or originate in the marrow. In addition, pancytopenia may be seen with hemophagocytic syndrome, a rare condition that occurs secondary to infectious, neoplastic, or metabolic diseases and is characterized by the proliferation of benign histiocytic cells that phagocytize hematopoietic precursors.

Animals with nonregenerative anemia in conjunction with normal neutrophil and platelet concentrations may have an intrinsic marrow defect (pure red cell hypoplasia, aplasia, or apparent erythroid maturation defect), or they may have a disorder that is extrinsic to the bone marrow but results in defective or decreased erythropoiesis. Pure red cell aplasia also may be either reversible or irreversible, and it usually is immune mediated or caused by viral (FeLV) damage. Extrinsic causes of nonregenerative anemia include anemia of inflammatory disease, anemia of renal failure, anemias associated with endocrine disorders, and rarely, nutritional deficiencies.

APLASTIC ANEMIA (APLASTIC PANCYTOPENIA)

Drugs, Chemicals, Toxins, and Estrogen

Antineoplastic and immunosuppressive drugs, such as doxorubicin, cyclophosphamide, cytosine arabinoside, vincristine, hydroxyurea, and azathioprine, probably are the most commonly used agents that cause reversible stem cell damage in dogs. These drugs are used for brief periods of time, however, and usually result in a neutropenia and thrombocytopenia rather than a significant nonregenerative anemia. Drugs that have been associated with stem cell injury in animals include estrogen (dogs and ferrets), phenylbutazone (dogs and possibly horses), meclofenamic acid (dogs), griseofulvin (cats), phenobarbital (dogs), phenytoin (dogs), colchicine (dogs), azidothymidine (a reverse transcriptase inhibitor; cats), chloramphenicol (dogs and cats), thiacetarsamide (dogs), and albendazole (a broad-spectrum anthelmintic; dogs and cats). Some drugs may induce stem cell destruction by immune-mediated mechanisms. In dogs, trimethoprim-sulfadiazine, cephalosporin, and phenobarbital have been associated with pancytopenia that may be immune-mediated. Drug-induced immune-mediated stem cell injury usually responds to discontinuation of the drug. Idiopathic immune-mediated stem cell injury often responds to immunosuppressive therapy, but these injuries may take several weeks to respond and often require long-term treatment for resolution. *Table 7.1* summarizes drugs and chemicals that may cause aplastic anemia in domestic animals.

Estrogen toxicosis may occur in bitches given exogenous estrogen for mismating, termination of pseudo-pregnancy, or urinary incontinence. Myelosuppression may result from the administration of excessive amounts of estrogen or from an idiosyncratic sensitivity to estrogen. Endogenous estrogen, resulting either from Sertoli cell tumors in male dogs or from cystic ovaries or granulosa cell tumors in female dogs, also may result in bone marrow suppression. Because ferrets are induced ovulators, marrow suppression from endogenous estrogen is a common—and potentially fatal—disorder in this species. The mechanism of estrogen toxicosis is unclear, but it is thought to result from the secretion (by thymic stromal cells) of an estrogen-induced substance that inhibits stem cells. Marrow suppression is preceded by an initial thrombocytosis and neutrophilia.

Aplastic anemia in cattle has been associated with grazing on bracken fern and ingestion of soybean meal contaminated with the solvent trichloroethylene. Benzene, a commonly used solvent, may cause aplastic anemia as well as leukemia. Mycotoxins have been associated with bone marrow suppression in horses and cattle, and experimental aflatoxin B_1 toxicity has been reported to cause aplastic anemia in pigs.

Infectious Agents

Feline leukemia virus can result in anemia by many mechanisms, one of which is induction of aplastic anemia. In addition, FeLV is associated with anemia that manifests as pure red cell aplasia or hypoplasia, myeloproliferative disorders (see Chapter 13), anemia of inflammatory disease, and hemolysis. Hemolytic anemias that may be associated with FeLV infection include Heinz-body anemia, immune-mediated hemolytic anemia, and feline infectious anemia (see Chapter 8). Before widespread use of the FeLV vaccine, approximately 70% of anemic cats were infected with FeLV. Anemia caused by FeLV often is macrocytic, or a subpopulation of the erythrocytes is macrocytic in the absence of reticulocytosis. This may be caused by prolonged dysplastic erythrocyte production resulting from FeLV-induced myelodysplasia (see Chapter 13).

Ehrlichia canis may result in pancytopenia by two mechanisms: immune-mediated destruction of circulating cells, or aplastic anemia (which also may be an immune-mediated mechanism). In addition, dogs with ehrlichiosis may present with only one decreased cell line (e.g., thrombocytopenia), may have a lymphocytosis, and commonly have hyperglobulinemia. The organism rarely is seen on blood films.

Equine infectious anemia virus (a lentivirus) causes anemia by a number of mechanisms, one of which is bone marrow suppression (possibly immune mediated). Parvovirus infection in dogs and cats causes acute bone marrow necrosis, but these animals usually recover—or die—before the anemia becomes significant.

TABLE 7.1 DRUGS, CHEMICALS, PLANTS, AND HORMONES ASSOCIATED WITH NONREGENERATIVE ANEMIA IN DOMESTIC ANIMALS

Dogs
  Albendazole
  Estrogen
  Cephalosporins
  Chemotherapeutic agents
  Colchicine
  Meclofenamic acid
  Phenobarbital
  Phenylbutazone
  Phenytoin
  Quinidine
  Thiacetarsamide
Cats
  Albendazole
  Azidothymidine
  Griseofulvin
Cattle
  Bracken fern
  Mycotoxins
  Trichlorethylene
Horses
  Mycotoxins
  Phenylbutazone

PURE RED CELL APLASIA

Pure red cell aplasia is characterized by a markedly decreased concentration of erythroid precursors in the bone marrow in the face of normal granulopoiesis and thrombopoiesis, resulting in a severe nonregenerative anemia with normal neutrophil and platelet concentrations. In dogs, pure red cell aplasia almost always is caused by immune-mediated destruction of erythroid precursors, and it often responds to immunosuppressive therapy. Spherocytes and agglutination may be present, and approximately half the affected dogs are Coombs' positive. Bone marrow examination usually reveals an apparent arrest at some stage of erythroid precursor maturation, ranging from the rubriblast to the metarubricyte stage. Phagocytosis of rubricytes or metarubricytes may be seen. Occasionally, however, erythroid precursors are completely absent.

Some dogs and horses treated with recombinant human erythropoietin developed an immune response against the recombinant as well as endogenous erythropoietin, resulting in a reversible pure red cell aplasia. Recombinant, species-specific erythropoietin does not produce this syndrome but is not yet commercially available.

Finally, certain strains of FeLV virus (subgroup C) cause pure red cell aplasia.

RED CELL HYPOPLASIA

Nonregenerative anemia may result from abnormalities that are extrinsic to the marrow, including anemia of inflammatory disease, anemia of chronic renal failure, and anemia associated with endocrine disease, and rarely, anemia associated with nutritional deficiencies. Other laboratory findings, such as an inflammatory leukogram, azotemia, other biochemical profile abnormalities or endocrine panel abnormalities, usually are key to establishing the diagnosis of these types of anemias.

Anemia of Inflammatory Disease

Anemia of inflammatory disease (anemia of chronic disease) is the most common anemia in domestic animals, but it usually is mild and clinically insignificant. This type of anemia is associated with various types of inflammatory processes, including infections, trauma, and neoplasia, and usually is mild to moderate, nonregenerative, and normocytic. The pathogenesis of anemia of inflammatory disease is not completely understood but is thought to be multifactorial. Laboratory findings include a decreased serum iron concentration, normal or decreased total iron-binding capacity, normal or increased serum ferritin, and normal or increased stainable iron stores in the bone mar-

row. An inflammatory leukogram commonly is present as well. Very rarely, animals may have a microcytic anemia, which makes anemia of inflammatory disease difficult to distinguish from iron-deficiency anemia; in these cases, serum ferritin or bone marrow stainable iron must be used to differentiate the two disorders.

Iron metabolism in patients with anemia of inflammatory disease has been extensively studied. Although the serum iron concentration is decreased, the iron stores are increased, and the assumption has long been that the anemia results from the unavailability of iron to erythroid precursors. Apolactoferrin (an iron-transport protein) is increased in inflammatory conditions and is induced by interleukin-1 and tumor necrosis factor-α. Macrophages then internalize lactoferrin-bound iron, which is transferred to ferritin for iron storage. Iron absorption by the gastrointestinal tract also is decreased because of reduced synthesis of transferrin. A decreased serum iron concentration presumably is advantageous to patients with inflammatory disease, because it reduces the availability of iron for bacterial growth. Increased erythrocyte destruction by activated macrophages also may play a role in the pathogenesis of anemia. Erythropoietin is thought to play a particularly large role in the pathogenesis of anemia of inflammatory disease. Erythropoietin secretion is decreased, and marrow response to erythropoietin is diminished, presumably because of inflammatory cytokines. Treatment is aimed at alleviating the underlying disease. Iron therapy, either oral or parenteral, has no benefit, but treatment with recombinant erythropoietin usually results in an increased hematocrit.

Anemia of Chronic Renal Failure

Anemia associated with chronic renal failure usually is moderate to severe, nonregenerative, and normocytic. The severity of the anemia correlates with the severity of the renal failure as evidenced by the degree of azotemia. The primary cause for this anemia is lack of production of erythropoietin by the kidney, and treatment with recombinant canine erythropoietin effectively increases the hematocrit. Other factors, such as increased bleeding tendencies, also may play a role in this type of anemia but likely are comparatively minor in importance. Increases in serum parathyroid hormone and phosphorus concentrations and increased erythrocyte osmotic fragility have not been found to correlate significantly with the degree of anemia.

Anemia Associated with Endocrine Disease

Hypothyroid dogs almost always have a mild, nonregenerative, normocytic anemia, usually with a hematocrit of approximately 30%. This anemia responds to therapy for hypothyroidism and may simply be a manifestation of the lowered metabolic rate. Some dogs with hypoadrenocorticism, particularly those with glucocorticoid deficiency, have a mild, nonregenerative, normocytic anemia that often is masked by dehydration.

Anemia Associated with Nutritional Deficiencies

Iron-deficiency anemia is the most common anemia associated with a nutritional deficiency. This type of anemia usually is regenerative (unless complicated by anemia of inflammatory disease) and is discussed in Chapter 8. Other types of anemia related to nutritional deficiency are diagnosed very infrequently.

Cobalamin deficiency is very rare in dogs and cats (unlike in humans) and usually results from a hereditary absence of intrinsic factor cobalamin receptors in ileal enterocytes, which is inherited as an autosomal recessive trait. This anemia is nonregenerative and normocytic (unlike the human counterpart, which is macrocytic) and has been reported in a Border collie, a beagle, giant schnauzers, and cats. Affected puppies fail to thrive. Other findings include neutropenia with hypersegmentation, anemia with anisocytosis and poikilocytosis, megaloblastic changes of the bone marrow, decreased serum cobalamin concentrations, methylmalonic aciduria, and homocystinemia. Parenteral, but not oral, cyanocobalamin administration eliminates all abnormalities except the decreased serum cobalamin concentration. Cobalt deficiency in ruminants results in a normocytic, nonregenerative anemia and is caused by grazing on cobalt-deficient soil. Cobalt is required for synthesis of cobalamin by rumen bacteria.

SUGGESTED READINGS

Drugs, Chemicals, Toxins, and Endogenous Estrogen

Alleman AR, Harvey JW. The morphologic effects of vincristine sulfate on canine bone marrow cells. Vet Clin Pathol 1993;22:36–41.

Berggren PC. Aplastic anemia in a horse. J Am Vet Med Assoc 1981;179:1400–1402.

Bernard SL, Leather CW, Brobst DF, et al. Estrogen-induced bone marrow depression in ferrets. Am J Vet Res 1983;44:657–661.

Bloo JC, Theim PA, Sellers TS, et al. Cephalosporin-induced immune cytopenia in the dog: demonstration of erythrocyte-, neutrophil-, and platelet-associated IgG following treatment with cefezedone. Am J Hematol 1988;28:71–78.

Bowen RA, Olson PN, Behrendt MD, et al. Efficacy and toxicity of estrogens commonly used to terminate canine pregnancy. J Am Vet Med Assoc 1985;186:783–788.

Brockus CW. Endogenous estrogen myelotoxicosis associated with functional cystic ovaries in a dog. Vet Clin Pathol 1998;27:55–56.

Deldar A, Lewis H, Bloom J, et al. Cephalosporin-induced changes in the ultrastructure of canine bone marrow. Vet Pathol 1988;25:211–218.

Farris GM, Benjamin SA. Inhibition of myelopoiesis by conditioned medium from cultured canine thymic cells exposed to estrogen. Am J Vet Res 1993;54:1366–1373.

Fox LE, Ford S, Alleman AR, et al. Aplastic anemia associated with prolonged high-dose trimethoprim-sulfadiazine administration in two dogs. Vet Clin Pathol 1993;22:89–92.

Giger U, Werner LL, Millichamp NJ, et al. Sulfadiazine-induced allergy in six Doberman pinschers. J Am Vet Med Assoc 1985;186:479–484.

Holland M, Stobie D, Shapiro W. Pancytopenia associated with administration of captopril to a dog. J Am Vet Med Assoc 1996;208:1683–1687.

Jeffeers M, Lenghaus C. Granulocytopenia and thrombocytopenia in dairy cattle—a suspected mycotoxicosis. Aust Vet J 1986;63:262–264.

Lavoie JP, Morris DD, Zinkl JG, et al. Pancytopenia caused by bone marrow aplasia in a horse. J Am Vet Med Assoc 1987;191:1462–1464.

McCandish IAP, Munro CD, Breeze RG, et al. Hormone producing ovarian tumors in the dog. Vet Rec 1979; 105:9–11.

Morgan RV. Blood dyscrasias associated with testicular tumors in the dog. J Am Anim Hosp Assoc 1982;18:970–975.

Pritchard WR, Rehfeld CE, Sauter JH. Aplastic anemia of cattle associated with trichloroethylene-extracted soybean oil meal. J Am Vet Med Assoc 1952;121:1–8.

Reagan WJ. A review of myelofibrosis in dogs. Toxicol Pathol 1993;21:164–169.

Rinkardt NE, Kruth SA. Azathioprine-induced bone marrow toxicity in four dogs. Can Vet J 1996;37:612–613.

Sherding RG, Wilson GP, Kociba GJ. Bone marrow hypoplasia in eight dogs with Sertoli cell tumor. J Am Vet Med Assoc 1981;178:497–500.

Sippel WL. Bracken fern poisoning. J Am Vet Med Assoc 1952;121:9–13.

Stokol T, Randolph JF, Nachbar S, et al. Development of bone marrow toxicosis after albendazole administration in a dog and cat. J Am Vet Med Assoc 1997;12:1753–1756.

Watson ADJ. Further observation on chloramphenicol toxicosis in cats. Am J Vet Res 1980;41:239–294.

Watson ADJ, Wilson JT, Turner OM, et al. Phenylbutazone-induced blood dyscrasias suspected in three dogs. Vet Rec 1980;107:239–241.

Weiss DJ. Idiopathic aplastic anemia in the dog. Vet Clin Pathol 1985;14:23–25.

Weiss DJ, Adams LG. Aplastic anemia associated with trimethoprim-sulfadiazine and fenbendazole administration in a dog. J Am Vet Med Assoc 1987;191:1119–1120.

Weiss DJ, Evanson OA, Sykes J. A retrospective study of canine pancytopenia. Vet Clin Pathol 1999;28:83–88.

Weiss DJ, Klausner JS. Drug-associated aplastic anemia in dogs: eight cases (1984–1988). J Am Vet Med Assoc 190;196:472–475.

Infectious Agents

Boosinger TR, Rebar AH, Denicola DB, et al. Bone marrow alterations associated with canine parvoviral enteritis. Vet Pathol 1982;19:558–561.

Dornsife RE, Gasper PW, Mullins JI, et al. Induction of aplastic anemia by intra-bone marrow inoculation of molecularly cloned feline retrovirus. 1989;13:745–755.

Kuehn NF, Gaunt SF. Clinical and hematologic findings in canine ehrlichiosis. J Am Vet Med Assoc 1985;186:355–358.

McGuire TC, Henson JB, Quist SE. Impaired bone marrow response in equine infectious anemia. Am J Vet Res 1969;30:2099–2104.

Reardon MJ, Pierce KR. Acute experimental canine ehrlichiosis. I. Sequential reaction of the hemic and lymphoreticular systems. Vet Pathol 1981;18:48–61.

Wardrop KJ, Bazzler TV, Relich E, et al. A morphometric study of bone marrow megakaryocytes in foals infected with equine infectious anemia virus. Vet Pathol 1996;33:222–227

Pure Red Cell Aplasia

Abkowitz JL, Holly RD, Grant CK. Retrovirus-induced feline pure red cell aplasia. J Clin Invest 1987;80:1056–1063.

Jonas RD, Thrall MA, Weiser MG. Immune-mediated hemolytic anemia with delayed erythrogenesis in the dog. J Am Anim Hosp Assoc
1987;23:201–204.

Piercy RJ, Swardson CJ, Hinchcliff KW. Erythroid hypoplasia and anemia following administration of recombinant human erythropoietin
to two horses. J Am Vet Med Assoc 1998;212:244–247.

Randolph JF, Stokol T, Scarlett JM, MacLeod JN. Comparison of bio-
logical activity and safety of recombinant canine erythropoietin
with that of recombinant human erythropoietin in clinically normal
dogs. Am J Vet Res 1999;60:636–642.

Stockham SL, Ford RB, Weiss DJ. Canine autoimmune hemolytic disease with a delayed erythroid regeneration. J Am Anim Hosp Assoc
1980;16:927–931.

Stokol T, Blue JT. Pure red cell aplasia in cats: nine cases (1989–1997).
J Am Vet Med Assoc 1999;214:75–79.

Stokol T, Blue JT, French TW. Idiopathic pure red cell aplasia and
nonregenerative immune-mediated anemia in dogs: 43 cases
(1988–1999). J Am Vet Med Assoc 2000;216:1429–1436.

Stokol T, Randolph J, MacLeod JN. Pure red cell aplasia after recombinant human erythropoietin treatment in normal beagle dogs. Vet
Pathol 1997;34:474. (Abstract 12.)

Anemia of Inflammatory Disease

Feldman BF, Kaneko JJ. The anemia of inflammatory disease in the dog.
I. The nature of the problem. Vet Res Commun 1981;4:237–252.

Feldman BF, Kaneko JJ, Farver TB. Anemia of inflammatory disease in
the dog: availability of storage iron in inflammatory disease. Am J
Vet Res 1981;42:586–589.

Feldman BF, Kaneko JJ, Farver TB. Anemia of inflammatory disease in
the dog: clinical characterization. Am J Vet Res 1981;42:1109–1113.

Feldman BF, Kaneko JJ, Farver TB. Anemia of inflammatory disease in
the dog: ferrokinetics of adjuvant-induced anemia. Am J Vet Res
1981;42:583–585.

Means RT Jr. Advances in the anemia of chronic disease. Int J Hematol 1999;70:7–12.

Weiss DJ, McClay CB. Studies on the pathogenesis of the erythrocyte
destruction associated with the anemia of inflammatory disease. Vet
Clin Pathol 1988;17:90–93.

Anemias Associated with Endocrine Disease

Lifton SJ, King LG, Zerbe CA. Glucocorticoid-deficient hypoadrenocorticism in dogs: 18 cases (1986–1995). J Am Vet Med Assoc
1996;209:2076–2081.

Panciera DL. Conditions associated with canine hypothyroidism. Vet
Clin North Am Small Anim Pract 2001;31:935–950.

Anemia Associated with Chronic Renal Failure

Cowgill LD. Pathophysiology and management of anemia in chronic
progressive renal failure. Semin Vet Med Surg (Small Anim) 1992;
7:175–182.

King LG, Giger U, Diserens D, Nagode LA. Anemia of chronic renal
failure in dogs. J Vet Intern Med 1992;6:264–270.

Cobalamin Deficiency

Fordyce HH, Callan MB, Giger U. Persistent cobalamin deficiency
causing failure to thrive in a juvenile beagle. Nutr J Small Anim
Pract 2000;41:407–410.

Fyfe JC, Giger U, Hall CA, et al. Inherited selective intestinal cobalamin
malabsorption and cobalamin deficiency in dogs. Pediatr Res
1991;29:24–31.

Fyfe JC, Giger U, Jezyk PF. Cobalamin metabolism. J Am Vet Med
Assoc 1992;201:202–204.

Morgan LW, McConnell JJ. Cobalamin deficiency associated with eryth-
roblastic anemia and methylmalonic aciduria in a Border collie.
J Am Anim Hosp Assoc 1999;35:392–395.

Ruaux CG, Steiner JM, Williams DA. Metabolism of amino acids in
cats with severe cobalamin deficiency. Am J Vet Res 2001;62:
1852–1858.

Simpson KW, Fyfe J, Cornetta A, et al. Subnormal concentrations of
serum cobalamin (vitamin B_{12}) in cats with gastrointestinal disease.
J Vet Intern Med. 2001;15:327–328.

Vaden SL, Wood PA, Ledley FD, Cornwell PE, Miller RT, Page R.
Cobalamin deficiency associated with methylmalonic acidemia in a
cat. J Am Vet Med Assoc 1992;200:1101–1103.

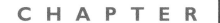

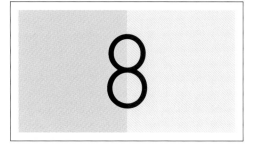

REGENERATIVE ANEMIA

Regenerative anemia is caused by either blood loss or blood destruction or may be seen in the recovery phase of marrow dysfunction. Blood loss may be external or internal, and may be acute or chronic. Causes of acute blood loss include trauma; bleeding lesions, such as tumors or large ulcers; and hemostatic disorders. Examples of hemostatic disorders include thrombocytopenia, inherited coagulopathies, and acquired coagulopathies, such as warfarin toxicosis or disseminated vascular coagulopathy. Common causes of chronic blood loss include bleeding lesions, particularly within the gastrointestinal tract, and gastrointestinal or external parasites.

Blood destruction (hemolysis) may be either intravascular or extravascular, and may be due to intrinsic (primary) defects, such as hereditary membrane defects or enzyme deficiencies, or extrinsic (secondary) causes, such as erythrocyte parasites or immune-mediated destruction. Intravascular hemolysis is the actual lysis of erythrocytes within the vascular system. Extravascular hemolysis occurs when abnormal erythrocytes are phagocytized by macrophages, usually within the spleen or liver. Common causes of erythrocyte destruction include immune mediated mechanisms, erythrocyte parasites, and drugs and chemicals that produce oxidative damage resulting in Heinz body formation. Less common causes include hypophosphosphatemia, water intoxication in young ruminants, bacteria (*Leptospira, Clostridium*), heparin overdose, and hereditary erythrocyte enzyme deficiencies and membrane defects.

BLOOD LOSS

If blood is lost outside of the body, including loss into GI tract, components of the blood such as iron and plasma protein are lost. On the other hand, if bleeding occurs within a body cavity, the protein is reabsorbed within hours, and most of the erythrocytes are reabsorbed by lymphatics within a few days. The remaining cells are lysed or phagocytized, and iron is reutilized.

Acute Blood Loss

If blood loss is acute, the PCV initially remains normal because both cells and plasma are lost. However, within a few hours the PCV and plasma protein decrease as a result of dilution, as interstitial fluid is added to blood. By 72 hours post-bleed, polychromatophilic erythrocytes (reticulocytes) should begin to appear in blood, and their concentration usually peaks within approximately one week. Plasma protein should return to normal within about one week, unless blood loss is recurrent or ongoing. Examples of disorders causing acute blood loss include trauma and surgical procedures, coagulation disorders, thrombocytopenia, and bleeding tumors.

Thrombocytopenia may result in bleeding when the platelet concentration is less than 25,000/µl; blood loss does not cause platelet concentrations to drop below 1000,000/µl. Platelet concentration can usually be estimated from the blood film. The combination of reticulocytosis (or increased polychromasia) and hypoproteinemia is indicative of blood loss anemia, unless hypoproteinemia is coincidental to a regenerative anemia. Causes of hypoproteinemia other than blood loss include decreased intake (malabsorption, maldigestion, starvation), decreased production (liver failure), or other types of protein loss (glomerulonephropathy, protein losing enteropathy).

Blood loss outside of the body is usually easy to diagnose, since the source of blood loss is usually apparent, unless it is being lost via the gastrointestinal tract. Blood loss within a body cavity is more difficult to diagnose, and thoracic or abdominal fluid evaluation may be necessary to confirm the diagnosis.

Erythrocyte morphology is usually normal with acute blood loss, with the exception of blood loss from hemangiosarcoma, one of the most common tumors of middle-aged to older dogs, especially large breeds such as German shepherds and golden retrievers. Hemangiosarcomas have been reported in cats, but are rare. They are malignant vascular tumors typically found in the spleen, liver, and right atrium of the heart, and most have metastasized to the lungs or other organs by the time the diagnosis is made. Many dogs present due to acute signs associated with anemia as a result of rupture of the tumor, with blood loss into the abdominal cavity. Some affected dogs have a history of intermittent weakness, as a result of multiple events involving tumor rupturing and bleeding, followed by absorption of blood from the abdominal cavity.

Acanthocytes and schistocytes are seen in the majority of dogs with hemangiosarcoma *(Fig. 8.1)*; these morphologic changes are helpful in making the diagnosis (see Chapter 5), and may also be observed in the erythrocytes in blood aspirated from the abdominal cavity *(Fig. 8.2)*.

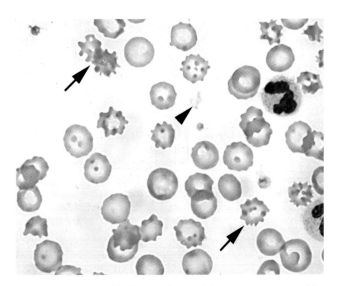

Figure 8.1 Blood film from a dog with hemangiosarcoma of the spleen. Note the acanthocytes (arrows) and schistocyte (arrowhead). Wright stain.

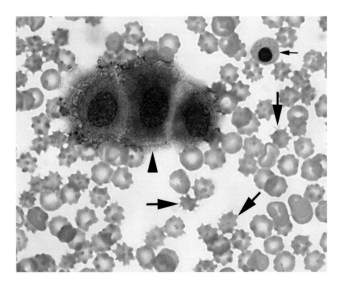

Figure 8.2 Abdominal fluid from a dog with ruptured splenic hemangiosarcoma and resultant hemoabdomen. Although morphology of erythrocytes is usually insignificant in body cavity effusions, animals with hemoabdomen resulting from hemangiosarcoma may have acanthocytes (large arrows) that are diagnostically useful. Mesothelial cells (arrowhead) and a nucleated erythrocyte are also present (small arrow). Wright stain.

Other common laboratory findings include reticulocytosis (increased polychromasia), transient hypoproteinemia, and thrombocytopenia, usually mild to moderate, as a result of localized microangiopathy within the tumor, or disseminated intravascular coagulation. Dogs that are treated with surgical resection alone have a mean survival time of approximately 2 to 3 months, and dogs that are treated with a combination of surgical resection and chemotherapy have a mean survival time of approximately 4 to 10 months, depending on the protocol used.

Chronic Blood Loss (Iron Deficiency Anemia)

Chronic blood loss results in iron deficiency anemia. Iron deficiency anemia in adults is almost always due to chronic blood loss. Conversely, iron deficiency anemia commonly occurs in neonates of all domestic animal species due to inadequate iron intake, since milk contains little iron and growth rates are high. Anemia is particularly severe in baby pigs that have no access to iron-containing soil, but also occurs in kittens, puppies, foals, and calves. When blood loss is ongoing, iron stores are depleted relatively quickly. One ml of blood contains 0.5 mg of iron; normally 1 mg of iron is absorbed and excreted daily. Iron deficiency anemia is quite common in dogs, less common in ruminants, and relatively rare in cats and horses.

Causes of chronic blood loss include gastrointestinal, as well as external, bloodsucking parasites, GI ulcers and neoplasms, inflammatory bowel disease, and rarely, thrombocytopenia or inherited hemostatic defects. In dogs, the source of blood loss is most commonly the gastrointestinal tract. Overuse of blood donors may also lead to features of severe iron deficiency anemia, although the degree of anemia may be very mild. A relatively large amount of blood may be present in feces without being noticed. Clinical signs of chronic blood loss include those of anemia, such as pallor, lethargy, and weakness, and are somewhat variable, depending on the underlying cause of the blood loss.

Laboratory Findings

The hallmark of iron deficiency anemia is a decreased MCV (see Chapters 1 and 6). Microcytosis occurs because erythrocyte precursors continue to divide in an attempt to reach their full hemoglobin content. Additional divisions result in smaller than normal erythrocytes. Examination of the erythrocyte histogram or computer graphic generated by the electronic cell counter is often useful, because sub-populations of microcytic erythrocytes can be observed, even when the MCV is within the reference interval (See Chapter 6). The MCV of reticulocytes is also decreased, since even immature iron deficient erythrocytes are smaller than normal. The red cell distribution width (RDW), which describes the width of the size distribution, is usually increased when sub-populations of microcytic erythrocytes are present, and will often be increased before the MCV decreases below the reference interval. Although one might expect the MCHC to be decreased in these patients, since the cells contain less hemoglobin than normal, it is commonly within the reference interval.

Blood film examination is diagnostically useful, particularly in the late stages of iron deficiency anemia. Erythrocytes of most species, other than cats, may appear pale, with increased central pallor, and sometimes only a thin rim of hemoglobin is present *(Fig. 8.3)*. Membrane abnormalities are common, including keratocyte and schistocyte formation, presumably due to increased susceptibility to oxidative damage (see Chapter 5). Initially the RBC develops what appears to be a blister or vacuole where inner membrane surfaces are cross-linked across the cell. These lesions subsequently enlarge, break open to form "apple-stem cells" and keratocytes, spiculated red cells with two or more pointed projections. The projections from the keratocytes then fragment from the cell, forming schistocytes. Erythrocytes are thin, and folded cells may be seen, particularly in llamas *(Fig. 8.4)*.

The anemia is usually regenerative, but may become non-regenerative in the late stages. Occasionally, the bone marrow response may be inappropriate due to underlying anemia of inflammatory disease, since many of these animals have concurrent inflammation related to bleeding lesions. Thrombocytosis is present in approximately 50%

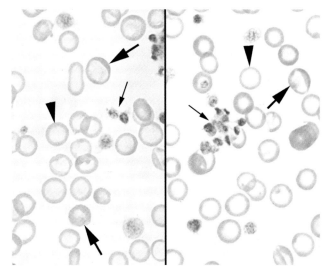

Figure 8.3 Blood film from a dog with iron deficiency anemia and hypochromic erythrocytes (arrowheads). Note the presence of polychromatophilic erythrocytes (large arrows), indicating that the anemia is regenerative. Animals with iron deficiency anemia commonly have increased platelets (small arrows), some of which may be large. Wright stain.

of iron deficient patients. The mechanism for the increased platelet concentration is not well understood, but may be due to increased erythropoietin or other cytokines. Approximately one-third of animals with chronic blood loss become hypoproteinemic, as protein production sometimes cannot keep pace with blood loss.

Other laboratory findings in patients with iron deficiency include decreased serum iron concentration,

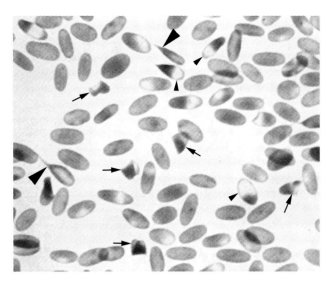

Figure 8.4 Blood film from a llama with iron deficiency anemia. Typical morphologic abnormalities associated with iron deficiency in llamas include dacryocytes (large arrowhead), folded erythrocytes (arrows), and eccentric pallor (small arrowheads). Wright stain.

decreased transferrin (a glycoprotein in plasma that transports iron between compartments) saturation, and low storage iron. Total iron binding capacity, a test for measuring the amount of transferrin available to transport iron, is usually normal in iron deficient dogs and cats, although it is usually increased in other species with iron deficiency. Iron is stored as either ferritin or hemosiderin. Although ferritin is primarily an intracellular iron storage compound, it can be detected in serum. Hemosiderin, on the other hand, is insoluble, and can only be detected by staining cells and tissues. Thus, storage iron can be evaluated by measuring serum ferritin, or by examining a bone marrow aspirate and noting lack of hemosiderin in macrophages. Serum ferritin is difficult to measure, is species-specific, and since it is an acute phase reactant protein, tends to increase when inflammation or liver disease are present. Special iron stains, such as Prussian blue, are not necessary in order to visualize hemosiderin in the bone marrow (see Chapter 13). The absence of hemosiderin in feline bone marrow aspirates is not significant, since hemosiderin is rarely seen in aspirates of bone marrow from normal cats.

For practical purposes, low serum iron in a patient with a decreased MCV and anemia is usually adequate to diagnose iron deficiency anemia, and to trigger additional diagnostic procedures to determine the source of blood loss, such as testing the feces for occult blood.

Therapy

Treatment consists of finding and treating the source of blood loss. Iron supplementation with intramuscular injectable iron in iron deficient neonates is useful, especially baby pigs, which are usually given 200 mg iron as iron dextran. Although oral iron supplementation is commonly used to treat iron deficiency, it is likely of little value, particularly in dogs and cats, because commercial pet food usually contains more iron than can be absorbed by the intestine. However, intestinal absorption of iron increases dramatically when animals are iron deficient. Oral iron should not be given to neonatal animals, especially kittens, since it can be toxic.

Differential Diagnoses

Other causes of microcytosis include portosystemic shunts, which are vascular connections between the portal and systemic circulation that divert portal blood around the liver. The cause of the microcytosis in these animals is not well understood, but is associated with abnormal iron metabolism, and some of these patients may actually have iron deficiency anemia, usually as a result of gastrointestinal hemorrhaging secondary to pressure changes in the liver. The anemia, if present, is usually mild, and although serum iron may be decreased, storage iron is usually normal to slightly increased. Approximately two thirds of dogs and one-third of cats with portosystemic shunts have microcytosis.

Animals with anemia of inflammatory disease usually have normocytic anemias, but occasionally the MCV will fall below the reference interval. While serum iron is decreased in these animals, storage iron is normal to increased.

Finally, some dogs of the Japanese Shiba and Akita breeds normally have microcytosis. These animals are not anemic, and their iron metabolism is normal.

BLOOD DESTRUCTION (INTRAVASCULAR OR EXTRAVASCULAR HEMOLYSIS)

Immune-Mediated Hemolytic Anemia

Immune-mediated hemolytic anemia (IMHA) is a consequence of increased red cell destruction, either as a result of antibody directed against erythrocytes, or immune complexes attaching to erythrocytes. Immune mediated hemolytic anemia is usually a markedly regenerative anemia, with increased polychromasia (reticulocytosis). However, in some instances, the anemia is non-regenerative as a result of antibody formation against RBC precursors, with destruction of polychromatophilic erythrocytes or earlier red cell precursors. The onset may be acute or gradual. Immune mediated hemolytic anemia is sometimes classified as primary (idiopathic), or secondary, if concurrent disease is present. However, this classification is somewhat meaningless, since "secondary" immune mediated hemolytic anemia may be coincidental to the concurrent disorder. Often the cause is never determined, but in some instances can be related to other disorders or events, such as infections, other immune-mediated disorders, modified live virus vaccination, neoplasia, particularly of the lymphoid system, bee stings, zinc toxicosis, and administration of drugs. Drugs that have been associated with IMHA are numerous and include penicillin, cephalosporins, trimethoprim-sulfamethoxazole, levamisole, and amiodarone; in these cases, immune mediated destruction occurs due to either the drug binding directly to erythrocytes (penicillin), or by the formation of drug-antibody immune complexes, which also may bind to red blood cells.

Immune mediated hemolytic anemia is the most common cause of hemolytic anemia in the dog, and has been described in horses, cattle, and cats. Breeds of dogs more commonly affected include cocker spaniels, poodles, and collies, and the disorder is slightly more common in females than in males. In horses, IMHA has been associated with penicillin and other antibiotic administration, clostridial infections, and neoplasia. In cats, IMHA has been most commonly associated with *Haemobartonella felis* (*Mycoplasma haemofelis*) infection, feline leukemia virus, and lymphoproliferative and myeloproliferative disease. Immune mediated hemolytic anemia has been reported in cattle with anaplasmosis, which is not surprising, since antibody is likely to be directed against the erythrocyte parasite.

Mechanisms of red cell destruction can be due to either erythrophagocytosis or intravascular hemolysis. Macrophages have receptors for antibody as well as complement (C_3b), and removal of erythrocytes by macrophages occurs in multiple organs, including the spleen, bone marrow, and liver. Rarely, monocytes that have phagocytized erythrocytes may be observed on blood films *(Fig. 8.5)*. Partial erythrophagocytosis by macrophages results in the formation of spherocytes, the hallmark of IMHA. Spherocytes appear small, although their volume is normal, and because they are sphere-shaped, lack central pallor and appear to be dense *(Fig. 8.6)*. They have a shortened half-life because they are not as deformable as normal biconcave disk-shaped erythrocytes. They exhibit increased saline fragility, which may be diagnostically useful. Spherocytes are difficult to detect in species in which the red cells normally lack central pallor. They are, however, readily detectable in dogs, although imperfect spherocytes, which have a small amount of central pallor, are sometimes missed. If complement fixation goes to completion, resulting in membrane attack complex formation, intravascular lysis occurs. In these instances, ghost erythrocytes are occasionally observed on blood films *(Fig. 8.7)*. Hemo-

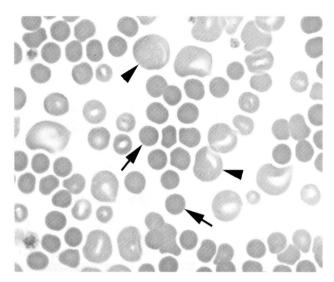

Figure 8.6 Blood film from a dog with immune mediated hemolytic anemia. The polychromatophilic erythrocytes (arrowheads) indicate that the anemia is regenerative; numerous spherocytes (arrows) are present, as is agglutination. Wright stain.

globinemia, hemoglobinuria, hyperbilirubinemia, and bilirubinuria are often present.

Antibodies associated with IMHA are usually IgG or IgM, but IgA has also been reported to bind to erythrocytes. Usually the antibody is attached to erythrocyte membrane glycoproteins. If IgM is involved, agglutination of erythrocytes can usually be observed on the blood film, and may be grossly evident in the blood tube. IgG is sometimes referred to as an incomplete antibody, since it usually does not result in intravascular hemolysis or

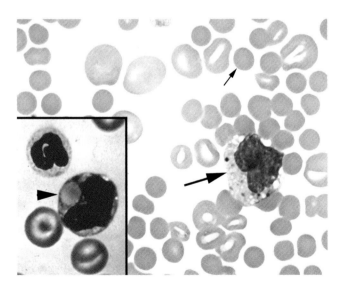

Figure 8.5 Blood film from a dog with immune mediated hemolytic anemia. Numerous spherocytes (small arrow) are present. Rarely, monocytes may be observed that contain hemosiderin (large arrow) or phagocytized erythrocytes (inset, arrowhead). Wright stain.

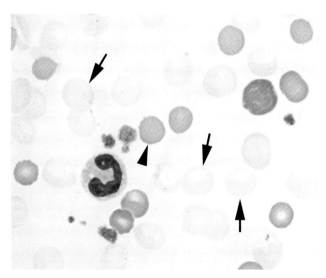

Figure 8.7 Blood film from dog with intravascular hemolysis secondary to immune mediated hemolytic anemia. Numerous spherocytes (arrowhead) and lysed "ghost" erythrocytes (arrows) are present. Wright stain.

agglutination, but rather predisposes to erythrocyte phagocytosis by macrophages. The presence of antibody can be detected by performing a Coombs' test (see Chapter 1). A species-specific antiglobulin reagent (Coombs' serum) is added to a saline-washed suspension of the patient's erythrocytes. Agglutination results if the red cells are coated with autoantibody. However, if agglutination is already present, a Coombs' test is not indicated. In some cases in which agglutination is observed, the Coombs' test is falsely negative, presumably because the IgM antibody is eluted from the erythrocytes during the washing process. The Coombs' test was first developed for use in humans in 1945 by R. R. A. Coombs, a veterinary immunologist in the Department of Pathology at Cambridge University, who hypothesized that antibody to human globulin could be synthesized by rabbits inoculated with human globulin, and this sera could then attach to globulin binding to erythrocytes, resulting in agglutination. This test is also known as the direct antiglobulin test (DAT). The Coombs' test has numerous limitations in domestic animals because of false-negative and false-positive results, both of which are common. False-negative results occur due to the following: low concentration of antibody bound to erythrocytes, improper antiglobulin to antibody ratio, not incorporating the drug that is suspected of inducing the antibody response, and improper temperature. False positive results occur when various types of disease cause immune complexes or complement to bind to erythrocytes, without resulting in anemia. False positives are particularly common in cats. Previous treatment with glucocorticosteroids may cause a negative result, and previous blood transfusion may cause a positive result. A more sensitive enzyme linked immunosorbent assay (ELISA) to detect immunoglobulins bound to erythrocytes has fewer false-negative results. However, this direct enzyme-linked antiglobulin test (DELAT) may also be falsely positive, is laborious, and not available in most laboratories. Direct immunofluorescence (DIF) flow cytometry is more sensitive (but less specific) than the Coombs' test, can be used to determine the class of antibody present, detects the percentage of erythrocytes bound with antibody, and can thus be used to monitor response to therapy.

Antibodies against erythrocytes are sometimes classified as either warm, which is common, or cold reactive, which is rare. Warm antibodies react most strongly at body temperature, and cold antibodies react more strongly at cold temperatures. Cold agglutinin disease may result in red blood cell agglutination in distal extremities such as the tips of the ear pinnae, tail tip, nose, and digits, with subsequent obstruction of small vessels and necrosis. Hemolytic anemia is sometimes associated with this syndrome, which has been described in the dog and cat.

Clinical Signs and Laboratory Findings

Clinical signs are variable and often include lethargy, splenomegaly, fever, and icterus, as well as other general signs associated with anemia, such as pale mucous membranes, dyspnea, tachycardia, and systolic heart murmur if the anemia is severe. If the anemia is acute, animals may present in a state of collapse, whereas animals with a more chronic onset may accommodate to the anemia, and show much less severe clinical signs.

Laboratory findings vary, but always include a decreased packed cell volume, red blood cell count, and hemoglobin concentration. If intravascular hemolysis is present, hemoglobinemia, hemoglobinuria, hyperbilirubinemia, and bilirubinuria may be present. Additionally, the hemoglobin concentration may be falsely increased relative to the packed cell volume, thus falsely increasing the MCHC. Blood film examination almost always reveals spherocytosis, which is the most diagnostically useful laboratory finding in these patients.

Agglutination may be present, and platelet concentration is commonly decreased because of concurrent immune mediated destruction (Evans Syndrome) or secondary disseminated intravascular coagulopathy (DIC). Agglutination may be differentiated from rouleaux formation by mixing a small quantity of blood with a drop of isotonic saline; agglutination will persist in the presence of saline while rouleaux formation will disperse. Agglutination may be so marked that it can be seen grossly on the blood film or on the side of the EDTA tube. If agglutination is present, the MCV may be falsely increased, since agglutinated red cells (doublets and triplets) may be counted as large cells (see Chapter 1). The MCV may also be increased if reticulocytosis is present.

The leukogram is almost always inflammatory, with a mature neutrophilia, increased bands, and monocytosis. This inflammatory response was once thought to be due to release of colony stimulating factors from activated macrophages. More recently, the degree of neutrophilia, as well as increased immature neutrophils, has been found to correlate with the amount of tissue damage secondary to hypoxia and thromboembolic disease.

Azotemia may be present, either pre-renal, or if intravascular hemolysis is severe, renal. Free hemoglobin binds to haptoglobin, but when the available haptoglobin is saturated, hemoglobinuria secondary to hemoglobinemia occurs. Acute renal failure may be due to either erythrocyte membrane antigen-antibody complex deposition or direct toxicity of free hemoglobin to renal tubular cells.

Bone marrow aspiration is usually not indicated in IMHA, but may be performed in patients in which the anemia is non-regenerative. In these cases, an apparent maturation arrest of the erythroid series, often at the rubricyte stage, may be present, presumably due to destruction of more mature forms of erythrocytes. Metarubricytes and polychromatophilic erythrocytes are often decreased to absent in the marrow from such patients, and occasionally, increased erythrophagocytosis and phagocytosis of nucleated erythrocytes may be observed.

Because both subclinical and clinical DIC are commonly associated with IMHA, other laboratory tests that may be abnormal are those that are used to diagnose DIC, including a prolonged activated partial thromboplastin time, prolonged one-stage prothrombin time, decreased antithrombin activity, increased fibrin(ogen) degradation products concentration, and increased D-dimer concentration.

Differential Diagnoses

Immune mediated hemolytic anemia can usually be easily differentiated from other types of hemolytic anemia by the presence of spherocytes in IMHA. However, spherocytes occasionally may be seen in dogs with rattlesnake envenomation *(Fig. 8.8)*. Although spheroechinocytes and type III echinocytes are seen commonly in dogs with rattlesnake envenomation (see Chapter 5), rarely, spherocytes may be present after the echinocytic changes have disappeared. It is unclear whether the rattlesnake envenomated dogs with spherocytes have immune mediated hemolytic anemia, or if the spherocyte formation is simply a result of membrane alterations secondary to the phospholipase present in the snake venom. Spherocytes, along with spheroechinocytes

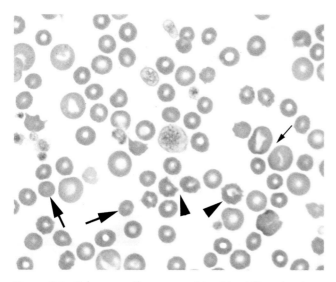

Figure 8.8 Spherocytes (large arrows) in a blood film taken from a dog several days following rattlesnake envenomation. The dog previously had echinospherocytes and some spiculated erythrocytes remain (arrowheads). The anemia is regenerative, as indicated by the polychromatophilic erythrocytes (small arrow). The dog is recovering from thrombocytopenia; a giant "young" platelet is in the center of the field. Wright stain.

and type III echinocytes, may also be observed in horses with clostridial infections presumably as a result of the bacterial phospholipase hydrolyzing erythrocyte membrane phospholipids (sphingomyelin and lecithin), producing lysolecithin, an echinogenic agent. These cases may be confusing, as clostridial infections in horses have been associated with immune mediated hemolytic anemia, diagnosed by the presence of spherocytes, autoagglutination, and positive Coombs' test. However, clostridial organisms also can directly induce hemolysis through the release of toxins. It is also possible that phospholipases may be able to induce immune-mediated hemolysis, likely as a result of attachment of antibody to altered erythrocyte membranes.

Immune mediated hemolytic anemia may be mistakenly diagnosed in horses with Heinz body anemia, possibly because collapse of the erythrocyte membrane following eccentrocyte formation results in erythrocytes that appear similar to spherocytes. However, an alternative explanation is that immune mediated destruction of erythrocytes with spherocyte formation may actually occur, since Heinz body formation may result in band-3 clustering with secondary antibody attachment. Spherocyte formation in cases of bee sting envenomation may be due to mellitin, a band-3 clustering agent, or phospholipase, both of which are present in bee venom. Band-3 clustering probably plays a significant role in immune mediated destruction of erythrocytes and spherocyte formation in these patients. Spherocyte formation secondary to band-3 clustering is also seen in dogs with zinc toxicosis. Interestingly, dogs with zinc toxicosis are Coombs' negative, and it has been hypothesized that during the erythrocyte washing process, zinc is removed, band 3 is returned to a dispersed distribution, and antibodies are eluted, resulting in a negative test. Finally, animals that have had incompatible blood transfusions may develop some degree of IMHA and spherocytosis, and animals that have fragmentation of erythrocytes may have spherocytosis, as the fragments may "round-up" and appear to be small spherocytes.

Prognosis

Mortality rates vary, and are reported to range from 25% to 50%. Although some reports suggest that dogs that are auto-agglutinating or have intravascular hemolysis have the highest mortality, this is controversial. Thromboembolism is a common finding in dogs that die. Recurrence of IMHA, or other immune mediated disorders such as immune mediated thrombocytopenia, is relatively common.

Therapy

Treatment of dogs consists of glucocorticosteroids (usually prednisone, 1–2 mg/kg per os every 12 hours), which decreases antibody production, T-cell activity, and diminishes macrophage function. Dexamethasone is often used in horses, and has been reported to be effective in cattle. Disadvantages of glucocorticoids include predisposing patients to infection, thromboembolic disease, and polyuria and polydipsia. Combination treatment may be warranted in dogs that are not responsive to or are intolerant of glucocorticoids. Therapeutic modalities may include azathioprine, danazol, cyclosporine, cyclophosphamide, bovine hemoglobin solution, or human immunoglobulin. However, in one retrospective study, no difference in mortality was detected between the use of multiple immunosuppressive agents and the use of glucocorticoids alone, and in fact the risk of death was slightly lower (30%) with glucocorticoids alone than the overall mortality rate of 50%. In addition, the use of cyclophosphamide and bovine hemoglobin solution has been associated with increased risk of death, and may be contraindicated. Danzol, a synthetic androgen, and cyclosporine, an immune response inhibitor, have been reported to be of no benefit with respect to reducing mortality. Some immunosuppressive drugs, other than the glucocorticoids, may injure marrow, resulting in a transient loss of regenerative response, and some drugs may not be effectively metabolized with severe anemia, making them more toxic than usual. Fluid therapy is indicated, particularly in patients with intravascular hemolysis, and lactic acidosis secondary to anemia should be corrected. Dogs usually respond to glucocorticoid therapy within one week, although anecdotal information suggests that dogs with antibody directed against erythrocyte precursors may take longer to respond. The dosage of glucocorticoids is gradually decreased once the PCV increases, and can sometimes be discontinued two or three months after the PCV returns to normal. In some cases, however, low dose therapy (0.5 mg/kg per os every other day) with prednisone or prednisolone may be required indefinitely. Blood transfusions should be given only when absolutely necessary, due to a life-threatening anemia. Splenectomy is usually not helpful long term, and removal of the spleen results in decreased erythropoietic tissue and may predispose dogs to *Mycoplasma haemocanis* infection.

Neonatal Isoerythrolysis

Neonatal isoerythrolysis (NI) is a form of immune mediated hemolytic anemia that occurs in newborn animals secondary to maternal antibodies against the neonate's blood-group antigen attaching to the neonate's erythrocytes, with subsequent erythrocyte hemolysis. The maternal antibodies are usually produced after sensitization of the mother with blood-group-incompatible erythrocytes, usually from the blood of a previous fetus gaining access to maternal circulation, but sometimes from vaccinations that contain erythrocytes or from mismatched blood transfusions. The disorder is most common in horse and mule foals, but occurs in less than 1% of thoroughbreds. The disorder rarely occurs in puppies, kittens, piglets, and calves. Cats are unique, in that antibodies against kitten erythrocytes can be produced with no previous exposure of the queen to incompatible erythrocytes. In domestic animals, the maternal antibody gains access to the neonate's blood following ingestion of antibody containing colostrum. Hemolytic anemia has been reported in lambs fed bovine colostrum during the first few days of life, and the anemia appears to be immune-mediated.

Affected animals are normal at birth, but within 24 to 48 hours they become weak, lethargic, pale, and anemic, with icterus and dyspnea. Hemoglobinemia and hemoglobinuria may be present, as well as splenomegaly and hepatomegaly. Thrombocytopenia and DIC may also occur.

In foals, approximately 90% of all cases of NI are attributable to the Aa or Qa antigen, but other antigens may be involved. The occurrence in mule foals may be due to a xenoantigen. It is possible that all mule pregnancies (donkey sire × horse dam) are incompatible with regard to this factor and a potential for NI exists in all cases.

Laboratory Diagnosis.

Diagnosis is usually made by confirming the presence of maternal antibodies on the neonate's erythrocytes by a Coombs' or a hemolytic test. Blood from pregnant mares can be tested 2 weeks prior to foaling for the presence of antibodies in order to predict the likelihood of neonatal isoerythrolysis in the foal. If the dam is sensitized, then her colostrum can be withheld from the foal for the first 48 hours of life, substituting another mare's colostrum.

Treatment

Treatment consists of blood transfusion if the animal is severely anemic. If the mare's blood is used, the erythrocytes must be washed extensively to remove antibody-containing plasma. Glucocorticoids may be helpful in reducing the rate of clearance of antibody coated erythrocytes.

Erythrocyte Parasites

Microorganisms that directly infect erythrocytes may result in intravascular hemolysis or extravascular hemolysis, and some may not cause hemolytic anemia. Traditionally, hemoparasites have been detected by examination of blood films. However, the development of highly sensitive and specific polymerase chain reaction (PCR) assays to detect small quantities of organisms has made diagnosis much more accurate for many of these diseases, in some cases even before the onset of clinical signs. The majority of the hemoparasites cause anemia by immune mediated extravascular hemolysis. Antibody against the organism, immune complexes, or complement bind to erythrocytes resulting in phagocytosis by macrophages. However, *Babesia* and *Theileria* species cause intravascular hemolysis. Specific hemoparasites are discussed below.

Hemotrophic Mycoplasmas (*Haemobartonella* and *Eperythrozoon* spp)

Haemobartonella and *Eperythrozoon* spp are pleomorphic bacteria that parasitize erythrocytes of many domestic animal species. These organisms are small, lack a cell wall, and stain gram-negatively. They adhere loosely to the surface of the erythrocyte membrane, and in many species, fall off easily, therefore appearing in the plasma. They were originally assigned either to the genus *Haemobartonella* or *Eperythrozoon* on the basis of whether they occurred more commonly as "ring forms," and whether they were found free in the plasma. If they fulfilled both of the previous criteria, they were assigned to the genus *Eperythrozoon*. These characteristics are now considered to be weak and arbitrary. These organisms were formerly classified as rickettsia, but based on sequence analysis of the 16S rRNA gene, they have been reclassified as members of the genera *Mycoplasma*.

Two strains of the organisms previously called *Haemobartonella felis* have been recognized; the large Ohio strain, which is considered most pathogenic, and a smaller California strain, the pathogenicity of which remains unclear. The Ohio strain has been renamed *Mycoplasma haemofelis*, and the smaller California strain has been named *Candidatus Mycoplasma haemominutum*. *Haemobartonella canis* has been renamed *Mycoplasma haemocanis*. *Eperythrozoon suis*, *E. wenyoni*, and *E. ovis* have been renamed *Mycoplasma haemosuis*, *M. wenyonii*, and *Candidatus Mycoplasma ovis*, respectively. The eperythrozoon in alpacas, previously not named, has been named *Candidatus Mycoplasma haemolamae*. It is presumed that this is the same organism that occurs in llamas (personal communication, Dr. Joanne Messick). The designation *Candidatus* is reserved for incompletely described members of taxa, to give them provisional status, and is eventually dropped.

Mycoplasma haemofelis. *Mycoplasma haemofelis*, formerly known as *Haemobartonella felis*, appears as small (0.5 µm) dark blue rods or ring forms on the surface of erythrocytes; it is more easily seen at the feathered edge of the blood film where the erythrocytes are flattened *(Fig. 8.9)*. Agglutination of erythrocytes may be present, as the presence of the organism on erythrocytes results in an immune mediated hemolytic anemia. *Mycoplasma haemofelis* is

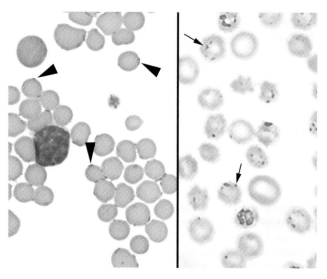

Figure 8.9   Left panel: Blood film from an anemic cat with *Mycoplasma haemofelis* (arrowheads), previously known as *Haemobartonella felis*. Right panel: Erythrocyte parasites are sometimes mistakenly diagnosed when artifacts are on erythrocytes (arrows). Artifacts may be caused by stain precipitate or staining the blood film before it is dry. Wright stain.

quite pathogenic, and can cause severe, sometimes fatal, hemolytic anemia. It is transmitted through infected blood, presumably by blood feeding arthropods such as fleas and ticks, cat bites, and iatrogenic exposure, and is present throughout the world. The organism is also transmitted from queens to kittens, either in utero, at birth, or by nursing. The parasitemia is intermittent, making diagnosis by blood film examination sometimes difficult. A PCR assay is available that is more diagnostically sensitive than blood film examination.

Clinical signs include those of anemia, splenomegaly, fever, lethargy, and sometimes icterus. Concurrent disease, immunosuppression, or splenectomy may predispose animals to acute infection. The anemia is regenerative unless underlying disease, often related to feline leukemia virus, is present that would inhibit erythropoiesis. Infected cats should be examined for the presence of feline leukemia virus and Feline Immunodeficiency Virus.

Treatment consists of blood transfusion if the anemia is severe. Prednisone (2 mg/kg per os every 12 hours) will suppress the immune mediated destruction of erythrocytes. Doxycycline (2–5 mg/kg per os every 12 hours for three weeks) is effective against the organism, but cats that recover often become latent carriers. Toxicity of doxycycline may include fever, gastrointestinal disturbances, and rarely, esophageal stricture formation. Enrofloxacin (5–10 mg/kg per os every 24 hours) a fluoroquinolone anti-*Mycoplasma* antibiotic, has been shown to be effective against *Mycoplasma haemofelis*, but a rare complication is acute blindness.

Mycoplasma haemocanis. *Mycoplasma haemocanis,* formerly known as *Haemobartonella canis,* is an opportunistic organism, usually causing disease only in splenectomized or severely immunosuppressed dogs. It is closely related phylogenetically to *Mycoplasma haemofelis,* with 99% homology of the 16SrRNA gene. Dogs that are splenectomized develop active infections if they are transfused with infected blood, or if they have latent infections. Active infection may manifest days to weeks after splenectomy. The microorganism appears somewhat different than *Mycoplasma haemofelis,* in that they appear as small chains of cocci across the surface of the erythrocyte. The chain commonly branches, and appears Y-shaped *(Fig. 8.10).* Clinical signs include those of anemia, and icterus is rarely present. Treatment consists of 5 mg/kg doxycycline orally twice daily for 3 weeks.

Haemoplasmas of Ruminants

Mycoplasma wenyonii, formerly known as *Eperythrozoon wenyonii,* also occurs worldwide, and similar to *Mycoplasma haemocanis* in dogs, usually only causes severe anemia in immunosuppressed or splenectomized cattle. The organism may be transmitted iatrogenically, by using the same syringe and needle in multiple animals in feedlot situations. Very large numbers of organisms can be seen on blood films, many of which are free in the plasma, in cattle that are not anemic *(Fig. 8.11).* However, a syndrome has been recognized in cattle that are heavily parasitized, which includes dependent edema and lymphadenopathy. Although the haemoplasma of sheep and goats, formerly known as *Eperythrozoon ovis*

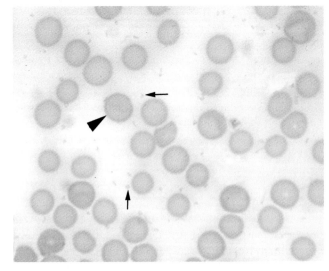

Figure 8.11 Blood film from a cow with hind limb and teat edema. Many *Mycoplasma wenyonii* (previously *Eperythrozoon wenyonii*) organisms are present in the background (small arrows). Polychromasia (arrowhead) is present, indicating regeneration. Wright stain.

(Fig. 8.12) is generally considered nonpathogenic in adults, its role as a cause of anemia in lambs is controversial. It will be renamed *Mycoplasma ovis.*

Mycoplasma haemosuis. *Mycoplasma haemosuis,* formerly known as *Eperythrozoon suis,* is pathogenic in very young pigs, as well as pigs that have been splenectomized, causing severe hemolytic anemia and sometimes death. In older animals, infection is associated with poor weight

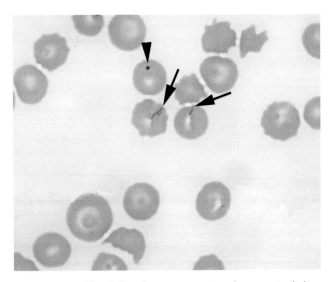

Figure 8.10 Blood film from an anemic splenectomized dog. Note the presence of *Mycoplasma haemocanis* (arrows) (previously *Haemobartonella canis*). Howell-Jolly bodies (arrowhead) are usually increased in splenectomized animals. Wright stain.

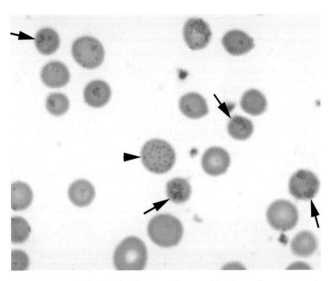

Figure 8.12 Blood film from a sheep with *Eperythrozoon ovis* (arrows). This organism will be renamed *Mycoplasma ovis.* Wright stain.

gain. The organisms appear similar to those in cattle, with many free organisms present on blood films *(Fig. 8.13)*. Baby pigs are usually treated with a single dose of long acting oxytetracycline (25 mg). Tetracycline is sometimes added to hog food to prevent the acute form of the disease.

Candidatus mycoplasma haemolamae. Haemoplasmas in llamas and alpacas appear to be opportunists that proliferate in animals doing poorly, and usually only cause a mild anemia. The organism appears similar to that in cattle *(Fig. 8.14)*.

Anaplasmosis

Bovine anaplasmosis caused by the intraerythrocytic rickettsia *Anaplasma marginale* is the most prevalent tickborne disease of cattle worldwide. *Anaplasma centrale* occurs in south America, the Middle East, and South Africa, and is less pathogenic. *A. marginale* has also been reported in deer, elk, and bison. *Anaplasma ovis* has been reported in goats and sheep, and causes hemolytic anemia. The organism appears similar to *A. marginale*. The organisms are transmitted by ticks, biting flies, and iatrogenically. *Anaplasma marginale* appears as a small (0.5–1 μm) dark blue inclusion on the margin of erythrocytes *(Fig. 8.15)*. *Anaplasma centrale* appears similar, but is located in a more central appearing location on erythrocytes. Infection with the organism can cause a fatal hemolytic anemia; older animals are usually more severely affected. The mechanism of anemia may be immune mediated. Untreated cattle that survive may become chronic carriers. Diagnosis can be made by PCR assays, as well as examination of blood films. Therapy consists of long acting

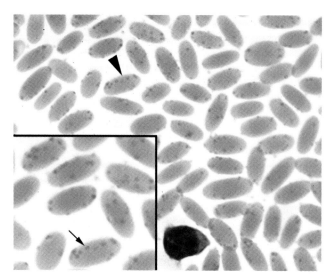

Figure 8.14 Blood film from a poor-doing llama with *Candidatus Mycoplasma haemolamae* (arrowheads), formerly *Eperythrozoon spp.* Higher magnification of the organisms (arrow) is shown in inset. Wright stain.

oxytetracycline, but. the most efficient method to control anaplasmosis is by vaccination using live *Anaplasma centrale*, which is capable of inducing significant protection against the more virulent *A. marginale*.

Babesiosis

Several species of *Babesia* cause hemolytic anemia and thrombocytopenia in domestic animals. *Babesia canis* and *B. gibsoni* are pathogenic in dogs, *B. bovis* and *B. bigemina* as well as other less important babesia infect cattle,

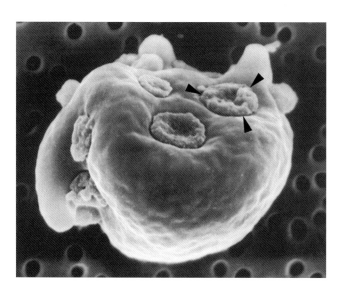

Figure 8.13 Electron micrograph of *Mycoplasma haemosuis* (arrowheads), formerly *Eperythrozoon suis*. Photograph provided by Dr. Joanne Messick.

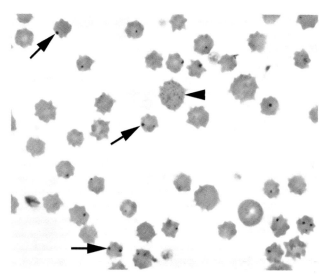

Figure 8.15 Blood film from an anemic cow with *Anaplasma marginale* (arrows). Note the basophilic stippling in the large polychromatophilic erythrocyte (arrowhead). Wright stain.

B. equi and *B. caballi* occur in horses, *B. ovis* and *B. motasi* infect sheep, and *B. cati*, *B. felis*, *B. herpailuri*, and *B. pantherae* infect cats. The disease is usually referred to as piroplasmosis in horses. Babesia are hemoprotozoan organisms, many of which are in the process of being reclassified based on PCR assays and gene sequencing. Some organisms previously thought to be *Babesia* appear to be more closely related to *Theileria* spp., including the California isolate of *Babesia gibsoni*, and *B. equi*. Babesia are transmitted by various types of ticks, most cause intravascular and extravascular hemolysis, and pathogenicity is variable. Other mechanisms of transmission include transplacental transmission and blood contamination. *Babesia* spp. vary in appearance; both large forms and small forms have been described. Large forms of babesia include *B. canis*, *B. caballi*, and *B. bigemina*. The other babesia are small forms. Large forms (2–5 μm) appear as single, paired, or tetrad oval inclusions that stain lightly basophilic with an eccentric nucleus *(Fig. 8.16)*. Small forms (1–3 μm) of babesia appear as round organisms *(Figs. 8.17 and 8.18)*. Usually only a few erythrocytes on blood films contain organisms, and they tend to be concentrated at the feathered edge of the blood film.

Canine babesiosis is becoming more common in the United States. *B canis vogeli* is endemic in the southeastern United States, particularly in greyhounds, but it usually only causes severe hemolytic anemia and life-threatening disease in young dogs or dogs that are heavily parasitized. Another subspecies, *B. canis rossi*, is more pathogenic, and is in South Africa. A third subspecies, *B. canis canis,* is found in Europe and parts of Asia, and is intermediate in pathogenicity. *B gibsoni* is endemic in northern Africa, the Middle East, and southern Asia. A small babesia, originally thought to be *B. gibsoni,* was described in California dogs in 1991. This organism causes

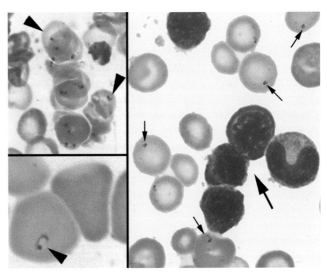

Figure 8.17 *Babesia gibsoni* in a bone marrow aspirate from a severely anemic Pit bull terrier from Kentucky. Aspirate provided by Antech Diagnostics, Inc. Wright stain.

severe disease, including hemolytic anemia, icterus, vasculitis, thrombocytopenia, hepatitis, glomerulonephritis, and reactive lymphadenopathy.

Since 1999 *B. gibsoni* has been reported in multiple states east of the Mississippi river, including North Carolina, Alabama, Georgia, Indiana, Wisconsin, Michigan, and Florida. At least some of these organisms have been distinct from the California organism. The disease is primarily seen in American pit bull terriers and Staffordshire terriers. Many dogs survive the acute phase and become chronic carriers. Prevention includes aggressive tick control. The high prevalence in the pit bull breed

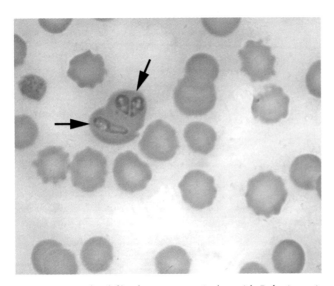

Figure 8.16 Blood film from an anemic dog with *Babesia canis* (arrows). Wright stain.

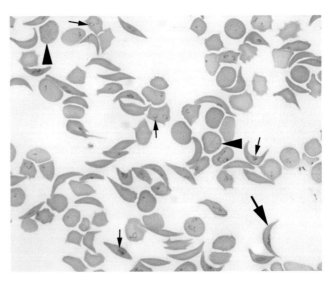

Figure 8.18 Babesia organisms in a deer (small arrows). Note that the erythrocytes have become sickle-shaped, which occurs in vitro (large arrow). Basophilic stippling is also present (arrowhead). Wright stain.

may be due to direct blood transmission. Babesiosis may be diagnosed by blood film or buffy coat film examination, but PCR is more sensitive and specific. Because most dogs are Coombs' positive, and many exhibit autoagglutination, a differential diagnosis is IMHA. Hyperglobulinemia, thrombocytopenia, and neutropenia are commonly observed, therefore ehrlichiosis must also be considered as a differential diagnosis, as these are common laboratory findings in that disease as well.

Treatment consists of imidocarb dipropionate (Imizol, Schering-Plough, Union, New Jersey). The recommended dosage is 6.6 mg/kg IM, repeated in two weeks. Diminazine aceturate is also effective, but is not available in the United States. Most dogs remain chronic carriers after therapy.

Theileriosis

Theileria parva, the cause of East Coast fever in Africa, and *T. annulata* are protozoans that may cause hemolytic anemia in cattle. The organisms are transmitted by ticks. Lymphocytes are first infected by sporozoites, which form schizonts *(Fig. 8.19)* from which the merozoites are released that infect erythrocytes. The organisms are small (1μm) and appear signet-ring or comma shaped. *Theileria lestoquardi* causes hemolytic anemia in sheep and goats of southern Europe, the Middle East, and northern Africa. Other, less pathogenic, species of *Theileria* may infect cattle, deer, and elk in North America.

Feline Cytauxzoonosis

Cytauxzoon felis is a protozoan that is classified within the same family as theileria. Like theileria, merozoites (piroplasms) infect erythrocytes, while a tissue phase, the schizonts, infect and fill macrophages within and surrounding blood vessels throughout the body. The disease was first described in 1948 in African ungulates, and was initially reported in cats from Missouri in 1976.

The disease is usually fatal, resulting in thrombosis of numerous vessels as a result of distended macrophages occluding vessels. Clinical findings include acute lethargy, anorexia, fever, and icterus. Although the organism causes a hemolytic anemia, the anemia is often non-regenerative, and may be accompanied by leukopenia and thrombocytopenia. Diagnosis is made by finding the signet-ring shaped piroplasms in erythrocytes in blood films relatively late in the course of the disease or by finding the schizonts in macrophages by cytologic examination of spleen, liver, lymph node or bone marrow aspirates *(Fig. 8.20)*. Several cats have survived *C. felis* infection; these cats were from the same geographic area and may have been infected with a less virulent strain.

The organism is transmitted by ticks; although erythroparasitemia may occur following blood inoculation, the tissue phase of the organism and disease do not develop. Bobcats, panthers, and cougars, which serve as natural reservoirs, usually have persistent asymptomatic infections, although bobcats occasionally have fatal disease. Fatal cytauxzoonosis has also been described in a Bengal tiger and White tiger. Anti-protozoal drugs such as dipropionate (Imizol) and diminazine aceturate (Ganaseg, Berenil) are occasionally effective against the organism, but diminazine is not available in the United States.

Heinz Body Anemia

Erythrocytes are particularly susceptible to oxidative damage, both because they carry oxygen and because

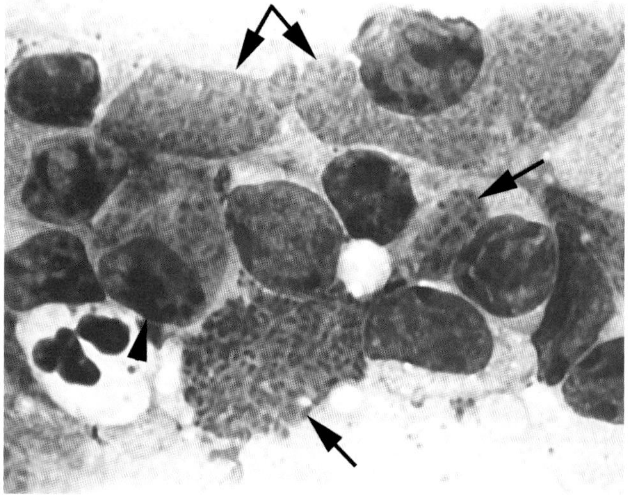

Figure 8.19 Lymph node aspirate from a cow with Theileriosis. Lymphocytes are filled with schizonts (arrows). Wright stain.

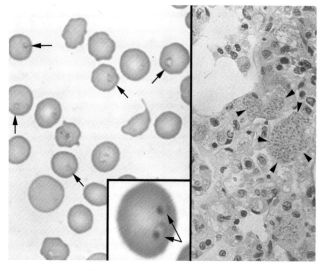

Figure 8.20 Left panel: Feline blood film with Cytauxzoon piroplasms in erythrocytes (arrows). Wright stain. Right panel: Cytauxzoon schizonts in macrophages of the same cat. H & E stain.

they may be exposed to various chemicals in plasma. Oxidants that are constantly generated include hydrogen peroxide (H_2O_2), superoxide free radical (O_2^-) and hydroxyl radicals (OH). When oxyhemoglobin is converted to methemoglobin (ferric state to ferrous state), superoxide radicals react with hydrogen peroxide, producing hydroxyl radicals. Formation of reversible and irreversible hemichromes then occurs. Reversible hemichromes include hemoglobin hydroxide and dihistidine ferrihemochrome. These reversible hemichromes can be converted back to methemoglobin and reduced hemoglobin. If irreversible hemichromes are formed, the hemoglobin denaturation continues, and aggregates of irreversible hemichromes are formed. These aggregates are called Heinz bodies, first recognized by Heinz in 1890 in humans and animals exposed to coal-tar drugs. Heinz bodies appear as small eccentric pale structures within the red cell and may protrude slightly from the red cell margin on Wright's stained blood films *(Fig. 8.21)*. They are usually large and single in cat erythrocytes *(Fig. 8.22)*, and small and multiple in dogs. When stained with vital stains such as new methylene blue or brilliant cresyl blue, Heinz bodies appear as blue structures (see Chapter 5).

The sulfhydryl groups on the globin portion of the molecule are also susceptible to oxidative damage, and although Heinz bodies may form by oxidation of these sulfhydryl groups, hemichrome formation is likely more important. Hemichromes have an affinity for membrane protein band 3. The protein band 3-hemichrome complex causes membrane protein band 3 to form clusters, both on

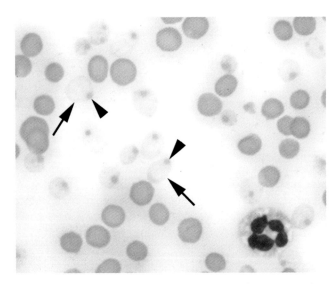

Figure 8.22 Blood film from an anemic cat with acetaminophen toxicosis. Note the lysed "ghost" erythrocytes (arrows). The Heinz bodies (arrowheads) are very apparent in the ghost cells. The pink background is due to hemoglobinemia. Wright stain.

the inside and outside of the erythrocyte membrane. This external clustering of protein band 3 creates a recognition site for auto-antibodies. Erythrocytes with attached antibody are then phagocytized by macrophages. The clustering of protein band 3 and associated auto-antibodies may be the best explanation for why animals with Heinz body formation may also have spherocyte formation and agglutination, such as has been described in zinc toxicosis and methylene blue toxicosis in dogs, and red maple leaf toxicosis in horses. Alternately, erythrocytes may have a spherocyte-like appearance because of collapse of the erythrocyte membrane following eccentrocyte formation. Some oxidants may affect the erythrocyte cytoskeleton, resulting in eccentrocyte formation without Heinz body formation. Features of eccentrocytes include shifting of hemoglobin to one side of the cell, loss of normal central pallor, and a clear zone outlined by a membrane *(Fig. 8.23)*.

In addition to formation of protein band 3-hemichrome complexes, spectrin-hemoglobin cross-linking also occurs, increasing erythrocyte membrane rigidity and decreasing deformability, ultimately making the erythrocyte more susceptible to removal. Heinz bodies may also be removed by the spleen, with the remaining portion of the erythrocyte returning to circulation. Hemichrome binding to the erythrocyte membrane also may stimulate proteolysis, contributing to breakdown of erythrocyte membrane integrity.

Oxidative injury occurs when enzymes and substrates used in the pathway to reverse oxidative processes are depleted, absent, or inhibited. Normally approximately three percent of the hemoglobin is oxidized to methemoglobin

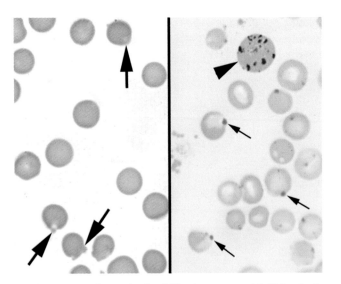

Figure 8.21 Left panel. Blood film from a cat with Heinz body anemia. Heinz bodies appear pale and are more apparent when they protrude from the edges of the erythrocytes (arrows). Wright stain. Right panel: Brilliant cresyl blue-stained blood film. Heinz bodies appear as medium-blue structures on the edges of the erythrocytes (arrows). A reticulocyte is also present (arrowhead).

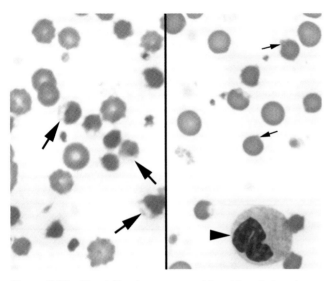

Figure 8.23 Blood film from a cow with oxidant-induced anemia. Note the eccentrocytes (large arrows), and Heinz bodies (small arrows). A neutrophil is present (arrowhead).

daily, but even that small amount is constantly being reduced back to hemoglobin by a reduced nicotinamide-adenine dinucleotide (NADH) dependent methemoglobin reductase enzyme within erythrocytes. Methemoglobin forms at higher concentrations when oxidative compounds are increased. Other enzymes also protect against oxidative damage to erythrocytes. These include superoxide dismutase (SOD), a zinc and copper containing enzyme that converts superoxide to hydrogen peroxide and water. Nicotinamide-adenine dinucleotide phosphate (NADPH) maintains glutathione in the reduced state, and glucose–6-phosphate dehydrogenase plays an important role in the initial steps of the pathway. Glutathione has an easily oxidizable sulfhydryl group that acts as a free-radical acceptor to counteract oxidant damage. Glutathione peroxidase catalyzes the conversion of hydrogen peroxide to water, producing oxidized glutathione, which is in turn reduced by glutathione reductase. Selenium is an important component of glutathione peroxidase. Finally, catalase is an enzyme that converts hydrogen peroxide to water and O_2 and may be more important than glutathione peroxidase.

Cats are considered to be more susceptible to Heinz body formation than other domestic species for a number of reasons, including differences in their hemoglobin structure, and normal cats commonly have a small percentage of circulating erythrocytes that contain Heinz bodies. Feline hemoglobin has eight sulfhydryl groups, compared with four in dogs and two in most other species. Many causes of oxidative damage to erythrocytes resulting in Heinz body or eccentrocyte formation have been reported, including oxidant drugs and chemicals, oxidant-containing plants, inherited enzyme deficiencies, and nutritional defi-

ciencies. Treatment depends on predisposing cause of Heinz body formation. Most of the oxidative compounds that result in Heinz body formation also cause methemoglobinemia, which when severe is characterized by brown discoloration of blood and cyanosis. These oxidants are discussed in more detail below.

Plants

Allium family (onions and garlic). Onion and garlic ingestion may result in Heinz body anemia and eccentrocyte formation in most species of domestic animals. Sources of onions and garlic include the feeding of cull onions to cattle and sheep, ingestion of wild onions by horses, and ingestion of raw, cooked, dehydrated onions, and baby food containing onion or garlic powder, by dogs and cats. The oxidative compounds in onions and garlic are aliphatic sulfides, specifically allyl and propyl di-, tri-, and tetrasulfides, with the allyl compounds being more potent than the propyl. These compounds decrease glucose-6 phosphate dehydrogenase activity in erythrocytes, which in turn curtails the regeneration of reduced glutathione needed to prevent oxidative denaturation of hemoglobin. Interestingly, the allyl derivatives are also thought to be effective in increasing tissue activities of cancer-protective enzymes such as quinone reductase (QR) and glutathione S-transferase (GST), thus decreasing the risk of cancer in humans who ingest these vegetables. Moreover, aged garlic extract is used to treat sickle cell anemia, because the extract is thought to contain antioxidants that prolong the life of sickle red blood cells.

Although the feeding of cull domestic onions (*Allium cepa*) appears to be reasonably safe in sheep, cattle may develop onion toxicosis. Sheep have been fed an exclusive onion diet, and although they initially developed a Heinz body hemolytic anemia with approximately 25% reduction in packed cell volume, there was no significant decrease in pregnancy or lambing rate, body condition, or fleece weight. Adaptation to an exclusive onion diet in sheep is thought to be due to a strong marrow response to the anemia, as well as modification of rumen metabolism of sulfoxides; one study showed that there was a marked increase in the number of sulfide-metabolizing bacteria (*Desulfovibrio spp*). Conversely, rumen microorganisms that convert sulfur containing amino acids to oxidants have been reported to exacerbate onion and *Brassica*-induced Heinz body anemia. One study showed that sheep fed onions (50 g/kg body weight/day) for 15 days developed more severe Heinz body hemolytic anemia than did the sheep fed the equivalent amount of onions with 5 g/day ampicillin sodium salt.

Feedlot cattle, on the other hand, can be fed a diet containing up to 25% cull onions on a dry-matter (DM) basis. Although a decrease in PCV occurs due to Heinz body-related hemolysis, the PCV returns to normal within 30 days after onion feeding is discontinued. Average daily gain and feed conversion ratios are not affected. It is thought, however, that the 25% (DM) probably approaches the toxic threshold for onion consumption in cattle. Onions should be mixed in a balanced ration, and cattle should not be allowed free access to the onions, as they may eat them preferentially.

Onion ingestion is the most common cause of Heinz body and eccentrocyte formation in dogs, and is a relatively common cause of clinical and subclinical anemia. In one study in which dogs were fed 5.5 g/kg body weight dehydrated onions, 70% of the erythrocytes contained Heinz bodies at 24 hours, and eccentrocytes were also common. Packed cell volume dropped approximately 20% by day 5. There appears to be some variation in individual susceptibility to the effects of onion ingestion in dogs. Erythrocytes with high concentrations of reduced glutathione, such as is seen in some Japanese shiba dogs, may be more susceptible to oxidative damage produced by onions. Garlic will also induce Heinz body and eccentrocyte formation in dogs.

Ingestion of onion soup and baby food containing onion powder has also been shown to produce Heinz body anemia in cats. In one study, as little as 0.3% onion powder significantly increased Heinz body formation; some commercial baby food may contain up to 1.8% onion powder on a dry weight basis.

Brassica (cabbage, kale, rape). Ingestion of plants belonging to *Brassica* species may result in Heinz body anemia in ruminants. These plants contain S-methyl-L-cysteine sulfoxide, which is metabolized to the oxidant dimethyl disulfide by rumen bacteria. *Brassica* species not only have a high sulfur content, which reduces copper availability, but also are low in copper and zinc concentration. While this copper deficiency may play a role in oxidative hemoglobin damage. Copper deficiency has not been shown to exacerbate susceptibility of lambs to brassica anemia. As with onion toxicosis, the severity of the Heinz body anemia is proportional to the quantity of *Brassica* in the diet. A maximum concentration of 30% DM for *Brassica* species consumption is recommended to avoid significant anemia.

Wilted red maple leaves (*Acer rubrum*). Severe Heinz body anemia and death in horses and zebras may be caused by ingestion of wilted or dried (not fresh) red maple leaves. Eccentrocyte formation and hemolysis may occur without concurrent Heinz body formation. Other findings commonly include methemoglobinemia, hemoglobinuria, hemoglobinuric nephrosis, and hepatic necrosis. The oxidative compound, which has not been discovered, causes a rapid depletion of glutathione; leaves are toxic when administered at doses of 1.5 gm/kg of body weight or more. Therapy consists of ascorbic acid, fluids, and blood transfusions, if necessary.

Drugs and Chemicals

Acetaminophen (paracetamol). Acetaminophen (Tylenol) ingestion is probably the most common cause of Heinz body anemia in cats. Owners, unaware of its toxic effects, often give the anti-inflammatory human drug to cats. Acetaminophen is metabolized in part by glucuronide conjugation; cats have limited ability to form acetaminophen glucuronides, probably due to very low activity of the liver enzyme acetaminophen UDP-glucuronosyltransferase, thus resulting in increased oxidant metabolites of acetaminophen. As a result, glutathione concentration is decreased and oxidative damage to erythrocytes occurs. Other findings commonly include methemoglobinemia, with associated brown discoloration of blood and cyanosis, and hepatic necrosis. The toxic dose of acetaminophen in cats is 50 to 60 mg/kg body weight. (One Extra Strength Tylenol Gelcap contains 500 mg acetaminophen, and one Extra Strength Excedrin contains 250 mg acetaminophen.) To confirm the diagnosis, acetaminophen concentrations can be determined on serum. Treatment consists of providing glutathione donors, such as N-acetylcysteine, orally. Acetaminophen-induced Heinz body anemia also occurs in dogs; the toxic dose is approximately 150 mg/kg body weight.

Propylene glycol. Propylene glycol, sometimes used as an additive in semi-moist pet food, causes Heinz body formation in cats, but does not cause an anemia when ingested in those small quantities. However, cats eating such diets may be more susceptible to other additional causes of oxidative injury. Even though overt anemia may not occur, red cells with Heinz bodies have a reduced life span.

Zinc. Ingestion of zinc containing materials, including pennies, which are 98% zinc by weight, other metal objects such as nuts and bolts in animal carriers, and zinc oxide containing ointments, have been reported to cause Heinz body anemia in dogs. The mechanisms by which zinc results in oxidative damage and Heinz body formation are unclear, but zinc is known to play a role in band-3 clustering. As a result of this clustering, opsonization of antibody and spherocyte formation may occur, resulting in the misdiagnosis of immune mediated hemolytic anemia.

Copper. Copper toxicosis in ruminants, especially sheep, results in Heinz body hemolytic anemia *(Fig. 8.24)*. Copper accumulates in the liver of animals ingesting high concentrations of copper. This copper is released follow-

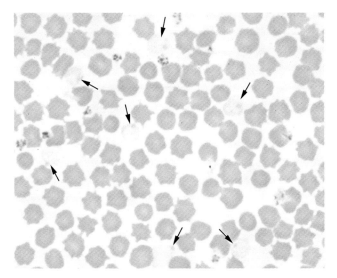

Figure 8.24 Blood film from a sheep with copper toxicosis. Note the Heinz bodies (arrows), which can be seen within "ghost" erythrocytes.

ing stress, resulting in a hemolytic crisis. Copper deficiency has also been associated with Heinz body formation.

Selenium deficiency. Selenium deficiency in ruminants, associated with grazing on selenium deficient soils in certain parts of the world, including New Zealand and the Florida everglades, has been associated with Heinz body anemia. Selenium deficiency has also been associated with reduced activity of glutathione peroxidase in erythrocytes of humans that live in selenium deficient areas, including New Zealand and Finland. It is speculated that reduced glutathione peroxidase activity may be the mechanism of the Heinz body anemia in selenium deficient cattle.

Methylene blue. Methylene blue was historically used as a urinary antiseptic in cats, and commonly resulted in Heinz body anemia with chronic administration. More recently, it has been associated with Heinz body anemia in river otters that were fed bait fish that had been kept in water containing methylene blue, which is used to detoxify ammonia in fish tanks. Interestingly, methylene blue is the drug of choice in the treatment of methemoglobinemia in humans and most domestic animals. There is no evidence to suggest that single therapeutic doses of methylene blue cause hemolytic anemia, even in cats.

Crude oil. Ingestion of crude oil by marine birds results in Heinz body anemia, one of the primary mechanisms of toxicity associated with the ingestion of crude oil by birds.

Other chemicals. Multiple other chemicals, such as naphthalene, a moth ball ingredient; propofol, an intravenous anesthetic; phenazopyridine, a urinary analgesic; pheno-

thiazine, an anthelmintic; ecabapide, a gastroprokinetic drug; benzocaine, a local anesthetic; and phenylhydrazine, an oxidative compound commonly used to experimentally induce hemolytic anemia, have been reported to cause Heinz body anemia.

Diseases

Heinz body formation is increased in specific disease states in cats and may contribute to anemia. Diabetes mellitus, hyperthyroidism, and lymphoma have been correlated with Heinz body formation. Diabetic cats in particular may have marked Heinz body formation. In one study, these diseases together accounted for nearly 40% of cats with Heinz body formation. Ketoacidotic cats had significantly more Heinz bodies than nonketotic diabetic cats. Percent Heinz bodies in diabetic cats is directly correlated with plasma beta-hydroxy-butyrate concentration, suggesting that ketones are associated with oxidative hemoglobin damage in cats. This may be a potential source of in vivo oxygen radical generation in animals with ketosis, such as may be seen in post parturient cattle.

Hypophosphatemia Induced Hemolysis

Severe hypophosphatemia, usually less than 1 mg/dl, has been reported to induce hemolysis in several species of animals, as well as humans. Erythrocyte glycolysis is inhibited by hypophosphatemia, primarily by decreasing intracellular phosphorus that is required for the enzyme glyceraldehyde phosphate dehydrogenase. This results in decreased glycolysis, leading to decreased erythrocyte ATP concentrations, and subsequent hemolysis. In some cases, this appears to be due to decreased glutathione, and increased susceptibility to oxidative injury. The most well recognized syndrome of hypophosphatemia induced hemolysis is post-parturient hemoglobinuria in cattle. Causes in small animals include hypophosphatemia related to diabetes, and enteral alimentation. Severe hypophosphatemia can be life-threatening, not only because of hemolysis, but also owing to depression of myocardial function, rhabdomyopathy, seizures, coma, and acute respiratory failure.

Post Parturient Hemoglobinuria

Post parturient hemoglobinuria in cattle is a sporadic disease of multiparous, high producing dairy cows characterized by intravascular hemolysis, anemia, and hemoglobinuria. It usually occurs within four weeks of calving. Most, but not all, cows with this syndrome are hypophosphatemic at the time of anemia. It is theorized that previous hypophosphatemia predisposes erythrocytes to injury and oxidative damage, primarily by decreasing

ATP and glutathione. Experimental hypophosphatemia (1 mg/dl) in post parturient cattle results in a decrease in erythrocyte ATP by 50% and a decrease in glutathione by 30%. The syndrome is complex, because some of the post parturient cattle with hemolytic anemia have Heinz body anemia, and some have ketoacidosis due to their nutritional status prior to and immediately following calving. Ketones are associated with oxidative hemoglobin damage, and may be a potential source of in vivo oxygen radical generation.

Hypophosphatemia in diabetic cats. Hypophosphatemia is sometimes present in diabetic animals, presumably because of phosphorus loss in the urine of polyuric animals. Several instances of hypophosphatemia-induced hemolysis have been reported in cats. Similar to the situation in cows with postparturient hemoglobinuria, diabetic cats may also be ketotic and have Heinz body anemia; in those cases, the hemolysis may be due to hypophosphatemia, ketosis, or a combination, since hypophosphatemia likely predisposes to Heinz body formation. Hypophosphatemia resulting in hemolytic anemia has also been reported in one cat with hepatic lipidosis.

Enteral alimentation in cats. A retrospective study of cats with hypophosphatemia revealed that hypophosphatemia can occur 12 to 72 hours after initiation of enteral alimentation. In this study, the nadir for phosphorus concentrations ranged from 0.4 to 2.4 mg/dl. Hemolysis occurred in 6 of the 9 cats that were hypophosphatemic. All cats had normal serum phosphorus concentrations prior to feeding. Hypophosphatemia also has been reported following oral tube feeding of human patients with anorexia nervosa.

Microorganisms (Other Than Erythrocyte Parasites)

Bacteria

Clostridial and leptospiral infections may result in hemolytic anemia. *Clostridium perfringens* Type A infection results in a hemolytic anemia in lambs and calves, sometimes referred to as "yellow lamb disease" or "enterotoxemic jaundice." The bacteria produces a phospholipase, which hydrolyses cell membrane phospholipids of erythrocytes, as well as those of other cells. Clinical signs include lethargy, fever, pale mucous membranes, anemia, hemoglobinuria, and icterus. Necropsy findings include evidence of intravascular hemolysis, renal hemoglobin casts, intestinal mucosal necrosis, hepatic necrosis, and petechial and ecchymotic hemorrhages. *Clostridium perfringens* has been associated with immune mediated hemolytic anemia in horses.

Clostridium haemolyticum and *C. novyi* Type D cause hemolytic anemia in cattle that is sometimes referred to as "bacillary hemoglobinuria" or "red water disease," which is acutely fatal. The disease occurs in summer and early fall, is associated with liver fluke migration, and is endemic in swampy areas of numerous countries, including the United States. The disease is rarely recognized antemortem. Clinical signs include those of anemia, lethargy, arched back, bloody diarrhea, fever, dyspnea, and occasionally hemoglobinuria. Bacterial spores are ingested and reside in macrophages of the liver. Anaerobic conditions within the liver, resulting from liver fluke migration, result in growth of the bacteria and production of toxic enzymes, including lecithinase, that metabolize lipids and protein in cell walls. Hemolysis and necrosis of other cells, including endothelial cells and hepatocytes, result in death. Necropsy findings include pale and icteric mucous membranes, foci of hepatic necrosis, hemorrhages, thoracic and abdominal effusion, hemoglobinuria, renal hemoglobin casts, and edema.

Leptospirosis (*Leptospira pomona*) may cause hemolytic anemia in young calves and lambs, but is almost never a feature of the disease in adult animals, nor does leptospirosis cause hemolytic anemia in dogs. The mechanism of the anemia may be toxins produced by the bacteria which act as hemolysins, but is more likely an immune mediated hemolytic anemia, probably IgM mediated. Necropsy findings in lambs include icterus, hemoglobinuria, renal tubular necrosis with hemoglobin casts, and hepatocellular necrosis.

Viruses

The equine infectious anemia (EIA) virus may result in hemolytic anemia in the acute stage of the disease. The anemia is likely immune mediated as a result of the virus binding with the erythrocyte membrane and activating complement. Later in the disease the anemia is nonregenerative, and may be similar to anemia of inflammatory disease. Equine infectious anemia is also referred to as "swamp fever." Diagnosis is made by detecting antibody against the EIA virus, using a Coggins test or a competitive ELISA test.

Water Intoxication Induced Hemolysis In Calves

Water intoxication resulting in hemolysis, hemoglobinuria, pulmonary edema, brain edema, convulsions, coma, and death may occur in calves that have unlimited access to water following its unavailability. Water intoxication may cause death within two hours, but most calves survive with no permanent ill effects. Cause of hemolysis is decreased osmolality of plasma. It has been theorized that water intoxication induced hemolysis occurs in calves from 4 to 5 months of age because osmotic fragility of their erythrocytes is greatest at that age, possibly related to the residual presence of iron deficient erythrocytes.

Hereditary Membrane Defects and Metabolic Disorders

Either inherited membrane defects or enzyme deficiencies leading to metabolic disorders may result in hemolytic anemia. Inherited erythrocyte membrane defects reported in domestic animals include hereditary spherocytosis, hereditary elliptocytosis, hereditary stomatocytosis, and membrane transport defects. However, hereditary elliptocytosis in dogs, which is caused by a hereditary protein 4.1 deficiency, results in increased osmotic fragility, elliptocytosis, membrane fragmentation, microcytosis, and poikilocytosis, but does not result in anemia.

Membrane Defects

Hereditary spherocytosis results in hemolytic anemia, spherocytosis, and splenomegaly. Hereditary spherocytosis has been reported in people, mice, and cattle. In cattle, HS is due to hereditary band 3 deficiency, an autosomal dominant trait that has been reported in Japanese black cattle. Band 3 protein is the most abundant protein in mammalian erythrocyte membranes, and functions include anion exchange across the membrane, as well as maintenance normal erythrocyte shape. Cattle homozygous for the trait lack band 3 protein in their erythrocyte membranes, have a mild anemia, spherocytosis, hyperbilirubinemia, splenomegaly, and growth impairment. The disease is more severe in calves; adults are relatively normal. Heterozygotes have a partial deficiency of band 3, mild spherocytosis, and compensate for their hemolytic anemia with increased erythrocyte regeneration.

Hereditary stomatocytosis has been reported in miniature schnauzers, chondrodysplastic Alaskan malamutes, and in the Drentse partrijshond breed of dogs that also have hypertrophic gastritis (see Chapter 5). These disorders have different underlying causes in these three breeds, and the schnauzers do not have anemia, although their red cell survival time is slightly shortened.

A Coombs' negative chronic intermittent hemolytic anemia has been reported in Abyssinian and Somali cats. Clinical signs and laboratory findings include mild to severe anemia, splenomegaly, increased MCV, and the presence of a few stomatocytes. Osmotic fragility of erythrocytes is markedly increased. Some of the cats improved following splenectomy. The specific cause of the hemolytic anemia is not known, but a membrane defect is suspected.

Animals with erythrocyte membrane transport defects, especially those with defects in transport of amino acids involved in glutathione metabolism, may develop hemo-

lytic anemia (Heinz body anemia) when exposed to oxidants. Some Finnish Landrace sheep have red cell glutathione deficiency, inherited as autosomal recessive. Cysteine uptake and glutathione synthesis are impaired, and glutathione concentration in erythrocytes is only 30% of normal. A similar defect is thought to be common in thoroughbred horses, but does not cause anemia. Some Japanese Shiba and Akita dogs have erythrocytes with high potassium, low sodium concentrations, due to retention of NA,K-ATPase in mature erythrocytes, inherited as an autosomal recessive trait. Some of these dogs have an increased concentration of reduced glutathione in their erythrocytes, which protects the cells against oxidative damage by acetylphenylhydrazine, but increases the risk of oxidative damage by onions (see Heinz body anemia).

Metabolic Disorders

Inherited erythrocyte enzyme defects result in abnormalities in metabolic pathways, often resulting in hemolytic anemia. Energy in mature mammalian erythrocytes is generated exclusively by anaerobic glycolysis, also known as the Embden-Meyerhof (EM) pathway, since they have lost their mitochondria, and thus their oxidative phosphorylation capabilities. Briefly, metabolism of glucose produces adenosine triphosphate (ATP), which is used to maintain erythrocyte shape, deformability, membrane transport, and synthesis of purines, pyrimidines, and glutathione. Many enzymes are involved in anaerobic glycolysis, including phosphofructokinase and pyruvate kinase. Deficiencies of both of these enzymes have been described in domestic animals.

Pyruvate kinase deficiency. Pyruvate kinase (PK) deficiency is the most common enzymopathy in humans, and was first recognized in Basenji dogs in 1971. Since that time, it has been reported in beagles, West Highland white terriers, Cairn terriers, miniature poodles, and various other breeds. Clinical signs include those of anemia, such as exercise intolerance. The anemia is very regenerative, and half or more of the erythrocytes on the blood film may be reticulocytes. The MCV may be markedly increased due to the reticulocytosis. Hepatosplenomegaly may be present. Affected dogs die of myelofibrosis or hepatic failure by 3 to 5 years of age. Myelofibrosis and osteosclerosis are a consistent finding in PK-deficient dogs, but do not develop in PK deficient people or cats. In certain breeds (Basenjis, West Highland white terriers) in which the mutation is specific, diagnosis can be made by PCR-based tests. Bone marrow transplantation has been shown to correct the disorder and prevent the development of osteosclerosis. Pyruvate kinase deficiency in cats has been described in various breeds, including Abyssinian, Somali, and domestic short hair cats. The anemia is mild to moderate, slightly to strongly regenerative; splenectomy reduces the severity of hemolytic anemia. Cats live to advanced age since osteosclerosis does not develop.

Phosphofructokinase deficiency. Phosphofructokinase (PFK) deficiency is a rare genetic disorder in humans, and has been described in English springer spaniels, an American cocker spaniel, and a mixed breed dog. The cocker spaniel had an ancestor that was bred in a kennel that also had English springer spaniels, and the mixed breed dog was thought to be part English springer spaniel. The mutation in all of these dogs was identical. It is inherited as an autosomal recessive trait, and is also referred to as glycogen storage disease type VII, since the enzyme deficiency also results in a lack of lactate production and accumulation of sugar phosphates and glycogen in muscle. Intermittent severe intravascular hemolysis is triggered by mild alkalemia; even mild respiratory alkalosis caused by hyperventilation and panting may precipitate a hemolytic crisis. Moreover 2,3-diphosphoglycerate (2,3-DPG), a compound that decreases the oxygen affinity for hemoglobin, thus making oxygen more available to tissues, is generated in the EM pathway. PFK deficiency results in a deficiency of 2,3-DPG, which results in tissue hypoxia of affected dogs. However, this tissue hypoxia stimulates erythropoietin production, and thus, except when in hemolytic crisis, these dogs are not anemic. Clinical signs include excitement or exercise-induced hemolytic anemia and occasional mild muscle cramping. Life expectancy can be normal if hemolytic crises are avoided. The disorder can be identified in affected dogs, as well as carriers, by a PCR-based DNA test that is specific for the English springer spaniel mutation.

Glucose-6-phosphate dehydrogenase deficiency. The pentose phosphate pathway (PPP) generates reduced nicotine adenine dinucleotide phosphate (NADPG), which is protective against mechanical and metabolic insults, particularly oxidants. Glucose 6-phosphate dehydrogenase (G6PD) is the rate-limiting enzyme in the PPP. In humans, G6PD deficiency is inherited as an X-linked disorder, which causes hemolytic anemia, particularly following exposure to oxidants. Hemolytic anemia caused by G6PD deficiency has been described in an American saddle bred colt, as well as a dog. Morphologic abnormalities in the colt included eccentrocytosis, and the colt's dam, which was a heterozygote for the disorder, also had eccentrocytes on her blood film.

Hereditary methemoglobinemia. Methemoglobin is not able to bind oxygen because the iron moiety of the heme group has been oxidized to the ferric state (see Heinz body anemia). Approximately 3% of hemoglobin is oxidized to methemoglobin each day, but this methemoglobin is reduced back to hemoglobin, primarily by the enzyme NADH-methemoglobin reductase. Inherited deficiencies of this enzyme have been described in numerous breeds of dogs and cats. This disorder does not cause significant problems in dogs and cats, other than increased risk associated with anesthesia. Glutathione reductase deficiency has been described in horses, and even in the absence of oxidants, resulted in a mild hemolytic anemia with eccentrocyte formation and methemoglobinemia. Horses in one report had normal methemoglobin reductase activity, but activity was reduced in a separate case.

Porphyrias. Hemoglobin synthesis occurs in erythroid precursors, where protoporphyrin, iron, and globin molecules are brought together and assembled into functional hemoglobin. Synthesis of the heme portion of the molecule is complex, and requires numerous enzymes. Inherited deficiencies of these enzymes result in an accumulation of porphyrin precursors, as well as a failure to adequately synthesis hemoglobin, and the disorders are known as erythropoietic porphyrias, which have been described in humans, cattle, swine, and cats. Some of the erythropoietic porphyrias result in hemolytic anemia. Hepatic porphyrias are caused by different enzyme deficiencies, and to date have been discovered only in humans; the liver is the site of synthesis for enzymes containing heme, such as catalase, cytochromes, and peroxidase.

Another inherited disorder, erythropoietic protoporphyria, is due to a defect of the enzyme heme synthetase (ferrochelatase). This disorder has been described in Limousin and Blonde d'Aquitaine cattle, and the only clinical manifestation is severe photosensitivity with intense pruritus. Anemia, porphyrinuria, and discolored teeth are not observed. Inheritance of erythropoietic protoporphyria is recessive in cattle and only occurs in homozygotes, unlike in humans in whom the heterozygous condition results in clinical signs.

Toxins, especially lead, may destroy many of the enzymes involved in the synthesis of heme. These toxicoses lead to a decrease in heme synthesis, as well as an excess of heme precursors, which are eliminated in increased concentration in the urine. These toxicoses are referred to as porphyrinurias.

Clinical signs associated with porphyrias vary, depending on the specific enzyme abnormality, and the amount of residual activity of the affected enzyme. Porphyrins are reddish-brown in color, have a characteristic red fluorescence when exposed to ultraviolet light, and stain various tissues, including teeth and bones; congenital erythropoietic porphyria in cattle was called "Pink Tooth" at one time. The porphyrins in these animals are excreted excessively in all body fluids, including urine, feces, saliva, sweat, and tears. One of the most common abnormalities is photosensitivity resulting in photodermatitis, particularly evident on light colored areas of the skin. This is due to excitation of porphyrins by ultraviolet light, and subsequent transfer of oxygen to tissues, causing oxidation of cellular lipids, proteins, and organelles.

Bovine congenital erythropoietic porphyria. Bovine congenital erythropoietic porphyria has been reported in Holsteins and Shorthorns, and is caused by a partial deficiency of uroporphyrinogen III cosynthetase (UROgenIII Cosyn), resulting in an accumulation of uroporphyrin I and coproporphyrin I, which accumulate in tissues, and are excreted in urine and feces in increased quantities. Clinical signs include pigmentation of tissues including teeth, anemia, and photosensitization. The disorder is inherited as an autosomal recessive trait. Affected animals have hemolytic anemia that is regenerative, and blood film findings are those of a regenerative anemia in cattle, including polychromasia, macrocytosis, anisocytosis, basophilic stippling, and increased nucleated erythrocytes. Affected calves have a particularly striking regenerative response, with many nucleated erythrocytes present. Erythrocyte life span is shortened, due to both the heme synthesis disorder, as well as the porphyrin-related damage to erythrocyte membrane lipids. Ultraviolet light may increase severity of hemolysis, due to exposure of erythrocytes while in surface capillaries. The disease has been almost completely eliminated in cattle.

Porphyria of cats. Two forms of porphyria have been described in cats. One type, described in a family of Siamese cats, is due to a partial deficiency of uroporphyrinogen III cosynthetase, and is similar to the disorder in humans and cattle. Affected cats had photosensitivity and severe hemolytic anemia, as well as renal disease. The renal disease was characterized by mesangial hypercellularity and proliferation and ischemic tubular injury. Membrane-enclosed lamellar bodies were present in cytoplasmic and extracellular locations of various tissues, similar to those seen in lysosomal storage disorders.

A second type of porphyria has been described in domestic cats in which the clinical signs are only discoloration of teeth and urine due to the presence of uroporphyrin, coproporphyrin, and porphobilinogen. Anemia and photosensitization are not present. The disorder in domestic cats is inherited as autosomal dominant.

Porphyria of swine. Porphyria of swine has been described in affected swine which have discoloration of teeth and excessive uroporphyrin in the urine. Affected swine are not anemic and photosensitization is not present. The specific defect is not known, and no animals are available for study. The disorder is inherited as autosomal dominant.

SUGGESTED READINGS

BLOOD LOSS

Acute Blood Loss

Gelberg H, Stackhouse LL. Three cases of canine acanthocytosis associated with splenic neoplasia. Vet Med Small Anim Clin 1977; 72:1183–1184.

Hirsch VM, Jacobsen J, Mills JH. A retrospective study of canine hemangiosarcoma and its association with acanthocytosis. Can Vet J 1981;22:152–155.

Ng CY, Mills JN. Clinical and haematological features of haemangiosarcoma in dogs. Aust Vet J 1985;62:1–4.

Rebar AH, Hahn FF, Halliwell WH, et al. Microangiopathic hemolytic anemia associated with radiation-induced hemangiosarcomas. Vet Pathol 1980;17:443–454.

Weiss DJ, Kristensen A, Papenfuss N. Qualitative evaluation of irregularly spiculated red blood cells in the dog. Vet Clin Pathol 1993; 22:117–121.

Chronic Blood Loss

Brommer H, van Oldruitenborgh-Oosterbaan MM. Iron deficiency in stabled Dutch warmblood foals. J Vet Intern Med 2000;15:482–485.

Bunch SE, Jordan HL, Sellon RK, et al. Characterization of iron status in young dogs with portosystemic shunt. Am J Vet Res 1995; 56:853–858.

Degen M. Pseudohyperkalemia in Akitas. J Am Vet Med Assoc 1987; 190:541–543.

Duval D, Mahaffey E. Predicted mean corpuscular volume as an indicator of bone marrow iron in anemic dogs. Vet Clin Pathol 1996; 25:95–98.

Easley JR. Erythrogram and red cell distribution width of Equidae with experimentally induced anemia. Am J Vet Res 1985;46:2378–2384.

Fulton R, Weiser MG, Freshman JL, et al. Electronic and morphologic characterization of erythrocytes of an adult cat with iron deficiency anemia. Vet Pathol 1988;25:521–523.

Gookin JL, Bunch SE, Rush LJ, et al. Evaluation of microcytosis in 18 Shibas. J Am Vet Med Assoc 1998;212:1258–1259.

Harvey JW, Asquith RL, Sussman WA, et al. Serum ferritin, serum iron, and erythrocyte values in foals. Am J Vet Res 1987;48:1348–1352.

Laflamme DP, Mahaffey EA, Allen SW, et al. Microcytosis and iron status in dogs with surgically induced portosystemic shunts. J Vet Int Med 1994;8:212–216.

Meyer DJ, Harvey JW. Hematologic changes associated with serum and hepatic iron alterations in dogs with congenital portosystemic vascular anomalies. J Vet Int Med 1994;8:55–56.

Morin DE, Garry FB, Weiser MG, et al. Hematologic features of iron deficiency anemia in llamas. Vet Pathol 1992;29:400–404.

Morin DE, Garry FB, Weiser MG. Hematologic responses in llamas with experimentally-induced iron deficiency anemia. Vet Clin Pathol 1993;22:81–86.

Murray SL, Lau KW, Begg A, Jacobs K. Myelodysplasia, hypophosphataemia, vitamin D and iron deficiency in an alpaca. Aust Vet J 2000;79:328–331.

Nathanson MH, Muir A, McLaren GD. Iron absorption in normal and iron-deficient beagle dogs: mucosal iron kinetics. Am J Physiol 1985;249:G439–448.

Ristic JM, Stidworthy MF. Two cases of severe iron-deficiency anaemia due to inflammatory bowel disease in the dog. J Small Anim Pract 2002;43:80–83.

Simpson KW, Meyer DJ, Boswood A, et al. Iron status and erythrocyte volume in dogs with congenital portosystemic vascular anomalies. J Vet Int Med 1997;11:14–19.

Weiser G, O'Grady M. Erythrocyte volume distribution analysis and hematologic changes in dogs with iron deficiency anemia. Vet Pathol 1983;20:230–241.

Weiser MG, Kociba GJ. Sequential changes in erythrocyte volume distribution and microcytosis associated with iron deficiency in kittens. Vet Pathol 1983;20:1–12.

BLOOD DESTRUCTION

Immune mediated hemolytic anemia

Breitschwerdt EB, Armstrong PJ, Robinette CL, et al. Three cases of acute zinc toxicosis in dogs. Vet Hum Toxicol 1986;28:109–117.

Brown DE, Meyer DJ, Wingfield WE, et al. Echinocytosis associated with rattlesnake envenomation in dogs. Vet Pathol 1994;31:654–657.

Burgess K, Moore A, Rand W, et al. Treatment of immune-mediated hemolytic anemia in dogs with cyclophosphamide. J Vet Int Med 2000;14:456–462.

Carr AP, Panciera DL, Kidd L. Prognostic factors for mortality and thromboembolism in canine immune-mediated hemolytic anemia: a retrospective study of 72 dogs. J Vet Intern Med 2002;16: 504–509.

Christian JA. Red blood cell survival and destruction. In: Feldman BF, Zinkl JG, Jain NC, Eds. Schalm's Veterinary Hematology, 5th ed. Philadelphia: Lippincott Williams & Wilkins, 2001;117–124.

Coombs RRA. History and evolution of the anti-globulin reaction and its application in clinical and experimental medicine. Am J Clin Path 1970;53:131–135.

Day TK, Macintire DK, Murtaugh RJ, et al. Differing opinions on treatment of immune-mediated hemolytic anemia. J Am Vet Med Assoc 2001;218:1414–1415.

Day MJ. Serial monitoring of clinical, haematological, and immunological parameters in canine autoimmune haemolytic anaemia. J Sm Anim Pract 1996;37:523–524.

Duval D, Giger U. Vaccine-associated immune-mediated hemolytic anemia in the dog. J Vet Int Med 1996;10:290–295.

Grundy SA. Barton C. Influence of drug treatment on survival of dogs with immune-mediated hemolytic anemia: 88 cases(1989–1999). J Am Vet Med Assoc 2001;218:536–543.

Jonas RD, Thrall MA, Weiser MG: Immune mediated hemolytic anemia with delayed erythrogenesis in the dog. J Am Anim Hosp Assoc 1987;23:201–204.

Klag AR, Giger U, Shofer FS. Idiopathic immune-mediated hemolytic anemia in dogs: 42 cases (1986–1990). J Am Vet Med Assoc 1993; 202:783–788.

Klein MK, Dow SW, Rosychuk RA. Pulmonary thromboembolism associated with immune-mediated hemolytic anemia in dogs: ten cases (1982–1987). J Am Vet Med Assoc 1989;195:246–250.

Latimer KS, Jain A, Inglesby HB, et al. Zinc-induced hemolytic anemia caused by ingestion of pennies by a pup. J Am Vet Med Assoc 1989; 195:77–80.

McManus PM, Craig LE. Correlation between leukocytosis and necropsy findings in dogs with immune-mediated hemolytic anemia: 34 cases (1994–1999). J Am Vet Med Assoc 2001;218:1308–1313.

Messer NT IV, Arnold K. Immune-mediated hemolytic anemia in a horse. J Am Vet Med Assoc 1991;198:1415–1416.

Mills JN, Day MJ, Shaw SE, et al. Autoimmune haemolytic anaemia in dogs. Aust Vet J 1985;62:121–123.

Noble SJ, Armstrong PJ. Bee sting envenomation resulting in secondary immune-mediated hemolytic anemia in two dogs. J Am Vet Med Assoc 1999;214:1026–1027.

Porter RE, Weiser MG. Effect of immune-mediated erythrocyte agglutination on analysis of canine blood using a multichannel blood cell counting system. Vet Clin Path 1990;19:45–50.

Reef VB. *Clostridium perfringins* cellulitis and immune-mediated hemolytic anemia in a horse. J Am Vet Med Assoc 1983;182:251–254.

Reimer ME, Troy GC, Warnick LD. Immune-mediated hemolytic anemia: 70 cases (1988–1996). J Am Anim Hosp Assoc 1999;35: 384–391.

Scott-Moncrieff JC, Reagan WJ, Snyder PW, et al. Intravenous administration of human immune globulin in dogs with immune-mediated hemolytic anemia. J Am Vet Med Assoc 1997;210:1623–1627.

Scott-Moncrieff JC, Treadwell NG, McCullough SM, et al. Hemostatic abnormalities in dogs with primary immune-mediated hemolytic anemia. J Am Anim Hosp Assoc 2001;37:220–227.

Stokol T, Blue JT, French TW. Idiopathic pure red cell aplasia and nonregenerative immune-mediated anemia in dogs: 43 cases (1988–1999). J Am Vet Med Assoc 2000;216:1429–1436.

Swenson C, Jacobs R. Spherocytosis associated with anaplasmosis in two cows. J Am Vet Med Assoc 1986;188:1061–1063.

Walton RM, Brown DE, Hamar DW, et al. Mechanisms of echinocytosis induced by *Crotalus atrox* venom. Vet Pathol 1997;34(5): 442–449.

Weiser MG, Thrall MA. Immune-mediated hemolytic anemia in dogs (letter). J Am Vet Med Assoc 1993;202:1786–1788.

Weiss DJ, Moritz A. Equine immune-mediated hemolytic anemia associated with *Clostridium perfringens* infection. Vet Clin Pathol 2003; 32:22–26.

Wilkerson MJ, Davis E, Shuman W, et al. Isotype-specific antibodies in horses and dogs with immune-mediated hemolytic anemia. J Vet Int Med 2000;14:190–196.

Wysoke JM, Bland van-den Berg P, Marshall C. Bee sting-induced haemolysis, spherocytosis and neural dysfunction in three dogs. J S African Vet Assoc 1990;61:29–32.

Neonatal isoerythrolysis

MacLeay JM. Neonatal isoerythrolysis involving the Qc and Db antigens in a foal. J Am Vet Med Assoc 2001;219:79–81.

McClure JJ, Koch C, Traub-Dargatz J. Characterization of a red blood cell antigen in donkeys and mules associated with neonatal isoerythrolysis. Anim Genet 1994;25:119–120.

Smith JE, Dever M, Smith J, et al. Post-transfusion survival of 50Cr-labeled erythrocytes in neonatal foals. J Vet Intern Med 1992; 6:183–185.

Traub-Dargatz JL, McClure JJ, Koch C, et al. Neonatal isoerythrolysis in mule foals. J Am Vet Med Assoc 1995;206:67–70.

Erythrocyte parasites

Haemotrophic mycoplasmas

Alleman AR, Pate MG, Harvey JW, et al. Western immunoblot analysis of the antigens of *Haemobartonella felis* with sera from experimentally infected cats. J of Clin Micro 1999;37:1474–1479.

Austerman JW. Haemobartonellosis in a nonsplenectomized dog. Vet Med Sm Anim Clin 1979;74:954.

Bellamy JE. MacWilliams PS. Searcy GP. Cold-agglutinin hemolytic anemia and *Haemobartonella canis* infection in a dog. J Am Vet Med Assoc 1978;173:397–401.

Berent LM, Messick JB, Cooper SK. Detection of *Haemobartonella felis* in cats with experimentally induced acute and chronic infections, using a polymerase chain reaction assay. Am J Vet Res 1998; 59:1215–1220.

Berent LM, Messick JB, Cooper SK, et al. Specific in situ hybridization of *Haemobartonella felis* with a DNA probe and tyramide signal amplification. Vet Pathol 2000;37:47–53.

Bobade PA, Nash AS, Rogerson P. Feline haemobartonellosis: clinical, haematological and pathological studies in natural infections and the relationship to infection with feline leukaemia virus. Vet Record 1988;122:32–36.

Brinson JJ, Messick JB. Use of a polymerase chain reaction assay for detection of *Haemobartonella canis* in a dog. J Am Vet Med Assoc 2001;218:1943–1945.

Carney HC, England JJ. Feline hemobartonellosis. Vet Clin of N Am—Sm Anim Pract 1993;23:79–90.

Dowers KL, Olver C, Radecki SV, et al. Use of enrofloxacin for treatment of large-form *Haemobartonella felis* in experimentally infected cats. J Am Vet Med Assoc 2002;221:250–253.

Foley JE, Harrus S, Poland A, et al. Molecular, clinical, and pathologic comparison of two distinct strains of *Haemobartonella felis* in domestic cats. Am J Vet Res 1998;59:1581–1588.

Grindem CB, Corbett WT, Tomkins MT. Risk factors for *Haemobartonella felis* infection in cats. J Am Vet Med Assoc 1990;196: 96–99.

Jensen WA, Lappin MR, Kamkar S, et al. Use of a polymerase chain reaction assay to detect and differentiate two strains of *Haemobartonella felis* in naturally infected cats. Am J Vet Res 2001; 62: 604–608.

Krakowka S. Transplacentally acquired microbial and parasitic diseases of dogs. J Am Vet Med Assoc 1977;171:750–753.

Lester SJ, Hume JB, Phipps B. *Haemobartonella canis* infection following splenectomy and transfusion. Can Vet J 1995;36:444–445.

MacWilliams PS. Erythrocytic rickettsia and protozoa of the dog and cat. Vet Clin N Am—Sm Anim Pract 1987;17:1443–1461.

Maede Y. Sequestration and phagocytosis of *Haemobartonella felis* in the spleen. Am J Vet Res 1979;40:691–695.

Messick JB, Cooper SK, Huntley M. Development and evaluation of a polymerase chain reaction assay using the 16S rRNA gene for detection of *Eperythrozoon suis* infection. J Vet Diag Invest 1999; 11:229–236.

Messick JB, Berent LM, Cooper SK. Development and evaluation of a PCR-based assay for detection of *Haemobartonella felis* in cats and differentiation of *H. felis* from related bacteria by restriction fragment length polymorphism analysis. J Clin Micro 1998;36:462–466.

Neimark H, Johansson KE, Rikihisa Y, et al. Proposal to transfer some members of the genera *Haemobartonella* and *Eperythrozoon* to the genus *Mycoplasma* with descriptions of 'Candidatus Mycoplasma haemofelis,' 'Candidatus Mycoplasma haemomuris,' 'Candidatus Mycoplasma haemosuis' and 'Candidatus Mycoplasma wenyonii.' Internat J Systemic Evolutionary Micro 200;51:891–899.

Pospischil A. Hoffmann R. Eperythrozoon suis in naturally infected pigs: a light and electron microscopic study. Vet Pathol 1982;19: 651–657.

Reagan WJ, Garry F, Thrall MA, et al. The clinicopathologic, light, and scanning electron microscopic features of eperythrozoonosis in four naturally infected llamas. Vet Pathol 1990;27:426–231.

Shelton GH, Linenberger ML. Hematologic abnormalities associated with retroviral infections in the cat. Sem Vet Med Surg (Sm Anim) 1995;10:220–233.

Smith JA, Thrall MA, Smith JL, et al. Eperythrozoon wenyonii infection in dairy cattle. J Am Vet Med Assoc 1990;196:1244–1250.

Stevenson M. Treatment for *Haemobartonella felis* in cats. Vet Record 1997;140:512.

Tasker S, Helps CR, Belford CJ, et al. 16S rDNA comparison demonstrates near identity between a United Kingdom *Haemobartonella felis* strain and the American California strain. Vet Micro 2001;81: 73–78.

VanSteenhouse JL, Taboada J, Dorfman MI. *Hemobartonella felis* infection with atypical hematological abnormalities. J Am Anim Hosp Assoc 1995;31:165–169.

Zulty JC. Kociba GJ. Cold agglutinins in cats with haemobartonellosis. J Am Vet Med Assoc 1990;196:907–910.

Babesiosis

Conrad PA, Thomford J, Yamane I, et al. Hemolytic anemia caused by *Babesia gibsoni* infection in dogs. J Am Vet Med Assoc 1991;199: 601–605.

Gaunt SD. Hemolytic anemias caused by blood rickettsial agents and protozoa. In: Feldman BF, Zinkl JG, Jain, NC eds. Schalm's Veterinary Hematology, 5th ed. Philadelphia: Lippincott Williams & Wilkins, 2001;154–162.

Irizarry-Rovira AR, Stephens J, Christian J, et al. *Babesia gibsoni* infection in a dog from Indiana. Vet Clin Pathol 2001;30:180–188.

Jacobson LS, Clark IA. The pathophysiology of canine babesiosis: new approaches to an old puzzle. J South African Vet Assoc 1994;65: 134–145.

Macintire DK, Boudreaux MK, West GD, et al. *Babesia gibsoni* infection among dogs in the southeastern United States. J Am Vet Med Assoc 2002;220:325–329.

Meinkoth JH, Kocan AA, Loud SD, et al. Clinical and hematologic effects of experimental infection of dogs with recently identified *Babesia gibsoni*-like isolates from Oklahoma. J Am Vet Med Assoc 2002;220:185–189.

Stegeman JR, Birkenheuer AJ, Kruger JM, et al. Transfusion-associated *Babesia gibsoni* infection in a dog. J Am Vet med Assoc 2003;222: 959–963.

Anaplasmosis

Shkap V, Molad T, Fish L, et al. Detection of the *Anaplasma centrale* vaccine strain and specific differentiation from *Anaplasma marginale* in vaccinated and infected cattle. Parasitol Res 2002;88:546–552.

Swenson C, Jacobs R. Spherocytosis associated with anaplasmosis in two cows. J Am Vet Med Assoc 1986;188:1061–1063.

Theileriosis

Stockham SL, Kjemtrup AM, Conrad PA, et al. Theileriosis in a Missouri beef herd caused by *Theileria buffeli*: case report, herd investigation, ultrastructure, phylogenetic analysis, and experimental transmission. Vet Pathol 2000;37:11–21.

Cytauxzoonosis

Garner MM, Lung NP, Citino S, et al. Fatal cytauxzoonosis in a captive-reared white tiger (*Panthera tigris*). Vet Pathol 1996;33:82–86.

Greene CE, Latimer K, Hopper E, et al. Administration of diminazene aceturate or imidocarb dipropionate for treatment of cytauxzoonosis in cats. J Am Vet Med Assoc. 1999;215:497–500.

Hoover JP, Walker DB, Hedges JD. Cytauxzoonosis in cats: eight cases (1985–1992). J Am Vet Med Assoc 1994;205:455–460.

Jakob W, Wesemeier HH. A fatal infection in a Bengal tiger resembling cytauxzoonosis in domestic cats. J Comp Pathol 1996;114:439–444.

Meier HT, Moore LE. Feline cytauxzoonosis: a case report and literature review. J Am Anim Hosp Assoc 2000;36:493–496.

Meinkoth J, Kocan AA, Whitworth L, et al. Cats surviving natural infection with *Cytauxzoon felis*: 18 cases (1997–1998). J Vet Intern Med 2000;14:521–525.

Nietfeld JC, Pollock C. Fatal cytauxzoonosis in a free-ranging bobcat (Lynx rufus). J Wildl Dis 2002;38:607–610.

Rotstein DS, Taylor SK, Harvey JW, et al. Hematologic effects of cytauxzoonosis in Florida panthers and Texas cougars in Florida. J Wildl Dis 1999;35:613–617.

Walker DB, Cowell RL. Survival of a domestic cat with naturally acquired cytauxzoonosis. J Am Vet Med Assoc 1995;206:1363–1365.

Heinz body anemia

Andress JL, Day TK, Day D. The effects of consecutive day propofol anesthesia on feline red blood cells. Vet Surg 1995;24(3):277–282.

Bauer MC, Weiss DJ, Perman V. Hematologic alterations in adult cats fed 6 or 12% propylene glycol. Am J Vet Res 1992;53(1):69–72.

Bauer MC, Weiss DJ, Perman V. Hematological alterations in kittens induced by 6 and 12% dietary propylene glycol. Vet Hum Toxicol 1992;34(2):127–131.

Christopher MM, Broussard JD, Peterson ME. Heinz body formation associated with ketoacidosis in diabetic cats. J Vet Int Med 1995; 9:24–31.

Christopher MM, Perman V, Eaton JW. Contribution of propylene glycol-induced Heinz body formation to anemia in cats. J Am Vet Med Assoc 1989;194:1045–1056.

Christopher MM, Perman V, White JG, et al. Propylene glycol-induced Heinz body formation and D-lactic acidosis in cats. Prog Clin Biol Res 1989;319:69–87.

Christopher MM, White JG, Eaton JW. Erythrocyte pathology and mechanisms of Heinz body-mediated hemolysis in cats. Vet Pathol 1990;27:299–310.

Christopher MM. Relation of endogenous Heinz bodies to disease and anemia in cats: 120 cases (1978–1987). J Am Vet Med Assoc 1989; 194:1089–1095.

Fallin CW, Christopher MM. In vitro effect of ketones and hyperglycemia on feline hemoglobin oxidation and D- and L-lactate production. Am J Vet Res 1996;57:463–467.

Gardner DE, Martinovich D, Woodhouse DA. Haematological and biochemical findings in bovine post-parturient haemoglobinuria and the accompanying Heinz-body anaemia. New Zealand Vet J 1976;24:117–122.

George LW, Divers TJ, Mahaffey EA, et al. Heinz body anemia and methemoglobinemia in ponies given red maple (*Acer rubrum L.*) leaves. Vet Pathol 1982;19:521–533.

Harvey JW, French TW, Senior DF. Hematologic abnormalities associated with chronic acetaminophen administration in a dog. J Am Vet Med Assoc 1986;189:1334–1335.

Harvey JW, Rackear D. Experimental onion-induced hemolytic anemia in dogs. Vet Pathol 1985;22:387–392.

Hickman MA, Rogers QR, Morris JG. Effect of diet on Heinz body formation in kittens. Am J Vet Res 1990;51:475–478.

Hill AS, O'Neill S, Rogers QR, et al. Antioxidant prevention of Heinz body formation and oxidative injury in cats. Am J Vet Res. 2001; 62:370–374.

Houston DM, Myers SL. A review of Heinz-body anemia in the dog induced by toxins. Vet Hum Toxicol 1993;35:158–161.

Kinuta M, Matteson JL, Itano HA. Difference in rates of the reaction of various mammalian oxyhemoglobins with phenylhydrazine. Arch Toxicol 1995;69:212–214.

Knight AP, Lassen D, McBride T, et al. Adaptation of pregnant ewes to an exclusive onion diet. Vet Hum Toxicol 2000;42:1–4.

Lee K-W, Yamato O, Tajima M, et al. Hematologic changes associated with the appearance of eccentrocytes after intragastric administration of garlic extract to dogs. Am J Vet Res 2000;61:1446–1450.

Leighton FA, Peakall DB, Butler RG. Heinz-body hemolytic anemia from the ingestion of crude oil: a primary toxic effect in marine birds. Science 1983;220(4599):871–873.

Lincoln SD, Howell ME, Combs JJ, et al. Hematologic effects and feeding performance in cattle fed cull domestic onions (*Allium cepa*). J Am Vet Med Assoc 1992;200:1090–1094.

Luttgen PJ, Whitney MS, Wolf AM, et al. Heinz body hemolytic anemia associated with high plasma zinc concentration in a dog. J Am Vet Med Assoc 1990;197:1347–1350.

McConnico RS, Brownie CF. The use of ascorbic acid in the treatment of 2 cases of red maple (Acer rubrum)-poisoned horses. Cornell Vet 1992;82(3):293–300.

Morris JG, Cripe WS, Chapman HL Jr, et al. Selenium deficiency in cattle associated with Heinz bodies and anemia. Science 1984; 223(4635):491–493.

Munday R, Munday JS, Munday CM. Comparative effects of mono-, di-, tri-, and tetrasulfides derived from plants of the Allium family: redox cycling in vitro and hemolytic activity and Phase 2 enzyme induction in vivo. Free Radic Biol Med 2003;34:1200–1211.

Narurkar NS, Thomas JS, Phalen DN. Heinz-body hemolytic anemia associated with ingestion of methylene blue in a river otter. J Am Vet Med Assoc 2002;220:363–366.

Ohno H, Tojo H, Kakihata K, et al. Heinz body hemolytic anemia induced by DQ-2511, a new anti-ulcer drug, in dogs. Fund Appl Toxicol 1993;20:141–146.

Prache S. Haemolytic anaemia in ruminants fed forage brassicas: a review. Vet Res 1994;25:497–520.

Reagan WJ, Carter C, Turek J. Eccentrocytosis in equine red maple leaf toxicosis. Vet Clin Path 1994;23:123–127.

Robertson JE, Christopher MM, Rogers QR. Heinz body formation in cats fed baby food containing onion powder. J Am Vet Med Assoc 1998;212(8):1260–1266.

Rumbeiha WK, Oehme FW. Methylene blue can be used to treat methemoglobinemia in cats without inducing Heinz body hemolytic anemia. Vet Hum Toxicol 1992;34(2):120–122.

Soli NE, Froslie A. Chronic copper poisoning in sheep. I. The relationship of methaemoglobinemia to Heinz body formation and haemolysis during the terminal crisis. Acta Pharm Toxicol 1977; 40:169–177.

Suttle NF, Jones DG, Woolliams C, et al. Heinz body anaemia in lambs with deficiencies of copper or selenium. Br J Nutr. 1987;58:539–548.

Taljaard TL. Cabbage poisoning in ruminants. J S Afr Vet Assoc 1993; 64:96–100.

Tennant B, Dill SG, Glickman LT, et al. Acute hemolytic anemia, methemoglobinemia, and heinz body formation associated with ingestion of red maple leaves by horses. J Am Vet Med Assoc 1981; 179:143–150.

Torrance AG, Fulton RB Jr. Zinc-induced hemolytic anemia in a dog. J Am Vet Med Assoc 1987;191:443–444.

Villar D, Buck WB, Gonzalez JM. Ibuprofen, aspirin and acetaminophen toxicosis and treatment in dogs and cats. Vet Hum Toxicol 1998; 40:156–162.

Wallace KP, Center SA, Hickford FH, et al. S-adenosyl-L-methionine (SAMe) for the treatment of acetaminophen toxicity in a dog. J Am Anim Hosp Assoc 2002;38:246–254.

Weiss DJ, McClay CB, Christopher MM, et al. Effects of propylene glycol-containing diets on acetaminophen-induced methemoglobinemia in cats. J Am Vet Med Assoc 1990;196:1816–1819.

Yamato O, Hayashi M, Yamasaki M, et al. Induction of onion-induced haemolytic anaemia in dogs with sodium n-propylthiosulphate. Vet Rec 1998;142:216–219.

Yamoto O, Maede Y. Susceptibility to onion-induced hemolysis in dogs with hereditary high erythrocyte reduced glutathione and potassium concentrations. Am J Vet Res. 1992;53:134–137.

Yamato O, Goto I, Maede Y. Hemolytic anemia in wild seaducks caused by marine oil pollution. J Wildl Dis 1996;32:381–384.

Hypophosphatemia

Adams LG, Hardy RM, Weiss DJ, et al. Hypophosphatemia and hemolytic anemia associated with diabetes mellitus and hepatic lipidosis in cats. J Vet Intern Med 1993;7:266–271.

Jubb TF, Jerrett IV, Browning JW, et al. Haemoglobinuria and hypophosphataemia in postparturient dairy cows without dietary deficiency of phosphorus. Aust Vet J 1990;67:86–89.

Justin RB, Hohenhaus AE. Hypophosphatemia associated with enteral alimentation in cats. J Vet Intern Med 1995;9:228–233.

Melvin JD, Watts RG. Severe hypophosphatemia: a rare cause of intravascular hemolysis. Am J Hematol. 2002;69:223–224.

Ogawa E, Kobayashi K, Yoshiura N, et al. Bovine postparturient hemoglobinemia: hypophosphatemia and metabolic disorder in red blood cells. Am J Vet Res 1987;48:1300–1303.

Ogawa E, Kobayashi K, Yoshiura N, et al: Hemolytic anemia and red blood cell metabolic disorder attributable to low phosphorus intake in cows. Am J Vet Res 1989;50:388–392.

Wang XL, Gallagher CH, McClure TJ, et al. Bovine post-parturient haemoglobinuria: effect of inorganic phosphate on red cell metabolism. Res Vet Sci. 1985;39:333–339.

Willard MD, Zerbe CA, Schall WD, et al: Severe hypophosphatemia associated with diabetes mellitus in six dogs and one cat. J Am Vet Med Assoc 1987;190:1007–1010.

Microorganism induced anemia

Decker MJ, Freeman MJ, Morter RL. Evaluation of mechanisms of leptospiral hemolytic anemia. Am J Vet Res 1970;31:873–878.

McGuire TC, Henson JB, Quist SE. Viral-induced hemolysis in equine infectious anemia. Am J Vet Res 1969;30:2091–2097.

Olander HJ, Hughes JP, Biberstein EL. Bacillary hemoglobinuria: induction by liver biopsy in naturally and experimentally infected animals. Pathologia Veterinaria 1966;3:421–450.

Reef VB. *Clostridium perfringens* cellulitis and immune-mediated hemolytic anemia in a horse. J Am Vet Med Assoc 1983;182:251–254.

Sellon DC. Equine infectious anemia. Vet Clin North Am Equine Pract 1993;9:321–336.

Stockham SL. Anemia associated with bacterial and viral infections. In: Feldman BF, Zinkl JG, Jain, NC, Eds. Schalm's Veterinary Hematology, 5th ed. Philadelphia: Lippincott Williams & Wilkins, 2001; 163–168.

Water intoxication induced hemolysis

Gibson EA, Counter DE, Barnes EG. An incident of water intoxication in calves. Vet Rec 1976;98:486–487.

Gilchrist F. Water intoxication in weaned beef calves. Can Vet J 1996; 37:490–491.

Kirkbride CA, Frey RA. Experimental water intoxication in calves. J Am Vet Med Assoc 1967;151:742–746.

INHERITED MEMBRANE DEFECTS

Brown DE, Weiser MG, Thrall MA, et al. Erythrocyte indices and volume distribution in a dog with stomatocytosis. Vet Pathol 1994;31:247–250.

Fletch SM, Pinkerton PH, Brueckner PJ. The Alaskan malamute chondrodysplasia (dwarfism-anemia) syndrome-in review. J Am Anim Hosp Assoc 1975;11:353–361.

Inaba M, Yawata A, Koshino I, et al. Defective anion transport and marked spherocytosis with membrane instability caused by hereditary total deficiency red cell band 3 in cattle due to a nonsense mutation. J Clin Invest 1996;97:1804–1817.

Inaba M. Red blood cell membrane defects. In: Feldman BF, Zinkl JG, Jain, NC eds. Schalm's Veterinary Hematology, 5th ed. Philadelphia: Lippincott Williams & Wilkins, 2001;1012–1019.

Kohn B, Goldschmidt MH, Hohenhaus AE, et al. Anemia, splenomegaly, and increased osmotic fragility of erythrocytes in Abyssinian and Somali cats. J Am Vet Med Assoc 2000;217:1483–1490.

Pinkerton PH, Fletch SM, Brueckner PJ, et al. Hereditary stomatocytosis with hemolytic anemia in the dog. Blood 1974;44:557–567.

Slappendel RJ, Renooij W, de Bruijne JJ. Normal cations and abnormal membrane lipids in the red blood cells of dogs with familial stomatocytosis-hypertrophic gastritis. Blood 1994;84:904–909.

Slappendel RJ, van der Gaag I, van Nes JJ, et al. Familial stomatocytosis—hypertrophic gastritis (FSHG), a newly recognized disease in the dog (Drentse patrijshond). Vet Quarterly 1991;13(1):30–40.

Smith JE, Moore K, Arens M, et al. Hereditary elliptocytosis with protein band 4.1 deficiency in the dog. Blood 1983;61:373–377.

Tucker EM, Young JD, Crowley C. Red cell glutatathione deficiency: clinical and biochemical investigations using sheep as an experimental model system. Br J Haematol 1981;48:403–415.

Yamoto O, Maede Y. Susceptibility to onion-induced hemolysis in dogs with hereditary high erythrocyte reduced glutathione and potassium concentrations. Am J Vet Res 1992;53(1):134–137.

INHERITED METABOLIC DISORDERS

Dixon PM, McPherson EA, Muir A. Familial methaemoglobinaemia and haemolytic anemia in the horse associated with decreased erythrocytic glutathione reductase and glutathione. Equine Vet J 1977;9:198–201.

Fine DM, Eyster GE, Anderson LK, et al. Cyanosis and congenital methemoglobinemia in a puppy. J Am Anim Hosp Assoc. 1999;35:33–35.

Giger U. Erythrocyte phosphofructokinase and pyruvate kinase deficiencies. In: Feldman BF, Zinkl JG, Jain, NC eds. Schalm's Veterinary Hematology, 5th ed. Philadelphia: Lippincott Williams & Wilkins, 2001;1020–1025.

Harvey JW. Hereditary Methemoglobinemia. In: Feldman BF, Zinkl JG, Jain, NC eds. Schalm's Veterinary Hematology, 5th ed. Philadelphia: Lippincott Williams & Wilkins, 2001;1008–1011.

Harvey JW, Dahl M, High ME. Methemoglobin reductase deficiency in a cat. J Am Vet Med Assoc 1994;205:1290–1291.

Harvey JW. Congenital erythrocyte enzyme deficiencies. Vet Clin N Am—Small Anim Pract 1996;26:1003–1011.

Skibild E, Dahlgaard K, Rajpurohit Y, et al. Haemolytic anaemia and exercise intolerance due to phosphofructokinase deficiency in related springer spaniels. J Small Anim Pract 200;42:298–300.

Smith JE. Animal models of human erythrocyte metabolic abnormalities. Clin Haemat 1981;10:239–251.

Smith JE, Ryer K, Wallace L. Glucose-6-phosphate dehydrogenase deficiency in a dog. Enzyme 1976;21:379–382.

Srivastava S, Alhomida AS, Siddiqi NJ, et al. Methemoglobin reductase activity and in vitro sensitivity towards oxidant induced methemoglobinemia in Swiss mice and beagle dogs erythrocytes. Mol Cell Biochem. 2002;232:81–85.

Stockham SL, Harvey JW, Kinden DA. Equine glucose-6-phosphate dehydrogenase deficiency. Vet Pathol 1994;31:518–527.

Zaucha JA, Yu C, Lothrop CD Jr, et al. Severe canine hereditary hemolytic anemia treated by nonmyeloablative marrow transplantation. Biol Blood Marrow Transplant 2001;7:14–24.

PORPHYRIAS

Bloomer JR, Morton KO, Reuter RJ, et al. Bovine protoporphyria: documentation of autosomal recessive inheritance and comparison with the human disease through measurement of heme synthetase activity. Hum Genet 1982;34:322–330.

Giddens WE Jr, Labbe RF, Swango LJ, et al. Feline congenital erythropoietic porphyria associated with severe anemia and renal disease. Clinical, morphologic, and biochemical studies. Am J Pathol 1975;80:367–386.

Glenn B L, Glenn HG, Omtvedt IT. Congenital porphyria in the domestic cat (Felis catus): preliminary investigations on inheritance pattern. Am J Vet Res 1968;29:1653–1657.

Healy PJ, Dennis JA. Inherited enzyme deficiencies in livestock. Vet Clin North Am Food Anim Pract 1993;9:55–63.

Johnson LW, Schwartz S. Isotopic studies of erythrocyte survival in normal and porphyric cattle: influence of light exposure, blood withdrawal, and splenectomy. Am J Vet Res 1970;31:2167–2177.

Kaneko JJ. The porphyrias and the porphyrinurias. In: Feldman BF, Zinkl JG, Jain, NC Eds. Schalm's Veterinary Hematology, 5th ed. Philadelphia: Lippincott Williams & Wilkins, 2001;1002–1007.

Kaneko JJ, Mills R. Erythrocytic enzyme activity, ion concentrations, osmotic fragility, and glutathione stability in bovine erythropoietic porphyria and its carrier state. Am J Vet Res 1969;30:1805–1810.

Kaneko JJ, Mills R. Hematological and blood chemical observations in neonatal normal and porphyric calves in early life. Cornell Vet 1970;60:52–60.

Kaneko JJ, Zinkl JG, Keeton KS. Erythrocyte porphyrin and erythrocyte survival in bovine erythropoietic porphyria. Am J Vet Res 1971;32:1981–1985.

Moore WE, Stephenson BD, Anderson AS, et al. Detection of the heterozygous state in bovine porphyria: analysis of urinary coproporphyrin isomers. Proc Soc Exp Biol Med 1970;134:926–929.

Moore WE. Metabolic acidosis in bovine erythropoietic porphyria during the neonatal period. Am J Vet Res 1970;31:1561–1567.

Pence ME, Liggett AD. Congenital erythropoietic protoporphyria in a Limousin calf. J Am Vet Med Assoc 2002;221:277–279.

Rudolph WG, Kaneko JJ. Kinetics of erythroid bone marrow cells of normal and porphyric calves in vitro. Acta Haematol 1971;45:330–335.

Ruth GR, Schwartz S, Stephenson B. Bovine protoporphyria: the first nonhuman model of this hereditary photosensitizing disease. Science 1977;198:199–201.

Schelcher F, Delverdier M, Bezille P, et al. Observation on bovine congenital erythrocytic protoporphyria in the blonde d'Aquitaine breed. Vet Rec 1991;129:403–407.

Scott DW, Mort JD, Tennant BC. Dermatohistopathologic changes in bovine congenital porphyria. Cornell Vet. 1979;69:145–158.

CHAPTER

9

CLASSIFICATION OF AND DIAGNOSTIC APPROACH TO POLYCYTHEMIA

Polycythemia refers to an increase in the concentration of erythrocytes in the blood as evidenced by an increased packed cell volume (PCV; or hematocrit), red-blood-cell count, or hemoglobin concentration. Because the term *polycythemia* implies that all blood cells, including leukocytes, are increased in concentration, the term *erythrocytosis* is sometimes preferred when only the erythrocytes are increased.

Polycythemia may be either relative or absolute. Relative polycythemia may occur due to decreased plasma volume or erythrocyte redistribution. Examples of the former include dehydration and body fluid shifts. The latter is the result of splenic contraction seen most commonly in excitable animals such as cats and horses. Absolute polycythemia is caused by an actual increase in the red cell mass and may be primary or secondary. Secondary absolute polycythemia results from overproduction of erythrocytes secondary to increased erythropoietin concentration, which in turn is secondary to either generalized hypoxia, localized renal hypoxia, or overproduction of erythropoietin by a tumor. Primary absolute polycythemia (i.e., polycythemia vera) is consid-

ered to be a well-differentiated myeloproliferative disorder in which erythropoiesis occurs independent of the erythropoietin concentration. Whereas primary polycythemia is rare, it is still more common than secondary polycythemia. Primary polycythemia usually is diagnosed by excluding relative and secondary polycythemia.

RELATIVE POLYCYTHEMIA

Relative Polycythemia Caused by Fluid Shifts or Dehydration

Patients with relative polycythemia caused by a reduction in plasma volume usually have a concurrent increase in plasma protein. In addition, clinical evidence of dehydration usually is present. Some dehydrated animals, however, may have normal or decreased plasma protein concentration resulting from decreased protein intake, decreased protein production by the liver, or increased protein loss via the kidney, gastrointestinal tract, or cutaneous lesions (see Chapter 26). Moreover, fluid shifts may

121

occur so rapidly, such as in patients with acute gastrointestinal disease or severe acute hyperthermia, that the classic clinical signs of dehydration may not be apparent. Relative polycythemia is treated by diagnosis of and therapy for the underlying disease and by replacement of fluids and electrolytes.

Relative Polycythemia Caused by Transient Increase in Red Cell Mass Secondary to Splenic Contraction

Splenic contraction causes only a modest increase in PCV, usually to no greater than 60%. Polycythemia as a result of splenic contraction typically is seen only in animals that normally have a high PCV, such as some poodles, greyhounds, and dachshunds. Splenic contraction may occur secondary to exercise, or it may be a response to epinephrine release in animals that are excited or in pain. Plasma protein concentration is not increased, and the presence of fear, pain, or excitement at the time of blood collection usually is apparent. An excitement leukogram also may be present, as evidenced by a mature neutrophilia and lymphocytosis; occasionally, mild thrombocytosis also is noted. Transient polycythemia has no clinical significance, and the red cell concentration reverts to normal in a short period of time.

ABSOLUTE POLYCYTHEMIA

Absolute polycythemia can be either secondary or primary.

Secondary Absolute Polycythemia

Secondary Absolute Polycythemia Caused by Generalized Hypoxia or Hypoxemia (Physiologically Appropriate Polycythemia)

Physiologically appropriate polycythemia is observed when inadequate tissue oxygenation triggers an increase in erythropoietin production, which in turn stimulates erythrocyte production and release so that more oxygen can be carried to the tissues. Generalized hypoxia and hypoxemia (reduced PaO_2) may be seen in animals with severe chronic heart or lung disease. Congenital heart disorders that result in shunting of blood away from the lungs are associated more often with polycythemia than in acquired heart disease. Severe lung disease also may result in hypoxemia, but it must be of chronic duration to induce polycythemia. Other causes of hypoxemia include living at very high altitude, alveolar hypoventilation, and severe obesity. Polycythemia associated with hypoxia without hypoxemia occurs in people with certain rare, inherited hemoglobinopathies, but these conditions have not been reported in domestic animals. Acquired chronic hemoglobinopathies (e.g., carboxyhemoglobinemia secondary to carbon monoxide poisoning or methemoglobinemia) may induce polycythemia as well.

Secondary absolute polycythemia caused by hypoxemia is diagnosed by detecting decreased PaO_2 and oxygen saturation. The reference interval for PaO_2 varies somewhat with the altitude. At sea level, the lower end of the reference interval is 80 mm Hg, and oxygen saturation is 92%; at approximately 6000 feet above sea level, the lower end of the reference interval is 74 mm Hg. Usually, the PaO_2 must be less than 60 mm Hg to induce polycythemia. Imaging of the heart and lungs as well as other diagnostic procedures to detect cardiopulmonary disease can then be used to establish a more definitive diagnosis.

Secondary Absolute Polycythemia Caused by Increased Erythropoietin Production (Physiologically Inappropriate Polycythemia)

Physiologically inappropriate polycythemia occurs when erythropoietin production is increased in the absence of generalized tissue hypoxia. Erythropoietin production may be increased in patients with renal lesions (usually tumors that induce localized renal hypoxia). Increased production of erythropoietin or of an erythropoietin-like substance by nonrenal tumors also may occur, but this is rare. Animals with physiologically inappropriate polycythemia have normal to slightly decreased PaO_2 and oxygen saturation. Mild hypoxemia may be present as a result of poor perfusion, and patients usually have increased serum erythropoietin concentration. Other diagnostic procedures to evaluate the kidneys, such as imaging, renal aspiration cytology or biopsy, and urinalysis, should be performed.

Primary Absolute Polycythemia

Primary absolute polycythemia (i.e., polycythemia vera) is a well-differentiated myeloproliferative disorder in which erythrocytes proliferate uncontrollably, producing an increased hematocrit. Unlike most other types of hematopoietic neoplasia, the neoplastic erythroid cells appear to be normal and to have a normal maturation sequence. In humans with polycythemia vera, an abnormal proliferation of neutrophils and platelets often accompanies erythrocyte proliferation, resulting in leukocytosis and thrombocytosis. An abnormal proliferation of cells other than red blood cells is rarely observed in domestic animals; thus, in dogs and cats, the disorder probably should be referred to as *primary erythrocytosis* rather than as *primary polycythemia* or *polycythemia vera*. The pathophysiology is thought to involve the presence of an abnormal clone of erythroid precursors that is either capable of proliferating independent of erythropoietin concentrations or hyperresponsive to erythropoietin. The disorder usually is diagnosed by excluding other causes of polycythemia. Most cases of primary polycythemia in domestic animals have been reported in dogs and cats, but a few have been reported in horses, cattle, and a llama.

CLINICAL FINDINGS

Clinical findings may be secondary to the underlying cause of the polycythemia or may result from the increased number of erythrocytes per se. In animals with relative polycythemia, dehydration or excitement may be clinically evident. In animals with secondary absolute polycythemia caused by hypoxia, clinical signs associated with congenital heart disease (e.g., murmurs, cyanosis) or with pulmonary disease (e.g., cyanosis, dyspnea, abnormal lung sounds) may be observed. In animals with secondary absolute polycythemia caused by inappropriate erythropoietin production, clinical signs associated with renal disease often are not apparent.

Clinical signs associated with erythrocytosis are secondary to increased blood volume and viscosity. They include deep-red mucous membranes, sometimes with slight cyanosis. Increased blood viscosity may result in sluggish blood flow and subsequent decreased tissue perfusion and oxygen transport as well as hemorrhage and thrombosis. Mild to severe central nervous system signs associated with decreased oxygen transport, such as lethargy, ataxia, blindness, or seizures, also may be observed. Polyuria and polydipsia occasionally are reported and are thought to result from impaired release of vasopressin release. Splenomegaly rarely is observed in domestic animals; however, human patients commonly have splenomegaly, may have generalized pruritis, and eventually may develop marrow fibrosis and lymphoid neoplasia.

DIAGNOSTIC APPROACH

When PCV is increased, one should consider if the patient is excited or dehydrated and then perform a second complete blood count to confirm that the finding is repeatable. If the total protein concentration also is increased, the polycythemia likely is relative, secondary to dehydration and decreased plasma volume. Sometimes, however, animals with rapid fluid shifts, such as those with gastrointestinal disease, may not have an increased total protein. Moreover, total protein may be decreased or normal in dehydrated animals that have decreased protein intake, production, or increased loss.

If relative polycythemia is excluded, secondary absolute polycythemia due to hypoxemia from congenital heart disease or pulmonary disease should be considered. Hypoxemia is best diagnosed by performing an arterial blood gas analysis to determine the PaO_2 and oxygen saturation. If the PaO_2 is less than 60 mm Hg, then hypoxemia likely is the cause of polycythemia. Imaging using thoracic radiographic and ultrasonic examination will provide additional information.

If hypoxemia is excluded, secondary absolute polycythemia caused by increased erythropoietin production should be considered. Tumors of the kidney are the most common cause of increased erythropoietin production. In these cases, imaging with renal ultrasonography or intravenous urography is indicated. Serum erythropoietin concentration usually is increased in animals with hypoxemia or inappropriate erythropoietin production and is normal to decreased in animals with primary polycythemia (*Table 9.1*). Erythropoietin concentrations appear to be more useful in dogs than in cats. If secondary polycythemia caused by inappropriate erythropoietin production is excluded, then the likely diagnosis is polycythemia vera.

Other laboratory findings are not particularly helpful. Affected humans commonly have neutrophilia and thrombocytosis, but these findings are rare in domestic animals. Neutrophilia associated with stress or inflammation is a more likely finding. Other than mild increased cellularity and mild erythroid hyperplasia, bone marrow aspirates usually are normal in appearance. Measuring total red cell mass with a dye technique or radioisotope-labeled erythrocytes, though infrequently performed, can help to establish a more definitive diagnosis.

THERAPY

Relative polycythemia is treated by therapy for the underlying disease and correction of dehydration with fluid

---

TABLE 9.1 PaO_2 AND ERYTHROPOIETIN IN ANIMALS WITH POLYCYTHEMIA

Polycythemia	PaO_2	Erythropoietin
Relative	Normal	Normal
Secondary		
Caused by hypoxemia	Decreased	Increased
Caused by inappropriate erythropoietin production	Normal	Increased
Primary	Normal	Normal or decreased

therapy. The underlying disorder also is treated in animals with secondary polycythemia caused by hypoxemia or inappropriate erythropoietin production. Phlebotomy may be contraindicated in animals with hypoxemia, because the erythrocytosis is physiologic. If the PCV is very high in these patients, however, then tissue perfusion may be impaired, and phlebotomy may be helpful.

Primary polycythemia most commonly is treated—and often with long-term success—by performing repeated phlebotomy to maintain the PCV in the high-normal range. Injectable iron may need to be given to avoid iron-deficiency anemia. Chemotherapy to decrease red cell production also may be used; oral hydroxyurea is the most common such treatment. Dose and frequency are variable, depending on the response. A reported complication in cats is methemoglobinemia and Heinz-body anemia. Alternately, radioactive phosphorus has been used with success in some cases. A veterinary oncologist should be consulted for up-to-date treatment options.

SUGGESTED READINGS

Beech J, Bloom JC, Hodge TG. Erythrocytosis in a horse. J Am Vet Med Assoc 1984;18:986–989.

Berlin NI, Lewis SM. Measurement of total RBC volume relative to lean body mass for diagnosis of polycythemia. Am J Clin Pathol 2000;114:922–926.

Campbell KL. Diagnosis and management of polycythemia in dogs. Compend Small Anim 1990;12:543–550.

Cook G, Divers TJ, Rowland PH. Hypercalcemia and erythrocytosis in a mare associated with a metastatic carcinoma. Equine Vet J 1995; 27:316–318.

Cook SM, Lothrop CD Jr. Serum erythropoietin concentrations measured by radioimmunoassay in normal, polycythemic, and anemic dogs and cats. J Vet Intern Med 1994;8:18–25.

Couto CG, Boudrieau RJ, Zanjani ED. Tumor-associated erythrocytosis in a dog with nasal fibrosarcoma. J Vet Intern Med 1989;3:183–185.

Crow SE, Allen DP, Murphy CJ, et al. Concurrent renal adenocarcinoma and polycythemia in a dog. J Am Anim Hosp Assoc 1995; 31:29–33.

Foster ES, Lothrup CD. Polycythemia vera in a cat with cardiac hypertrophy. J Am Vet Med Assoc 1988;192:1736–1738.

Gavaghan BJ, Kittleson MD, Decock H. Eisenmenger's complex in a Holstein-Friesian cow. Aust Vet J 2001;79:37–40.

Gentz EJ, Pearson EG, Lassen ED, et al. Polycythemia in a llama. J Am Vet Med Assoc 1994;204:1490–1492.

Gorse MJ. Polycythemia associated with renal fibrosarcoma in a dog. J Am Vet Med Assoc 1988;192:793–794.

Hasler AH, Giger U. Serum erythropoietin values in polycythemic cats. J Am Anim Hosp Assoc 1996;32:294–301.

Kaneko JJ, Zinkl J, Tennant BC, et al. Iron metabolism in familial polycythemia of Jersey calves. Am J Vet Res 1968;29:949–952.

Khanna C, Bienzle D. Polycythemia vera in a cat: bone marrow culture in erythropoietin-deficient medium. J Am Anim Hosp Assoc 1994; 30:45–49.

Kirby D, Gillick A. Polycythemia and tetralogy of Fallot in a cat. Can Vet J 1974;15:114–119.

Lane VM, Anderson BC, Bulgin MS. Polycythemia and cyanosis associated with hypoplastic main pulmonary segment in the bovine heart. J Am Vet Med Assoc 1983;183:460–461.

Legendre AM, Appleford MD, Eyster GE, et al. Secondary polycythemia and seizures due to right-to-left shunting patent ductus arteriosus in a dog. J Am Vet Med Assoc 1974;164:1198–1201.

Lennox TJ, Wilson JH, Hayden DW, et al. Hepatoblastoma with erythrocytosis in a young female horse. J Am Vet Med Assoc 2000; 216: 718–721.

McFarlane D, Sellon DC, Parker B. Primary erythrocytosis in a 2-year-old Arabian gelding. J Vet Intern Med 1998;12:384–388.

McGrath CJ. Polycythemia vera in dogs. J Am Vet Med Assoc 1974; 164:1117–1122.

Nelson RW, Hager D, Zanjani ED. Renal lymphosarcoma with inappropriate erythropoietin production in a dog. J Am Vet Med Assoc 1983;182:1396–1397.

Page RL, Stiff M, McEntee MC, et al. Transient glomerulonephropathy associated with primary erythrocytosis in a dog. J Am Vet Med Assoc 1990;196:620–622.

Peterson ME, Randolph JF. Diagnosis of canine primary polycythemia and management with hydroxyurea. J Am Vet Med Assoc 1982; 180:415–418.

Peterson ME, Zanjani ED. Inappropriate erythropoietin production from a renal carcinoma in a dog with polycythemia. J Am Vet Med Assoc 1981;179:995–996.

Reed C, Ling GV, Gould D, et al. Polycythemia vera in a cat. J Am Vet Med Assoc 1970;157:85–91.

Roby KA, Beech J, Bloom JC, et al. Hepatocellular carcinoma associated with erythrocytosis and hypoglycemia in a yearling filly. J Am Vet Med Assoc 1990;196:465–467.

Scott RC, Patnaik AK. Renal carcinoma with secondary polycythemia in the dog. J Am Anim Hosp Assoc 1972;8:275–283.

Smith M, Turrell JM. Radiophosphorus (^{32}P) treatment of bone marrow disorders in dogs: 11 cases (1970–1987). J Am Vet Med Assoc 1989;194:98–102.

Swinney G, Jones BR, Kissling K. A review of polycythemia vera in the cat. Aust Vet Pract 1992;22:60–66.

Tennant B, Harrold D, Reina-Guerra M, et al. Arterial pH, P_{O_2} and P_{CO_2} of calves with familial bovine polycythemia. Cornell Vet 1969; 59:594–604.

Thiele J, Kvasnicka HM, Muehlhausen K, et al. Polycythemia rubra vera versus secondary polycythemias. A clinicopathological evaluation of distinctive features in 199 patients. Pathol Res Pract 2001; 197:77–84.

Thiele J, Kvasnicka HM, Zankovich R, et al. The value of bone marrow histology in differentiating between early stage polycythemia vera and secondary (reactive) polycythemias. Haematologica 2001; 86:368–374.

Van Vonderen IK, Meyer HP, Kraus JS, Kooistra HS. Polyuria and polydipsia and disturbed vasopressin release in two dogs with secondary polycythemia. J Vet Intern Med 1997;11:300–303.

Waters DJ, Preuter JC. Secondary polycythemia associated with renal disease in the dog: two case reports and review of the literature. J Am Anim Hosp Assoc 1988;24:109–114.

Watson ADJ, Moore AS, Helfand SC. Primary erythrocytosis in the cat: treatment with hydroxyurea. J Small Anim Pract 1994;35:320–325.

Weller RE. Paraneoplastic disorders in dogs with hematopoietic tumors. Vet Clin North Am Small Anim Pract 1985;15:805–816.

INTRODUCTION TO LEUKOCYTES AND THE LEUKOGRAM

Interpretation of leukocyte concentrations in blood provides insight regarding potential processes that may be occurring in the patient. The complete set of numeric data in the leukocyte profile, along with any noted morphologic abnormalities, is known as the *leukogram.* An abnormal leukogram usually leads to identification of a pathologic process (e.g., inflammation), but not to establishment of a specific diagnosis. Interpretation of leukocyte abnormalities into a process coupled with clinical findings, however, may lead to a diagnosis.

To interpret leukocyte patterns in disease, one must first learn the normal characteristics of the leukogram as a basis for recognizing abnormal patterns. This chapter presents background information regarding the normal leukogram that is necessary for building skills in its interpretation.

COMMON BLOOD LEUKOCYTES: GENERAL FUNCTIONS AND MORPHOLOGY

This section reviews pertinent characteristics of blood leukocytes, such as general functions and morphologic features, including species variations in morphology.

Neutrophils

Neutrophils participate in inflammatory responses by means of chemoattraction into tissue sites of inflammation and phagocytosis of organisms and other foreign material. After phagocytosis, lysosomal granules fuse with phagosomes to kill organisms and then degrade the material by enzymatic digestion.

Neutrophil morphology is introduced in *Figure 10.1.* The neutrophilic metamyelocyte is not present in normal blood. It has a bean-shaped nucleus that, as it matures, changes to the horseshoe shape that is characteristic of the band neutrophil. The band nucleus has smooth, parallel sides and no constrictions in the nuclear membrane. The band neutrophil may be present in normal blood at small concentrations. Segmented neutrophils have a horseshoe-shaped nucleus with variable degrees of indentation and constriction along its perimeter (Fig. 10.1). As the nucleus develops constrictions, it may fold into various shapes (*Fig. 10.2*). Neutrophils have numerous small, very poorly stained granules. These vary among individual animals from colorless, invisible granules to lightly staining granules. Neutrophilic granules of the cow often stain faintly pink, giving the cytoplasm a slightly orange-pink tint overall (*Fig. 10.3*).

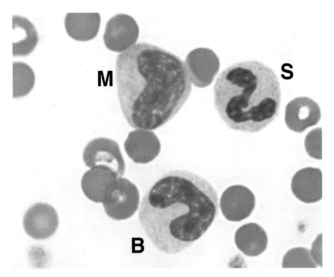

Figure 10.1 Neutrophil maturation sequence commonly seen in blood. The segmented or mature neutrophil (S) has an irregular nuclear membrane, with one or more constrictions. Note the small, faintly staining neutrophilic granules in the cytoplasm. The neutrophilic granules vary in prominence from animal to animal. The band neutrophil (B) has a horseshoe-shaped nucleus with smooth, parallel sides. The metamyelocyte (M) has a bean-shaped nucleus. (Wright's Giemsa stain, high magnification.)

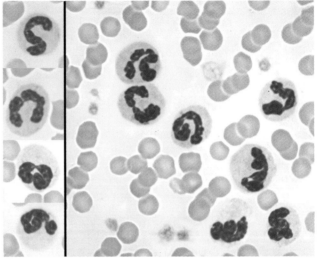

Figure 10.2 Representative segmented neutrophils illustrating variation in nuclear shape. Segmented neutrophils start with the horseshoe-shaped nucleus of the band cell. As the neutrophil nucleus develops more constrictions, it may more easily fold into various shapes. Note the "S"- and horseshoe-shaped nuclei in the upper left. Then, note the various nuclear shapes that result from folding and superimposition of the folded nucleus on itself. Cells are arranged in this figure with greater degrees of folding moving toward the bottom. (Wright's Giemsa stain, high magnification.)

Lymphocytes

Blood lymphocytes represent a diverse set of lymphocyte subpopulations, but these subpopulations cannot be distinguished at blood-film examination or by techniques routinely used in clinical veterinary laboratories. The subpopulations include B lymphocytes, which are responsible for humoral immunity, and T lymphocytes, which are responsible for cell-mediated immunity and cytokine responses. T lymphocytes may be further classified as T-inducer (i.e., helper; CD4-bearing) cells and T-cytotoxic/suppressor (CD8-bearing) cells. Null cells are a third population present at small concentrations. Null cells consist of at least several lymphocyte subtypes, including large granular lymphocytes, natural killer cells, and other cells with killer activity. Lymphocyte subtypes may be differentiated by surface immunoglobulin and cluster designation (i.e., CD) markers; however, this technology is not yet routine in veterinary clinical laboratories. Some laboratories may provide special procedures for quantitation of certain subpopulations (e.g., B- and T-cell concentrations).

Lymphocytes are recognized by a round-to-oval nucleus and a minimal amount of clear, almost colorless cytoplasm. The amount of cytoplasm may be variable, as illustrated in Figure 10.3. Normal circulating lymphocytes have smaller diameters than those of neutrophils. In ruminants, lymphocytes may be more irregular in size and have diameters equal to those of neutrophils (Fig. 10.3).

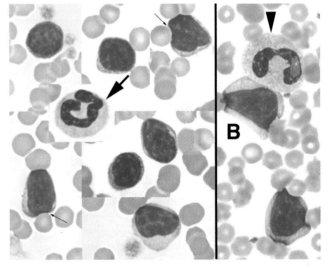

Figure 10.3 Variation in normal lymphocyte morphology in comparison to neutrophils. In the left panel, note that the lymphocyte nucleus may vary from round to oval. The cell shape, including the nucleus, may be indented by adjacent erythrocytes (thin arrows). The amount of cytoplasm varies from virtually none to a modest amount. Lymphocytes in most species are smaller than adjacent neutrophils (thick arrow). The exception is indicated in the right panel: Bovine lymphocytes (B) are larger than the lymphocytes of most other common species and may have the same diameter as that of the bovine neutrophil (arrowhead). Note that the bovine neutrophil has slightly pink neutrophilic granules. (Wright's Giemsa stain, high magnification.)

Less common forms of lymphocytes include reactive lymphocytes and granular lymphocytes (*Fig. 10.4*). Reactive forms likely are B cells capable of producing immunoglobulin. They have intensely basophilic cytoplasm, and the nucleus may be more irregularly shaped. In addition, the nucleus may have a cleft or an amoeboid shape. Granular lymphocytes have a small number of pink-purple granules. These are large granular lymphocytes, some of which are thought to be natural killer or T cells. Large granular lymphocytes are most commonly observed in ruminant blood.

Monocytes

Monocytes also participate in inflammatory responses. Monocytes in blood are regarded as intermediate on a continuum of maturation. Monocytes migrate into tissues, where they continue to develop into macrophages. Mononuclear phagocytes may phagocytize bacteria, larger complex organisms (e.g., yeast and protozoa), injured cells, cellular debris, and foreign particulate debris. These cells play an important immunoregulatory function by presenting processed antigen to T lymphocytes. These cells are also responsible for normal erythrocyte destruction, associated metabolic iron recycling, and most pathologic erythrocyte destruction.

Monocytes are the most misidentified cell on blood films, particularly in the veterinary hospital laboratory.

The nucleus may be of almost any shape, including oval, bean, or segmented (like that of neutrophils). The chromatin pattern may be slightly less condensed than that of neutrophils. The key distinguishing features are a larger diameter and more grayish coloration to the cytoplasm compared with adjacent neutrophils (*Fig. 10.5*). The cytoplasm may contain extremely fine, light-purple granules. When uncertainty exists regarding monocyte identification, view at low power to make cell-to-cell comparisons (*Fig. 10.6*). At low power, monocytes will stand out as larger cells. Species differences in monocyte morphology are not remarkable.

Eosinophils

The functions of eosinophils are not well understood, even though a considerable number of studies and observations have been reported. Eosinophils contain proteins that bind to and damage parasite membranes, and they are responsible for providing a defense mechanism against larval stages of parasitic infestation. They are also involved in the modulation of allergic inflammation and immune-complex reactions.

Eosinophils vary in morphology among species (*Fig. 10.7*). The nucleus is segmented (like that of neutrophils).

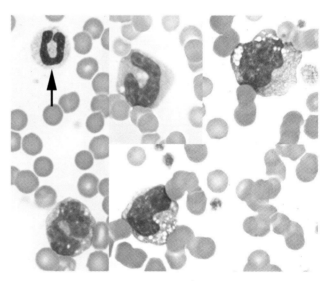

Figure 10.5 Variation in blood monocyte morphology; note the cells *not* marked by an arrow. Monocytes are typically larger than neutrophils (arrow). Monocytes may have cytoplasmic vacuoles, but this is not consistent. The monocyte nucleus is highly variable in shape: It may be round to bean shaped to amoeboid shaped, or it may be horseshoe shaped and even segmented (like the nuclei of neutrophils). Inexperienced observers frequently confuse monocytes with horseshoe-shaped nuclei for neutrophils. The consistent features of monocytes are larger diameter than an adjacent neutrophil (arrow) and darker blue-gray cytoplasm compared with neutrophils. (Wright's Giemsa stain, high magnification.)

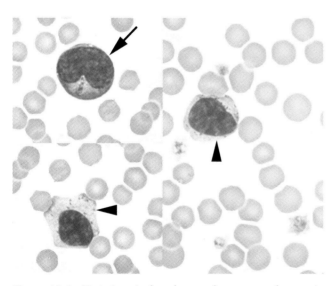

Figure 10.4 Variations in lymphocytes less commonly seen in blood. The reactive lymphocyte (arrow) is characterized by royal-blue cytoplasm. Its nuclear shape may be irregular, often with an indentation or cleft. Large granular lymphocytes (arrowheads) have an increased amount of light-staining cytoplasm, with a sparse sprinkling of azurophilic granules. The granules may vary in size. Large granular lymphocytes are most frequently seen in normal ruminants. (Wright's Giemsa stain, high magnification.)

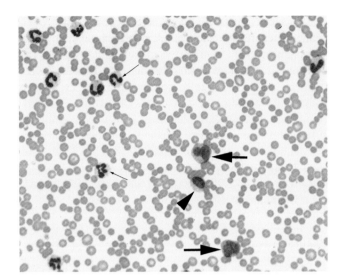

Figure 10.6 Low-magnification comparison of neutrophils and monocytes. When in doubt regarding identification of monocytes, use a lower magnification to make cell-to-cell comparisons that may be difficult at higher magnification. Note that the two monocytes (thick arrows) have larger diameters than the representative neutrophils indicated by thin arrows. A lymphocyte (arrowhead) is smaller than the adjacent neutrophils. (Wright's Giemsa stain, low magnification.)

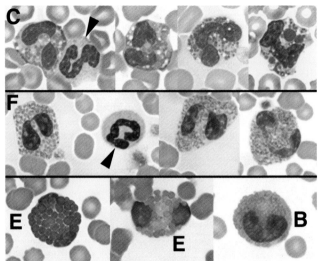

Figure 10.7 Species variation in eosinophil morphology. Representative neutrophils are shown for comparison (arrowheads). Eosinophils are typically larger in diameter than neutrophils. Canine eosinophils are shown in the top band (C). Note the variation in eosinophil granule size in dogs, which also may have eosinophil granules that appear to dissolve during the staining process, leaving a clear space that resembles a cytoplasmic vacuole. Feline eosinophils are shown in the middle band (F). Eosinophil granules of the cat are shaped like barrels or short rods. The density of the granularity may vary as shown. Large animal eosinophils are indicated in the bottom band. Equine eosinophils (E) have large, brightly staining granules that may obscure the nucleus, whereas bovine eosinophils (B) have smaller, brightly staining granules that are densely packed within the cytoplasm. (Wright's Giemsa stain, high magnification.)

The hallmark feature of eosinophils are prominent, red-orange granules that are tinctorally similar to erythrocytes. Canine eosinophils have highly variable granule size and number per cell. On rare occasions, a few large granules the size of erythrocytes may be present. Eosinophil granules also may wash out during the staining process, leaving what appears to be an empty vacuole; this observation is most pronounced in greyhound dogs. Feline eosinophils are densely packed, with uniform, rod- or barrel-shaped granules. Equine eosinophils have a raspberry appearance because of numerous round, very large granules that usually obscure the nucleus. Ruminant eosinophils have uniform, numerous round granules.

Basophils

The function of basophils is, basically, unknown. Basophils contain histamine and heparin. The cytoplasmic membrane has bound immunoglobulin E, like mast cells; however, their pathophysiologic role in the circulation is unknown. No convincing evidence has been reported that blood basophils migrate into tissues and become tissue mast cells. Concentrations of basophils in the circulation are very low, and they usually are not encountered in the routine differential count.

Basophils are larger in diameter than neutrophils. The nucleus is segmented (like those of other granulocytes). The granule morphology varies among species (*Fig. 10.8*). Dogs have a small number of dark-violet granules. Cats have large, faint-gray granules that form a pavement-stone arrangement. Large animal basophils are packed with dark-violet granules that are so numerous they often obscure portions of the nucleus.

REFERENCE VALUES: THE NORMAL LEUKOGRAM

The approach to interpretation of the leukogram involves a series of steps to arrive at a conclusion regarding what is normal or abnormal. Interpretive attention should focus only on the absolute values within the differential count (see Chapter 1). When examining the hematology report, one should look first at the total leukocyte concentration. The total leukocyte count is only used to calculate absolute differential concentrations; it is not directly inter-

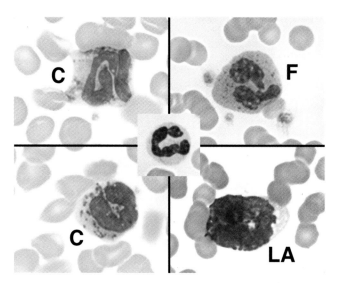

Figure 10.8 Species variation in basophil morphology. A representative neutrophil is shown in the center for comparison. Basophils are larger in diameter than neutrophils. Canine basophils (C) are poorly granulated. Note the sprinkling of basophilic granules in the cytoplasm. Feline basophils (F) have cytoplasm packed with large, poorly staining gray granules that are arranged like pavement stones. Large animal basophils (LA) have numerous dark-staining granules that often obscure the nucleus. (Wright's Giemsa stain, high magnification.)

preted. If the total count is decreased, examine the absolute concentration of each cell type to determine which are deficient. If the total count is increased, examine the absolute concentration of each cell type to determine which are present in excess. Even if the total concentration is normal, examine the absolute concentration of each cell type to determine if any abnormalities in distribution are present. Identified abnormalities in the absolute concentrations of individual leukocyte types are then interpreted into processes (see Chapter 12).

Reference values are given in *Table 10.1*. These values are patterned after general guidelines that that have been used for decades (from the original work of Schalm) and are similar to those used by most veterinary laboratories. A more comprehensive, population-based set of reference ranges generated by newer technology for automated cell counting is needed. This has been done in some teaching hospital laboratories for specific automated systems used in the respective settings. Improved precision of automated cell counting as well as improved procedures for statistical analysis may provide more useful interpretive guidelines in the future.

The clinician interprets leukocyte abnormalities by learning to examine the individual differential leukocyte concentrations and then noting any morphologic abnormalities or abnormal cell types currently present that

TABLE 10.1   REFERENCE RANGES FOR ABSOLUTE LEUKOCYTE CONCENTRATIONS OF COMMON DOMESTIC ANIMAL SPECIES

Leukocytes	Dog	Cat	Horse	Cow	Sheep	Pig
Total WBC (cells/µl)	6000–17,000	5500–19,500	5500–12,500	4000–12,000	4000–12,000	11,000–22,000
Differential WBC						
Band neutrophils (cells/µl)	0–300	0–300	0–100	0–100	0–100	0–800
Segmented neutrophils (cells/µl)	3000–11,500	2500–12,500	2700–6700	600–4000	700–6000	3200–10,000
Lymphocytes (cells/µl)	1000–5000	1500–7000	1500–5500	2500–7000	2000–9000	4500–13,000
Monocytes (cells/µl)	0–1200	0–800	0–800	0–800	0–800	200–2000
Eosinophils (cells/µl)	100–1200	0–1500	0–900	0–2400	0–1000	100–2000
Basophils (cells/µl)	Rare, 0–100	Rare, 0–100	0–200	0–200	0–300	0–400

WBC, white blood cell.

should not be present in normal blood. Differential leukocyte concentrations are reported in cells per microliter for each cell type. Abnormal nucleated cells include blasts, nucleated erythrocytes, mast cells, and immature granulocytes. Morphologic abnormalities include inherited and transiently acquired morphologic changes. Abnormal morphology is presented in Chapter 12.

SUGGESTED READING

Feldman BF, Zinkl JG, Jain NC, eds. Section 5: leukocytes—nonlymphoid leukocytes. In: Schalm's veterinary hematology. 5th ed. Baltimore: Lippincott Williams & Wilkins, 2000:281–433.
Lee GR, Bithell TC, Foerster J, Athens JW, Lukens JN, eds. Wintrobe's clinical hematology. 9th ed. Philadelphia: Lea & Febiger, 1993.

NEUTROPHIL PRODUCTION, TRAFFICKING, AND KINETICS

General trends regarding the trafficking and kinetics of neutrophils in blood have been observed. Although species differences are not well characterized, they appear to be unimportant. An understanding of these behaviors by neutrophils helps to interpret the timing of responses to disease and the sequential changes between hemograms.

PRODUCTION OF GRANULOCYTES

Neutrophils are produced exclusively in the active bone marrow of healthy, adult domestic animals. Some production may be found in extramedullary sites, most notably the spleen, in juvenile animals. With long-standing increased demand for neutrophils (e.g., in chronic inflammatory disease), extramedullary production may be observed in adult animals. This will be most prominent in the spleen, but it may also be seen in the liver and lymph nodes.

Neutrophils originate from the pluripotential stem cell system, which system gives rise to a more differentiated stem cell that has the capacity to create granulocytes and monocytes (GM stem cells). A subpopulation of these GM stem cells enters a pathway of committed differentiation of blood granulocytes, consisting of neutrophils, eosinophils, and basophils. The stem cells are not morphologically distinct, because they are present in small numbers and are probably indistinguishable from lymphocytes. Once a cell makes this entry commitment, it undergoes both proliferative and maturational events to propagate blood granulocytes. These proliferative and maturational events are associated with morphologically recognized stages of granulocytes. Recognition of these stages is important in the evaluation of bone marrow samples and the identification of cells in blood in response to disease. The morphologic stages of granulocytes are indicated in *Figure 11.1*.

The myeloblast is the first recognizable cell that is committed to granulocyte production. Myeloblasts are difficult to distinguish from primitive blasts of other lineages. Once committed, the myeloblast produces primary (i.e., azurophilic) granules, the presence of which identifies the progranulocyte stage. At subsequent stages of maturation, the primary granules change their staining character and become indistinguishable in conventional blood stains. In the next stage, the myelocyte begins to produce secondary (i.e., specific) granules that identify whether the cell will be a neutrophil, eosinophil, or basophil. Historically, the naming of the specific granules and the cell type has related to the dye component of the polychrome blood stains taken up by the specific granule. Neutrophil granules have neutral staining affinity; because of poor dye affinity, the granules are very faint or not visible. Eosinophil granules have an affinity for the orange-red dye and stain intensely orange-red. Basophil granules have affinity for basic dyes and stain intensely dark violet. Myeloblasts, progranulocytes, and myelocytes have the ability to undergo cell division as well as

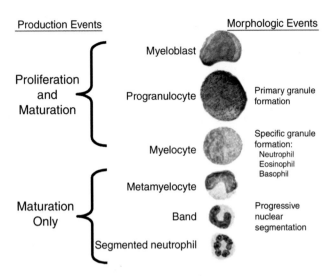

Figure 11.1   Morphologic features of stages of neutrophil maturation. Six morphologic stages are identified on a continuum of maturation, as indicated by the named cells. Cells capable of both cell division and maturation are at the top; cells capable of maturation only are at the bottom. Major changes associated with maturation are indicated in the right. (See text for a more complete description.)

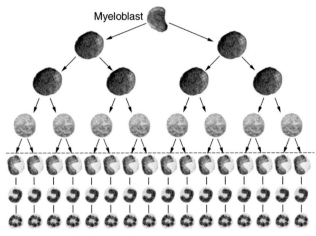

Figure 11.2   Orderly production of neutrophils in bone marrow. Note the progressive increase in relative cell numbers as maturation progresses. The myeloblast may give rise to approximately 16 to 32 cells before proliferative ability is lost. Cell stages above the dashed line are capable of cell division; cell stages below the dashed line are only capable of maturation. Please refer to Figure 11.1 for reference to cell stages.

to mature from one stage to the next. These stages are relatively rich in ribosomes, giving the cytoplasm a bluish tint. Nuclear features include round to oval shape and relatively fine chromatin pattern.

More mature stages are characterized by the loss of ability to undergo cell division and include metamyelocytes, bands, and segmented neutrophils. Maturation consists mostly of progressive nuclear condensation and change in shape. The cytoplasm loses most or all of its bluish tint as the ribosome content decreases. The metamyelocyte has a nucleus that has developed an indentation. The band cell nucleus forms a horseshoe shape and has smooth, parallel nuclear membranes. The segmented or mature neutrophil progressively develops indentations or constrictions in the nuclear membrane.

MATURATION AND ORDERLY PRODUCTION

Production normally results in a progressive increase in the relative numbers of more mature stages, as indicated in *Figure 11.2*. This results from the combined events of proliferating early forms, which amplify both the number of cells and the progress toward more mature stages. In the process, each myeloblast may produce approximately 16 to 32 segmented neutrophils. The pattern of production seen in the marrow is a mixture of a relatively small number of primitive cells, a larger number of intermedi-

ate stages, and numerous more mature stages. This progression of a few immature cells to many more mature cells is described as *orderly production*. Both normal production and accelerated production in response to increased granulocyte demand have this orderly appearance. Cells are also delivered to the blood in this orderly fashion (see the discussion of left shift in Chapter 12). *Disorderly production* is characterized by a disproportionate relative number of primitive forms and a relative decrease or absence of more mature forms. Disorderly production is one of the features used to identify certain pathologic patterns (e.g., myeloproliferative disorders).

NEUTROPHIL POOLS AND TRAFFICKING

To understand neutrophil responses in disease, it is helpful to visualize a set of compartments and pools consisting of bone marrow, blood, and tissues, as depicted in *Figure 11.3*. The bone marrow compartment may be conceptually divided into a stem cell pool, a proliferative pool, and a maturation and storage pool. The proliferative pool consists of neutrophils at stages during which they still have the ability to undergo cell division and is largely responsible for the amplification of cell numbers. The maturation and storage pool consists of cells having no ability to divide and that are completing morphologic maturation. These cells may accumulate to create a modest storage reserve that is variable in size, which depends on the species. The storage capacity is greatest in dogs, least in ruminants, and intermediate in cats and horses.

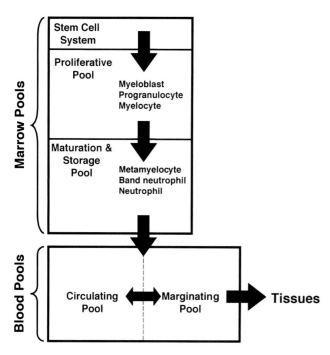

Figure 11.3 Bone marrow and blood neutrophil pools. Single arrows indicate unidirectional movement of cells; double arrow indicates bidirectional movement of cells. (See text for description of various compartments and progress through them.)

Neutrophils make a unidirectional migration to the blood compartment, which is divided into the circulating and margination pools. The circulating pool is located in large vessels in which no interaction normally occurs between neutrophils and the endothelial lining of the vessel. Blood samples taken by venipuncture are from the circulating pool. The margination pool consists of the microcirculation. Cells may move bidirectionally between the circulating and margination pools. Neutrophils interact with the endothelial lining of small vessels and capillaries by their property of stickiness. Neutrophils may then unidirectionally migrate into adjacent tissue spaces (i.e., the tissue compartment). It is in the tissue compartment that neutrophils participate in their host-defense purposes.

All neutrophil responses in disease may be understood as being mechanisms and disturbances occurring in this set of pools. They are discussed in detail in Chapter 12.

GROWTH FACTORS AND REGULATION OF PRODUCTION AND BLOOD CONCENTRATION

In health, the concentration of neutrophils in the blood is regulated to stay within a relatively narrow range compared with the range that is possible in disease. Regulation of production is mediated by a complicated set of

cytokines and growth factors, a simplified version of which is shown in *Figure 11.4*. The family of cytokines and growth factors depicted in Figure 11.4 work in concert at various stages to regulate neutrophil production. Colony-stimulating factor (CSF) is a group of characterized molecules; most notable are granulocyte-CSF and GM-CSF. These factors originate from numerous and diverse sites, including mononuclear cells, endothelium, fibroblasts, and other cell types. Mononuclear cells are probably the most important source of CSF and may modulate the release of CSFs from the other cell types. Interleukins (ILs) also participate in stimulation of production. The release of neutrophils from the marrow space to blood may be accelerated by IL-1, tumor necrosis factor (TNF), and leukocytosis-inducing factor (LIF). Because of variation in experimental conditions and methods, LIF may be the same as IL-1 and TNF.

In the normal steady state, production is balanced by the transendothelial migration of neutrophils into tissues. This balance yields blood neutrophil concentrations in the normal range. Increased levels of growth factors and cytokines are responsible for marked acceleration of the events to produce neutrophils in response to inflammation. This may result in a dramatic increase in neutrophil production and delivery to blood. Migration into the site of inflammation is accelerated and focused by chemoattractants that are released in the inflammatory lesion. The net result is an increase in the flux of neutrophils from the bone marrow to the inflammatory lesion. After resolution of the inflammatory lesion, blood neutrophil concentrations return to normal. This suggests the presence

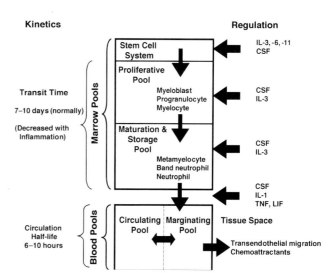

Figure 11.4 Bone marrow and blood neutrophil pools. Kinetic information is given on the left and regulation information on the right. Neutrophil production is regulated by a concert of growth factors and cytokines that act at multiple sites. The transit time is normally 7 to 10 days but may be shortened with increased demand. The circulation half-life is approximately 6 to 10 hours.

of some negative-feedback mechanism, but its nature is currently unknown.

NEUTROPHIL KINETICS

Some basic information about the kinetics of neutrophils in various pools is helpful in the interpretation of sequential changes in the leukogram. The transit time for production and the circulation time in blood are the two key benchmarks for neutrophil kinetics.

The transit time is the amount of time needed for the myeloblast to complete the maturational events and become a segmented neutrophil in blood (see Fig. 11.4). In the normal steady state, the transit time is approximately 7 days. When the bone marrow is stimulated by the inflammatory response, the transit time may become as short as 2 to 3 days.

The circulation time is the amount of time between release of the neutrophil to the blood and its subsequent egress into tissues. Neutrophils randomly migrate into tissues, so their circulation time is variable and not related to cell age. The circulation time is approximately 6 to 10 hours, encompassing some species variation. This means that the blood neutrophil pools are renewed approximately two to three times per day. The circulation time may be shortened considerably when neutrophils are consumed at a more rapid rate (e.g., at a site of inflammation). Given the rapid rate of blood neutrophil renewal in blood, marked changes in the blood neutrophil concentration may occur very rapidly in response to disease. The magnitude of these changes in the cell concentration that may be observed on hemograms sampled only hours apart is often dramatic and surprising.

SUGGESTED READINGS

Athens JW. Granulocytes—neutrophils. In: Lee GR, et al. Wintrobe's clinical hematology. 9th ed. Philadelphia: Lea & Febiger, 1993: 223–266.

Feldman BF, Zinkl JG, Jain NC. Schalm's veterinary hematology. 5th ed. Baltimore: Lippincott Williams & Wilkins, 2000.

Quesenberry PJ, Colein GA. Hematopoietic stem cells, progenitor cells, and cytokines. In: Beutler E, et al. William's hematology. 6th ed. New York: McGraw-Hill, 2001:153–174.

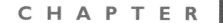

CHAPTER

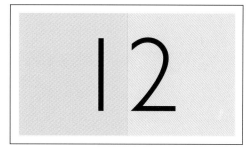

INTERPRETATION OF

LEUKOCYTE RESPONSES

IN DISEASE

To communicate about leukocyte responses, one must first become familiar with the descriptive terminology associated with abnormal patterns of cell concentrations in blood. To identify and interpret leukocyte responses, the rules for interpreting abnormal concentration patterns as indicators of disease processes must be learned. This chapter presents terminology, abnormal morphologic features encountered in the laboratory, and guidelines for interpretation of leukocyte patterns.

TERMINOLOGY OF ABNORMAL LEUKOCYTE CONCENTRATION PATTERNS

Suffixes

Abnormal concentrations are described using a variety of suffixes attached to the name of the cell type(s) involved.

The suffix *-penia* refers to a decreased concentration of the cell type in blood. A general term, *cytopenia,* refers to a decrease in cell concentration in a nonspecific manner. Cytopenias that are important for interpretation include neutropenia, lymphopenia, and eosinopenia. Cytopenia does not apply to monocytes, because a decreased concentration of this cell type is not important. It also does not apply to band neutrophils, metamyelocytes, basophils,

and metarubricytes, because the absence of these cells is normal.

The suffixes *-philia* or *-cytosis* refer to an increased concentration of the cell type in blood. Examples include:

- Neutrophilia or neutrophilic leukocytosis
- Eosinophilia
- Basophilia
- Monocytosis
- Lymphocytosis
- Metarubricytosis

Left Shift

Left shift refers to an increased concentration of immature neutrophils in blood. This usually indicates band neutrophils, but metamyelocytes and earlier forms may accompany increased bands. (See Fig. 10.1 for neutrophil and left-shift morphology.) A left shift may occur with neutrophilia. A left shift also may occur with neutropenia; this indicates a more severe consumption of neutrophils by a more aggressive inflammatory lesion. An orderly left shift suggests an inflammatory stimulus; in this case, the term *orderly* means that the concentration of each cell stage decreases with the degree of immaturity of the cell stage.

135

Leukemia

Leukemia refers to the presence of neoplastic cells in the circulation. The type of leukemia is designated by the type of neoplastic cell that is present if its morphologic features of differentiation are sufficient for identification. Examples include myelomonocytic leukemia and lymphocytic leukemia. The concentration of neoplastic cells may vary from detectable by extensive scanning of the blood film to extremely high.

Proliferative Disorder

Proliferative disorder is a nonspecific term for a hematopoietic cell neoplasm that is distributed in blood, bone marrow, other tissues, or a combination of sites. Proliferative disorders are classified into lymphoproliferative and myeloproliferative categories. The distinction between the lymphoid and bone marrow stem cell systems is somewhat artificial, but these two classes of proliferative disorders have different biologic behavior. Proliferative disorders are discussed separately in Chapter 13.

Lymphoproliferative Disorders

Lymphoproliferative disorders, which are characterized in *Figure 12.1*, are neoplastic processes with lymphoid cell differentiation. If the neoplasm is confined to solid tissues, it is termed *lymphosarcoma* or *lymphoma*. If it involves blood and/or bone marrow, it is termed *lymphocytic leukemia*. A specific form with plasma cell differentiation is termed *myeloma*, which is usually associated with production of a monoclonal immunoglobulin usually detected in blood. Immunoglobulin components also are usually detected in urine. More extensive and detailed classifications of lymphoproliferative disorders based on cellular morphology and immunophenotyping are available (see Chapter 13 and *Suggested Readings*).

Myeloproliferative Disorders

Myeloproliferative disorders arise from the bone marrow stem cell system. More extensive and detailed classifica-

tions of myeloproliferative disorders based on cellular morphology are available (see Chapter 13 and *Suggested Readings*). The recognized lines of differentiation and associated terminology for specific myeloproliferative disorders are detailed in *Figure 12.2*. Note that more differentiation pathways are recognized for myeloproliferative disorders than for lymphoproliferative disorders. Granulocytic, monocytic, and erythroid differentiations are the most common myeloproliferative disorders; the others are rare.

ACQUIRED CHANGES IN LEUKOCYTE MORPHOLOGY

Neutrophil Toxic Change

Neutrophil toxic change may be observed in association with inflammatory responses. The term *toxic change* is unfortunate, because it originated from early observations that these alterations in cell morphology were associated with toxemia in human patients, which implies that the cells are impaired. Today, however, we understand that the morphologic change is attributable to altered bone marrow production and that the cells have normal function. When an inflammatory stimulus is delivered to the bone marrow (see Fig. 11.4), neutrophils are produced at an accelerated rate. As a result, the cells may have increased amounts of certain organelles that are present during early development. The principal manifestation is cytoplasmic basophilia (*Fig. 12.3*). This is attributable to a larger-than-normal complement of ribosomes. Other, less common manifestations accompanying

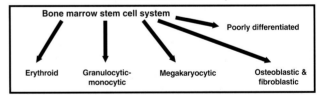

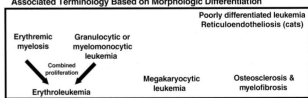

Figure 12.2 Organization and general terminology for myeloproliferative disorders. The top box shows general differentiation pathways based on morphologically recognized cell lineages. The bottom box shows historical and commonly applied terminology for the myeloproliferative disorders based on morphologic identity. See text for discussion.

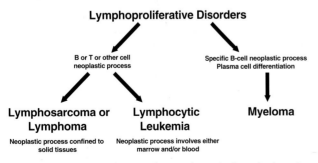

Figure 12.1 Organization and general terminology for lymphoproliferative disorders. See text for discussion.

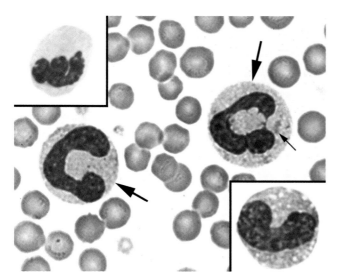

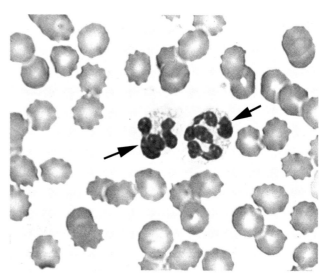

Figure 12.3 Neutrophils with marked toxic change (arrows). Note prominent cytoplasmic basophilia. A Döhle body is indicated by the thin arrow. A toxic neutrophil with fine cytoplasmic vacuolation is shown in the lower right inset. For comparison, a normal neutrophil is shown in the upper left inset. Wright-Giemsa stain, high magnification.

Figure 12.4 Neutrophils with hypersegmentation (arrows). Note the nuclear constrictions to a filament of chromatin that separates approximately five to seven chromatin lobes. Wright-Giemsa stain, high magnification.

cytoplasmic basophilia include Döhle bodies and cytoplasmic vacuolation. Döhle bodies are aggregates of endoplasmic reticulum and appear as gray-blue cytoplasmic precipitates and is seen more commonly in cats. (Fig. 12.3).

The interpretation of toxic change is that neutrophils are made under conditions of accelerated production that occurs as part of the inflammatory response. As a result, toxic change often accompanies other quantitative changes in the inflammatory leukogram presented later in this chapter.

Neutrophil Hypersegmentation

Neutrophil hypersegmentation is the normal progression of nuclear maturation in the neutrophil. The progression from band shape to segmentation to hypersegmentation is a continuum that occurs in a matter of hours. Normally, the process of continued segmentation and, finally, pyknosis occurs in neutrophils after egression to tissues. Hypersegmentation observed on the blood film results from longer-than-normal retention of neutrophils in the circulation (*Fig. 12.4*). The interpretation of hypersegmentation is relatively unimportant (it is usually associated with steroid effect on the leukogram presented in this chapter).

Neutrophil Degeneration

Neutrophil degeneration is a description ordinarily applied to neutrophils from samples other than blood (e.g., cytopathologic specimens). Neutrophils exposed to an unhealthy environment outside of blood may rapidly

degenerate. This is accelerated in cytopathologic specimens, which either have a bacterial component or are from epithelial surfaces such as skin, airways, and the gastrointestinal tract (*Fig. 12.5*). Features include cytoplasmic vacuolation and nuclear swelling seen as a loss of chromatin pattern and light staining. These changes may progress to cell lysis. It is an artifact in blood seen on the blood film if that film is made from blood that has aged for 12 hours or longer after collection from the animal (Fig. 12.5). In blood, it therefore is interpreted as an artifact of improper sample handling.

Leukocyte Agglutination

Leukocyte agglutination is an immunoglobulin-mediated agglutination of leukocytes in vitro. It may affect either neutrophils or lymphocytes. This phenomenon does not occur in the animal at body temperature, and it likely has no pathologic consequence in vivo. It is thought to be attributable to a cold-reacting immunoglobulin that acts at temperatures well below body temperature. When the blood cools to room temperature or below, this abnormal immunoglobulin binds to its leukocyte target and bridges cells into agglutinated particles. It therefore occurs in the blood tube after collection from the patient. Its importance is that it may result in a falsely low total white-blood-cell concentration, because agglutinated leukocytes are not counted by instruments. It is observed on scanning the blood film (*Fig. 12.6*).

Lymphocyte Vacuolation

Lymphocyte vacuolation may be an acquired change associated with ingestion of certain plants containing the

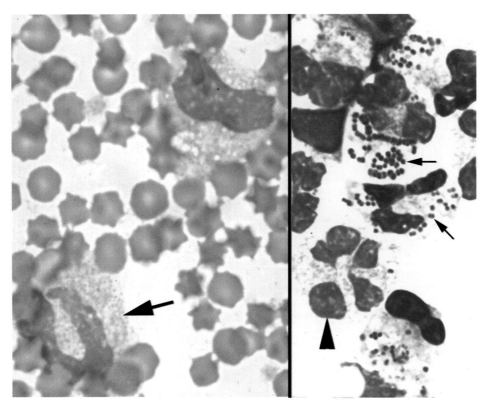

Figure 12.5 Neutrophil degeneration. The left panel shows neutrophil (arrow) degeneration on a blood film that is an artifact of aging in the collection tube before blood-film preparation. Note the swollen chromatin that results in lighter staining and loss of chromatin detail. The right panel shows neutrophils in various stages of degeneration in a cytologic preparation. This results from an unhealthy environment that is created, in part, by numerous bacteria (thin arrows). A neutrophil with chromatin swelling and loss of detail is indicated by the arrowhead. Wright-Giemsa stain, high magnification.

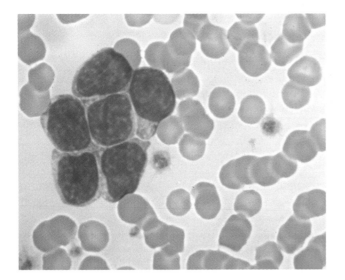

Figure 12.6 Leukoagglutination involving lymphocytes. Note the tight adherence of cells in a cluster. Multiple clusters are observable at low magnification. These cell clusters result in falsely low white-blood-cell counts when present in the counting fluid diluent (see text). Wright-Giemsa stain, high magnification.

toxic substance swainsonine. An example is locoweed ingestion in horses or cattle. The appearance is similar to that of lymphocyte vacuolation associated with inherited storage disorders (discussed later; see Fig. 12.11).

INHERITED ABNORMALITIES OF LEUKOCYTE MORPHOLOGY

Inherited Abnormalities of Neutrophil Morphology

Inherited abnormalities of neutrophil morphology include Pelger-Huët anomaly, Birman cat neutrophil granulation anomaly, mucopolysaccharidoses, and Chédiak-Higashi syndrome.

Pelger-Huët Anomaly

Mature, hyposegmented neutrophils are seen in heterozygotes for Pelger-Huët anomaly. These cells have an immaturely shaped nucleus (i.e., band or myelocyte form) but a coarse, mature chromatin pattern (*Fig. 12.7*). Neutrophils function normally, and affected animals are healthy. Typically, no segmented neutrophils are seen in blood films from these animals. Eosinophils are also affected and appear as band forms. The importance of recognizing Pelger-Huët anomaly is to prevent misidentification of a left shift and misinterpretation as an inflammatory response in an otherwise apparently healthy, affected individual.

Birman Cat Neutrophil Granulation Anomaly

Neutrophils from affected cats contain fine eosinophilic to magenta-colored granules (*Fig. 12.8*). This anomaly is inherited in an autosomal recessive manner. Neutrophil function is normal, and cats are healthy. This granulation must be distinguished from toxic granulation, which is rare, and from that seen in neutrophils from cats with mucopolysaccharidosis, which usually is more coarse.

Mucopolysaccharidoses

Neutrophils from animals with mucopolysaccharidosis (MPS) typically contain numerous distinct, dark-purple or magenta-colored granules (*Fig. 12.9*). Lymphocytes also usually contain granules and vacuoles.

Mucopolysaccharidosis is a group of heritable, lysosomal storage disorders caused by a deficiency of lysosomal enzymes needed for the stepwise degradation of glycosaminoglycans (i.e., mucopolysaccharides). Common features include dwarfism (except feline MPS I), severe

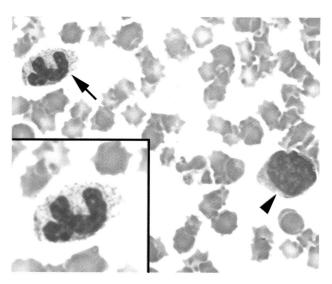

Figure 12.8 Granulated neutrophil from a cat with Birman cat neutrophil granulation anomaly (arrow). The lower left inset shows an enlarged view of the same cell. Note the fine granulation as compared with mucopolysaccharidosis (see Fig. 12.9). Lymphocytes (arrowhead) are not affected. Wright-Giemsa stain, high magnification.

bone disease, degenerative joint disease including hip subluxation, facial dysmorphia, hepatomegaly (except feline MPS VI), corneal clouding, enlarged tongue (canine MPS), heart-valve thickening, excess urinary excretion of glycosaminoglycans, and metachromatic granules (i.e., Alder-Reilly bodies) in blood leukocytes. These

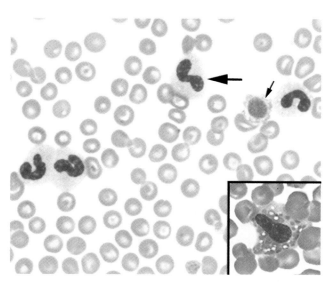

Figure 12.7 Granulocytes from a dog with Pelger-Huët anomaly. Four hyposegmented neutrophils (thick arrow) are present. The lower right inset shows a hyposegmented eosinophil. A macroplatelet, present by coincidence, is indicated by the thin arrow. Wright-Giemsa stain, high magnification.

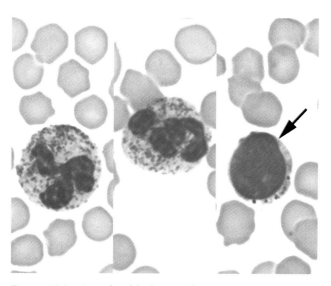

Figure 12.9 Granulated leukocytes from a cat with mucopolysaccharidosis VI. Note the prominently granulated neutrophils at the left and center. A lymphocyte with sparse granulation is typical of mucopolysaccharidosis (arrow). Wright-Giemsa stain, high magnification.

granules are more distinct in MPS VI and VII than in MPS I. Granules usually are not apparent when stained with Diff-Quik. The disease is progressive, with clinical signs becoming apparent at 2 to 4 months of age. Affected animals may live several years, but locomotor difficulty is progressive.

Chediak-Higashi Syndrome

Neutrophils in cats affected by Chediak-Higashi syndrome have large, fused, 2.0-μm lysosomes that stain lightly pink or eosinophilic within the cytoplasm (*Fig. 12.10*). Approximately one in three or four neutrophils contain one to four fused lysosomes. Eosinophilic granules appear slightly plump and large. These cats have a slight tendency to bleed, because platelet function is abnormal. Although neutrophil function is also abnormal, cats are generally healthy. The syndrome had been reported in cats of Persian ancestry and is inherited in an autosomal recessive manner.

Inherited Abnormalities of Lymphocyte Morphology

Cytoplasmic vacuolization is the most significant inherited abnormality of lymphocytes and usually is associated with lysosomal storage disorders (*Fig. 12.11*). Those lysosomal storage diseases described in domestic animals that result in vacuoles within the cytoplasm of lymphocytes include the MPS (also have granules in neutrophils); G_{M1} and G_{M2} gangliosidosis (G_{M2} gangliosidosis also has granules in lymphocytes and neutrophils) (*Fig. 12.12*); alpha-mannosidosis; Niemann-Pick types A, B, and C;

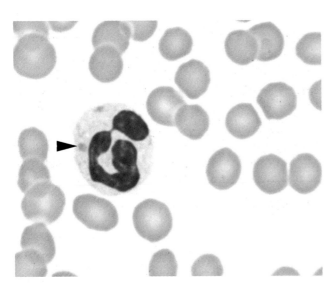

Figure 12.10 Neutrophil from a cat with Chédiak-Higashi syndrome. Note the large eosinophilic granule in the cytoplasm (arrowhead). Wright-Giemsa stain, high magnification.

acid-lipase deficiency; and fucosidosis. All these disorders, except for MPS and acid-lipase deficiency, result in severe, progressive neurologic disease that is ultimately fatal.

INTERPRETATION OF LEUKOCYTE RESPONSES

Perspective

Most leukocyte response patterns are not interpreted into specific diagnoses, although leukemias may be an exception. Instead, responses are interpreted into basic processes occurring in the animal. These processes must then be coupled with other clinical information to determine a clinical diagnosis.

Hematologic Response to Inflammation

Inflammation is the most important—and one of the most common—blood leukocyte responses. The nature of the response is best understood by considering a modified neutrophil trafficking model (*Fig. 12.13*). It also may be helpful to review the steady-state neutrophil trafficking model in Chapter 11 (see Fig. 11.3). When inflammation is established, an orchestra of chemical mediators modulates many events. Vasodilation and chemotactic substances work to increase the egress of neutrophils from the local marginated pool into the inflammatory lesion. Cytokines released from local mononuclear cells (see Fig. 11.4) make their way to the bone marrow, where they increase the rate of release of maturing neutrophils and the rate of production by increasing stem-cell entry, proliferative events, and maturation events. The net result is that the marrow response dramatically increases the delivery rate of neutrophils to blood. In summary, a complete cycle of consumption, production, and release is activated, with the goal of delivering a supply of neutrophils to the inflammatory lesion until it resolves.

The pattern of neutrophil concentrations seen in blood may vary from severely decreased to markedly increased. It is helpful to think of the pattern being dependent on a balance between consumption by the lesion and production and release by the marrow (*Fig. 12.14*). All neutrophil concentration patterns encountered during inflammation may be explained by this balance. Most inflammatory processes result in some degree of neutrophilia, indicating that marrow releases more cells to blood than are consumed at the site of inflammation. This is illustrated using the neutrophil trafficking model in *Figure 12.15*. Inflammatory patterns manifesting in neutrophilia may be regarded as mild to severe responses that are managing the lesion. The severity of the process may be roughly predicted by the magnitude of the left shift and the presence of toxic change in neutrophils.

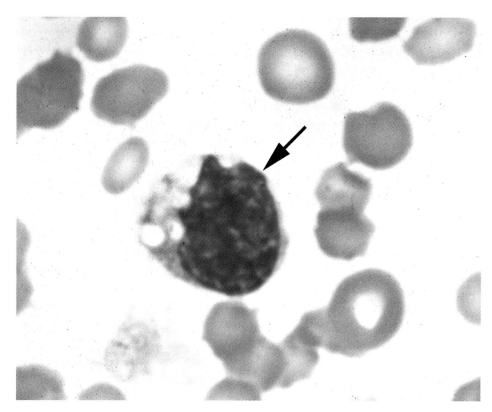

Figure 12.11   Cytoplasmic vacuolation of a lymphocyte (arrow) from a cat with a lysosomal storage disorder (alpha-mannosidosis). Wright-Giemsa stain, high magnification.

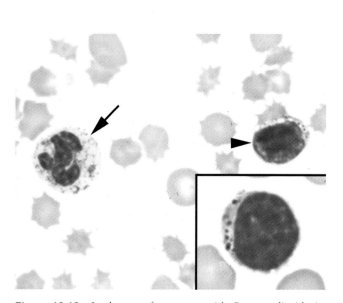

Figure 12.12   Leukocytes from a cat with G_{M2} gangliosidosis. Neutrophils (arrow) may have granulation similar to that seen with mucopolysaccharidosis. Lymphocytes (arrowhead) also have small numbers of granules with some degree of cytoplasmic vacuolation. The lower right inset shows an enlarged lymphocyte. Wright-Giemsa stain, high magnification.

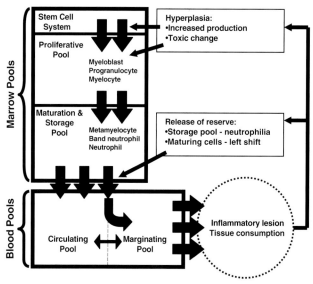

Figure 12.13   Modified neutrophil trafficking model illustrating effects of the inflammatory response on blood and bone marrow. Note the cycle of events leading to increased neutrophil delivery to blood and tissues at the inflammatory site: release of mediators from an inflammatory lesion, increased marrow hyperplasia, increased delivery from marrow to blood, and increased consumption to the site of inflammation.

Balance of Dynamics Determining Blood Neutrophil Concentration

Marrow Delivery Rate

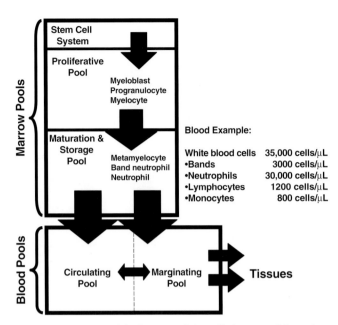

Balance between production and consumption. All inflammatory processes may be understood as a balance between marrow delivery and inflammatory-site consumption. When marrow delivery exceeds consumption, blood neutrophilia develops. When tissue consumption exceeds marrow delivery, neutropenia with a left shift develops.

Very severe—and typically acute—inflammatory lesions, on the other hand, may consume neutrophils more rapidly than the neutrophils can be delivered to blood. When this occurs, neutropenia develops, as shown in the neutrophil trafficking model in *Figure 12.16*. In this case, a left shift is expected. At one or more time points, the concentration of bands may be greater than that of segmented neutrophils.

The balance between neutrophil consumption and delivery by bone marrow is affected by species differences, as outlined in *Table 12.1*. Species may vary in the amount of neutrophil reserve and in the proliferative capacity of the marrow. Dogs have the largest reserve and the greatest ability to produce neutrophils; cows and other ruminants form the other extreme. Cats and horses are somewhat intermediate in their capacities to deliver cells to blood.

These differences translate into magnitudes of neutrophilia that can occur with inflammatory disease in each species. They also influence how neutrophil concentrations are interpreted with respect to chronicity and severity of the process in various species. For example, in chronic, closed-cavity inflammatory processes, neutrophilia may go as high as 100,000 cells/µL in dogs, but a corresponding process in cows will result in a maximum of approximately 25,000 cells/µL. Cats and horses will be intermediate, as indicated in Table 12.1.

Similarly, bone marrow behavior influences how neutropenia is interpreted during acute inflammation. Because of the canine ability to deliver cells to blood, neutropenia only occurs with inflammatory states involving severe con-

Modified neutrophil trafficking model used to illustrate a moderate inflammatory response. Also illustrated is an example of the balance between production and consumption. Note that in this case, marrow delivery exceeds tissue consumption. The example is described as leukocytosis caused by neutrophilia (30,000 cells/µL) and a left shift (3000 bands/µL). The neutrophil pattern is interpreted as inflammation.

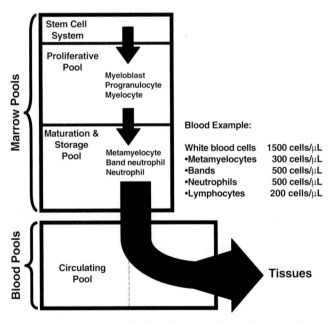

Modified neutrophil trafficking model used to illustrate a severe inflammatory response. Also illustrated is an example of the balance between production and consumption. Note that in this case, tissue consumption exceeds marrow delivery. The example is described as leukopenia caused by neutropenia (500 cells/µL) and a left shift (300 metamyelocytes/µL and 500 bands/µL). The neutrophil pattern is interpreted as severe, acute inflammation.

TABLE 12.1 COMPARATIVE BONE MARROW CONTRIBUTION TO NEUTROPHIL TRAFFICKING AND RELATIONSHIP TO RANGES OF NEUTROPHILIA SEEN WITH THE INFLAMMATORY RESPONSE IN VARIOUS SPECIES

Species	Marrow Reserve	Regenerative Capacity
Dog	Relatively high	Rapid
Cat	Intermediate	Intermediate
Horse	Intermediate	Intermediate
Cow	Relatively low	Slow

Species	Range of Possible Neutrophilia (neutrophils/μL)
Dog	20,000–100,000
Cat	20,000–60,000
Horse	15,000–30,000
Cow	10,000–25,000

Species	Interpretation of Neutropenia During Acute Inflammation
Dog	Very severe lesion
Cat	Very severe lesion
Horse	Probable severe lesion
Cow	Usual findings, regardless of severity

sumption. Neutropenia caused by inflammation may be regarded as a medical emergency in dogs; to some extent, this is also true in cats and horses. Neutropenia in cows is interpreted differently. Because of the minimal neutrophil reserve in this species, the expected response in the acute bovine inflammatory leukogram is neutropenia. Acute inflammatory lesions in cows consume neutrophils from the blood and marrow within a matter of hours. The result may be profound neutropenia that lasts for a few days. After that time, repopulation of blood with neutrophils, with a left shift, occurs as the marrow production increases.

Factors Modulating the Magnitude of Neutrophilia in the Inflammatory Response

The type of inflammatory lesion may influence the balance between consumption and marrow release. Acute inflam-

mation is a lesion with increased local blood flow and swelling. This results from inflammatory mediators that promote local vascular dilation. Chemotactic factors released within the lesion in conjunction with the vascular events have ample opportunity to promote consumption of neutrophils. An example is cellulitis associated with a bite wound, which results in a balance between consumption and production that is reasonably well matched. The blood inflammatory pattern then consists of mild to moderate neutrophilia with a variable left shift, depending on the severity of the lesion. Acute peritonitis is an example of a major consumer of neutrophils that may exceed the marrow capacity for production; in this example, it is possible to see neutropenia with a prominent left shift.

Chronic, walled-off inflammatory lesions, on the other hand, may result in very high neutrophil concentrations. Examples include pyometra in dogs or a chronic, walled-off abscess that does not resolve. These are also known as closed-cavity inflammatory lesions (as opposed to diffuse inflammation; discussed above). These lesions continue to stimulate the marrow to achieve maximal production; however, the rate of consumption is curtailed by the nature of the lesion, thus tipping the balance toward production exceeding consumption. In these cases, neutrophil concentrations may approach 100,000 cells/μL in dogs.

Excitement Response: Epinephrine Release

The excitement response is an immediate change associated with epinephrine release and is also known as the "fight-or-flight" response. Epinephrine release results in cardiovascular events that, in turn, result in increased blood flow through the microcirculation, particularly in muscle. Strenuous exercise just before bleeding may have the same effect. This results in a shift of leukocytes from the marginated pool to the circulating pool, as depicted in the neutrophil trafficking model (*Fig. 12.17*). On the leukogram, this manifests as an approximate doubling of leukocytes and is noted in the neutrophils and/or lymphocytes. Within the neutrophil population, no left shift occurs, because the neutrophilia is caused by mature cells in the microcirculation being flushed to the circulating pool.

The excitement response is recognized most frequently in cats. Lymphocytosis up to a maximum of approximately 20,000 cells/μL is the prominent feature of the feline excitement response. Mature neutrophilia may occur if the resting neutrophil concentration was at the upper end of normal before initiation of the excitement response. In large animals, the excitement response is recognized in association with exercise before bleeding or events that may induce excitement, such as trucking or movement through chutes for blood collection. The excitement response is least common in dogs, because this species is

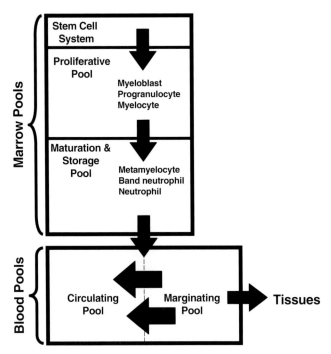

Figure 12.17 Modified neutrophil trafficking model used to illustrate the excitement response. Note that the change involves cell movement from the marginating pool to the circulating pool, resulting in an approximate doubling of resting leukocyte concentrations. Marrow delivery and tissue consumption are unchanged.

usually accustomed to physical handling related to blood collection.

Stress Response: Corticosteroid Release or Administration

Physiologic stress is a body response mediated by release of adrenocorticotropic hormone by the pituitary gland and resultant release of cortisol by the adrenal gland. This occurs in response to major systemic illnesses, metabolic disturbances, and pain. Examples of conditions eliciting the stress response include renal failure, diabetic keto-acidosis, dehydration, inflammatory disease, and pain associated with trauma. The response may be detected in the leukogram by changes in multiple cell types.

The most consistent change is lymphopenia. Steroids may induce lymphocyte apoptosis and may alter patterns of recirculation. The second most consistent change is an approximate doubling of the circulating neutrophils. Steroids cause decreased stickiness and margination, resulting in slightly longer-than-normal retention in the circulation. As a result, hypersegmentation may be observed. When the resting neutrophil concentration is in the upper 50th percentile of the normal range, neutrophilia is expected. A left shift will not occur unless inflammation is superimposed. Eosinopenia is the next most consistent change. Monocytosis is variable but oc-

curs most consistently in dogs. The importance of interpreting the steroid leukogram is to look for an underlying physiologic disturbance (if it has not yet been recognized) and to avoid interpreting a simple steroid pattern as inflammation.

Lastly, it is important to note that a steroid response not being present in a very sick animal should prompt the consideration of hypoadrenocorticism (i.e., Addison disease).

Summary: Approach to Neutrophilia

In summary, neutrophilia has three causes. Thus, it is useful to develop an orderly approach to looking at the leukogram to rapidly arrive at the proper interpretation of the neutrophilia. The flowchart in *Figure 12.18* develops this approach. When neutrophilia is identified, one should next examine the leukogram for the presence of a left shift. If a left shift is present, the interpretation is inflammation. If a left shift is not present, the lymphocyte concentration should be examined. If lymphopenia is found with a neutrophilia and no left shift, the interpretation is steroid response. If the lymphocyte concentration is upper normal or increased within certain limits, the interpretation of excitement response should be considered. Keep in mind that clear neutrophilia with a left-shift inflammatory pattern may have a superimposed steroid response; this is identified by the presence of lymphopenia in conjunction with the neutrophil pattern.

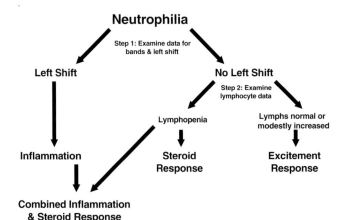

Figure 12.18 Summary flow chart for interpretation of neutrophilias. When neutrophilia is seen, the observer should examine the data for a left shift (Step 1). If a left shift is present, then the interpretation is inflammation. If no left shift is present, then the observer should examine the lymphocyte data (Step 2). Lymphopenia in conjunction with a mature neutrophilia indicates a steroid response. If the lymphocyte concentration is normal to increased, an excitement response should be considered. Also, note that an inflammatory pattern may have a superimposed steroid response that is recognized as lymphopenia occurring in conjunction with the inflammatory pattern.

Lymphocytosis

Lymphocytosis has two common causes. The first is the excitement response (discussed above), and the second is lymphocytic leukemia. The approach to interpreting lymphocytosis involves analysis of both concentration and cell morphology (*Fig. 12.19*). The lymphocyte morphology should be critically examined when lymphocytosis is present. If the cell concentration is only modestly increased and the cells are morphologically small, normal-appearing lymphocytes, then an excitement response should be considered. As a guideline, this modest increase is suggested to be a lymphocyte concentration of up to approximately 12,000 and 20,000 cells/µL in dogs and cats, respectively. If the concentrations exceed this guideline or the animal was not excited, then a lymphocytic leukemia should be considered. Repeating the hemogram the next day while making note of the possibility of excitement during blood collection also may be helpful. The higher the concentration, the greater the probability that the cause is a lymphoproliferative disorder with leukemia.

A common misconception is that lymphocytosis may occur with chronic inflammatory diseases. This concept likely is extrapolated from the knowledge that inflammatory disease results in an immune system response that includes lymphoid hyperplasia. This process does occur, but the expansion is confined to lymphoid tissues and rarely manifests as lymphocytosis in blood. An exception is the chronic form of canine ehrlichiosis, which has been documented to result in lymphocytosis and also monoclonal gammopathy. The monoclonal gammopathy is expected to be superimposed on an underlying polyclonal gammopathy. When the lymphocytosis is examined, a high proportion of large granular lymphocytes (see Fig. 10.4) may

be observed. In dogs, chronic ehrlichiosis should be considered with lymphocyte concentrations up to 30,000 or 40,000 cells/µL.

Abnormal lymphocyte morphology in the interpretation of lymphocytosis usually relates to features of neoplastic cells by virtue of cell types that do not belong in the circulation of the normal animal. These cells have one or more features of a cell undergoing proliferation, as opposed to the small, resting lymphocyte that is ordinarily seen in blood (*Fig. 12.20*). These features may include a diameter larger than that of adjacent neutrophils, a fine chromatin pattern resulting in a lighter-staining nucleus, a visible nucleolus, and increased cytoplasm (*Figs. 12.20 and 12.21*). If cells with abnormal features are present in the circulation, leukemia is a diagnostic consideration with normal to mildly increased lymphocyte concentrations. Lymphoproliferative disorders and lymphocytic leukemia are presented in more detail in Chapter 13.

Bovine persistent lymphocytosis may occur in cattle infected with bovine leukemia virus (BLV). Persistent lymphocytosis is defined as a lymphocyte concentration of greater than 7500 cells/µL on two or more hemograms. The morphology may be normal. Persistent lymphocytosis is part of a continuum in BLV-infected cows that eventually may progress to a diagnosis of lymphocytic leukemia or lymphosarcoma. Historically, hemograms, with an emphasis on the lymphocyte concentration, have been used as a screening test for BLV infection.

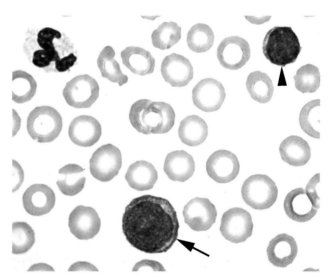

Figure 12.20 Lymphocyte morphology in relationship to evaluation of lymphocytosis. Normal blood lymphocyte morphology consists of small, resting lymphocytes (arrowhead). Note that the diameter is less than that of adjacent neutrophils, the chromatin is condensed, and cytoplasm is scant. An abnormal lymphocyte (arrow) in blood suggests a lymphoproliferative disorder involving blood. Note the increased size, increased cytoplasm, and more fine chromatin pattern. This cell also has a visible nucleolar ring in the nucleus. Wright-Giemsa stain, high magnification.

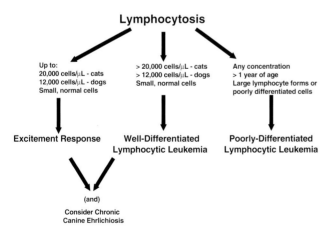

Figure 12.19 Summary approach to interpretation of lymphocytosis. This flow chart may be useful for distinguishing the excitement response from lymphocytic leukemias based on lymphocyte concentration and morphology guidelines. Inflammatory disease is rarely associated with lymphocytosis; however, chronic canine ehrlichiosis is an exception. See text for discussion.

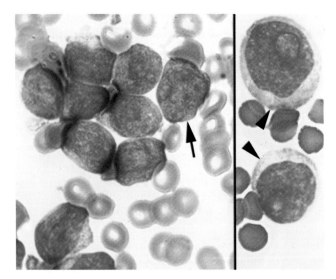

Figure 12.21 The left pane shows large, abnormal lymphocytes (arrow) from a dog with lymphoblastic leukemia (~70,000 lympho-cytes/μL). Note the fine, granular chromatin pattern as well as the occasional, faint nucleoli and the large size. The right panel shows two lymphoblasts (arrowheads) from a cat with lymphoblastic leukemia. Note the large cell size, fine chromatin pattern, and prominent nucleolar rings. Wright-Giemsa stain, high magnification.

Neutropenia

Neutropenia Resulting from Acute Inflammatory Consumption

Neutropenia resulting from overwhelming consumption by an inflammatory lesion was discussed earlier (with the inflammatory response). Neutropenia resulting from consumption is associated with a left shift in dogs and cats. Toxic changes are also expected within a few days of the onset of the process. An alternative form of consumptive neutropenia is immune-mediated neutropenia, in which immunoglobulin that recognizes epitope(s) on the neutrophil surface or adsorbed onto the surface results in destruction of both circulating neutrophils and late stages of maturation within the marrow. This may result in profound neutropenia not associated with a demonstrable inflammatory lesion.

Neutropenia Resulting from Stem Cell Injuries

The various stem cell injuries may be considered modifications of the neutrophil trafficking model in *Figure 12.22*. Stem cell injuries have numerous causes, ranging from very acute, transient injury of variable duration to permanent, irreversible injuries. Stem cell injuries are nonspecific in that all cell lines of marrow are involved. Evidence of marrow failure manifested in blood is related to the duration of the injury in relationship to the circulating time or life span of various cell types. Because neu-

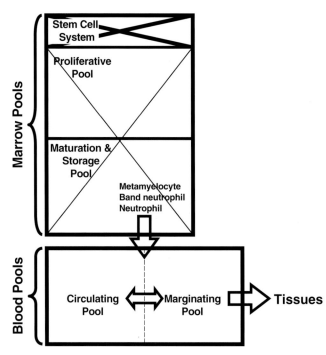

Figure 12.22 Modified neutrophil trafficking model used to illustrate neutropenias caused by stem cell injury. Injury occurs to the stem cell system, which results in a lack of recruited cells to proceed through the proliferative and maturation stages. The end result is interruption in the supply of neutrophils to blood. Because tissue consumption is not interrupted, profound neutropenia in the blood pools may occur within a few days or less.

trophils are renewed in blood most rapidly, neutropenia develops first with a stem cell injury. Thrombocytopenia is seen second, because platelets last approximately 7 days in the circulation. Nonregenerative anemia occurs last because of the long erythrocyte life span.

Neutropenia Caused by Reversible Stem Cell Injuries

Several acute, transient stem cell injuries are caused by the tropism of viruses for rapidly dividing cells. Canine parvovirus and feline panleukopenia are notable examples; these result in injury to intestinal lining, lymphoid cells, and the bone marrow stem cell system. Profound neutropenia is attributable to two mechanisms. First, stem cell injury results in transient failure of production. Second, neutrophil consumption increases at the site of gastrointestinal injury. The stem cell injury involves all marrow cell lines but is so transient that marrow repopulation occurs before thrombocytopenia and nonregenerative anemia can develop. If anemia is observed, it likely is caused by blood loss into the gastrointestinal tract. Acute neutropenia persists for only 24 to 48 hours. During the short period of neutropenia, a left shift is not observed. As the marrow repopulates, a left shift with progressively increasing neutrophil concentrations is observed. An inflammatory pattern, consisting of neutrophilia and left shift, is usually observed during recovery.

Reversible stem cell injury of varying duration also has numerous causes. These generally are present for days or longer; thus, varying degrees of thrombocytopenia and nonregenerative anemia accompany the neutropenia. One group of causes are chemicals or drugs that injure rapidly dividing cells. Most chemotherapeutic drugs are in this category. Estrogen overdosage and phenylbutazone administration are characterized toxicities in dogs. Very high, repeated doses of estradiol may cause stem cell injury in dogs but not in cats. Historically, an alternate form of a long-acting, potent estrogen—estradiol cypionate—has been used to prevent unwanted pregnancies in dogs. This drug is used safely in small doses to treat incontinence. Naturally occurring estrogen toxicity may occur in ferrets if ovulation is not stimulated. Phenylbutazone, a common medication for pain and lameness that is used safely in horses, may cause marked stem cell injury in dogs. An example of an infectious cause is ehrlichiosis in dogs; ehrlichiosis may induce cytopenias by an immune-mediated mechanism that appears to act on cells in the marrow.

Neutropenia Caused by Irreversible Stem Cell Injuries

This category of stem cell injury may be regarded as a continuum of proliferative abnormalities of the bone marrow stem cell system. The underlying nature and mechanism of these injuries are poorly understood. Causes include infection with feline leukemia virus, idiopathic hypoproliferative disorders, myelodysplasias, and myeloproliferative disorders. Because these are long-standing disorders, any combination of neutropenia, nonregenerative anemia, and thrombocytopenia may occur. These relatively irreversible stem cell injuries are considered in detail in Chapter 13.

Approach to Neutropenia

The approach to interpretation of neutropenia is summarized in *Figure 12.23*. The observer should first determine if the neutropenia is associated with a left shift. If a prominent left shift is observed with toxic change, then the neutropenia is caused by an inflammatory disease. If no left shift is seen, then the other cell lines should be assessed. If any combination of thrombocytopenia, nonregenerative anemia, or evidence of hematopoietic cell neoplasia is found, then marrow injury should be considered.

Lymphopenia

Lymphopenia is usually attributable to a steroid response; other causes are uncommon to rare. Lympholytic acute

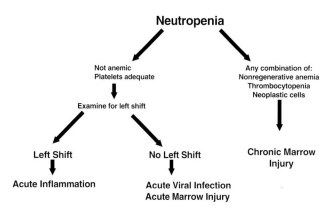

Figure 12.23 Summary approach to interpretation of neutropenia. This flow chart may be useful for distinguishing the various causes of neutropenia. When confronted with neutropenia, the observer should first examine the platelet and erythrocyte data for evidence of production problems. If these cell lines appear to have normal production, then a selective neutropenia is present. The observer should next examine the data for a left shift. If a left shift is found, then the interpretation is severe, acute inflammation (e.g., see Fig. 12.16). If no left shift is found, then an acute failure to produce neutrophils should be considered (as in Fig. 12.22). If the neutropenia is accompanied by evidence of failure to produce other cell lines (e.g., platelets and/or erythrocytes), then a more chronic marrow injury should be considered. The presence of neoplastic cells may indicate an underlying hematopoietic cell neoplasm and is also a possible cause of marrow failure. See text for discussion.

viral infections induce lymphopenia that is accompanied by neutropenia; however, neutropenia is the more important finding. Combined immunodeficiency syndrome of Arabian foals is an inherited disorder with severe deficiency of both T- and B-cell lymphocyte functions. The lymphocyte concentration may be used as a screening test for this disorder in newborn Arabian foals. A lymphocyte concentration of greater than 1000 cells/μL is a finding that rules out the disease. If lymphopenia is found, more confirmatory tests may be performed.

Monocytosis

Monocytosis is a relatively unimportant change. It may accompany both acute and chronic inflammatory responses. Monocytosis in this situation is interpreted as a response to increased demand for mononuclear cells in tissues. Monocytes in blood are regarded as immature cells that become macrophages after migration to tissue sites. Monocytosis also may occur in the steroid response, particularly in dogs.

Eosinophilia

Eosinophilia is interpreted as a nonspecific response that requires consideration of parasitism, hypersensitivity, or an unusual lesion producing eosinophil chemoattractants. Tissue-invading parasitisms are frequently associated with eosinophilia. Notable examples include heartworm disease and hookworm infestation in dogs. Inflammation at epithelial surfaces rich in mast cells (e.g., skin, respiratory tract, gastrointestinal tract) may be associated with eosinophilia, particularly if a component of hypersensitivity is present. Examples include flea-bite allergic dermatitis, inhalant allergen disease or asthma-like syndromes, feline hypereosinophilic syndromes, and poorly characterized gastroenteritis that may have an allergic component.

Basophilia

Basophilia is uncommon. In fact, basophils are so rare in normal animals that they usually are not encountered in the 100-cell microscopy differential. The interpretation of basophilia is unknown or not clear. It most frequently accompanies eosinophilia. When this happens, it is described as eosinophilia and basophilia, but it is eosinophilia that is interpreted as indicated earlier.

SUGGESTED READINGS

General
Feldman BF, Zinkl JG, Jain NC, eds. Schalm's veterinary hematology. 5th ed. Baltimore: Lippincott Williams & Wilkins, 2000.

Leukemia and Proliferative Disorders
Jain NC. Classification of myeloproliferative disorders in cats using criteria proposed by the Animal Leukaemia Study Group: a retrospective study of 181 cases (1969–1992). Comp Haematol Int 1993;1: 125–134.

Jain NC, Blue JT, Grindem CB, et al. Proposed criteria for classification of acute myeloid leukemias in dogs and cats—a report of the animal leukemia study group. Vet Clin Pathol 1991;20:63–82.

Leifer CE, Matus RE. Lymphoid leukemia in the dog: acute lymphoblastic leukemia and chronic lymphocytic leukemia. Vet Clin North Am Small Anim Pract 1985;15:723–739.

MacEwen G. Hematopoietic tumors. Feline lymphoma and leukemias. In: Withrow SJ, MacEwen EG, eds. Small animal clinical oncology. 2nd ed. Philadelphia: WB Saunders, 1989:479–495.

MacEwen EG, Young KM. Hematopoietic tumors. Canine lymphoma and lymphoid leukemias. In: Withrow SJ, MacEwen EG, eds. Small animal clinical oncology. 2nd ed. Philadelphia: WB Saunders, 1989: 451–477.

Madewell BR. Hematological and bone marrow cytological abnormalities in 75 dogs with malignant lymphoma. J Am Anim Hosp Assoc 1986;22:235–240.

Morrison WB. Plasma cell neoplasms. In: Morrison WB. Cancer in dogs and cats: medical and surgical management. Baltimore: Williams & Wilkins, 1998:697–704.

Thrall MA. Lymphoproliferative disorders. Vet Clin North Am 1981; 11:321–347.

Young KM, MacEwen EG. Hematopoietic tumors. Canine myeloproliferative disorders. In: Withrow SJ, MacEwen EG, eds. Small animal clinical oncology. 2nd ed. Philadelphia: WB Saunders, 1989: 495–505.

Pelger-Huët Anomaly
Latimer KS, Duncan JR, Kircher IM. Nuclear segmentation, ultrastructure, and cytochemistry of blood cells from dogs with Pelger-Huët anomaly. J Comp Pathol 1987; 97:61–72.

Latimer KS, Rakich PM, Thompson DF. Pelger-Huët anomaly in cats. Vet Pathol 1985;22:370–374.

Birman Cat Anomaly
Hirsch VM, Cunningham TA. Hereditary anomaly of neutrophil granulation in Birman cats. Am J Vet Res 1984;45:2170–2174.

Chédiak-Higashi Syndrome
Kramer J, Davis WC, Prieur DJ, Baxter J, Norsworthy GD. An inherited disorder of Persian cats with intracytoplasmic inclusions in neutrophils. J Am Vet Med Assoc 1975;166:1103–1104.

MPS, alpha-Mannosidosis, and Related Anomalies
Alroy J, Freden GO, Goyal V, et al. Morphology of leukocytes from cats affected with alpha-mannosidosis and mucopolysaccharidosis VI (MPS VI). Vet Pathol 1989;26:294–302.

Haskins M, Giger U. Lysosomal storage diseases. In: Kaneko JJ, Harvey JW, Bruss ML, eds. Clinical biochemistry of domestic animals. 5th ed. New York: Academic Press, 1997:741–760.

Skelly BJ, Franklin RJM. Recognition and diagnosis of lysosomal storage diseases in the cat and dog. J Vet Intern Med 2002;16: 133–141.

Warren CD, Alroy J. Morphological, biochemical and molecular biology approaches for the diagnosis of lysosomal storage diseases. J Vet Diagn Invest 2000;12:483–496.

Canine Ehrlichiosis and Lymphocytosis
Weiser MG, Thrall MA, Fulton R, et al. Granular lymphocytosis and hyperproteinemia in dogs with chronic ehrlichiosis. J Am Anim Hosp Assoc 1991;27:84–88.

Neutropenias
Brown MR, Rogers KS. Neutropenia in dogs and cats: a retrospective study of 261 cases. J Am Anim Hosp Assoc 2001;37:131–139.

McManus PM, Litwin C, Barber L. Immune-mediated neutropenia in two dogs. J Vet Intern Med 1999;13:372–374.

C H A P T E R

13

LABORATORY EVALUATION

OF BONE MARROW

Cytologic evaluation of a bone marrow aspiration biopsy specimen is helpful in animals with unexplained hematologic abnormalities when a diagnosis cannot be established based on examination of the blood. Examples of such abnormalities include nonregenerative anemia, neutropenia, thrombocytopenia, gammopathy, and suspicion of neoplastic marrow disease (e.g., lymphoma). In horses, bone marrow aspirates are useful to determine if anemias are regenerative, because equine species do not release immature erythrocytes into the peripheral blood. Contraindications to bone marrow aspiration are few, but marrow aspirates from the ribs or sternum of horses with clotting disorders have resulted in death because of hemothorax or cardiac tamponade. Hemorrhage usually can be prevented in thrombocytopenic animals by applying pressure to the aspiration site for several minutes.

TECHNIQUE

The sites that most commonly are used for bone marrow aspiration in dogs are the proximal end of the femur at the trochanteric fossa, the iliac crest, and the proximal humerus *(Fig. 13.1)*. The trochanteric fossa and humerus are

the preferred sites in cats, and the ilium, ribs, or sternum usually are aspirated in horses, cattle, and camelids. If general anesthesia or sedation is not used, a local anesthetic is indicated. Both the subcutis and periosteum should be infiltrated with anesthetic. Bone marrow biopsy needles (16–22 G) are commercially available (Fig. 13.1); conventional hypodermic needles without stylets tend to plug with bone and are not suitable. After surgical preparation of the skin, the needle is introduced. In thick-skinned animals, the skin may be incised to facilitate introduction of the needle. Once the needle is against cortical bone, it should be rotated until firmly seated in the bone and then advanced a few more millimeters, all while keeping pressure on the stylet to prevent any backward movement and subsequent bone plugging *(Fig. 13.2)*. The stylet then is removed, the syringe attached, and negative pressure applied, but only until marrow becomes visible in the syringe barrel. Aspiration of a larger volume results in contamination of marrow with blood. Once the marrow is collected, it should be placed in an EDTA (disodium ethylenediaminetetraacetate) tube, or slides made very quickly, because clotted samples are nondiagnostic. Alternatively, two or three drops of 10% EDTA solution can be placed in the syringe before aspiration. Pull films are prepared

149

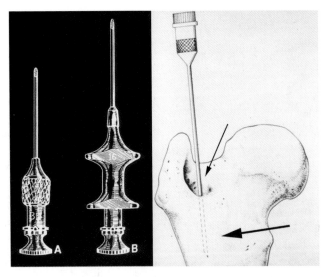

Figure 13.1   Left. Examples of commercially available bone marrow needles with stylets. **Right.** Correct placement of bone marrow needle in the trochanteric fossa.

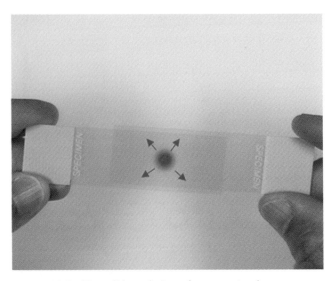

Figure 13.3   Two-slide technique for preparing bone marrow films. The drop of marrow is allowed to spread slightly before pulling the two glass slides apart.

by placing a drop of marrow on a glass slide, gently placing a spreader slide directly atop the drop with little or no manual pressure, briefly allowing the drop to spread, and then pulling the two glass slides apart *(Fig. 13.3)*. Slides are air-dried and then stained with a Romanowsky (i.e., Wright-type) stain. Because the preparations usually are quite cellular, staining time should be increased beyond that used for blood films.

If marrow cannot be aspirated even though multiple sites are attempted, a core biopsy is indicated. Core biopsies are collected using a Jamshidi marrow biopsy needle.

An infant- or pediatric-sized needle should be used for small animals. After collection, the core of marrow can be gently rolled onto the surface of a glass slide for cytologic evaluation before placing the core in formalin solution for fixation.

CELLS ENCOUNTERED IN BONE MARROW FILMS

Erythroid Series

Erythroid precursors tend to have round nuclei, coarse chromatin, and moderate to deep blue cytoplasm that becomes more pink in color as hemoglobin is produced by more-differentiated cells. The developmental stages of the erythroid series, from immature to mature, are the rubriblast, prorubricyte, rubricyte, metarubricyte, polychromatophilic erythrocyte, and mature erythrocyte *(Fig. 13.4)*.

Rubriblasts are the most immature cells that are recognizable in the erythroid series. These cells are relatively large, have round nuclei, slightly coarse chromatin, and nucleoli. The nucleus:cytoplasm ratio is high, with a scant amount of deeply basophilic cytoplasm. A clear Golgi zone may be present as well.

Prorubricytes, which are the next stage in erythrocyte maturation, have a round nucleus, slightly more coarse chromatin, and no visible nucleolus. The cytoplasm is slightly less blue, and it also is more abundant than that of the rubriblast.

Rubricytes are the most mature stage of maturation in which mitosis can still occur. These cells have smaller nu-

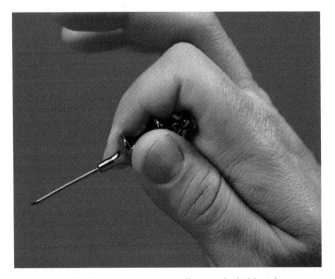

Figure 13.2   The bone marrow needle must be held with pressure against the stylet to keep the stylet in place within the needle, thus preventing bone plugs.

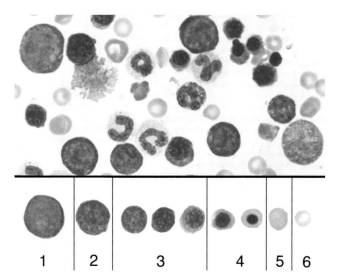

Figure 13.4   Top. Bone marrow aspirate from a dog showing numerous erythroid precursors with round nuclei, coarse chromatin, and blue- to hemoglobin-colored cytoplasm. **Bottom.** Maturation stages of erythroid precursors, from immature to mature. *1,* rubriblast; *2,* prorubricyte; *3,* rubricytes; *4,* metarubricytes; *5,* polychromatophilic erythrocyte; *6,* mature erythrocyte. Wright stain.

clei, very coarse chromatin, and blue to blue-pink (i.e., polychromatophilic) cytoplasm.

Metarubricytes are the most mature cells of the erythroid series that still contain a nucleus. The nucleus is very small, dark, and dense, and the cytoplasm is either polychromatophilic or the red-orange color of mature erythrocytes. Nuclei are extruded from metaruribicytes, thereby resulting in polychromatophilic erythrocytes.

Polychromatophilic erythrocytes are anucleate, blue-pink in color, and larger than mature erythrocytes. They also may contain nuclear remnants (i.e., Howell-Jolly bodies). When stained with supravital stains (e.g., new methylene or brilliant cresyl blue), their mRNA and organelles clump, thereby resulting in blue-staining dots and fibrils (i.e., reticulum) throughout the cells. When stained in this manner, polychromatophilic erythrocytes are termed *reticulocytes.*

Mature erythrocytes are red-orange in color. Evaluation of mature erythrocyte morphology in bone marrow preparations usually is not indicated, but it can be diagnostically useful in that abnormalities such as red cell parasites, spherocytes, or hypochromasia occasionally may be observed.

Granulocyte (Myeloid) Series

Granulocytic precursors tend to have irregularly shaped and, sometimes, eccentric nuclei, with fine to stippled chromatin patterns and abundant, lavender-colored cytoplasm. At certain stages of maturation, they contain azurophilic (i.e., red-purple) to pink granules within the

cytoplasm. As the cells mature, the nuclei elongate, from amoeboid or round in shape to kidney-bean or horseshoe shaped to segmented. The developmental stages of the myeloid series, from immature to mature, are the myeloblast, progranulocyte (promyelocyte), myelocyte, metamyelocyte, band granulocyte, and segmented granulocyte *(Fig. 13.5).* When the maturation process is hastened, whether resulting from inflammation or other causes, the cytoplasm of the myeloid precursors at all stages of maturation is more basophilic and, sometimes, is even vacuolated.

Myeloblasts are subclassified into type I and type II. Type I myeloblasts, which are the most immature cells that are still recognizable in the granulocytic series, are large cells with round to oval nuclei, finely stippled or smooth nuclear chromatin, one or more nucleoli, a small amount of moderately blue cytoplasm, and no azurophilic granules. The nucleus usually is centrally located, and the nuclear outline may be slightly irregular. The nucleus:cytoplasm ratio is high (>1.5), and the cell size is approximately 1.5- to 3.0-fold greater than the red cell diameter. The cytoplasm has a "ground-glass" appearance and, rarely, contains small vacuoles. Type II myeloblasts are very similar to type I, except that some small, azurophilic granules (primary granules) are scattered in the cytoplasm and the nucleus may be central or eccentric.

Promyelocytes are cells with smooth or slightly stippled nuclear chromatin, with or without a nucleolus, and many distinct azurophilic granules dispersed in slightly to moderately blue cytoplasm. The nucleus is central or

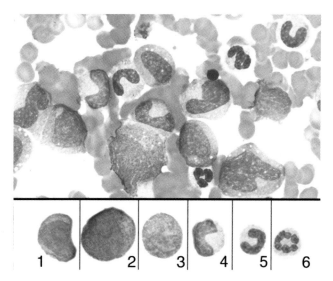

Figure 13.5   Top. Bone marrow aspirate from a dog showing numerous granulocytic (myeloid) precursors. Note the irregularly shaped nuclei, fine chromatin patterns, and lavender-colored cytoplasm. **Bottom.** Maturation stages of myeloid precursors, from immature to mature. *1,* myeloblast; *2,* promyelocyte; *3,* myelocyte; *4,* metamyelocyte; *5,* band neutrophil; *6,* segmented neutrophil. Wright stain.

eccentric. Prominent nucleoli may be present, even in cells with a high concentration of granules. A clear Golgi zone may be present as well.

Myelocytes, which are the last maturation stage in which mitosis can occur, are smaller than progranulocytes, have round to oval nuclei, light blue cytoplasm, and no primary granules within the cytoplasm. In these cells, the primary granules have been replaced by secondary (i.e., specific) granules, which are difficult to see in neutrophil precursors but are very distinct in eosinophil and basophil precursors. Eosinophil precursors contain pink (i.e., eosinophilic) granules, and basophil precursors contain azurophilic to dark purple granules *(Fig. 13.6)*.

Metamyelocytes have kidney bean–shaped nuclei. The cytoplasm is similar in appearance to that of myelocytes.

Band granulocytes have nuclei that are curved and elongated, with parallel sides. Some chromatin clumping is present, and the cytoplasm is similar to that of myelocytes and metamyelocytes.

Segmented granulocytes have lobulated or markedly constricted nuclei, with large and dense chromatin clumps. The cytoplasmic characteristics are generally similar to those of myelocytes, metamyelocytes, and bands.

Monocyte Series

Cells of the monocyte series are relatively few in concentration, and they are very difficult to distinguish from those of the myeloid series in normal marrow. A distinctive feature is their irregular nuclear outlines. Monoblasts appear similar to myeloblasts, and promonocytes

appear similar to myelocytes and metamyelocytes. Mature monocytes have the same appearance as monocytes in peripheral blood *(Fig. 13.7)*. Monocyte precursors usually are recognizable only in animals with monocytic leukemia.

Monoblasts are large cells with round, irregular or folded nuclei and finely reticular nuclear chromatin, one or more prominent nucleoli, and a moderate amount of basophilic, agranular cytoplasm. A Golgi zone often is prominent at the site of nuclear indentation. The nucleus : cytoplasm ratio usually is less than that of myeloblasts.

Promonocytes are large cells with cerebriform nuclei and prominent nuclear folds, stippled or lacy chromatin, and no distinct nucleolus. They also have more abundant and less basophilic "ground-glass" cytoplasm than that of monoblasts.

Megakaryocyte Series

Megakaryocytes are very large cells, and their cytoplasmic fragments become platelets, which are important in the clotting process. Although these cells undergo mitosis, they do not divide, thus becoming very large and multinucleated, with as many as 16 (or more) nuclei. The nuclei are not separate entities, however, and they appear as a large, multilobulated structure in the center of the cell. The developmental stages of the megakaryocyte series, from immature to mature, are the megakaryoblast, promegakaryocyte, and megakaryocyte *(Fig. 13.8)*.

Megakaryoblasts are first recognizable when their size exceeds that of other types of precursors. The nuclei usu-

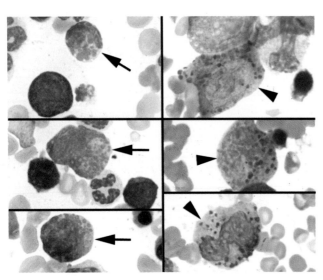

Figure 13.6 **Left.** Various maturation stages of eosinophil precursors (arrows). **Right.** Various maturation stages of basophil precursors (arrowheads). Granules may obscure the nucleus, thus making identification of specific maturation stage difficult. Wright stain.

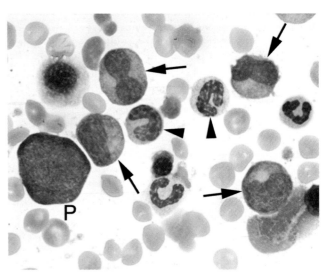

Figure 13.7 Bone marrow aspirate from dog with granulocytic and monocytic hyperplasia. Monocyte precursors (arrows) are difficult to distinguish from granulocytic precursors (arrowheads). Chromatin pattern is more coarse in granulocytic precursors. *P,* progranulocyte. Wright stain.

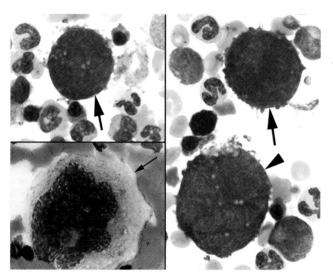

Figure 13.8 Various maturation stages of megakaryocyte series. *Large arrows*, megakaryoblasts; *arrowhead*, promegakaryocyte; *small arrow*, mature megakaryocyte. Wright stain.

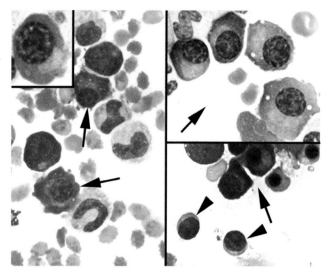

Figure 13.9 Plasma cells (arrows) have a variable appearance, depending on thickness of preparation and degree of flattening of the cells. Flattened plasma cells usually appear to have abundant cytoplasm and obvious, clear Golgi areas. **Inset.** Higher magnification of a plasma cell. Note the coarse chromatin and clear Golgi area. Lymphocytes (arrowheads) have a small amount of cytoplasm. Wright stain.

ally appear to be more dense than those of other types of blast cells, and the cytoplasm usually is deeply basophilic.

Promegakaryocytes have from two to four nuclei, which usually are connected by thin strands of nuclear material and deep blue agranular cytoplasm. They also usually are several-fold larger than rubriblasts or myeloblasts.

Megakaryocytes are very large (diameter, 50–200 µm), with numerous nuclei that form a lobulated mass of nuclear material. The cytoplasm stains more lightly than that of promegakaryocytes. As megakaryocytes mature, they become larger, gain more nuclei, and contain cytoplasm that becomes granular and, sometimes, light pink in color. Naked nuclei of megakaryocytes commonly are observed in bone marrow films.

Other Cells

Small lymphocytes in bone marrow appear as they do in peripheral blood, with a round and usually indented nucleus, a diffuse chromatin pattern without visible nucleoli, and scant, light blue cytoplasm. They are slightly smaller than neutrophils *(Fig. 13.9)*. Plasma cells are differentiated lymphocytes that produce immunoglobulin, and they are similar in size to neutrophils. The appearance of plasma cells is very similar to that of rubricytes, except that the cytoplasm of plasma cells is light blue and more abundant, with a clear Golgi zone adjacent to the often eccentric nucleus sometimes being apparent (Fig. 13.9). The nuclei are round, with very coarse and dense chromatin, and nucleoli are inapparent. The cytoplasm of plasma cells occasionally may contain either very eosinophilic material (i.e., "flame cells") or round, clear

to light blue structures that represent immunoglobulin (i.e., Russell bodies). Plasma cells that contain Russell bodies are called Mott cells *(Fig. 13.10)*.

Lymphoblasts rarely are seen in the bone marrow aspirates from normal animals, and their presence often is indicative of a lymphoproliferative disorder. Lymphoblasts are small to large cells with a round to oval nucleus,

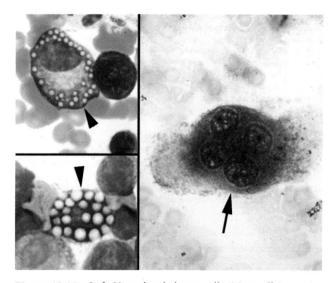

Figure 13.10 **Left.** Vacuolated plasma cells (Mott cells) containing packets of immunoglobulin (Russell bodies). **Right.** Osteoclast, which can be differentiated from a megakaryocyte because the osteoclast nuclei are separate rather than lobulated. Wright stain.

finely stippled to slightly course nuclear chromatin, one or more nucleoli, and a small to moderate amount of pale blue cytoplasm without azurophilic granules. The nuclear outline may appear to be slightly indented or irregular. The nucleus:cytoplasm ratio usually is greater than that of myeloblasts. Lymphoblasts are distinguished from myeloblasts by the slightly more coarse chromatin, less cytoplasm, and the absence of azurophilic granules. Lymphoblasts may appear similar to rubriblasts, but the nuclei of lymphoblasts are less perfectly round.

Macrophages derive from monocytes and are present at a low concentration in normal bone marrow. The appearance of macrophages is highly variable. The nuclei usually are round to slightly kidney bean in shape, and the nucleoli usually are small and inconspicuous. The cytoplasm is gray-blue and usually vacuolated; small, pink granules may be present in the cytoplasm as well. Macrophage nuclei may contain several small nucleoli. Macrophages commonly phagocytize cellular debris, including nuclei that have been extruded from metarubricytes, and they often contain hemosiderin, which is a red cell breakdown product containing iron.

Osteoblasts and osteoclasts may be seen in the bone marrow aspirates from young animals and from those in which bone remodeling is occurring. Osteoclasts are very large, multinucleated cells that may appear similar to megakaryocytes, but their nuclei are individual and not connected to each other (unlike those of megakaryocytes). The cytoplasm is basophilic, and may contain a few pink to azurophilic granules. Osteoclasts are specialized macrophages that derive from monocytes, and they function in the lysis of bone (Fig. 13.10). Osteoblasts are similar in appearance to plasma cells but are larger *(Fig. 13.11)*. They have eccentric, round to oval nuclei that appear to be falling out of one end of the cell; they also have abundant basophilic cytoplasm and a clear Golgi area. Small pink or azurophilic granules may be present in the cytoplasm as well.

Mast cells are easily recognized in the bone marrow, and although rarely observed, they normally are present at very low concentrations. Mast cells are large, round, and discrete cells with abundant small metachromatic granules in the cytoplasm (Fig. 13.11). They usually can be distinguished from basophil myelocytes, because mast cell granules are smaller and more numerous. Mast cells are more apparent and, possibly, increased in concentration in bone marrow that is hypocellular, such as that which may be seen with ehrlichiosis. When mast cells are abundant, infiltration by mast cell neoplasia is likely.

Fibrocytes and fibroblasts are seen only infrequently, even in aspirates from animals with myelofibrosis, because they do not exfoliate easily. The nuclei are round to oval, and the cytoplasm is lightly basophilic and spindle-shaped.

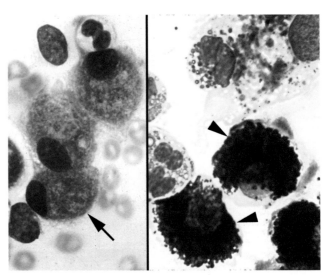

Figure 13.11 Left. Osteoblasts, which have a similar appearance to plasma cells but are larger, with a less condensed chromatin pattern and less distinct cytoplasmic margins (arrow). **Right.** Mast cells with abundant cytoplasmic granules that tend to obscure the round nucleus (arrowheads). Wright stain.

CYTOCHEMISTRY AND IMMUNOPHENOTYPING

Cytochemical reactions sometimes are useful in the process of cell identification. These stain reactions are based on various cell types having different amounts, distribution, and types of enzyme activities. The stains most commonly used include peroxidase, Sudan black B, chloroacetate esterase, α-naphthyl acetate esterase, α-naphthyl butyrate esterase, and alkaline phosphatase (ALP). Peroxidase, Sudan black B, and chloroacetate esterase are myeloid (i.e., granulocytic) markers. The non-specific esterases α-Naphthyl acetate esterase and α-naphthyl butyrate esterase, which can be inhibited by sodium fluoride, and are monocyte markers, but their staining patterns vary. Monocytes may have a few small, round granules that stain positive for Sudan black B. Reactivity for ALP is somewhat confusing, however, because ALP positivity is rare in the immature neutrophils of normal animals but ALP-positive myeloid cells are common in animals with acute myelogenous leukemia. Moreover, ALP activity is present in some types of lymphoid cells as well as in cells, with monocytic differentiation in animals with acute myelomonocytic leukemia. Cytochemical staining of blood and bone marrow films can facilitate the classification of neoplastic cells, but in many cases, negative staining occurs, perhaps because of abnormalities in hematopoietic differentiation that are associated with the neoplastic process.

Immunophenotypic analysis is based on using monoclonal antibodies that are directed against antigens on the surface of hematopoietic cells to determine the phenotypic profile of those cells, thus identifying the cell type. Very little sample quantity usually is necessary, and flow cytometric analysis using the antibodies makes the technique relatively simple to perform. Briefly, monoclonal antibodies directed against cell surface proteins are conjugated to fluorescent molecules and then mixed with the cells, after which the cells are analyzed by flow cytometry. Flow cytometry provides information regarding the size of the cells, expression of any particular surface protein, and concentration of the surface protein. Phenotypes of both normal and neoplastic cells are continuously being classified as more monoclonal antibodies become available. Immunophenotyping likely will eventually replace cytochemistry for use in the classification of hematopoietic cells.

EVALUATION AND INTERPRETATION OF BONE MARROW FILMS

Bone marrow films must be evaluated and interpreted in conjunction with the analysis of concurrent complete blood count (CBC) data. For example, if an animal has a decreased platelet concentration (i.e., thrombocytopenia), the megakaryocyte concentration is particularly important to evaluate.

Cellularity

The low-power (×10) objective should be used to scan the slide at ×100 magnification to assess the degree of cellularity and amount of fat that is present *(Fig. 13.12)*. Hemodiluted marrow samples are difficult to evaluate for cellularity. Normal marrow cellularity varies, but in general, approximately 50% of the marrow consists of fat and 50% of cells. Cellularity is increased when production in either the myeloid or the erythroid cell line is increased in response to cell loss, destruction, or consumption. Abnormal causes of increased cellularity include lymphoproliferative and myeloproliferative disorders as well as other neoplastic disorders. Overall cellularity may be decreased with disorders such as myelofibrosis, certain infectious agents (including *Ehrlichia* sp. in dogs and feline leukemia virus [FeLV]), estrogen toxicity (in dogs and ferrets), drug toxicities (including some commonly used chemotherapeutic agents), chemicals that are toxic to the marrow, radiation, and immune-mediated disorders in which stem cells are destroyed *(Fig. 13.13)*. A decrease in cellularity is termed *hypoplasia*, and a complete absence of cells is termed *aplasia*. Hypoplasia of only one cell line is relatively common, whereas aplasia usually involves all cell lines. Erythroid or myeloid aplasia is rare. Histopathologic evaluation of a core biopsy specimen is

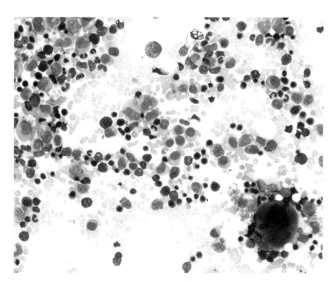

Figure 13.12 Bone marrow aspirate from a dog, low magnification. The degree of cellularity is adequate to increased. Cellularity is judged by the density of sheets of cells, as exemplified in this figure, or by estimating the ratio of fat to cells in particles. Wright stain, low power.

indicated when the cellularity cannot be determined by examination of the marrow aspirate.

Megakaryocytes

Using the low-power (10×) objective, the megakaryocyte concentration should be estimated as either increased (i.e., hyperplasia), decreased (i.e., hypoplasia), or adequate.

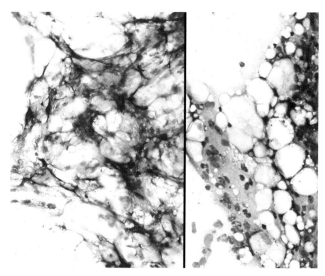

Figure 13.13 Bone marrow aspirate from a cat with generalized marrow hypoplasia, low magnification. **Right.** Numerous adipocytes are present, with very little hematopoietic cellularity. **Left.** Broken adipocytes and stroma are present, with few hematopoietic cells. Wright stain, low power.

Interpretation of this estimate depends on the platelet concentration in the peripheral blood. Areas with high cellularity normally contain at least a few megakaryocytes, and unless the sample is markedly hemodiluted, at least 5 to 10 megakaryocytes should be present on the slide. In animals with increased platelet consumption (e.g., animals with disseminated intravascular coagulopathy) or destruction (e.g., animals with immune-mediated thrombocytopenia), the megakaryocyte concentration in the marrow should be increased. Animals with megakaryocytic hyperplasia may have as many as 50 or more megakaryocytes in cellular areas of the slide. Increased concentrations of megakaryoblasts, promegakaryocytes, and smaller, more immature megakaryocytes typically are seen with megakaryocytic hyperplasia. In thrombocytopenic patients with megakaryocytic hyperplasia, the platelet size usually is increased because of the early release of platelets; this increase in size is analogous to the increased size of immature erythrocytes. Animals that are thrombocytopenic because of the lack of platelet production have very few—or even no—megakaryocytes in the marrow film. Megakaryocytic hypoplasia without erythroid and myeloid hypoplasia is rare and may be caused by immune-mediated destruction of megakaryocytes.

Myeloid : Erythroid Ratio

Using the ×10 objective, appropriate areas that are not too thick and in which cells are not broken can be chosen for further examination of the bone marrow using the ×50 or ×100 oil objectives (to magnify 500- and 1000-fold, respectively). At these higher magnifications, erythroid and myeloid precursors can be identified, and the myeloid:erythroid (M:E) ratio can be estimated *(Fig. 13.14)*. Usually, estimation of this ratio is just as informative as actual quantification. To quantify the M:E ratio, 300 to 500 nucleated cells are classified as being either myeloid or erythroid. This classification should be performed while examining several different areas, because some fields may be predominantly granulocytic and other areas predominantly erythroid.

Normal M:E ratios differ with the species, but in general, they range from 0.5:1 to 3:1. Decreased or increased production of either cell line shifts the M:E ratio, and such shifts must be interpreted in light of the CBC results, particularly the packed cell volume and the neutrophil concentration. For example, if the M:E ratio is increased, the animal is anemic, and the blood neutrophil concentration is normal, then the ratio is increased because of a decrease in red cell production rather than an increase in neutrophil production. Conversely, if the animal is not anemic and the neutrophil concentration is increased, then the increased M:E ratio results from an

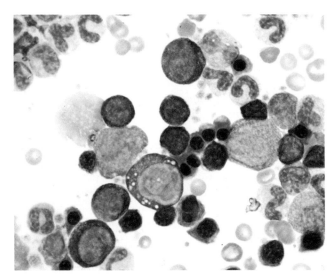

Figure 13.14 Bone marrow aspirate from a dog. Both myeloid and erythroid precursors are present, with a normal myeloid:erythroid ratio of approximately 1. Wright stain.

increased neutrophil production rather than a decreased erythrocyte production.

Decreased M : E Ratio

A decreased M:E ratio may be indicative of increased red cell production, such as that seen with a regenerative anemia (i.e., erythroid hyperplasia); a decreased neutrophil production (i.e., myeloid hypoplasia); or a combination of the two *(Fig. 13.15)*. Myeloid hypoplasia without erythroid hypoplasia is rare but, when present, usually

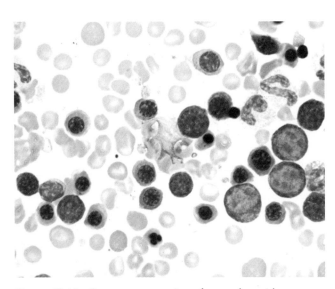

Figure 13.15 Bone marrow aspirate from a dog with regenerative anemia. The myeloid:erythroid ratio is decreased because of increased red cell production (erythroid hyperplasia). Wright stain.

is associated with myelodypslasia or myeloproliferative disorder.

Increased M:E Ratio

An increased M:E ratio may be indicative of increased granulocyte production (i.e., myeloid hyperplasia), decreased in red cell production (i.e., erythroid hypoplasia), or both *(Fig. 13.16)*. Granulocytic hyperplasia usually results from inflammation, but it also may be seen in animals with immune-mediated destruction of neutrophils and in those recovering from viral-induced marrow damage, such as parvovirus infections in dogs (i.e., parvoviral enteritis) and cats (i.e., panleukopenia). Causes of erythroid hypoplasia are discussed in Chapter 7 and include renal failure, endocrinopathies, and anemia of inflammatory disease. Anemia of inflammatory disease (i.e., anemia of chronic disease) is one of the more common causes of mild erythroid hypoplasia in domestic animals. Granulocytic hyperplasia and increased iron stores (i.e., hemosiderin) also usually are seen in the marrow from these patients. Pure red cell aplasia is rare but, when present, usually is caused by immune-mediated destruction of very early erythroid precursors.

Orderliness of Maturation

The orderliness and completion of maturation in erythroid and myeloid cells should be determined. Blast cells divide to ultimately produce 16 to 32 mature cells. Thus, approximately 80% to 90% of the cells should be more mature forms (i.e., metamyelocytes, bands, and neutro-

phils in the myeloid series, and rubricytes and metarubricytes in the erythroid series), and polychromatophilic erythrocytes should be present. Orderly progression of maturation usually is referred to as a "pyramid," with the few immature forms comprising the top and the numerous more mature forms comprising the broad bottom *(Fig. 13.17)*.

Disorderly maturation of erythroid and myeloid precursors commonly is seen in animals with leukemia and myelodysplasia, but it also may be seen in animals with nonneoplastic conditions. An apparent arrest in maturation of the erythroid series, often at the rubricyte stage of maturity, may be seen in animals with immune-mediated destruction of immature erythroid cells. These animals do not have a typical regenerative response, such as that usually seen in animals with immune-mediated hemolytic anemia. Metarubricytes and polychromatophilic erythrocytes often are decreased to absent in the marrow from such patients.

A similar apparent arrest of maturation in the granulocytic series, which often occurs in conjunction with marked myeloid hyperplasia, commonly is seen in marrow aspirates from animals with immune-mediated neutropenia *(Fig. 13.18)*. This "arrest" may appear at any stage of granulocytic maturity, but it often occurs at the metamyelocyte stage. Marrow from animals with immune-mediated destruction can appear similar to that from patients with granulocytic leukemia, but the concentration of myeloblasts usually is lower in those with immune-mediated disease. Other conditions that cause disorderly maturation of granulocytes include marked inflammatory

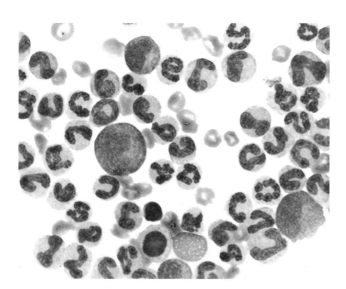

Figure 13.16 Bone marrow aspirate from a dog. The myeloid:erythroid ratio is markedly increased because of increased granulocyte production (myeloid hyperplasia). Wright stain.

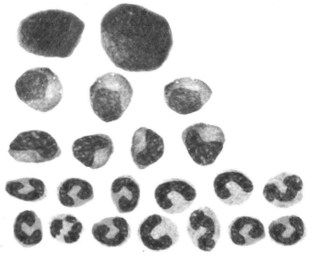

Figure 13.17 A normal "pyramid," illustrating an orderly maturation of myeloid precursors. A few very immature cells form the top of the pyramid, with numerous more mature cells forming the bottom.

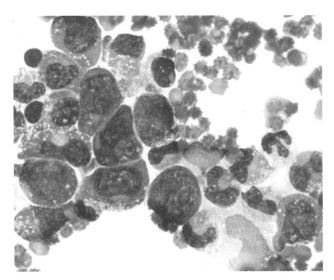

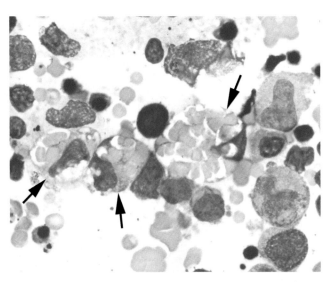

Figure 13.18 Bone marrow aspirate from a dog with immune-mediated neutropenia. Marked myeloid hyperplasia is evident, with an increased proportion of more immature granulocyte precursors and few mature granulocytes because of the immune-mediated destruction of more mature cells. Note that the cytoplasm is basophilic and vacuolated, likely because of the increased rate of cell production. Wright stain.

Figure 13.19 Bone marrow aspirate from a cat. Macrophages (arrows) are increased and have phagocytized many erythrocytes. This degree of phagocytic activity is abnormal and suggestive of either immune-mediated destruction of red cells or hemophagocytic syndrome. Wright stain.

disease (with consumption of more mature forms) and recovery from viral-induced neutropenia.

Macrophages and Iron Stores

Macrophages (i.e., histiocytes) normally are present in small concentrations (<1% of nucleated cells), and phagocytosis of red cells and nuclear debris by macrophages occasionally may be seen in normal animals. The concentration of macrophages may be increased in animals with immune-mediated disorders, and macrophages that have phagocytized nucleated red cells, platelets, and neutrophils occasionally are observed *(Fig. 13.19)*. Other causes of increased cell destruction, such as marrow necrosis secondary to drugs, toxins, or radiation, may result in increased macrophage concentration. In these cases, other morphologic evidence of necrosis, such as pyknosis and increased cytoplasmic vacuolation, usually is observed.

A marked increase in the concentration of macrophages may be seen in animals with hemophagocytic syndrome, which also is called hemophagocytic histiocytosis and is a rare condition characterized by a benign, histiocytic proliferation secondary to infectious, neoplastic, or metabolic diseases. This syndrome is associated with cytopenia of at least two cell lines, and it must be distinguished, on the basis of red cell morphology (i.e., lack of spherocytes and agglutination) and a negative Coombs' test, from the much more commonly occurring immune-mediated diseases. Macrophages are a prominent cellular component in the marrow from animals with hemopha-

gocytic syndrome, and they appear to be normal and well differentiated, with amoeboid nuclei and abundant, light blue cytoplasm. Many macrophages are observed with phagocytized hematopoietic cells within their cytoplasm *(Fig. 13.20)*. An increased concentration of macrophages also is seen in animals with malignant histiocytosis, which is a neoplastic proliferation of histiocytes.

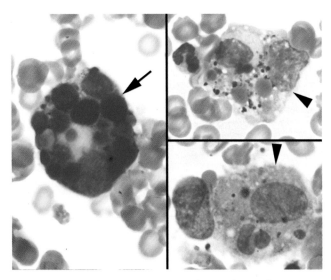

Figure 13.20 Bone marrow aspirate from a dog. **Left.** A macrophage (arrow) that has phagocytized erythrocytes as well as nucleated erythrocytes. **Upper right.** A macrophage (arrowhead) that has phagocytized erythrocytes, a large nucleated cell, platelets, and cellular debris. **Lower right.** A macrophage (arrowhead) that has phagocytized a neutrophil and contains hemosiderin. Phagocytosis of platelets and immature cells may be seen with immune-mediated disease and with hemophagocytic syndrome. Wright stain.

The presence or absence of hemosiderin (i.e., iron stores) in macrophages should be noted *(Fig. 13.21)*. Special stains for iron, such as a Prussian blue stain (Fig. 13.21), usually are not necessary, because hemosiderin can be readily visualized with use of Romanowsky stains. Hemosiderin rarely is seen in the marrow aspirates from normal cats, but it usually is abundant in that from normal dogs and horses. Animals with iron deficiency anemia lack iron stores in the marrow, and animals with anemia of inflammatory disease may have increased iron stores.

Other Cells

The presence and percentage of other types of cells, such as lymphocytes and plasma cells, should be noted as well. In animals that have been antigenically stimulated, the plasma cell concentration may be markedly increased, and the plasma cells may be present in small groups. Normally, approximately 2% or less of the marrow cells are plasma cells. Approximately 15% or less of the cells observed in a bone marrow film from healthy dogs may be lymphocytes, whereas as much as 20% of the cells may be lymphocytes in normal cats. The concentrations of plasma cells and lymphocytes in the bone marrow film usually vary from one area of the film to the next.

Microorganisms

Microorganisms occasionally may be found in bone marrow aspirates. Bacteria very rarely are seen, but *Histoplasma capsulatum* (Fig. 13.22), *Toxoplasma gondii* (Fig. 13.23), *Leishmania donovani* (Fig. 13.24), *Cytaux-*

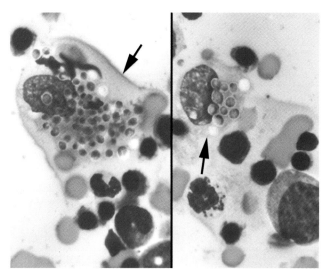

Figure 13.22 Bone marrow aspirate from a cat. Macrophages (arrows) contain numerous *Histoplasma capsulatum* organisms, which are round yeast cells with a well-defined, thin capsule. Wright stain. (Specimen courtesy of Antech Diagnostics.)

zoon felis, and rarely, *Ehrlichia* sp. can be observed. Red cell parasites such as *Hemobartonella* or *Babesia* sp. also may be observed in marrow aspirates.

STEM CELL DISORDERS OF MARROW

Reversible Stem Cell Injuries

Reversible injury is transient in nature and, therefore, usually manifests as neutropenia because of the short

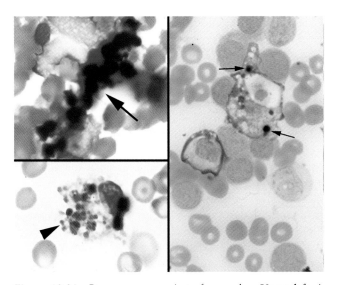

Figure 13.21 Bone marrow aspirate from a dog. **Upper left.** A clump of hemosiderin (storage iron; arrow) from a broken macrophage. Wright stain. **Lower left.** A macrophage (arrowhead) containing hemosiderin. Wright stain. Right. Prussian blue iron stain, showing the presence of blue-staining iron (small arrows).

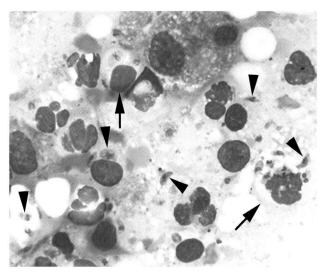

Figure 13.23 Bone marrow aspirate from a cat. Macrophages (large arrows) contain trophozoites of *Toxoplasma gondii*. Individual trophozoites (arrowheads) have a characteristic crescent shape and a central nucleus. Wright stain.

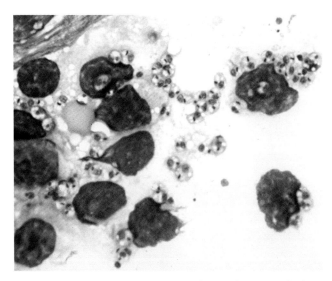

Figure 13.24 Bone marrow aspirate from a dog. Note the broken mononuclear cells with numerous *Leishmania donovani* organisms. These organisms are oval, with a typical, dark-staining, rod-shaped structure (kinetoplast). Wright stain.

half-life of neutrophils in blood (see Chapter 11). Causes include viral injury, drugs or chemicals, and chemotherapeutic drugs, such as doxorubicin, that injure rapidly dividing cells. Although neutropenia is recognized initially, thrombocytopenia and nonregenerative anemia may occur if the injury lasts for more than 1 to 2 weeks. In general, if the animal does not have complications associated with the cytopenias, the stem cell system can be expected to recover and repopulate the blood with normal concentrations of cells.

Some drugs and chemicals apparently are directly cytotoxic to stem cells. Drugs that have been associated with stem cell injury in animals include estrogen (in dogs and ferrets), phenylbutazone (in dogs), and albendazole, which is a broadspectrum anthelmintic (in dogs and cats). Estrogen toxicosis may occur in bitches given exogenous estrogen for mismating, termination of pseudopregnancy, or urinary incontinence. Myelosuppression may occur either from administration of excessive amounts of estrogen or from an idiosyncratic sensitivity to estrogen. Endogenous estrogen, either because of Sertoli cell tumors in male dogs or cystic ovaries in female dogs, also may result in bone marrow suppression. Because ferrets are induced ovulators, marrow suppression from endogenous estrogen is a common and potentially fatal disorder in this species. The mechanism of estrogen toxicosis is unclear but is thought to result from secretion, by thymic stromal cells, of an estrogen-induced substance that inhibits stem cells. Marrow suppression is preceded by an initial thrombocytosis and neutrophilia.

Other drugs may induce cell destruction by immune-mediated mechanisms. In dogs, trimethoprim-sulfadiazine, cephalosporin, and phenobarbital have been associated with pancytopenia that may be immune-mediated. Methimazole, which is used for treating cats with hyperthyroidism, is associated with neutropenia and thrombocytopenia in approximately 20% of the cats given this drug. Stem cell injury that is drug related and immune-mediated usually responds to discontinuation of the drug. Idiopathic immune-mediated stem cell injury usually responds to immunosuppressive therapy; however, it may take several weeks to respond and, often, requires long-term treatment for resolution.

Myelofibrosis may develop in response to various types of marrow injury. Any agent that is directly toxic to hematopoietic cells presumably may damage the microvasculature of the marrow, thereby leading to necrosis and subsequent fibrosis. Myelofibrosis also has been associated with myeloproliferative and lymphoproliferative disorders, other types of neoplasia, chronic hemolytic anemia secondary to pyruvate kinase deficiency, radiation, and other unidentified causes.

Irreversible Stem Cell Injuries

In contrast to reversible stem cell injuries, irreversible injuries result from an intrinsic defect in proliferative behavior or regulation of stem cell entry into differentiated hematopoiesis. These types of injuries generally are regarded as being irreversible, because they do not spontaneously correct themselves and therapeutic intervention almost never corrects the proliferative abnormality (with the exception of bone marrow transplantation, in which defective stem cells are replaced by normal donor stem cells). The causes of this form of stem cell injury are not well understood. The best-characterized causative association in domestic animals, however, is infection with the FeLV in cats. In other domestic animals, the cause almost always is unknown. Chronic exposure to benzene-related chemical compounds is an employment hazard in humans and, rarely, may cause similar injury in animals. Radiation also may induce such an injury in a number of species. Manifestations of stem cell injury are highly variable *(Fig. 13.25)*. These manifestations are best regarded as being a continuum, from lack of cell production on one extreme to uncontrolled, neoplastic proliferation at the other. In the middle of this continuum is dysplastic cell production, which usually is associated with one or more cytopenias and with subtle morphologic abnormalities of the blood cells. Many cases likely begin as dysplasia and then, with time, progress to either hypoplasia or neoplasia. The stage observed at the initial examination is variable, depending on when during the course of the disease the animal is presented to the veterinarian. (More detailed descriptions of the points on this continuum are presented later.)

Irreversible Stem Cell Injury

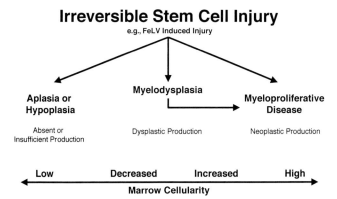

Figure 13.25 Organizational diagram of irreversible stem cell disorders. Myelodysplasia may progress to neoplasia over time. Expected cellularity of proliferative abnormalities are indicated at the bottom.

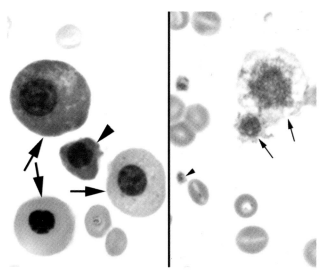

Figure 13.26 **Left.** Bone marrow aspirate from a cat with myelodysplasia. Note the three rubricytes with dysynchrony of nuclear and cytoplasmic maturation (arrows) and the more normal-appearing metarubricyte (arrowhead). **Right.** Blood film from a cat with myelodysplasia. Note the giant atypical platelets (small arrows) and the normal-appearing platelet (small arrowhead). Wright stain.

Aplasias or Hypoplasia

The hallmark feature of this manifestation is hypocellular to acellular marrow. The hematologic result may be either somewhat selective, severe, and nonregenerative anemia (i.e., pure red cell aplasia or hypoplasia) or pancytopenia in which neutropenia and thrombocytopenia accompany the anemia (i.e., aplastic anemia). Establishing the morphologic diagnosis depends on the examination of marrow particles or histopathology to distinguish the hypocellularity from a hemodiluted marrow sample. Most cases of pure red cell aplasia in dogs, as well as those that are not associated with FeLV in cats, likely are immune-mediated, and many respond to immunosuppresive therapy.

Myelodysplasia

Myelodysplasia is a variable manifestation with some subtle, morphologic changes in blood cells. The hematologic manifestations almost always involve some form of cytopenia, and this may include any single abnormality or combination of nonregenerative anemia, thrombocytopenia, and neutropenia. Cellularity of marrow is variable. The marrow may be hypocellular, of normal cellularity, or hypercellular, thereby making it difficult to distinguish this condition from a myeloproliferative disorder. Characteristic morphologic abnormalities include large, highly variable erythroid precursor size and dysynchrony of nuclear and cytoplasmic maturation events *(Fig. 13.26)*. The disturbed erythroid production in cats commonly leads to establishment of marked macrocytosis and increased erythrocyte volume heterogeneity (i.e., anisocytosis) seen as a widening of the erythrocyte histogram. Cats that are positive for FeLV infection may have mean red cell volumes of 70 fL or greater (reference range, 40–55 fL). Macrocytosis also has been reported in dogs with myelodyspla-

sia. Other features in blood may include extreme platelet macrocytosis (Fig. 13.26). Megakaryocyte differentiation may be altered as well, with both hypo- and hyperlobulation of nuclei *(Fig. 13.27)*. Neutrophils of unusually large diameter may be observed, with nuclear changes that may include both hyper- and hyposegmentation *(Fig. 13.28)*. Very early precursors are not found in blood.

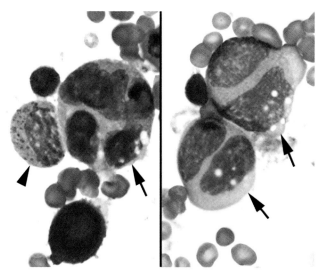

Figure 13.27 **Left.** Bone marrow aspirate from a cat with myelodysplasia. Note the dysplastic megakaryocyte (arrow) and the granulocytic precursor with retained primary granules (arrowhead). **Right.** Dysplastic megakaryocytes with hypolobulation of the nuclei (arrows). Wright stain.

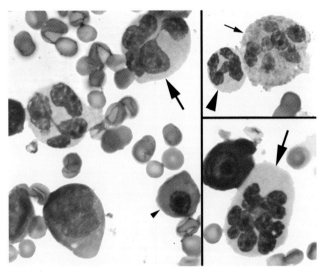

Figure 13.28   Bone marrow aspirate from a cat with myelodysplasia. **Left and lower right.** Note the giant hypersegmented neutrophils (arrows) and megaloblastic erythrocyte precursor (small arrowhead). **Upper right.** Note the giant hypersegmented neutrophil (small arrow) and the neutrophil of normal size (large arrowhead). Wright stain.

Myelodysplasia is easiest to recognize when a combination of hypo- or normocellular marrow is associated with the previously mentioned morphologic abnormalities. Myelofibrosis often is present as well. When the process is hypercellular, myelodysplasia may be difficult to distinguish from overt neoplastic disease, although most animals with myeloproliferative disorder have circulating blast cells. The diagnosis of myelodysplastic syndrome is established when blasts comprise less than 30% of all nucleated cells or nonerythroid cells and dysplastic changes in the erythroid, myeloid, or megakaryocytic lines are present. If the erythroid component is greater than 50% of all nucleated cells, the designation of MDS-Er may be used. Other differential diagnoses for hypercellular marrow and cytopenias include the recovery stage of marrow damage, such as might be seen with parvovirus infection; immune-mediated disease, with destruction of more mature cells; and consumption of neutrophils, such as might be seen with an overwhelming inflammatory process.

Myelodysplasia is most common in cats and quite rare in other domestic animals. Cats with myelodysplasia almost always are positive for FeLV. Clinical signs usually include lethargy, anorexia, and weight loss. Animals may die within weeks of diagnosis, without progression to myeloproliferative disease, but overt myeloproliferative disease is a common sequela.

Overview of Myeloproliferative and Lymphoproliferative Disorders (Leukemia)

Leukemia, which is a neoplastic proliferation of hematopoietic cells within the bone marrow, is defined by the presence of neoplastic blood cells in the peripheral blood or bone marrow, and it is classified broadly into myeloproliferative and lymphoproliferative disorders. The diagnosis of these disorders is established based on finding characteristic blast cells in the blood or bone marrow and on associated hematologic abnormalities. Specific cell types are identified by their morphologic appearance in Wright-stained blood and bone marrow films, cytochemical staining properties, electron microscopic appearance, and monoclonal antibody binding to surface antigens. In some cases, cells may appear so morphologically undifferentiated that classifying the disorder into either the myeloproliferative or the lymphoproliferative category may be difficult *(Fig. 13.29)*. Myeloproliferative leukemias include neoplastic proliferation of erythrocytes, granulocytes, monocytes, and megakaryocytes Multiple cell lines may be neoplastic if the affected stem cell is multipotential; an example is myelomonocytic leukemia, in which both neutrophils and monocytes have been neoplastically transformed. Lymphoproliferative disorders of the bone marrow include acute lymphoblastic leukemia, chronic lymphocytic leukemia, and multiple myeloma.

Leukemias are also classified according to the concentration of neoplastic cells that are circulating in the blood. With leukemic leukemias, many neoplastic cells are circulating, thereby resulting in a markedly increased nucleated cell count. In patients with subleukemic leukemias, however, the nucleated cell count is near normal, with only a few neoplastic cells circulating. No circulating cells are observed on blood films from patients with aleukemic leukemia. Establishing the diagnosis of leukemia when few or no cells are circulating usually is based on examination of the marrow aspirate.

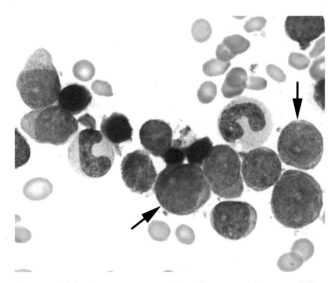

Figure 13.29   Bone marrow aspirate from a cat. Large undifferentiated cells (arrows) are difficult to classify based on their morphologic appearance. Cells may be lymphoblasts or type 1 myeloblasts. Wright stain.

Leukemias are further classified as either acute or chronic based primarily on the maturity or degree of neoplastic cell differentiation as well as by the clinical course. The neoplastic cells in acute leukemias are immature (i.e., blasts), and the patient survival time usually is quite short. By definition, 30% or more blast cells in the marrow is diagnostic of acute myeloid leukemia. The percentage of blast cells in the blood, however, is quite variable in these patients. Chronic leukemias are characterized by the predominance of mature, more well-differentiated cells in the blood and marrow, and the patient survival time usually is longer. Neoplastic cells commonly can be found in organs other than the bone marrow in patients with leukemia. The spleen commonly is involved, and the liver and lymph nodes also may contain neoplastic cells *(Fig. 13.30)*.

Myeloproliferative Disease

Myeloproliferative disease is characterized by bone marrow hypercellularity, loss of orderliness in maturation, and a tendency for abnormal (i.e., leukemic or neoplastic) cells to be released into the blood. Myeloproliferative disease is more common in cats than in other domestic animals and, as mentioned, usually is associated with FeLV. Hematopoietic precursors are infected by FeLV, and viral proteins are thought to interact with host cell products that are important in cell proliferation, thereby likely resulting in recombination or rearrangement events involving host gene sequences that encode products involved in the normal regulation of cell growth. Feline immunodeficiency virus (FIV) also appears to be associated with stem cell disorders of cats, although FIV does not directly

infect myeloid or erythroid precursors. The mechanism probably relates to infection of other cells in the bone marrow microenvironment or to the virus or viral antigen affecting hematopoiesis in some way.

Clinical signs usually relate to the crowding out of normal hematopoietic cells in the bone marrow, but they may also result from the infiltration of different organs by neoplastic cells. Lethargy, weakness, pallor, bleeding, shifting leg lameness, and bone pain frequently are seen, as are hepatomegaly and splenomegaly. Typical CBC findings include an increased nucleated cell count, neoplastic cells in the peripheral blood, nonregenerative anemia, and thrombocytopenia, although thrombocytosis may be present, particularly in cats. Other abnormal laboratory findings are variable, depending on the type and degree of organ dysfunction.

The response of myeloproliferative disorders in dogs and cats to therapy usually is disappointing, and the prognosis is poor, particularly in animals with acute myeloid leukemia. Chemotherapeutic drugs (e.g., cytosine arabinoside) may produce remissions of very short duration (e.g., usually a few weeks). Types of recommended chemotherapy differ with the type of leukemia and the species. A veterinary oncologist should be consulted for advice on new protocols for therapy. Bone marrow transplantation offers the potential for a complete cure, but this is expensive and requires intensive care. Cats that are negative for FeLV and FIV and have a sibling that can serve as a marrow donor are reasonably good candidates for bone marrow transplantation. Animals with chronic myelogenous leukemia (CML) have a longer survival time after the diagnosis is established, but they almost always eventually develop a terminal blast crisis and die. The most satisfactory therapy for CML at this time is oral hydroxyurea. The mean survival time of treated dogs is approximately 1 year.

Classification of Acute Myeloid Leukemias

Traditionally, myeloproliferative disorders in domestic animals have been characterized as being granulocytic (i.e., myeloid, neutrophilic), myelomonocytic (i.e., neutrophils and monocytes), monocytic, eosinophilic, basophilic, megakaryocytic, erythremic myelosis (i.e., erythrocytes), or erythroleukemia (i.e., erythrocytes and granulocytes). Diagnostic criteria have varied considerably, however, and agreement on nomenclature and classification of hematopoietic neoplasms has been lacking. Because of potential differences in response to various treatment protocols and prognosis, an animal leukemia study group standardized the definitions for acute myeloid leukemias by using a human classification scheme.

Myeloproliferative and myelodysplastic syndromes in humans are classified according to the French-American-British (FAB) criteria, which are based primarily on the

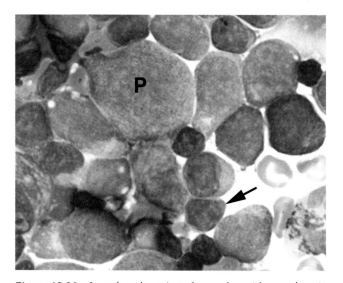

Figure 13.30 Lymph node aspirate from a dog with granulocytic leukemia (M2). Most of the large blast cells cannot be differentiated from lymphoblasts based on their morphology, but some are differentiating toward promyelocytes (P). Note the small lymphocyte (arrow). Wright stain.

number and morphology of blast cells in Wright-stained blood and bone marrow films. This classification scheme now has been adapted for use in dogs and cats. To classify a myeloproliferative or myelodysplastic disorder, 200 cells are differentiated to calculate an M:E ratio and to determine the percentages of blast and other cell types. Blast cell percentages in the bone marrow are calculated in relation to all nucleated cells as well as to nonerythroid cells. Lymphocytes, macrophages, mast cells, and plasma cells are excluded for all-nucleated-cell counts, and erythrocyte precursors are excluded for nonerythroid cell counts.

Cytochemical stains and immunophenotyping, as discussed earlier, may be useful adjuncts in the classification of leukemia *(Figs. 13.31 and 13.32)*. The clinical relevance of cytomorphologic, cytochemical, and immunophenotypic characterization of acute myeloproliferative diseases remains to be determined. Moreover, the classification of leukemia in a patient may change as the disease progresses; for example, erythremic myelosis may convert to erythroleukemia or acute myelogenous leukemia. A classification scheme showing historically used terminology, more current terminology, and a summary of bone marrow findings is presented in *Table 13.1*.

Undifferentiated Leukemia

The diagnosis of undifferentiated leukemia is established when approximately 100% of the cells in the bone marrow are blast cells that cannot be properly classified ac-

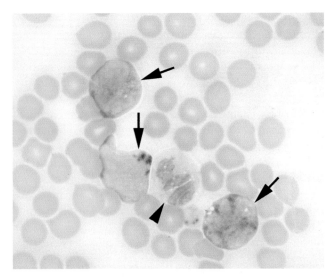

Figure 13.32 Blood film from dog with myelomonocytic leukemia (M4) stained with α-naphthyl butyrate esterase (ANBE), a monocyte marker. Note the brown-staining granules in the monocytes (arrows) and the neutrophil (arrowhead) that does not stain with ANBE. (Specimen courtesy of Dr. Wendy Sprague, Colorado State University.)

cording to the usual morphologic and cytochemical criteria. The diagnosis can be based on electron microscopy, ultrastructural cytochemistry, or immunophenotyping. Included in this category are cases of what previously were termed *reticuloendotheliosis*, in which a predominance of blast cells have pseudopodia, eccentric nuclei, and sometimes, features of both erythroblasts and myeloblasts *(Figs. 13.33 and 13.34)*. Some cells may contain azurophilic granules. If the neoplastic cells do not appear to be maturing toward erythroid or myeloid cells, they are categorized as being undifferentiated.

Myeloblastic Leukemia (M1)

The predominant cell in the bone marrow in animals with myeloblastic leukemia is the type I myeloblast; type II myeloblasts are only seen infrequently *(Fig. 13.35)*. Both types of blasts comprise more than 90% of all nucleated cells. Differentiated granulocytes (promyelocytes to neutrophils and eosinophils) comprise less than 10% of the nonerythroid cells.

Myeloblastic Leukemia with Maturation (M2)

Myeloblasts constitute from more than 30% to less than 90% of all nucleated cells, with a variable number of type II myeloblasts being present *(Figs. 13.36 and 13.37)*. Differentiated granulocytes comprise more than 10% of the nonerythroid cells, usually with a predominance of promyelocytes.

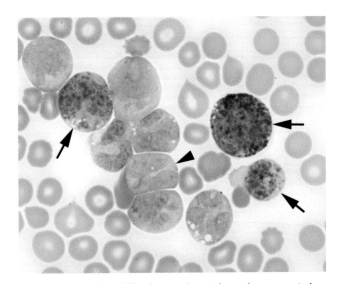

Figure 13.31 Blood film from a dog with myelomonocytic leukemia (M4) stained with chloracetate esterase (CAE), a granulocyte marker. Note the metamyelocyte and neutrophil with red-staining granules in the cytoplasm (arrows). Several monocytes (arrowhead) are present that do not stain positive with CAE. (Specimen courtesy of Dr. Wendy Sprague, Colorado State University.)

TABLE 13.1   CLASSIFICATION OF LEUKEMIAS

Historical Terminology	FAB Subtype	Description
Acute leukemias (≥30% blasts in marrow)		
Reticuloendotheliosis	AUL	Acute undifferentiated leukemia, myeloid and erythroid features
Granulocytic leukemia	M1	Myeloblastic leukemia with differentiation
Granulocytic leukemia	M2	Myeloblastic leukemia with neutrophilic differentiation
Myelomonocytic leukemia	M4	Combination of myeloblasts and monoblasts
Monocytic leukemia	M5a	Monocytic leukemia without differentiation
Monocytic leukemia	M5b	Monocytic leukemia with differentiation
Erythroleukemia	M6	Combination of myeloblasts and rubriblasts
Erythremic myelosis	M6Er	Erythroid leukemia
Megakaryoblastic leukemia	M7	Increased megakaryoblasts in blood and marrow
Chronic myeloid leukemias (<30% blasts in marrow)		
Chronic granulocytic leukemia		Mature neutrophilia, left shift, similar to granulocytic hyperplasia
Chronic myelomonocytic leukemia		Combination of mature neutrophilia, left shift, and monocytosis
Chronic monocytic leukemia		Mature monocytosis in blood and bone marrow
Chronic eosinophilic leukemia		Eosinophilia with left shift, eosinophilic predominance in marrow
Chronic basophilic leukemia		Basophilia with left shift, basophilic predominance in marrow
Essential thrombocythemia		Marked increase in platelets, megakaryocytic hyperplasia in marrow
Polycythemia vera		Mature erythroid proliferative disorder, erythroid hyperplasia
Lymphoid leukemias		
Acute lymphoblastic leukemia		Lymphoblasts in blood or bone marrow
Chronic lymphocytic leukemia		Lymphocytosis, >30% lymphocytes in marrow

FAB, French-American-British.

Myeloblastic Leukemia with Maturation and Atypical Granulation of Promyelocytes (M3)

Although myeloblastic leukemia with maturation and atypical granulation of promyelocytes is one of the classifications for human leukemia, no such cases have been reported in domestic animals. This type of myeloblastic leukemia is characterized by either hypergranular, hypogranular, or microgranular promyelocytes with folded, reniform, or bilobed nuclei.

Myelomonocytic Leukemia (M4)

Myeloblasts and monoblasts together constitute more than 30% of all nucleated cells, and differentiated granulocytes and monocytes comprise more than 20% nonerythroid cells *(Figs. 13.38 and 13.39).*

Monocytic Leukemia (M5)

The predominant population is monocytic, as determined by the characteristic nuclear morphology and confirmed by cytochemical staining for nonspecific esterase. Monoblasts and promonocytes constitute more than 80% of nonerythroid cells in M5a *(Figs. 13.40 and 13.41)*, while M5b has more than 30% to less than 80% monoblasts and promonocytes with prominent differentiation to monocytes *(Figs. 13.42 and 13.43)*. The granulocytic component is less than 20%.

Erythroleukemia (M6)

The erythroid compartment in M6 is more than 50%, and the myeloblasts and monoblasts combined are less than 30% of all nucleated cells. The M6 classification is

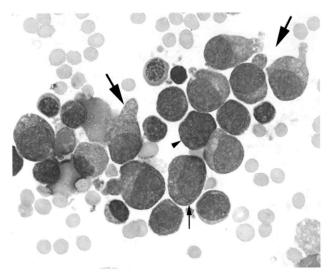

Figure 13.33 Bone marrow aspirate from a cat with undifferentiated leukemia. The cells have features of both erythroid and myeloid precursors. Cytoplasmic pseudopodia (large arrows) typically are present. Note the cell with obvious erythroid characteristics (arrowhead) and the cell with myeloid features and primary granules (small arrow). Wright stain.

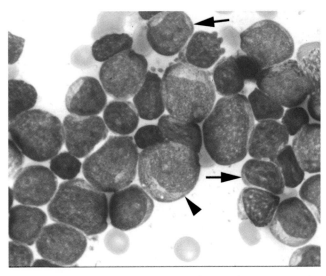

Figure 13.35 Bone marrow aspirate from a dog with granulocytic (myeloblastic) leukemia (M1). Almost all the cells present are type 1 myeloblasts (arrows). A type II myeloblast with cytoplasmic primary granules (arrowhead) is present as well. Type I myeloblasts are morphologically similar to lymphoblasts, and without the presence of more differentiated cells, immunophenotyping may be necessary to correctly classify the leukemia. Wright stain.

recognized when either of the following criteria are met: myeloblasts and monoblasts constitute more than 30% of non-erythroid cells, or blast cells (including rubriblasts) constitute more than 30% of all nucleated cells. An M6Er designation is used to define the latter situation when there is a predominance of rubriblasts in the erythroid compo-

nent. Erythremic myelosis, which is a myeloproliferative disorder of erythroid precursors, may fall under the designation of M6Er or MDS-Er, because the erythroid component constitutes more than 50% of all nucleated cells and the blast cell concentration, (including rubriblasts) may constitute more than 30% (i.e., M6ER) or less than 30% (i.e., MDS-Er) *(Figs. 13.44 and 13.45)*.

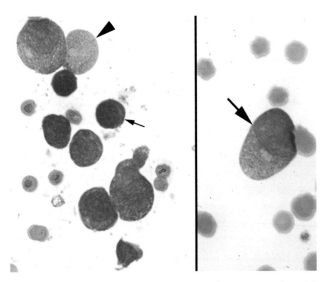

Figure 13.34 **Left.** Bone marrow aspirate from a cat with undifferentiated leukemia. Note the cytoplasmic pseudopodia that has detached from the cell (arrowhead). When present in blood, these cytoplasmic fragments may be mistaken for platelets. Note the rubricyte (small arrow) as well. **Right.** Blood film from a cat with undifferentiated leukemia. Note the typical undifferentiated cell with primary granules and an eccentric nucleus (large arrow). Wright stain.

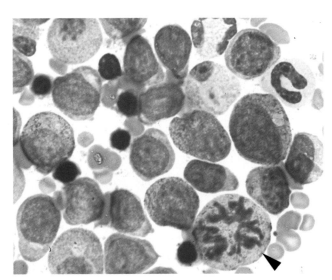

Figure 13.36 Bone marrow aspirate from a cat with granulocytic (myeloblastic) leukemia (M2). Numerous type II myeloblasts with cytoplasmic granules are present, as is a cell in mitosis (arrowhead). Note that cells are more differentiated than those seen in marrow aspirates of patients with M1. Wright stain.

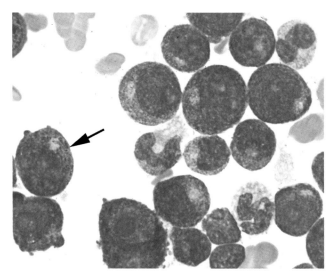

Figure 13.37   Bone marrow aspirate from a cat with granulocytic (myeloblastic) leukemia (M2). Note that most of the cells present are type II myeloblasts or progranulocytes (arrow). Most of these cells have clear Golgi areas. A few more differentiated myeloid precursors are present as well. Wright stain.

Megakaryoblastic Leukemia (M7)

More than 30% of all nucleated cells or nonerythroid cells is comprised of megakaryoblasts in the M7 stage. An increased concentration of megakaryocytes may be present as well, and megakaryoblasts usually are detected in the blood *(Fig. 13.46)*. Animals often are thrombocytopenic, although thrombocytosis has been reported. Immunohistochemical techniques to detect reactivity for factor VIII–related antigen and platelet glycoprotein IIIa sometimes are necessary to definitively identify megakaryoblasts. Primitive mega karyoblasts may also stain positive for

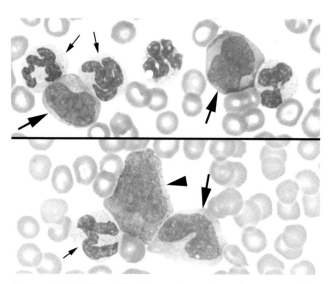

Figure 13.39   Blood film from a dog with myelomonocytic leukemia (M4). **Top.** Note the monoblasts (large arrows) and normal-appearing, segmented neutrophils (small arrows). **Bottom.** Note the segmented neutrophil (small arrow), monocyte (large arrow), and type II myeloblast (arrowhead). Wright stain.

acetylcholime esterase, a specific cytochemical marker for this cell line.

Chronic Myeloproliferative Disorders

Classification of chronic myeloproliferative disorders was not addressed by the animal leukemia study group. Chronic myeloproliferative disorders probably fall into the myelodysplasic syndrome category, however, based

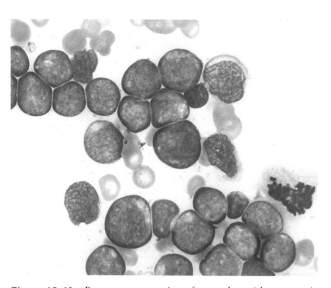

Figure 13.40   Bone marrow aspirate from a dog with monocytic leukemia (M5a). Almost all the cells present are undifferentiated monoblasts. These cells appear to be morphologically similar to lymphoblasts and type I myeloblasts, but immunophenotyping and cytochemistry determined this was a very undifferentiated type of monocytic leukemia. Wright stain.

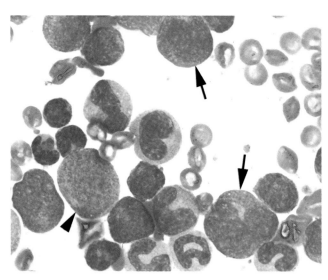

Figure 13.38   Bone marrow aspirate from a dog with myelomonocytic leukemia (M4). Both monocyte precursors (arrows) and myeloid precursors (arrowhead) are present. Wright stain.

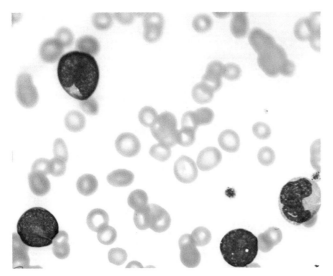

Figure 13.41 Blood film from a dog with monocytic leukemia (M5a). Cells were classified as monoblasts based on the presence of other cells that appeared to be differentiating to monocytes as well as on the results of cytochemical analysis and immunophenotyping. Wright stain.

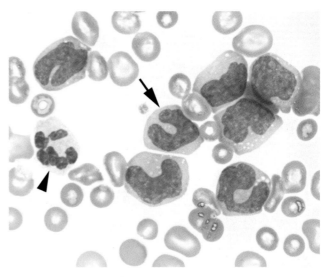

Figure 13.43 Blood film from a dog with monocytic leukemia (M5b). Note the numerous monocytes (large arrow), and compare the blue color of the cytoplasm and density of the nuclear chromatin with that of a segmented neutrophil, which has more dense nuclear chromatin and pink cytoplasm (arrowhead). Wright stain.

on marrow examination, because blast cell percentages usually are less than 30%. This section presents a brief discussion of these rare disorders; polycythemia vera, which is a chronic myeloproliferative disorder of erythrocytes, is discussed in Chapter 9.

Chronic Granulocytic (Myelogenous) Leukemia

Chronic myelogenous leukemia is extremely rare in domestic animals and is characterized by marked neutro-

philia, a left shift that often is disorderly, and anemia. A monocytosis may be present as well, in which case the disorder is termed *chronic myelomonocytic leukemia*. Chronic myelogenous leukemia has been reported more frequently in dogs than in cats. Based on marrow examination, chronic myeloid leukemia may be classified as a myelodysplastic syndrome, because the blast cell count in the marrow is less than 30% of all nucleated cells and the erythroid component less than 50% *(Fig. 13.47)*. This leukemia, however, can be differentiated from classic

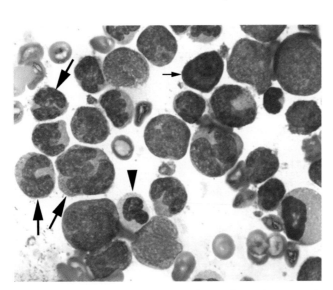

Figure 13.42 Bone marrow aspirate from a dog with monocytic leukemia (M5b). Note the numerous monocytes in various stages of maturation (large arrows), the segmented neutrophil (arrowhead), and the plasma cell (small arrow). Wright stain.

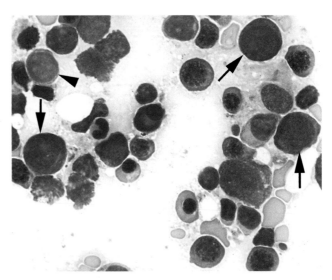

Figure 13.44 Bone marrow aspirate from a cat with erythremic myelosis (M6Er). Almost all the cells present are erythroid precursors. Note the rubriblasts (large arrows) and the nonerythroid blast (arrowhead), which probably is a myeloblast. Wright stain.

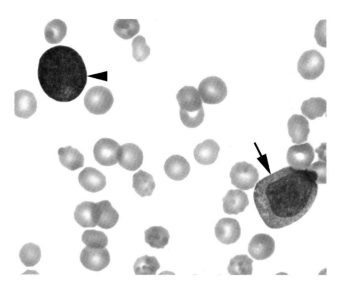

Figure 13.45   Blood film from a dog with erythroleukemia (M6). Note the rubriblast (arrowhead) and myeloblast (arrow). Also note the typical lack of polychromasia, because the erythroid precursors do not mature normally. Wright stain.

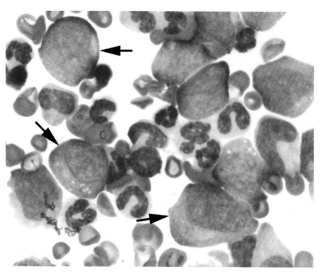

Figure 13.47   Bone marrow aspirate from a dog with chronic myelogenous leukemia. Note the increased concentration of myeloblasts (arrows). Although some degree of maturation to segmented neutrophils is occurring, the maturation appears to be disorderly. Very few erythroid precursors were present in the marrow, and none are present in this field. Wright stain.

myelodysplastic syndrome by the lack of prominent dysplastic changes in the marrow and by the marked leukocytosis in the blood. Inflammatory responses can mimic CML, and such "leukemoid reactions" often are misdiagnosed as leukemias. Marrow examination may not be helpful in distinguishing the two, because marked inflammatory leukograms can be associated with marked granulocytic hyperplasia and a pronounced increase in the M:E ratio and the orderliness of maturation may ap-

pear disrupted. Histopathologic evaluation of the spleen and liver is not always helpful, because these organs may exhibit marked granulopoiesis with some types of inflammatory disease. Animals with CML eventually develop a disorderly left shift, and they usually have a "blast crisis," during which myeloblasts appear in the blood *(Fig. 13.48)*. Animals with CML also usually develop much more severe anemia than animals with inflammatory

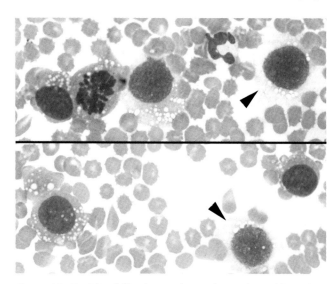

Figure 13.46   Blood film from a dog with megakaryoblastic leukemia (M7). **Top.** Note the numerous megakaryoblasts (arrowhead), one of which is in mitosis. Also note the abundant vacuolated cytoplasm with ruffled borders. **Bottom.** Note the broken megakaryoblast (arrowhead). Wright stain.

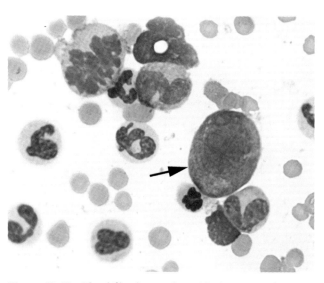

Figure 13.48   Blood film from a dog with chronic myelogenous leukemia in blast crisis. Note the cell in mitosis (upper left corner) and the myeloblast (arrow). The nucleated cell concentration in this dog was 150,000 cells/μL. Wright stain.

disease. Humans with CML almost always have a characteristic cytogenetic abnormality (i.e., the Philadelphia chromosome), but cytogenetic abnormalities have not been documented in other species.

Eosinophilic Leukemia

Eosinophilic leukemia is rare but has been reported primarily in FeLV-negative cats. It is characterized by eosinophilia, immature eosinophils in the blood, eosinophil predominance in the marrow *(Fig. 13.49)*, and infiltration of various organs with eosinophils. This disorder is difficult to differentiate from feline hypereosinophilic syndrome, in which the same characteristics can be seen, although the eosinophilic left shift may be more orderly with hypereosinophilic syndrome. Intestinal involvement is typical as well. Recent reports are suggestive that the separation between the two disorders may be artificial, and that they both may represent a neoplastic proliferation of eosinophils. Clinical signs are similar to those seen in animals with other myeloproliferative disorders. Typically, however, they also include thickened bowel loops, diarrhea, and vomiting, because the intestine usually is infiltrated. Most cats die within 6 months of the diagnosis being established, but hydroxyurea in combination with prednisone may prolong survival.

Chronic Basophilic Leukemia

Chronic basophilic leukemia is very rare but has been reported in dogs and cats. Abnormal blood findings include marked basophilia with an orderly left shift of the baso-

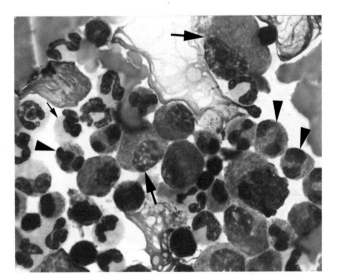

Figure 13.49 Bone marrow aspirate from a cat with eosinophilic leukemia or hypereosinophilic syndrome. Note the eosinophil precursors (large arrows) and the numerous, mature eosinophils (arrowheads). For comparison, note the neutrophil (small arrow). Wright stain. (Specimen courtesy of Antech Diagnostics.)

philic series, anemia, and occasionally, thrombocytosis. Multiple organ usually are infiltrated. Chronic basophilic leukemia must be differentiated from mast cell leukemia. Basophils have segmented nuclei, whereas mast cells have round nuclei. Basophilic myelocytes, however, may be difficult to differentiate from mast cells, and animals with systemic mast cell neoplasia may have a mild basophilia.

Essential Thrombocythemia

Essential thrombocythemia is a very rare chronic myeloproliferative disorder that is characterized by a marked increase in the platelet concentration. Platelets may appear atypical, with hypo- or hypergranularity, and giant forms may be present. The concentrations of megakaryocytes and megakaryoblasts usually are increased in the bone marrow as well. The platelet concentration may be increased secondary to many other disorders, such as iron deficiency anemia, inflammation, antineoplastic drug therapy, corticosteroids, and neoplasia (particularly lymphoma).

LYMPHOPROLIFERATIVE DISORDERS

Although the term *lymphoproliferative disorder* can be used to describe any abnormal proliferation of lymphoid cells, it more commonly is used to describe neoplastic proliferations. Tumors that derive from lymphocytes or plasma cells are classified as lymphoproliferative, or lymphoid neoplasms. Lymphoproliferative disorders are much more common than myeloproliferative disorders in domestic animals, and they are more common in cats than in any of the other domestic species. As with myeloproliferative disorders, cats with lymphoproliferative disorders usually test positive for FeLV, FIV, or both. Lymphoproliferative disorders generally are categorized as primary lymphoid leukemia, lymphoma, or plasma cell tumors, including multiple myeloma and solitary tumors. In turn, the leukemias can be classified as either acute or chronic, as discussed earlier, and are termed *acute lymphoblastic leukemia* or *chronic lymphocytic leukemia*. Use of polymerase chain reaction to detect antigen-receptor rearrangements can identify a clonal, neoplastic population of cells and differentiate non-neoplastic lymphoproliferative disorders from those that are neoplastic.

Lymphoid leukemia differs from malignant lymphoma primarily in the anatomic distribution. Solid neoplastic masses are present in lymphoma but are less common in patients with primary lymphoid leukemia. At least 10% to 25% of dogs and cats with lymphoma develop leukemia, however, and some investigators report that approximately 65% of dogs with multicentric lymphoma

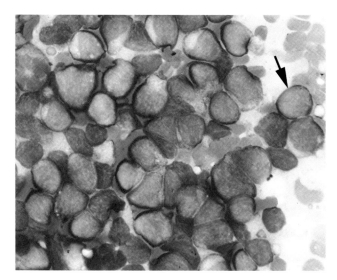

Figure 13.50 Bone marrow aspirate from a dog with acute lymphoblastic leukemia. Note that normal hematopoietic cells are absent, having been replaced by lymphoblasts (arrow). Wright stain.

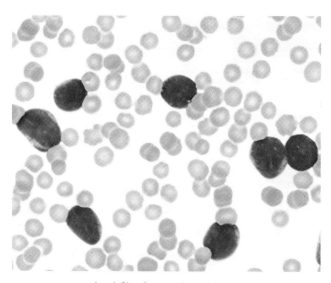

Figure 13.52 Blood film from a dog with acute lymphoblastic leukemia. Note the numerous large lymphoblasts. Wright stain.

are leukemic at the time of presentation (if the determination of leukemia is based on the evaluation of blood, bone marrow aspirates, and marrow core biopsy specimens). Lymphoproliferative disease that arises in the bone marrow rather than in the lymph nodes has a different biologic behavior, response to therapy, and prognosis.

Acute Lymphoblastic Leukemia

Acute lymphoblastic leukemia is characterized by the presence of lymphoblasts in the blood and bone marrow

(Figs. 13.50 through 13.53). In both acute lymphoblastic leukemia and the leukemic phase of lymphoma, however, lymphoblasts can be found in the blood and bone marrow, thereby making these two disorders difficult to differentiate. A general rule of thumb is that if lymphadenopathy is not present, the disorder most likely is acute lymphoblastic leukemia rather than lymphoma. Approximately half of the dogs with acute lymphoblastic leukemia, however, also have lymphadenopathy. As with the myeloproliferative disorders, clinical signs relate either to a lack of normal hematopoietic cells or to the infiltration of organs by neoplastic cells. Common findings include pale mucous membranes, splenomegaly, and hepatomegaly.

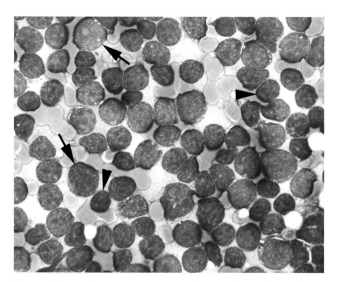

Figure 13.51 Bone marrow aspirate from a dog with acute lymphoblastic leukemia. Numerous intermediate-sized lymphoid cells are present and have completely replaced the normal marrow elements. Note the lymphoblasts (arrows) and lymphocytes (arrowheads). Wright stain.

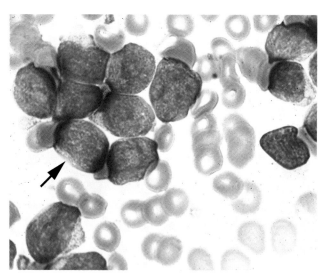

Figure 13.53 Blood film from a dog with acute lymphoblastic leukemia and a nucleated cell count of 300,000 cells/μL. All the cells present are lymphoblasts (arrow). Note the large size, high nucleus:cytoplasm ratio, and nucleoli with the nuclei. Wright stain.

Common CBC abnormalities include anemia, thrombocytopenia, lymphocytosis, and lymphoblasts in the blood.

Lymphoblasts usually can be differentiated from other types of immature cells based on their characteristic morphology, as described earlier. Occasionally, however, certain types of lymphoblasts (e.g., large granular lymphoblasts) may contain a few fine to coarse azurophilic granules *(Fig. 13.54)*. These cells may be difficult to distinguish from myeloblasts, in which case immunophenotyping (using monoclonal antibodies directed against proteins on the surface of leukocytes) may be very helpful. Cytochemical reactions also may be helpful, because lymphoblasts typically are negative for most of the cytochemical stains except nonspecific esterase. Chemotherapy, usually involving a combination of vincristine, cyclophosphamide, and prednisone, may result in remission, though usually of short duration.

Chronic Lymphocyte Leukemia

In animals with chronic lymphocytic leukemia, the lymphocytes are small and well-differentiated *(Fig. 13.55)*. Chronic lymphocytic leukemia is more common in dogs than in other domestic animals. This type of leukemia, however, must be differentiated from physiologic lymphocytosis in excited cats (usually kittens), in which the absolute lymphocyte count may reach 20,000 cells/μL. Other differential diagnoses include lymphocytosis induced by chronic antigenic stimulation, such as that seen in dogs with chronic ehrlichiosis. Lymphocytosis is rare and usually mild (<10,000 lymphocytes/μL) with other

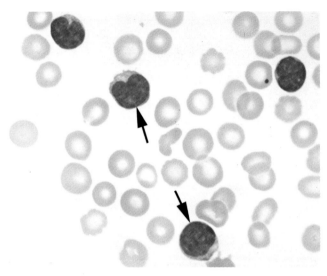

Figure 13.55 Blood film from a dog with chronic lymphocytic leukemia. Note the relatively small, normal-appearing lymphocytes (arrows). The diagnosis of leukemia was based on the high concentration of small lymphocytes in the blood (40,000 cells/μL) and by polymerase chain reaction results. Wright stain.

types of antigenic stimulation, however. Lymphocytosis predominated by large granular lymphocytes may be seen in animals with ehrlichiosis or chronic lymphocytic leukemia.

Clinical signs and abnormalities found on physical examination are similar to those seen in animals with other types of leukemia, including lethargy, anorexia, pale mucous membranes, lymphadenopathy, splenomegaly, and hepatomegaly. The most striking CBC abnormality is a marked lymphocytosis. Anemia and thrombocytopenia may be present, but the anemia usually is not as severe as that seen in animals with acute lymphoblastic leukemia. The concentration of small lymphocytes in the marrow is greater than normal, being reported to range from 25% to 93% of cells. Monoclonal gammopathies occasionally are seen in animals with chronic lymphocytic leukemia.

Therapeutic intervention is controversial, because untreated animals may live for months to years. Recommendations for chemotherapy in dogs and cats include a combination of chlorambucil and prednisone; long remissions and survival can be achieved. The median survival time for dogs is more than 1 year. Survival time has been reported to be significantly different in untreated dogs with chronic lymphocytic leukemia (~450 days), as compared to that of dogs with acute lymphoblastic leukemia (~65 days).

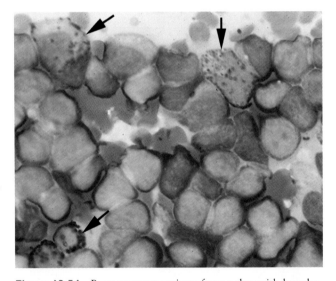

Figure 13.54 Bone marrow aspirate from a dog with lymphoblastic leukemia. Note the presence of a few cells with azurophilic granules within the cytoplasm (arrows), which are referred to as large granular lymphoblasts. These granules make this type of leukemia difficult to distinguish from M1 based on cell morphology alone. Wright stain.

Plasma Cell Myeloma (Multiple Myeloma)

Plasma cells derive from B lymphocytes and typically secrete immunoglobulins. Plasma cell myeloma is a rela-

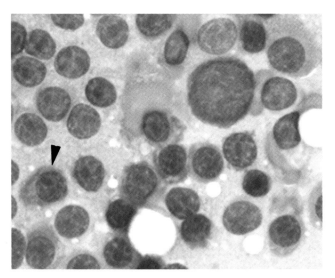

Figure 13.56 Bone marrow aspirate from a dog with plasma cell myeloma. Almost all the cells present are plasma cells. Note the more typical plasma cell with an eccentric nucleus and abundant cytoplasm (arrowhead). Wright stain.

tively rare lymphoproliferative neoplasm, in which plasma cells or their precursors proliferate abnormally *(Figs. 13.56 and 13.57).* As implied by the term *multiple myeloma,* plasma cells proliferate in the bone marrow at multiple sites. The incidence of multiple myeloma in cats is thought to be even less than that in dogs and usually is not associ-

ated with FeLV or FIV infections. These plasma cell proliferations may be detected on bone marrow films, but plasma cells only rarely are seen on blood films. When plasma cell leukemia is present, the survival time usually is less. Markedly increased plasma cell concentration in the bone marrow (>20 percent of all nucleated cells) often results from plasma cell neoplasia, but plasma cell proliferation also may occur secondary to chronic antigenic stimulation. Neoplastic plasma cells often are seen in large aggregates and, sometimes, appear slightly abnormal or immature, with occasional multinucleated plasma cells being present. Neoplastic cells may appear to be very well-differentiated, however, in which case they are difficult to distinguish from normal plasma cells. Plasma cells occasionally may have a ruffled eosinophilic cytoplasmic margin that appears similar to a flame; these are termed *flaming plasma cells* or *flame cells* (Fig. 13.57).

An important diagnostic and clinical manifestation of plasma cell myeloma is a monoclonal or biclonal gammopathy, usually immunoglobulin G or A but, occasionally, immunoglobulin M *(Fig. 13.58).* The immunoglobulins synthesized by malignant plasma cells also are known as paraproteins. Other diagnostic features include Bence-Jones protein (i.e., light chains of immunoglobulins) in the urine and radiographic evidence of osteolysis *(Fig. 13.59).* Two or three of these four features traditionally are considered to be essential for the diagnosis of plasma cell myeloma to be established. Dogs with chronic ehrlichiosis, however, may have a monoclonal gammopathy and a markedly increased concentration of plasma cells in the bone marrow. Other disorders in which monoclonal

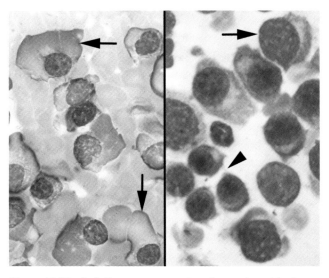

Figure 13.57 **Left.** Bone marrow aspirate from a dog with plasma cell myeloma. These plasma cells have eosinophilic-colored cytoplasm that is ruffled, and they sometimes are referred to as flame cells. The cytoplasm is filled with immunoglobulin. **Right.** Bone marrow aspirate from a dog with plasma cell myeloma. Note the variation in cell size, ranging from the large, immature plasma cell with loose chromatin (arrow) to the small cells with more condensed chromatin (arrowhead). Wright Stain.

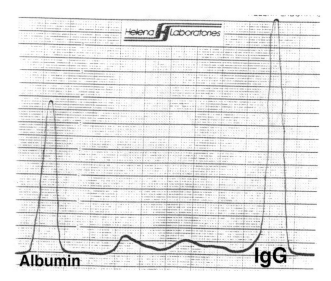

Figure 13.58 Protein electrophoretogram from a dog with plasma cell myeloma and monoclonal gammopathy. Note the monoclonal immunoglobulin (IgG) spike at the right. Albumin is represented by the smaller spike to the left. Wright stain.

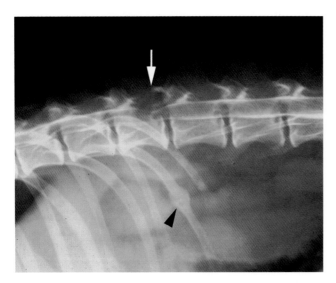

Figure 13.59 Thoracolumbar radiograph with contrast myelography of a dog with plasma cell myeloma. Cord compression results from extradural proliferative lesion and lysis of bone (white arrow). A proliferative lesion also is present on the rib (black arrowhead). Proliferative lesions are rare in animals with plasma cell myeloma; lytic lesions are more typical.

gammopathies may be seen include chronic lymphocytic leukemia, lymphoma, feline infectious peritonitis, and extramedullary plasmacytoma.

Clinical signs associated with multiple myeloma also usually are associated with plasma cell infiltration of the bone marrow and other organs or with increased concentration of circulating immunoglobulins, which may result in increased viscosity of the blood (i.e., hyperviscosity syndrome). Lethargy, anorexia, lameness, bleeding from the nares, paresis, polyuria, and polydipsia are relatively common. Fundoscopic changes such as retinal hemorrhages and engorged retinal blood vessels commonly are observed as well. Renal disease is relatively common and usually associated with the abnormal proteins interfering with tubular and glomerular function, but it sometimes occurs secondary to hypercalcemia with subsequent calcification of renal tissue. Central nervous system impairment may result from serum hyperviscosity and subsequent sludging of blood in small vessels. Bleeding diatheses, which are seen in approximately one-third of dogs with multiple myeloma, may result from thrombocytopenia, but it also can result from the abnormal immunoglobulins interfering with platelet function. Skeletal lesions are rare in cats with multiple myeloma.

Dogs with multiple myeloma that are treated with alkylating agents (e.g., melphalan or cyclophosphamide) often have survival times of from 1 to 2 years. Reported survival times in treated cats usually are less. Animals with multiple myeloma that are azotemic or have severe anemia, neutropenia, or thrombocytopenia usually have a poorer prognosis. Hypercalcemia, Bence-Jones proteinuria, plasma cell leukemia, and extensive bony lesions also are associated with a shorter survival time. In humans, stem cell transplantation offers significantly improved prognosis and survival rates.

OTHER NEOPLASTIC DISORDERS INVOLVING BONE MARROW

Mast cell leukemia may be seen in dogs and cats with systemic mastocytosis secondary to mast cell tumors *(Fig. 13.60)*. Although examinations of bone marrow aspirate commonly are performed to stage mast cell tumors, involvement of the marrow by mast cell tumors very rarely is observed. Buffy coat examination for mast cells also rarely is useful, because circulating mast cells occasionally may be seen in animals without mast cell tumors.

Malignant histiocytosis is a rapidly progressive—and ultimately fatal—proliferative disorder of the mononuclear phagocyte system that has been described in adult dogs, including Bernese mountain dogs and other breeds. An increased incidence of the disorder has been suggested to occur in the golden retriever and flat-coated retriever breeds. The disorder often is characterized by the systemic proliferation of large, pleomorphic, single and multinucle-

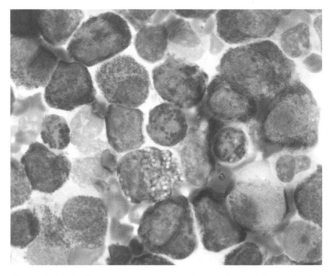

Figure 13.60 Bone marrow aspirate from a dog with poorly differentiated mast cell leukemia. Almost all the cells present are mast cells with metachromatic cytoplasmic granules. This dog also had mast cells on the blood film. Wright stain.

ated histiocytes with marked cellular atypia and phago-cytosis of erythrocytes and leukocytes. The bone marrow as well as lung, lymph nodes, liver, spleen, and central nervous system commonly are involved. Positive reactivity of neoplastic cells to histiocytic markers (e.g., lysozyme and α_1-antitrypsin) can be demonstrated by immunohisto-chemistry. This immunohistochemical reactivity aids in the differentiation of neoplastic histiocytic cells from lymphoid and epithelial neoplasms, and it is important for establishing a definitive diagnosis of the neoplasm. The cellularity of bone marrow aspirates containing neoplastic histiocytes is consistently very high. These histiocytes are pleomorphic, large, discrete, and markedly atypical mononuclear cells, and the nuclei are round to oval or reniform. Features of malignancy include marked aniso-cytosis and anisokaryosis, prominent nucleoli, bizarre mi-totic figures, marked phagocytosis of erythrocytes, leuko-cytes, other tumor cells, and moderate amounts of lightly basophilic, vacuolated cytoplasm *(Fig. 13.61)*. The presence of multinucleated giant cells also is supportive of the diagnosis. Other findings vary and may include erythroid hypoplasia, with prominent cytophagia of marrow elements, or generalized marrow hypoplasia, with neoplastic infiltration of atypical histiocytes and marked phago-cytosis. Hematologic abnormalities such as anemia and mild to marked thrombocytopenia also may be present, correlating with marrow changes.

Epithelial and mesenchymal tumors rarely metastasize to the bone marrow. Epithelial tumors (i.e., carcinomas) tend to form groups of cohesive cells that are easy to dis-

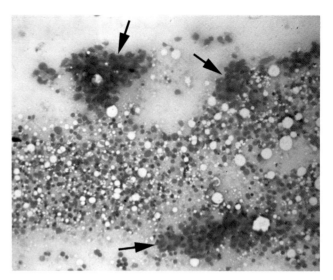

Figure 13.62 Bone marrow aspirate from a dog with metastatic mammary carcinoma, low magnification. The islands of cells (arrows) are neoplastic epithelial cells and can be differentiated from the normal hematopoietic cells by their tendency to adhere to each other. Wright stain. Low power.

tinguish from normal hematopoietic cells *(Figs. 13.62 and 13.63)*. Metastatic sarcomas are more difficult to diagnose, however, and are characterized by large, discrete, spindle-shaped cells that meet multiple criteria for malignancy *(Fig. 13.64)*. These cells must be distinguished from fibroblasts that may be observed in myelofibrosis.

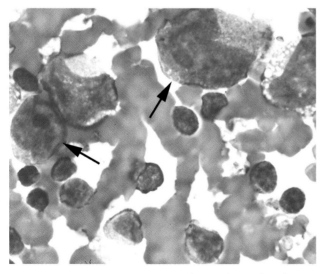

Figure 13.61 Bone marrow aspirate from a dog with malignant histiocytosis. Note the large, neoplastic histiocytic cells with prominent, irregularly shaped nucleoli (arrows). Most of the other nucleated cells in the field are small lymphocytes. Wright stain.

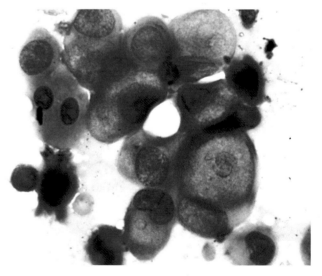

Figure 13.63 Bone marrow aspirate shown in Figure 13.62, high magnification. Note the large epithelial cells that exhibit numerous criteria of malignancy, including nuclear molding, binucleate cells, and prominent nucleoli. Wright stain.

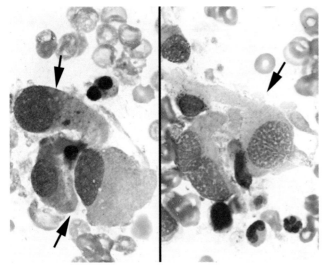

Figure 13.64 Bone marrow aspirate from a dog with metastatic hemangiosarcoma. Spindle-shaped neoplastic cells (arrows) exhibit numerous criteria of malignancy, including variability in nuclear size, variability in cell size, ropy chromatin, and prominent nucleoli. Note that some cells have fine, azurophilic granules in their cytoplasm. Wright stain. (Specimen courtesy of Dr. Kyra Somers, Colorado State University.)

SUGGESTED READINGS

General Approach to Bone Marrow Aspiration and Interpretation

Harvey JW. Canine bone marrow: normal hematopoiesis, biopsy techniques, and cell identification and evaluation. Comp Cont Educ Pract Vet 1984;6:909–927. (This manuscript also was published in The compendium collection: veterinary laboratory medicine. Trenton, NJ: Veterinary Learning Systems, 1993:208–225.

Latimer KS, Andreasen CB. Bone marrow. In: Cowell RI, Tyler RD, eds. Cytology and hematology of the horse. Goleta, CA: American Veterinary Publishing Company, 1992:209–219.

Lewis HB, Rebar AH. Bone marrow evaluation in veterinary practice. St. Louis: Ralston Purina, 1979.

Tyler RD, Cowell RL, Meinkoth JH. Bone marrow. In: Diagnostic cytology and hematology of the dog and cat. 2nd ed. St. Louis: Mosby, 1999:284–304.

Nonneoplastic Disorders of Bone Marrow

Bernard SL, Leather CW, Brobst DF, et al. Estrogen-induced bone marrow depression in ferrets. Am J Vet Res 1983;44:657–661.

Bloom JC, Theim PA, Sellers TS, et al. Cephalosporin-induced immune cytopenia in the dog: demonstration of erythrocyte-, neutrophil-, and platelet-associated IgG following treatment with cefazedone. Am J Hematol 1988;28:71–78.

Boosinger TR, Rebar AH, Denicola DB, et al. Bone marrow alterations associated with canine parvoviral enteritis. Vet Pathol 1982;19:558–561.

Bowen RA, Olson PN, Behrendt MD, et al. Efficacy and toxicity of estrogens commonly used to terminate canine pregnancy. J Am Vet Med Assoc 1985;186:783–788.

Brockus CW. Endogenous estrogen myelotoxicosis associated with functional cystic ovaries in a dog. Vet Clin Pathol 1998;27:55–56.

Deldar A, Lewis H, Bloom J, et al: Cephalopsorin-induced changes in the ultrastructure of canine bone marrow. Vet Pathol 1988;25:211–218.

Farris GM, Benjamin SA. Inhibition of myelopoiesis by conditioned medium from cultured canine thymic cells exposed to estrogen. Am J Vet Res 1993;54:1366–1373.

Fox LE, Ford S, Alleman AR, et al. Aplastic anemia associated with prolonged high-dose trimethoprim-sulfadiazine administration in two dogs. Vet Clin Pathol 1993;22:89–92.

Giger U, Werner LL, Millichamp NJ, et al. Sulfadiazine-induced allergy in six Doberman pinschers. J Am Vet Med Assoc 1985;186:479–484.

Hoff B, Lumsden JH, Valli VEO. An appraisal of bone marrow biopsy in assessment of sick dogs. Can J Comp Med 1985;49:34–42.

Holland M, Stobie D, Shapiro W. Pancytopenia associated with administration of captopril to a dog. J Am Vet Med Assoc 1996;208:1683–1687.

Jacobs G, Calvert C, Kaufman A. Neutropenia and thrombocytopenia in three dogs treated with anticonvulsants. J Am Vet Med Assoc 1998;212:681–684.

Jonas RD, Thrall MA, Weiser MG. Immune-mediated hemolytic anemia with delayed erythrogenesis in the dog. J Am Anim Hosp Assoc 1987; 23:201–204.

Kuehn NF, Gaunt SF. Clinical and hematologic findings in canine ehrlichiosis. J Am Vet Med Assoc 1985;186:355–358.

Morgan RV. Blood dyscrasias associated with testicular tumors in the dog. J Am Anim Hosp Assoc 1982;18:970–975.

Peterson ME, Kintzer PP, Hurvitz AI. Methimazole treatment of 262 cats with hyperthyroidism. J Vet Intern Med 1988;2:150–157.

Reagan WJ. A review of myelofibrosis in dogs. Toxicol Pathol 1993;21:164–169.

Rebar AH. General responses of the bone marrow to injury. Toxicol Pathol 1993;21:118–129.

Rinkardt NE, Kruth SA. Azathioprine-induced bone marrow toxicity in four dogs. Can Vet J 1996;37:612–613.

Sherding RG, Wilson GP, Kociba GJ: Bone marrow hypoplasia in eight dogs with Sertoli cell tumor. J Am Vet Med Assoc 1981;178:497–500.

Stochaus C, Slappendel RJ. Haemophagocytic syndrome with disseminated intravascular coagulation in a dog. J Small Anim Pract 1998;39:203–206.

Stokol T, Blue JT. Pure red cell aplasia in cats: 9 cases (1989–1997). J Am Vet Med Assoc 1999;214:75–79.

Stokol T, Blue JT, French TW. Idiopathic pure red cell aplasia and nonregenerative immune-mediated anemia in dogs: 43 cases (1988–1999). J Am Vet Med Assoc 2000;216:1429–1436.

Stokol T, Randolph JF, Nachbar S, et al. Development of bone marrow toxicosis after albendazole administration in a dog and cat. J Am Vet Med Assoc 1997;12:1753–1756.

Walker D, Cowell RL, Clinkenbeard KD, et al. Bone marrow mast cell hyperplasia in dogs with aplastic anemia. Vet Clin Pathol 1997;26:106–111.

Walton R, Modiano JF, Thrall MA, et al. Bone marrow cytologic findings in four dogs and one cat with hemophagocytic syndrome. J Vet Intern Med 1996;10:7–14.

Watson ADJ, Wilson JT, Turner OM, et al. Phenylbutazone-induced blood dyscrasias suspected in 3 dogs. Vet Rec 1980; 107:239–241.

Weiss DJ. Idiopathic aplastic anemia in the dog. Vet Clin Pathol 1985;14:23–25.

Weiss DJ. Histopathology of canine nonneoplastic bone marrow. Vet Clin Pathol 1985;15:7–11.

Weiss DJ, Adams LG. Aplastic anemia associated with trimethoprim-sulfadiazine and fenbendazole administration in a dog. J Am Vet Med Assoc 1987;191:1119–1120.

Weiss DJ, Armstrong PJ, Reimann K. Bone marrow necrosis in the dog. J Am Vet Med Assoc 1985;187:54–59.

Weiss DJ, Evanson OA, Sykes J. A retrospective study of canine pancytopenia. Vet Clin Pathol 1999;28:83–88.

Weiss DJ, Greig B, Aird B, et al. Inflammatory disorders of the bone marrow. Vet Clin Pathol 1992;21:79–84.

Weiss DJ, Klausner JS. Drug-associated aplastic anemia in dogs: eight cases (1984–1988). J Am Vet Med Assoc 1990;196:472–475.

Cytochemistry and Immunophenotyping

Cobbold S, Holmes M, Willett B. The immunology of companion animals: reagents and therapeutic strategies with potential veterinary and human clinical applications. Immunol Today 1994;15:347–352.

Dean GA, Groshek PM, Jain NC, et al. Immunophenotypic analysis of feline hemolymphatic neoplasia using flow cytometry. Comp Hematol 1995;5:84–92.

Facklan NR, Kociba GJ. Cytochemical characterization of feline leukemic cells. Vet Pathol 1986;23:155–161.

Facklan NR, Kociba GJ. Cytochemical characterization of leukemic cells from 20 dogs. Vet Pathol 1985;22:363–369.

Grindem CB. Blood cell markers. Vet Clin North Am Small Anim Pract 1996;26:1043–1064.

Grindem CB, Stevens JB, Perman V. Cytochemical reactions in cells from leukemic dogs. Vet Pathol 1986;23:103–109.

Groshek PM, Dean GA, Hoover EA. Monoclonal antibodies identifying feline hemopoietic cell lineages. Comp Hematol 1994;4:181–191.

Jain NC, Kono CS, Madewell BR. Cytochemical studies of normal feline blood and bone marrow cells. Blut 1989;58:195–199.

Jain NC, Madewell BR, Weller RE, et al. Clinical-pathological findings and cytochemical characterization of myelomonocytic leukemia in 5 dogs. J Comp Pathol 1981;91:17–31.

Momoi Y, Nagase M, Okamoto Y, et al. Rearrangements of immunoglobulin and T-cell receptor genes in canine lymphoma/leukemia cells. J Vet Med Sci 1993;55:755–780.

Myelodysplastic Syndrome

Baker RJ, Valli VE. Dysmyelopoiesis in the cat: a hematological disorder resembling refractory anemia with excess blasts in man. Can J Vet Res 1986;50:3–6.

Boone LI, Knauer KW, Rapp SW, et al. Use of human recombinant erythropoietin and prednisone for treatment of myelodysplastic syndrome with erythroid predominance in a dog. J Am Vet Med Assoc 1998;213:999–1001.

Breuer W, Hermanns W, Thiele J. Myelodysplastic syndrome (MDS), acute myeloid leukaemia (AML) and chronic myeloproliferative disorder (CMPD) in cats. J Comp Pathol 1999;121:203–216.

Linenberger ML, Abkowitz JL. Haematological disorders associated with feline retrovirus infections. Baillieres Clin Haematol 1995;8:73–112.

McManus PM, Hess RS. Myelodysplastic changes in a dog with subsequent acute myeloid leukemia. Vet Clin Pathol 1998;27:112–115.

Miyamoto T, Horie T, Shimada T, et al. Long-term case study of myelodysplastic syndrome in a dog. J Am Anim Hosp Assoc 1999;35:475–481.

Weiss DJ, Raskin R, Zerbe C. Myelodysplastic syndrome in two dogs. J Am Vet Med Assoc 1985;187:1038–1040.

Myeloproliferative and Lymphoproliferative Disorders (General)

Couto CG. Clinicopathologic aspects of acute leukemias in the dog. J Am Vet Med Assoc 1985;186:681–685.

Grindem CB. Ultrastructural morphology of leukemic cells from 14 dogs. Vet Pathol 1985;22:456–462.

Grindem CB, Perman V, Stevens JB. Morphological classification and clinical and pathological characteristics of spontaneous leukemia in 10 cats. J Am Anim Hosp Assoc 1985;21:227–236.

Grindem CB, Stevens JB, Perman V. Morphological classification and clinical and pathological characteristics of spontaneous leukemia in 17 dogs. J Am Anim Hosp Assoc 1985;21:219–226.

Hutson CA, Rideout BA, Pederson NC. Neoplasia associated with feline immunodeficiency virus infection in cats from Southern California. J Am Vet Med Assoc 1991;199:1357–1362.

Jain NC. The leukemias. In: Essentials of veterinary hematology. Philadelphia: Lea & Febiger, 1993:319–348.

Jain NC. The leukemias: general aspects. In: Essentials of veterinary hematology. Philadelphia: Lea & Febiger, 1993:307–318.

Jain NC, Madewell BR, Weller RE, et al. Clinical-pathological findings and cytochemical characterization of myelomonocytic leukaemia in 5 dogs. J Comp Pathol 1981;91:17–31.

Macy DW. Hematopoietic tumors. Feline retroviruses. In: Withrow SJ, MacEwen EG, eds. Small animal clinical oncology. 2nd ed. Philadelphia: WB Saunders, 1989:432–451.

Reagan WJ, DeNicola DB. Myeloproliferative and lymphoproliferative disorders. . In: Morrison WB. Cancer in dogs and cats: medical and surgical management. Baltimore: Williams & Wilkins, 1998:95–122.

Rinsky RA, Smith AB, Hornung R, et al. Benzene and leukemia. N Engl J Med 1987;316:1044–1050.

Savage CJ. Lymphoproliferative and myeloproliferative disorders. Vet Clin North Am Equine Pract 1998;14:563–578.

Shelton GH, Linenberger ML, Abkowitz JL. Hematologic abnormalities in cats seropositive for feline immunodeficiency virus. J Am Vet Med Assoc 1991;199:1353–1357.

Myeloproliferative

Blue JT. Myelofibrosis in cats with myelodysplastic syndrome and acute myelogenous leukemia. Vet Pathol 1988;25:154–160.

Blue JT, French TW, Kranz JS. Non-lymphoid hematopoietic neoplasia in cats: a retrospective study of 60 cases. Cornell Vet 1988;78:21–42.

Boudreaux MK, Blue JT, Durham SK, et al. Intravascular leukostasis in a horse with myelomonocytic leukemia. Vet Pathol 1984;21:544–546.

Clark P, Cornelisse CJ, Schott HC, et al. Myeloblastic leukaemia in a Morgan horse mare. Equine Vet J 1999;31:446–448.

Colbatzky F, Hermanns W. Acute megakaryoblastic leukemia in one cat and two dogs. Vet Pathol 1993;30:186–194.

Dunn JK, Heath MF, Jefferies AR, et al. Diagnostic and hematologic features of probable essential thrombocythemia in two dogs. Vet Clin Pathol 1999;28:131–138.

Durando MM, Alleman AR, Harvey JW. Myelodysplastic syndrome in a quarter horse gelding. Equine Vet J 1994;26:83–85.

Fine DM, Tvedten HW. Chronic granulocytic leukemia in a dog. J Am Vet Med Assoc 1999;214:1809–1812.

Gorman NT, Evans RJ. Myeloproliferative disease in the dog and cat: clinical presentations, diagnosis, and treatment. Vet Rec 1987;121:490–496.

Hammer AS. Thrombocytosis in dogs and cats: a retrospective study. Comp Haematol 1991;1:181–186.

Hammer AS, Cuoto CG, Getzy D, et al. Essential thrombocythemia in a cat. J Vet Intern Med 1990;4:87–91.

Harvey JW, Shields RP, Gaskin JM. Feline myeloproliferative disease. Changing manifestation in the peripheral blood. Vet Pathol 1978;15;437–448.

Hendrick M. A spectrum of hypereosinophilic syndromes exemplified by six cats with eosinophilic enteritis. Vet Pathol 1981;18:188–200.

Hopper PE, Mandell CP, Turrel JM, et al. Probable essential thrombocythemia in a dog. J Vet Intern Med 1989;3:79–85.

Huibregtse BA, Turner JL. Hypereosinophilic syndrome and eosinophilic leukemia: a comparison of 22 hypereosinophilic cats. J Am Anim Hosp Assoc 1994;30:591–599.

Jain NC. Classification of myeloproliferative disorders in cats using criteria proposed by the Animal Leukaemia Study Group: a retrospective study of 181 cases (1969–1992). Comp Haematol Int 1993;1:125–134.

Jain NC, Blue JT, Grindem CB, et al. Proposed criteria for classification of acute myeloid leukemias in dogs and cats—a report of the animal leukemia study group. Vet Clin Pathol 1991;20:63–82.

Leifer CE, Matus RE, Patnaik AK, et al. Chronic myelogenous leukemia in the dog. J Am Vet Med Assoc 1983;183:686–689.

Messick J, Carothers M, Wellman M. Identification and characterization of megakaryoblasts in acute megakaryoblastic leukemia in a dog. Vet Pathol 1090;27:212–214.

Miyamoto T, Hachimura H, Amimoto A. A case of megakaryoblastic leukemia in a dog. J Vet Med Sci 1996;58:177–179.

Ndikuwera J, Smith DA, Obsolo MJ, et al. Chronic granulocytic leukaemia/eosinophilic leukaemia in a dog? J Small Anim Pract 1992;33:353–357.

Neer TM. Hypereosinophilic syndrome in cats. Compend Cont Educ Pract Vet 1991;13:549–555.

Pucheu-Haston CM, Camus A, Taboada J, et al. Megakaryoblastic leukemia in a dog. J Am Vet Med Assoc 1995;207:194–196.

Puette M, Latimer KS. Acute granulocytic leukemia in a slaughter goat. J Vet Diagn Invest 1997;9:318–319.

Raskin RE. Myelopoiesis and myeloproliferative disorders. Vet Clin North Am Small Anim Pract 1996;26:1023–1042.

Ringger NC, Edens L, Bain P, et al. Acute myelogenous leukaemia in a mare. Aust Vet J 1997;75:329–331.

Shimada T, Matsumoto Y, Okuda M, et al. Erythroleukemia in two cats naturally infected with feline leukemia virus in the same household. J Vet Med Sci 1995;57:199–204.

Sykes GP, King JM, Cooper BC. Retrovirus-like particles associated with myeloproliferative disease in the dog. J Comp Pathol 1985;95:559–564.

Takayama H, Gejima S, Honma A, et al. Acute myeloblastic leukaemia in a cow. J Comp Pathol 1996;115:95–101.

Toth SR, Onions DE, Jarrett O. Histopathological and hematological findings in myeloid leukemia induced by a new feline leukemia virus isolate. Vet Pathol 1986;23:462–470.

Watanabe Y, Sekine T, Yabe M, et al. Myeloproliferative disease in a calf. J Comp Pathol 1998;119:83–87.

Young KM. Myeloproliferative disorders. Vet Clin North Am Small Anim Pract 1985;15:769–781.

Young KM, MacEwen EG. Hematopoietic tumors. Canine myeloproliferative disorders. In: Withrow SJ, MacEwen EG, eds. Small animal clinical oncology. 2nd ed. Philadelphia: WB Saunders, 1989:495–505.

Lymphoproliferative

Darbes J, Majzoub M, Breuer W, et al. Large granular lymphocyte leukemia/lymphoma in six cats. Vet Pathol 1998;35:370–379.

Couto CG, Ruehl W, Muir S. Plasma cell leukemia and monoclonal (IgG) gammopathy in a dog. J Am Vet Med Assoc 1984;184:90–92.

Hodgkins EM, Zinkl JG, Madewell BR. Chronic lymphocytic leukemia in the dog. J Am Vet Med Assoc 1980;177:704–707.

Leifer CE, Matus RE. Chronic lymphocytic leukemia in the dog: 22 cases (1974–1984). J Am Vet Med Assoc 1986;189:214–217.

Leifer CE, Matus RE. Lymphoid leukemia in the dog: acute lymphoblastic leukemia and chronic lymphocytic leukemia. Vet Clin North Am Small Anim Pract 1985;15:723–739.

Ludwig H, Meran J, Zojer N. Multiple myeloma: an update on biology and treatment. Annals Oncology 1999;10(Suppl 6):31–43.

MacEwen G. Hematopoietic tumors. Feline lymphoma and leukemias. In: Withrow SJ, MacEwen EG, eds. Small animal clinical oncology. 2nd ed. Philadelphia: WB Saunders, 1989:479–495.

MacEwen EG, Young KM. Hematopoietic tumors. Canine lymphoma and lymphoid leukemias. In: Withrow SJ, MacEwen EG, eds. Small animal clinical oncology. 2nd ed. Philadelphia: WB Saunders, 1989:451–477.

Madewell BR. Hematological and bone marrow cytological abnormalities in 75 dogs with malignant lymphoma. J Am Anim Hosp Assoc 1986;22:235–240.

Madewell BR, Munn RJ. Canine lymphoproliferative disorders. An ultrastructural study of 18 cases. J Vet Intern Med 1990;4:63–70.

Matus RE, Leifer CE, MacEwen G. Acute lymphoblastic leukemia in the dog: a review of 30 cases. J Am Vet Med Assoc 1983;183:859–862.

Matus Re, Leifer CE, MacEwen G, et al: Prognostic factors for multiple myeloma in the dog. J Am Vet Med Assoc 1986;188:1288–1292.

Morris JS, Dunn JK, Dobson JM. Canine lymphoid leukemia and lymphoma with bone marrow involvement: a review of 24 cases. J Small Anim Pract 1993; 34:72–79.

Morrison WB. Plasma cell neoplasms. In: Morrison WB. Cancer in dogs and cats: medical and surgical management. Baltimore: Williams & Wilkins, 1998:697–704.

Raskin RE, Krehbiel JD. Prevalence of leukemic blood and bone marrow in dogs with multicentric lymphoma. J Am Vet Med Assoc 1989; 193:1427–1429.

Schick RO, Murphy GF, Goldschmidt MH. Cutaneous lymphosarcoma and leukemia in a cat. J Am Vet Med Assoc 1994;204:606–609.

Thrall MA. Lymphoproliferative disorders. Vet Clin North Am Small Anim Pract 1981;11:321–347.

Thrall MA, Macy DW, Snyder SP, et al. Cutaneous lymphosarcoma and leukemia in a dog resembling Sezary syndrome in man. Vet Pathol 1984;21:182–186.

Vail DM. Hematopoietic tumors. Plasma cell neoplasms. In: Withrow SJ, MacEwen EG, eds. Small animal clinical oncology. 2nd ed. Philadelphia: WB Saunders, 1989:509–520.

Weiser MG, Thrall MA, Fulton R, et al: Granular lymphocytosis and hyperproteinemia in dogs with chronic ehrlichiosis. J Am Anim Hosp Assoc 1991;27:84–88.

Wellman ML, Couto CG, Starkey RJ, et al. Lymphocytosis of large granular lymphocytes in three dogs. Vet Pathol 1989;26:158–163.

Other Neoplastic Disorders Involving Bone Marrow

Boone L, Radlinsky MA. Bone marrow aspirate from a dog with anemia and thrombocytopenia. Vet Clin Pathol 2000;29:59–61.

Brown DE, Thrall MA, Getzy DM, et al. Cytology of canine malignant histiocytosis. Vet Clin Pathol 1994;23:118–122.

Court EA, Earnest-Koons KA, Carr SC, et al. Malignant histiocytosis in a cat. J Am Vet Med Assoc 1993;203:1300–1302.

McManus PM. Frequency and severity of mastocytemia in dogs with and without mast cell tumors: 120 cases (1995–1997). J Am Vet Med Assoc 1999;215:355–357.

Moore PF, Rosin A. Malignant histiocytosis of Bernese mountain dogs. Vet Pathol 1986;23:1–10.

Walton RM, Brown DE, Burkhard MJ, et al. Malignant histiostiocytosis in a domestic cat: cytomorphologic and immunohistochemical features. Vet Clin Pathol 1997;26:56–60.

Therapy for Neoplastic Bone Marrow Disorders

Cotter SM. Treatment of lymphoma and leukemia with cyclophosphamide, vincristine, and prednisone: II. Treatment of cats. J Am Anim Hosp Assoc 1983;19:166–172.

Gasper PW, Rosen DK, Fulton R. Allogeneic marrow transplantation in a cat with acute myeloid leukemia. J Am Vet Med Assoc 1996; 208:1280–1284.

Hamilton TA. The leukemias. In: Morrison WB, ed. Cancer in dogs and cats: medical and surgical management. Baltimore: Williams & Wilkins, 1998:721–729.

Hamilton TA, Morrison WB, DeNicola DB. Cytosine arabinoside chemotherapy for acute megakaryocytic leukemia in a cat. J Am Vet Med Assoc 1991;199:359–361.

Helfand SC. Low-dose cytosine arainsoide-induced remission of lymphoblastic leukemia in a cat. J Am Vet Med Assoc 1987;191:707–710.

Thrall MA, Haskins ME. Bone marrow transplantation. In: August JR, ed. Consultations in feline internal medicine. 3rd ed. Philadelphia: WB Saunders, 1997:514–524.

14

DIAGNOSIS OF DISORDERS
OF HEMOSTASIS

The cardiovascular system delivers blood to tissues throughout the body, and it is susceptible to injury of many types. Injury occurs to the vascular system on a daily basis, but normal individuals have a finely controlled system that prevents blood loss, maintains blood flow, and allows the healing and repair of injured vessels.

OVERVIEW OF HEMOSTASIS

The term *hemostasis* is defined as the arrest of bleeding, and defects of hemostasis include excessive hemostasis, with resulting intravascular thrombosis, and excessive bleeding. Both types of defects may be life-threatening, but intravascular thrombosis is more difficult to detect and manage. This chapter discusses a systematic approach for establishing an effective diagnosis of the commonly encountered disorders of hemostasis, and it emphasizes disorders that result in bleeding. Effective hemostasis after vascular injury reflects integrated responses by three major components: the soluble circulating coagulation factors (i.e., proteins) that form stable insoluble fibrin, circulating platelets, and the vessel wall formed by a matrix of endothelial cells, muscle cells, and fibroblasts.

Coagulation Factors

The term *coagulopathy* usually refers to excessive bleeding that results from the abnormal function or absence of one or more circulating coagulation factors. Coagulation factors are present in plasma at very small concentrations (μg/mL), and most are proteases *(Table 14.1)*. Coagulation factors are activated predominantly by exposure to tissue thromboplastin expressed on the surface of endothelial cells or extravascular fibroblasts. After the initial activation, coagulation factors are activated serially and by feedback amplification loops to enhance the initial stimulus. The culminating event of coagulation factor activation is the conversion of fibrinogen to fibrin and the formation of a stable fibrin clot in association with platelets. Defective coagulation factor activity or absence of factors will delay the formation of fibrin.

The coagulation cascade or "waterfall" sequential activation and amplification scheme of hemostasis traditionally has been divided into the intrinsic, extrinsic, and common pathways *(Fig. 14.1)*. This scheme implies two pathways of activation: by exposure to tissue thromboplastin, or by contact activation of basement membrane and collagen (or other negatively charged surfaces). The results of recent kinetic analyses of individual factors,

TABLE 14.1   PROCOAGULATION FACTORS

Factor	Trivial Name	Location of Synthesis	Molecular Weight	Plasma Concentration
I	Fibrinogen	Liver	340,000	0.1–2.5 gm/dL
II	Prothrombin	Liver, macrophage	72,000	—
III	Tissue thromboplastin	Lipoprotein, is a constituitent of fibroblasts and smooth muscle cell plasma membrane; lipoprotein can be induced in endothelium, monocytes, and macrophages.		
IV	calcium			
V	Proaccelerin	Liver, macrophages	350,000	—
VI	No factor			
VII	Proconvertin	Liver, macrophages	53,000	—
VIII:C	Antihemophiliac factor	Liver	Ambiguous	—
IX	Christmas factor (plasma thrombo- plastin component)	Liver	56,000	—
X	Stuart factor	Liver, macrophages	56,000	—
XI	Plasma thromboplastin antecedent	Liver (probably)	124,000	6 µg/mL
XII	Hageman factor	Liver (probably)	80,000	30 µg/mL
XIII	Fibrin-stabilizing factor	Liver (probably)	320,000	—
Prekallikrein	Fletcher factor	Liver (probably)	85,000	50 µg/mL
High-molecular- weight kininogen	Fitzgerald factor	Liver (probably)	110,000	70–90 µg/mL

auto. dom., autosomal dominant; *auto. rec.*, autosomal recessive; *X-linked rec.*, X-linked recessive.
[a] Severe in neonates, mild in adults.
[b] Severe bleeding may occur after major surgical procedures or trauma.
[c] Normally not present in marine mammals, most reptiles, and fowl.

however, suggest a scheme in which the initial activation by tissue thromboplastin forms small amounts of thrombin, which is then followed and amplified by subsequent loop activation of the intrinsic, extrinsic, and common pathways. Important in this loop activation is thrombin (factor IIa) activation of factor VII, XI, and the accelerators factor V and VIII *(Fig. 14.2)*. This implies that contact activation is not a significant contributor to coagulation factor activation, and that the intrinsic system primarily is an amplification loop that becomes activated after the initial thrombin generation by tissue thromboplastin. Evidence supporting this view exists in human patients who do not bleed when they are deficient in any of the contact activator proteins (factor XII, prekallikrein, or high-molecular-weight kininogen [HMWK]) This view may not be true in some domestic animals, however, because dogs and horses with prekallikrein deficiency have mild clinical bleeding tendencies.

Normal coagulation factor activity requires vitamin K, which serves as a cofactor for the carboxylation of coagulation factors II, VII, IX, and X as well as of anticoagulant proteins C and S. Vitamin K normally is oxidized during carboxylation and then reduced back to the active hydroquinone form in a two-step process involving the enzyme epoxide reductase. In the presence of vitamin K antagonists or the absence of vitamin K, the procoagulant and anticoagulant proteins are formed but lack activity. These nonfunctional proteins are designated PIVKA (i.e., proteins in vitamin K absence or antagonism), and they can be detected by immunologic methods.

Platelets

Platelets are cytoplasmic fragments of megakaryocytes with numerous cytosolic organelles *(Table 14.2)*, and they are shaped like a flat disk *(Fig. 14.3)*. Platelets are crucial to hemostasis and are responsible for the initial, temporary cessation of blood flow after injury to the microvascular bed. Platelets respond to vascular injury in a series of reactions that are divided into adhesion of platelets

Plasma Half-Life	Vitamin K Dep.	Species Affected	Inheritance/Disease Name	Clinical Disease
1.5–6.3 days	–	Man, goats, dogs	Autosomal	Severe
2.1–4.4 days	+	Man, dog	Auto. rec.	Mild
15–24 hours	–	Man	auto. rec., parahemophilia	Variable, mostly mild
1–6 hours	+	Man, dogs	Auto. dom. (auto rec. in man)	Mild
2.9 days	–	Man, dogs, cats, horses	X-linked rec., hemophilia A	Variable
24 hours	+	Man, dogs, cats	X-linked rec., hemophilia B	Often severe
32–48 hours	+	Man, dogs	Auto. dom.	Severe[a]
30 hours	–	Man, cattle, dogs	Auto. rec., hemophilia C	Mild[b]
48–52 hours	–	Man, cats[c]	Auto. rec., Hageman trait	None
4.5–7.0 days	–	Man		
35 hours	–	Man, dogs, horses	Auto. rec.	None to mild
6.5 days	–	Man		

to vessel wall, aggregation of platelets, and release reaction of platelets. Platelets can adhere to collagen in the basement membrane and extravascular stroma through a surface receptor (glycoprotein 1b) that binds plasma glycoprotein von Willebrand factor (vWF), which in turn binds collagen. Lack of the receptor (Bernard-Soulier syndrome) or vWF (von Willebrand disease) results in clinical bleeding. After adhesion, platelets adhere to one another by fibrinogen interacting with surface receptors (IIB and IIIa) induced to express by adenosine diphosphate. As platelets adhere to one another, they swell, centralize their organelles, and then form pseudopodia *(Fig. 14.4)*. Aggregation of platelets as well as recruitment of additional platelets are promoted by the release reaction that empties products in the platelet granules into plasma. Coagulation factors stored within granules ensure fibrin formation, which is necessary for platelet plug stabilization. Platelets furnish a phospholipid (platelet factor III), which acts as a receptor for coagulation factor adherence. Platelet granules empty their contents into the open canalicular system that communicates with the exterior. Platelets do not lyse during aggregation.

Vessels

Vessels contribute to the cessation of blood loss by reflex vasoconstriction of smooth muscle cells to reduce the vessel lumen diameter as well as by secretion of thrombogenic substances from the injured endothelial cells to promote clot formation. Damage or loss of endothelium also reduces the local secretion of mediators that downregulate the reactivity of platelets, thus enhancing platelet responsiveness at that site. Decreased perivascular collagen support in disease conditions such as Marfan syndrome, Ehlers-Danlos syndrome, scurvy, and steroid excess have been associated with increased vascular fragility and bleeding as well as with some evidence of defective platelet response to abnormal collagen. Vascular abnormalities, when compared with platelet and coagulation factor abnormalities, are the least frequent cause of excessive bleeding but the most difficult to evaluate.

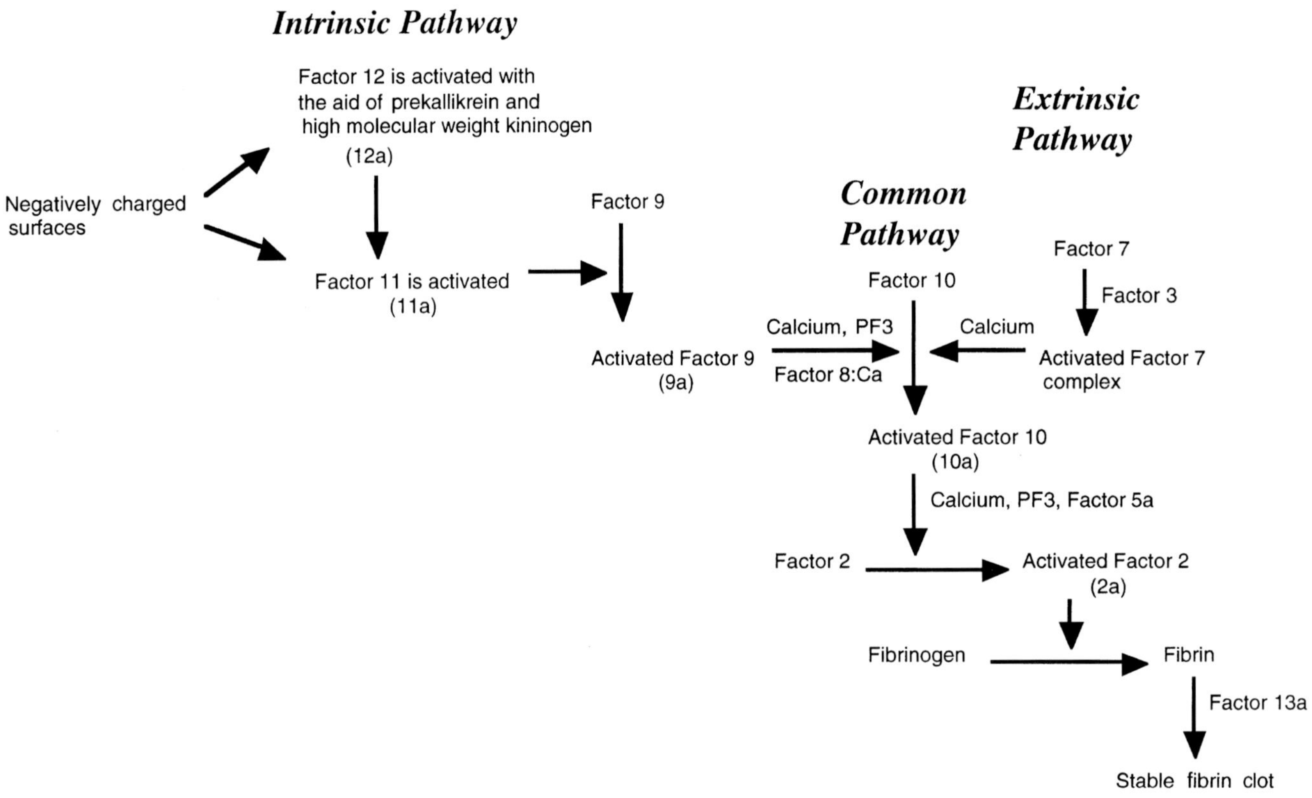

Intrinsic Pathway

Extrinsic Pathway

Common Pathway

Negatively charged surfaces

Factor 12 is activated with the aid of prekallikrein and high molecular weight kininogen (12a)

Factor 11 is activated (11a)

Factor 9

Activated Factor 9 (9a)

Calcium, PF3

Factor 8:Ca

Factor 10

Calcium

Factor 7

Factor 3

Activated Factor 7 complex

Activated Factor 10 (10a)

Calcium, PF3, Factor 5a

Factor 2

Activated Factor 2 (2a)

Fibrinogen

Fibrin

Factor 13a

Stable fibrin clot

Figure 14.1 The traditional activation cascade of the intrinsic system by contact activation of negatively charged surfaces. Activation of factor XI by thrombin (IIa), however, may be more important. Factor IX is activated by factor XIa (and activated factor VII), and it can activate factor X in the presence of calcium and platelet factor III. Factor VIII:C is not required for activation, but when factor VIII:Ca is present, the rate of factor Xa formation is increased. The designation "a" denotes an activated factor. The extrinsic system is thought to be the predominant method of coagulation activation, and this occurs when factor III (tissue thromboplastin) is in contact with factor VII, which then can activate factor X. Factor X is the first factor of common pathway and is activated by either factor IX or VII. The common pathway culminates in the formation of a stable fibrin clot. Activation of prothrombin to thrombin (IIa) does not require factor V, but it proceeds much faster with activated factor V.

Effective maintenance of the vascular integrity and perfusion of tissues requires the precise control of clot formation and resolution of the clot for re-establishing blood flow in tissues. Even as the clot forms, lysis of the clot occurs by plasmin, which is formed by the activation of plasminogen. In vivo activation of plasminogen to plas-

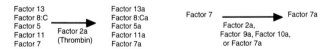

Figure 14.2 Thrombin activates many other factors of the coagulation cascade and amplifies the initial activation of prothrombin to form much more thrombin. Also, once factor VII has been activated, additional amplification loops generate more factor VIIa to enhance the overall activity of the coagulation cascade. Factor VIIa also activates factor IX to IXa to enhance the formation of factor Xa from X. The purpose of these activation loops is to fully activate the cascade and to generate much more thrombin to, ultimately, shorten the time needed to convert a critical mass of fibrinogen to fibrin for the formation of a stable fibrin clot.

min is done primarily by active factor XII and by tissue-plasminogen activator from endothelial cells. Factor XII activates plasminogen as well as factor XI, complement, and kinins by the scheme depicted in *Figure 14.5*. Patients who are deficient in factor XII do not bleed excessively, but they do have a tendency for thrombosis resulting from the insufficient resolution of fibrin clots by plasmin. Other activators of plasminogen are known (epithelial plasminogen activator, urokinase, bilokinase, streptokinase, staphylokinase), but these are not important in the normal regulation of intravascular clot resolution. Plasmin degrades fibrin and fibrinogen to small fragments and peptides *(Fig. 14.6)*. Detection of fibrin and fibrinogen (fibrin[ogen]) degradation by plasmin primarily is by the immunologic identification of fragment E in most species. Fibrin(ogen) degradation products (FDPs) normally are removed from the circulation by hepatocytes, and decreased removal results in increased circulating concentration of FDP. In the absence of liver disease, the usual clinical implication of an increased FDP concentration is

TABLE 14.2 ULTRASTRUCTURAL AND FUNCTIONAL ANATOMY OF PLATELETS

Anatomic-Structure	Constituents	Functions
Exterior coat	Fibrinogen	Platelet aggregation
	Glycoprotein	Platelet adhesion
Unit membrane	Arachidonic Acid	Prostaglandin synthesis
	Platelet factor III (phosphatidylserine)	Enhances coagulation
Microtubules	Tubulin	Provides cytoskeleton and contractile system
Microfilaments	Thrombosthenin	Shape change, clot retraction, platelet release
α-Granules	β-Thromboglobulin	Impedes prostacyclin production by endothelium
	von Willebrand factor	Platelet adhesion to subendothelial collagen
	Factor V (Platelet factor I)	
	Fibrinogen	
	Fibronectin	
	Growth factor(s)	Mitosis of fibroblasts, endothelium, smooth muscle
	High-molecular-weight kininogen	
	Platelet factor IV	Antiheparin activity
Dense bodies	Adenine nucleotides	Platelet metabolism and hemostasis
	Histamine	Increases vascular permeability
	Serotonin	Vasoconstriction and enhancement of aggregation
	Calcium	Necessary for platelet stimulation
Lysosomal granules	Acid hydrolases	proteolysis
Dense tubular system	Calcium	Necessary for platelet stimulation
	Enzymes for prostaglandin synthesis	Thromboxane A_2 is important in recruiting more platelets and mobilizing calcium
Open canalicular system	Extensive surface area	Route for exocytosis, endocytosis, phagocytosis

increased intravascular coagulation with subsequent clot resolution.

Anticoagulant Proteins

Anticoagulant proteins downregulate the coagulation cascade by inhibiting the procoagulant proteins of the intrin-
sic, extrinsic, and common pathways. This ensures that activation of coagulation does not exceed the immediate need for hemostasis at the site of vascular injury. These anticoagulant proteins are in balance with the procoagulant proteins, and deficient anticoagulant protein activity relative to the procoagulant protein concentration results in thrombosis. This balance can be shifted in favor of

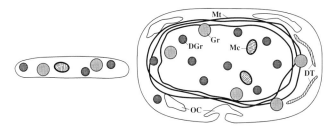

Figure 14.3 The disc shape of a platelet on end (*left*) and from above (*right*). *DGr*, dense granules; *DT*, dense tubular system; *Gr*, granules; *Mc*, mitochondria; *Mt*, microtubules around the margin; *OC*, open canilicular system.

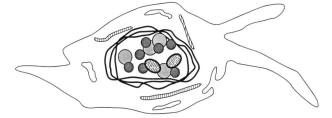

Figure 14.4 The centralization of platelet contents during activation, with pseudopodia formation and fusion of granules to the open canalicular system to release their contents into the extracellular milieu without lysis of the platelet membrane.

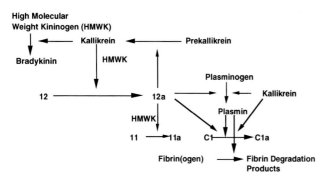

Figure 14.5 Factor XIIa can activate four protein cascades, but the only significant functional loss associated with decreased factor XII activity in plasma is thrombosis caused by reduced generation of plasmin from plasminogen.

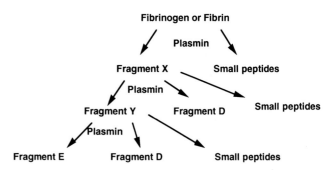

Figure 14.6 The degradation of fibrin and fibrinogen to smaller peptide fragments that can be used in anabolism by hepatocytes.

thrombosis by the loss of anticoagulant proteins or by selective, increased concentration of procoagulant proteins. Important anticoagulant proteins are listed in *Table 14.3*.

The most important circulating anticoagulant protein is antithrombin III (AT-III), which accounts for approximately 70% of the total antithrombin activity in plasma. Antithrombin III requires heparin for activity at the endothelial surface. Heparin allows AT-III to bind to thrombin in a 1:1 ratio and inactivates thrombin. The AT-III:thrombin complex subsequently is removed by hepatocytes. In addition to the inactivation of thrombin (IIa), AT-III also inactivates other serine proteases (IXa, Xa, XIa, and XIIa). Antithrombin III has a very low molecular weight (Table 14.3) and is lost in the urine of patients with severe glomerular nephritis or amyloidosis. Low AT-III activity in plasma, either through loss or hereditary deficiency, often is associated with clinical thrombosis. A deficiency of other anticoagulant proteins, such as proteins C and S, which inhibit factors Va and VIII:Ca, also may be associated with thrombosis. α_2-Macroglobulin

inhibits thrombin, plasmin, and kallikrein, and it accounts for another 20% of antithrombin activity in plasma. Extrinsic pathway inhibitor is a lipoprotein produced by the liver and endothelial cells that is thought to be the major regulator of extrinsic pathway activation. Extrinsic pathway inhibitor inactivates thromboplastin and factor VIIa, and it requires factor Xa for activation.

EVALUATION OF THE BLEEDING PATIENT

When an animal is suspected of having a hemostatic defect, the following case-analysis method may be used to accurately determine if a defect exists and, if so, to determine the nature of a defect.

Patient history is a very important component in the analysis of an animal suspected of having a hemostatic defect. Specific questions should be asked, such as:

1. Have there been large hemorrhages into the subcutaneous tissue?

TABLE 14.3 ANTICOAGULANT FACTORS

Factor	Trivial Name	Location of Synthesis	Molecular Weight
Antithrombin III	Heparin cofactor	Liver	62,000
C1 esterase inhibitor			
Extrinsic pathway inhibitor		Liver, endothelium (lipoprotein)	
α1-antitrypsin			
α2-antiplasmin			
Protein C			62,000
Thrombomodulin	Protein C cofactor	Endothelium	
Protein S	Cofactor for activated protein C		75,000

[a] Normally not present in marine mammals, most reptiles, and fowl.
[b] Severe in neonates, mild in adults.
[c] Severe bleeding may occur after major surgical procedures or trauma.

2. Have there been previous petechial or ecchymotic hemorrhages on the skin?
3. What has been the color of urine?
4. Does the animal have periodic lameness, suggesting intra-articular hemorrhage?
5. What is the color and the character of the fecal material?
6. Did the animal bleed excessively during previous surgery?
7. Has the animal been administered any drug and, if so, when?
8. What is the animal's environment?

Questions such as these should be asked to determine if the hemorrhage is appropriate for the degree of injury and if it resolves in an appropriate length of time. Persistent, recurrent hemorrhage at one site suggests a local vascular problem rather than a generalized homeostatic defect. Drugs and toxins, including rodenticides, may result in hemostatic defects, and possible access to such chemicals also is important information.

A careful physical examination to determine the nature and severity of the hemostatic defect provides useful information as well. For example, if evidence is found for underlying disease processes such as icterus, mass lesions, or fever, then disorders such as liver disease, hemangiosarcomas, or Rocky Mountain spotted fever, respectively, may be causing secondary bleeding disorders. Also, petechial and ecchymotic hemorrhages are characteristic of platelet abnormalities *(Fig. 14.7)* and generalized vascular abnormalities, whereas large hematomas, hemarthrosis, and deep muscle hemorrhages are characteristic of coagulopathies *(Figs. 14.8 and 14.9)*.

Appropriate laboratory evaluation is another important component in evaluation of hemostasis and should initially include a complete blood count (CBC), activated partial thromboplastin time (aPTT) or activated coagulation time (ACT), and prothrombin time (PT). The CBC provides information such as platelet concentration and packed cell volume. The aPTT or ACT and PT help to determine if the levels of coagulation factors (except factor XIII) are deficient. A bleeding time may be necessary if the platelet concentration is normal but the animal is still suspected of having a platelet-related problem. In addition, clinical chemistry, urinalysis, radiology, ultrasound, or isotope scanning may be helpful in evaluating other system functions in a patient with a hemostatic defect.

EVALUATION OF THE COMPONENTS OF HEMOSTASIS

Coagulation Factors

All circulating coagulation factors are produced by the liver, and hepatic insufficiency often is associated with clinical bleeding because of the decreased synthesis of one or more coagulation factors. The factors and some of their characteristics are listed in Table 14.1. Of the coagulation factors, only factors VIII:C and V are not proteases; these two factors increase the activity of other coagulation factors. Hereditary deficiencies of coagulation factors are uncommon in domestic animals, but hereditary deficiencies of most known factors have been described. The most frequent hereditary coagulation factor deficiency described in veterinary medicine involves factor VIII:C. Deficiencies of factors VIII:C and IX are sex-linked traits and occur more frequently in male patients; the remaining factors are coded on somatic chromosomes.

Evaluation of coagulation factors usually is not performed in the clinic setting but at local or regional laboratories, because the tests require infrequently used and often expensive equipment, which in turn require high

Plasma Concentration	Plasma Half-Life	Vitamin K Dep.	Species Affected	Inheritance	Clinical Disease
			Man	Autosomal	Thrombosis
	6–9 hours	+	Man		Thrombosis (purpura)
30 µm/mL		+	Man	Autosomal	Thrombosis (purpura)

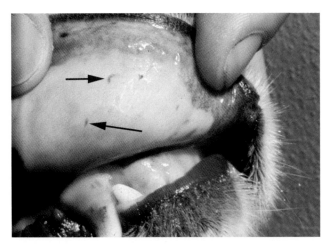

Figure 14.7 Petechial hemorrhages on the gingival surface of the lips are suggestive of a platelet function defect or of decreased numbers of platelets. (Courtesy of Dr. Ellen Miller.)

maintenance. The only exception to this generalization is the ACT test, which is easily performed and evaluates all coagulation factors (except factors VII and XIII). This test uses sterile, diatomaceous earth as a contact activator and has an end point of loose blood clot formation. An ACT also requires a minimum functional platelet concentration of 10^4 cell/mL (see Appendix 14.1 for specific details of the ACT test). If the ACT and platelet count are normal, then coagulation factor deficiencies are an unlikely cause of the hemostatic defect. Factor XIII deficiency has never been reported in animals, and factor VII deficiency is associated with mild clinical bleeding.

Selective evaluation of the coagulation cascade may be done by collecting blood in 3.8% sodium citrate in a volume of 1:9 anticoagulant:blood. Atraumatic venipuncture and collection of blood, first into a tube that is thrown away before collection into a sample vial to be sent

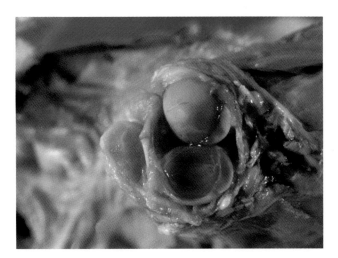

Figure 14.8 Hemorrhage into joints (as in this lamb with a carboxylation defect of coagulation factors) or body cavities suggests deficiency of coagulation factor (or factors).

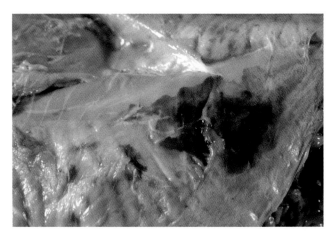

Figure 14.9 Subcutaneous hemorrhage suggestive of a coagulation factor deficiency.

to the laboratory, are important steps in proper blood collection. Blood is then sent to a laboratory for testing, optimally within 4 hours of collection. The aPTT uses one of several contact activators, and the PT uses tissue thromboplastin to activate coagulation. Phospholipid is added as a substitute for platelets in both tests. A prolonged aPTT results from one or more plasma concentrations of factors II, V, VIII:C, IX, X, XI, XII, prekallikrein, HMWK, or fibrinogen of less than 25% of normal activity or concentration. A prolonged PT results if there is less than 25% of normal activity or concentration of any of factors II, V, VII, X, or fibrinogen. A thrombin time also may be done, which essentially reflects fibrinogen concentration and may be modified to quantitate the actual fibrinogen level. Coagulation factor concentrations as well as activation kinetics to convert fibrinogen to fibrin vary between species, but these details are clinically unimportant. Submission of plasma for an aPTT or PT should be co-ordinated with the laboratory performing the evaluation order to optimize reliability of the results and to avoid any delay in testing. A similarly collected blood sample from a normal animal also may be required as an additional control for the patient's sample. If individual coagulation factor analysis is desired for a complete evaluation, it usually is referred to a specialized laboratory for determination. The clinician should consult with laboratory personnel before collection and delivery of the sample to enhance reliability of the results.

Platelets

Inadequate platelet concentration and, less commonly, abnormal platelet function can be responsible for excessive bleeding. Both platelet concentration and function can be assessed by several methods. Platelet concentration can be determined by counting platelets electronically or manually. The concentration can be estimated on a blood film; at least 5 to 10 platelets/oil immersion field

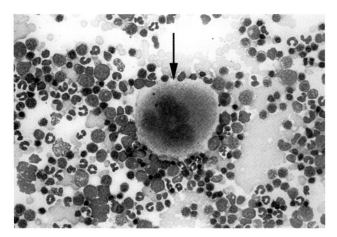

Figure 14.10 Bone marrow film showing a mature megakaryocyte. The cytoplasm is eosinophilic and granular, with a large, syncytial nucleus.

(magnification, ×1000) should be present. Normal platelet concentrations vary among animal species, but the range for all species is 100,000 to 800,000 platelets/μL or platelets/10^{-6}L, with horses having the lowest and cattle the highest concentrations. Animals do not spontaneously bleed because of low platelet concentration, however, until the concentration is ≤10,000 to 50,000. Platelet concentration can be decreased in blood because of decreased production by the bone marrow, increased removal from the blood (i.e., destruction), or activation (i.e., consumption). When the bone marrow production of platelets is decreased, the megakaryocyte concentration within the marrow is decreased; conversely, the bone marrow megakaryocytes concentration is increased when platelets are being destroyed or consumed *(Fig. 14.10)*. Platelets may appear to be larger than normal if production and release are accelerated *(Fig. 14.11)*.

If the platelet concentration is adequate, platelet function can be evaluated by performing a bleeding time or by measuring platelet response to specific agonists in vitro. In general, the bleeding time is the time that it takes blood to cease flowing from a shallow wound that causes injury to capillaries under a hairless skin surface. A bleeding time usually is done by creating a wound on the lip, gum, or nasal planum of an animal (see Appendix 14.1 for details). The time that it takes for blood to stop flowing initially is the bleeding time, and it reflects platelet plug formation stopping the capillary blood leakage. If coagulation factors are insufficient, the platelet plug still forms, but the wound begins bleeding again (i.e., rebleed phenomena) because fibrin has not been formed rapidly enough to stabilize the formed platelet plug. If the platelet concentration is decreased, the bleeding time is prolonged. If the platelet concentration is within the reference range but the bleeding time is prolonged, then platelets are not responding appropriately. Once an animal is thought to have a platelet defect, more sophisticated platelet function analysis can be performed by platelet aggregometry using a wide variety of chemical stimuli for platelets. The pattern of response to known platelet agonists suggests the type of platelet defect.

Thrombocytosis (i.e., a platelet concentration greater than the reference range) is a nonspecific disorder that usually is not associated with clinical signs. Thrombocytosis often is associated with iron deficiency anemia, inflammatory conditions, epinephrine release, and some forms of myeloproliferative disorders.

Vascular Abnormalities

Disorders of hemostasis resulting from defects or abnormalities in the vessel are uncommon. These patients may have a prolonged bleeding time with normal platelet function or a localized vascular injury resulting in bleeding. Evaluation of possible vascular causes of bleeding include tissue-incisional biopsy for histologic evaluation of vessel structure. Alternatively, a skin biopsy with biochemical evaluation of the collagen characteristics that would be altered in patient with a suspected hereditary collagen disorder may be appropriate in the evaluation of a bleeding patient. Depending on the species affected, clinical evaluation for scurvy or Cushing syndrome may be appropriate for increased fragility of the skin and collagen in a bleeding patient.

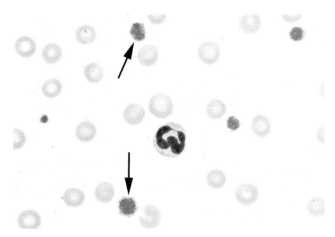

Figure 14.11 Large platelets (megaplatelets) in a thrombocytopenic dog infected with *Ehrlichia canis*. Large platelets suggest accelerated thrombocytopoiesis and early release of immature forms.

COMMONLY ENCOUNTERED DISORDERS OF HEMOSTASIS

Disseminated Intravascular Coagulation

Disseminated intravascular coagulation (DIC) is associated with many clinical diseases and is caused by excessive activation of coagulation, either regionally or throughout the entire body. Initiation of coagulation can vary from widespread tissue damage, as in heat stroke, to elaboration of procoagulant proteins by neoplastic cell populations, as in some leukemias. Diffuse thrombosis, especially in the microcirculation, is seen, with resulting exhaustion of coagulation factors and decreased platelet concentrations. In turn, this consumption of coagulation factors and platelets leads to bleeding. Disseminated intravascular coagulation often is life-threatening, and it is difficult to control. Effective control is not possible without determining what induced the DIC and then treating the underlying cause. During DIC, excessive activation of coagulation occurs, and whereas coagulation times initially may be shorter than normal, most animals present with clinical bleeding and prolonged coagulation times. Clear diagnostic parameters are not available to identify DIC, but many of the available tests have abnormal results in most patients with DIC. The aPTT commonly is prolonged, and other abnormalities include a prolonged PT, decreased fibrinogen concentration, decreased platelet concentration, presence of fragmented erythrocytes (i.e., schistocytes), and increased levels of FDPs. *Table 14.4* lists the frequency of coagulation abnormalities detected during DIC. No test directly evaluates increased coagulation, but an increased serum FDP concentration provides indirect evidence of increased intravascular coagulation. This is because plasmin simultaneously degrades

fibrin clots as they are being formed. Occasionally, FDP concentrations also are increased in patients with resolution of extensive hemorrhage into subcutaneous tissue or pleural or peritoneal spaces, such as might occur in patients with warfarin toxicosis.

Disseminated intravascular coagulation has been associated with many disease conditions, including a wide variety of neoplasms. Dogs with hemangiosarcoma often have associated DIC and thrombosis within the tumor mass. Some leukemias secrete procoagulant proteins that initiate DIC, and many other tumors are associated with DIC as well. Immune-mediated hemolytic anemia, incompatible blood transfusions, and endotoxin-related endothelial injury often initiate DIC. Physical and infectious causes of DIC include heat stroke, snake bite, pancreatitis, and infections with *Rickettsia rickettsii* and *Dirofilaria imitis.*

Hereditary Coagulopathies

Inherited coagulopathies and the domestic species in which they have been reported are summarized in Table 14.1. The most common hereditary coagulopathy in domestic animals is hemophilia A, which is a deficiency of coagulation factor VIII:C. Hemophilia A has been described in sheep, dogs, cats, and horses. This disorder is inherited in a recessive pattern, and the gene is located on the X chromosome. Hemophilia A often is confused with von Willebrand disease, because historically, both these conditions have been termed defects of factor VIII. Factor VIII:C and vWF circulate in plasma in close physical association with one another. Von Willebrand disease, which is the most common hereditary hemostatic defect in domestic animals, is strictly a defect of platelet function. Expected hematologic parameters in patients with hemophilia A and in patients with von Willebrand disease are given in *Table 14.5.* Whereas hemophilia A is a sex-linked trait and occurs more frequently in male patients, von Willebrand disease is an autosomally transmitted defect with an equal frequency of occurrence in male and female patients.

Other hereditary deficiencies of circulating coagulation factors are infrequent, but examples of all but factor XIII deficiency have been described at least once. Prekallikrein deficiency has been described in several dogs and horses with only mild bleeding tendencies. Deficiency of HMWK was suspected in one horse but was not proved. This horse did not have a bleeding tendency but did have a prolonged aPTT, a normal PT, and normal activity in plasma of other intrinsic coagulation factors. Factor XII deficiency has been described in cats and in dogs associated with prekallikrein deficiency or von Willebrand disease. Factor XII deficiency in cats and humans is not associated with bleeding, but in humans, it is associated with a ten-

TABLE 14.4 FREQUENCY OF ABNORMAL COAGULATION PARAMETERS DURING DISSEMINATED INTRAVASCULAR COAGULATION CAUSED BY A VARIETY OF DISEASES

Coagulation Parameter	Abnormality and % of Time Abnormal
Activated partial thromboplastin time	Prolonged, 87%
Antithrombin III activity	Decreased, 85%
Prothrombin time	Prolonged, 80%
Platelet numbers	Decreased, 80%
Fragmented red blood cells (schizocytes)	Increased, 71%
Fibrin(ogen) degradation products	Increased, 61%
Fibrinogen	Decreased, 61%
Plasminogen activity	Decreased, 49%
Factor 5 V activity	Decreased, 46%
Factor VIII:C activity	Decreased, 29%

From Feldman BF, Madewell BR, O'Neill S. Disseminated intravascular coagulation: antithrombin, plasminogen, and coagulation abnormalities in 41 dogs. J Am Vet Med Assoc 1981;179;151–154.

TABLE 14.5 EXPECTED COAGULATION PARAMETER RESULTS IN HEMOPHILIA A OR VON WILLEBRAND DISEASE

Test	Hemophilia A	von Willebrand Disease
Activated partial thromboplastin time	Prolonged	Normal to prolonged[a]
Prothrombin time	Normal	Normal
Activated coagulation time	Prolonged	Normal to prolonged
Bleeding time	Normal	Prolonged
Fibrinogen	Normal	Normal
Fibrin(ogen) degradation products	<10 µg/mL	<10 µg/mL
Platelet number	Normal	Normal
von Willebrand factor concentration	Normal	Decreased
Factor VIII:C activity	Decreased	Normal to decreased

[a] Some variable results (normal to decreased or normal to prolonged) reflect the physical relationship that factor VIII and von Willebrand factor have while cirulating in plasma together. Loss of von Willebrand factor may prolong the activated partial thromboplastin time, because factor VIII:C is not appropriately oriented physically but is present.

dency for thrombosis. Interestingly, factor 12 is not present in marine mammals, reptiles, or avian species. Factor XI deficiency has been described in cattle and dogs, with severe bleeding in Holstein cattle and milder bleeding tendencies in dogs. Factor IX deficiency (i.e., hemophilia B) has been demonstrated in dogs and cats and, like factor VIII:C, has a sex-linked inheritance pattern. Factor IX deficiency usually is associated with severe bleeding tendencies. Coagulation factors XII, XI, IX, VIII:C, HMWK, or prekallikrein deficiencies all produce a prolonged aPTT with a normal PT, regardless if these patients bleed clinically or not. Factor X deficiency has been described in dogs and cats with variable bleeding tendencies. Factor VII deficiency has been described in beagle dogs and usually is associated with mild clinical bleeding. These dogs have a prolonged PT and a normal aPTT or ACT. Factor II (i.e., thrombin) deficiency has been described in dogs. Fibrinogen deficiency has been described in dogs and goats and is associated with severe bleeding clinically. Animals with deficiencies of factor X, V, II, or fibrinogen have a prolonged PT, ACT, and aPTT. Animals with a deficiency of coagulation factor XIII deficiency do not have a prolonged aPTT or PT, because a stable fibrin clot is not necessary for these tests. Hereditary deficiencies of several coagulation factors simultaneously, because of several genetic defects, have been sporadically reported. In addition, hereditary deficiency of all vitamin K–dependent coagulation factors because of abnormal carboxylation has been reported in Devon Rex cats and Rambouillet sheep. *Figure 14.12* shows a simple algorithm to aid in establishing the diagnosis of common hereditary deficiencies of coagulation factors.

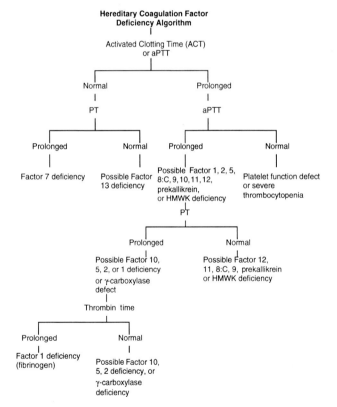

Figure 14.12 Specific coagulation factor deficiencies can be determined by mixing patient plasma with specific factor deficient plasma and then repeating the activated partial thromboplastin time (aPTT) or prothrombin time (PT). The factor-deficient plasma will correct the prolonged coagulation time for all deficiencies except the deficiency that is common to the patient's plasma and the specific factor-deficient plasma. The only exception is factor XIII deficiency, in which a clot urea solubility evaluation is done to determine if factor XIII is active.

Acquired Coagulopathies

A relatively common cause of acquired coagulopathy in both large and small animals is exposure to vitamin K antagonists that inhibit reduction of oxidized vitamin K back to the active hydroquinone form. Antagonists of vitamin K reduction include coumarin from moldy sweet clover, sulfaquinoxaline (a coccidiastat) that is added to water, and some rodenticides. Rodenticides containing indanedione-type active ingredients have a half-life of 15 to 20 days in the body, whereas warfarin-type rodenticides have a half-life of only 40 hours. Administration of vitamin K allows vitamin K epoxide to be reduced back to the active form through a second pathway, which operates at a much higher concentration of vitamin K than usually is present *(Fig. 14.13)*. Low availability of vitamin K also is associated with obstructive hepatopathy (i.e., lack of bile for absorption of vitamin K), malabsorption syndromes with an inability to absorb lipids, and low dietary levels of vitamin K. In small animals, administration of antibiotics that inhibit production of vitamin K by gut flora may result in deficiency. Severe liver disease commonly results in an acquired coagulopathy. Most coagulation factors are produced by hepatocytes; moreover, the liver is responsible for the removal of activated coagulation factors and FDPs from plasma.

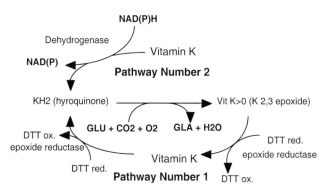

Figure 14.13 This figure depicts the two pathways that mediate the formation of reduced vitamin K_1H_2 (hydroquinone). Pathway number 1 is the physiologic pathway that is normally operative and cycles oxidized vitamin K_1 to the reduced form, but epoxide reductase can be inhibited by warfarin or newly manufactured long-acting antagonists. Pathway 2 is insensitive to warfarin, but requires supraphysiologic concentrations of vitamin K_1 for activity. Therapeutic administration of vitamin K_1 to a warfarin-poisoned patient uses this pathway, but administered vitamin K_1 is exhausted as it is reduced then subsequently oxidixed with accumulation of vatamin K_1 2,3 epoxide in the plasma and liver. Repeated administration of vitamin K1 is required as oxidized vitamin K_1 (2,3 epoxide) is not reduced by pathway 2. DTT = Dithiothreitol, a proposed electro donor, but other molecular species may be the actual electron donor. GLU = glutamic acid in the peptide sequence of the coagulation factor or anticoagulant protein, GLA = gamma-carboxyglutamic acid that has been transformed in the peptide sequence.

Uncommon causes of acquired coagulopathy include amyloidosis, which is associated with selective factor X deficiency because this factor is incorporated in the amyloid matrix, thereby depleting plasma factor X. Autoimmune disease, with an autoantibody directed against a coagulation factor, also has been described in domestic animals but occurs only rarely. *Figure 14.14* provides an algorithm to aid in establishing the diagnosis of acquired abnormalities and other defects of hemostasis that result in clinical bleeding.

Thrombocytopenia

Numerous conditions may cause decreased platelet production (see Chapter 13). Whole-body irradiation, drugs, toxins, infectious agents, neoplastic processes, or immune-mediated disorders may result in decreased production of platelets. Estrogen toxicosis is a common cause of decreased production in dogs and ferrets.

Increased platelet consumption is associated with DIC (discussed earlier), hemangiosarcoma in dogs, vasculitis, and other types of vascular injury. Blood loss does not result in significant thrombocytopenia; the platelet concentration rarely is less than 100,000 platelets/μL secondary to hemorrhage.

Increased platelet destruction commonly results from increased phagocytosis of platelets secondary to an overly active monocyte-macrophage system or immune-mediated mechanisms. Immune-mediated thrombocytopenia, which historically was referred to as idiopathic thrombocytopenia purpura, is one of the most common causes of thrombocytopenia in dogs. Antibodies may be directed specifically against platelet epitopes or may be against antigen (e.g., drugs or infectious agents)–antibody complexes absorbed to platelets. Administration of intravenous heparin may induce mild thrombocytopenia in some horses, and heparin overdose may result in severe thrombocytopenia in cats. Heparin-induced thrombocytopenia is thought to be immune-mediated in humans secondary to antibodies directed against a heparin–platelet component complex. Recently, better methods to determine if autoantibodies are present on the surface of platelets have been developed. These methods are either indirect (examining plasma) or direct (examining) patient platelets for the presence of autoantibodies. Direct methods are more sensitive but have less flexibility regarding both time and handling.

The most common infectious cause of thrombocytopenia in dogs is ehrlichiosis. Infection with *Ehrlichia canis* and, less commonly, *E. platys*, *E. ewingii*, and *E. equis* cause thrombocytopenia *(Figs. 14.15 through 14.17)*. *Ehrlichia canis* is thought to initially cause platelet destruction by immune-mediated mechanisms. Then, late in the disease, the agent causes bone marrow aplasia, with a subsequent decrease in platelet production. The marrow aplasia also may be immune-mediated.

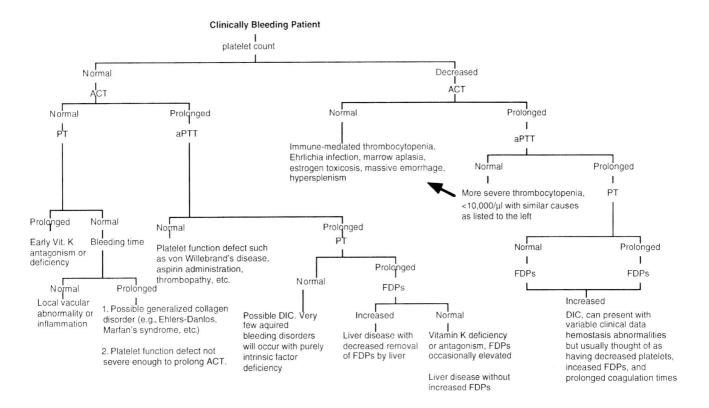

Figure 14.14 This algorithm provides a general guide for a diagnostic approach in clinical practice when presented with a bleeding patient, progressing from tests that can be done in most clinical settings to those that are more difficult to perform. The final diagnosis for each of these disease conditions relies on additional serum biochemical, hematologic, physical, serologic, and tissue evaluations or other specialized tests. This list is not all-inclusive, but it does include the most common clinical diseases in practice. *aPTT*, activated partial thromboplastin time; *FDP*, fibrinogen degradation products; *PT*, prothrombin time.

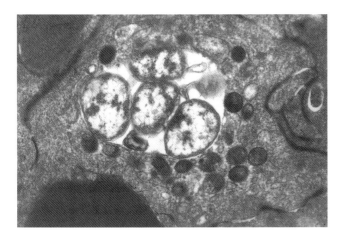

Figure 14.15 Transmission-electron micrograph of a platelet with a morula of *Ehrlichia platys*. The elementary bodies are surrounded and held together by another membrane.

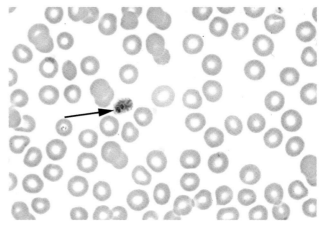

Figure 14.16 Wright-stained blood film from a dog with two *Ehrlichia platys* morulas in a platelet. (High magnification)

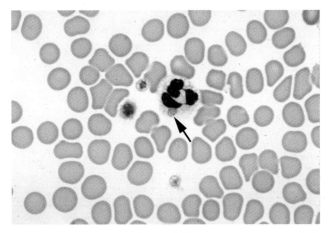

Figure 14.17 Peripheral blood film containing neutrophils with morula of *Ehrlichia ewingii* that appears identical to the *Ehrlichia equis* that may appear in the cytoplasm of neutrophils. (High magnification)

Defects of Platelet Function

Acquired

Platelet function can be inhibited by most nonsteroidal anti-inflammatory drugs, abnormal plasma proteins (myeloma paraproteins), proteins such as FDPs, autoantibodies that inhibit platelet function, phenothiazine tranquilizers, or plasma waste products that accumulate in patients with uremia.

Hereditary

Platelets may not function because of hereditary defects, such as von Willebrand disease, or various thrombasthenias (i.e., poor adhesion of platelets to one another) or thrombopathies (i.e., defective function of platelets) de-

scribed in domestic as well as laboratory animals with associated defects of platelet components or proteins important to platelet function. *Table 14.6* provides several specific examples of hereditary platelet defects that have been described. The most common hereditary platelet defect in domestic animals is von Willebrand disease.

Von Willebrand disease is associated with the lack of vWF, a glycoprotein that is synthesized and secreted by endothelial cells and megakaryocytes. Von Willebrand factor circulates in close physical association with factor VIII:C, and it is a heterogeneous glycoprotein of various-sized multimers of an identical 270-kDa polypeptide subunit linked to each other by disulfide bonds. Plasma concentrations of vWF can be measured by immunologic methods. Laurell rocket immunoelectrophoresis has been used in the past, and enzyme-linked immunosorbent assay has been used recently. Results usually are reported as a percentage of normal pooled plasma. Circulating multimers can be separated by sodium dodecyl sulfate–agarose electrophoresis and visualized with labeled antibody after electroblotting *(Fig. 14.18)*. These multimers range in size from 500 to 10^4 kDa. The higher-molecular-weight multimers are most effective in mediating platelet adherence and aggregation. Von Willebrand factor binds to surface glycoprotein 1b of platelets and also to IIb/IIIa that usually binds fibrinogen. If the level of vWF is deficient or the vWF itself is defective, platelets are not activated, because they do not recognize and respond to collagen in the basement membranes or extravascular tissue. Release of vWF can be stimulated by 1-desamino-8-D-arginine vasopressin (DDAVP) administration.

There are three types of von Willebrand disease. Type I has a decreased level of vWF:Ag (antigen), with levels of all plasma multimers decreased as well. This group includes the Welsh corgi (percentage of breed population

TABLE 14.6   HEREDITARY PLATELET FUNCTION DEFECTS IN DOMESTIC AND LABORATORY ANIMALS

Species/Breed Affected	Type of Defect
Basset hound, Spitz, Otterhounds, Great Pyrenees (Thrombasthenia)	α_{IIB} or β_3 surface membrane defect, with altered fibrinogen binding
Rats, mice	Various additional storage pool defects of α or δ granules in platelets
Chédiak-Higashi syndrome (cattle, cats, whales, beige mice, mink)	Storage pool granule defect
Simmental cattle	Cytoskeletal assembly
Fawn-hooded rats	Serotonin release
Pale ear mouse	Mouse counterpart to Hermansky-Pudlak syndrome (δ-granule defect)
Dogs	Arachidonate insensitivity
Cocker Spaniels	δ-Granule storage pool disease

Lanes

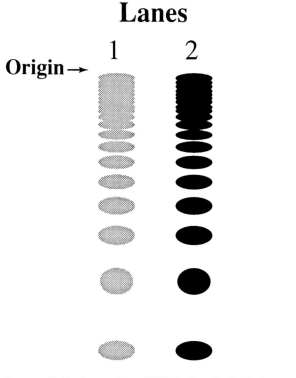

Low Molecular Weight Multimers

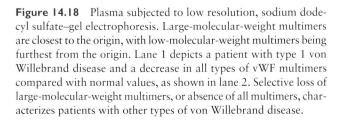

Figure 14.18 Plasma subjected to low resolution, sodium dode-cyl sulfate–gel electrophoresis. Large-molecular-weight multimers are closest to the origin, with low-molecular-weight multimers being furthest from the origin. Lane 1 depicts a patient with type 1 von Willebrand disease and a decrease in all types of vWF multimers compared with normal values, as shown in lane 2. Selective loss of large-molecular-weight multimers, or absence of all multimers, characterizes patients with other types of von Willebrand disease.

affected or carriers, 43%), Doberman pinscher (73%), German shepherd (35%), golden retriever (30%), and poodle (30%). Type I appears to have an autosomal dominant pattern with incomplete penetrance. Type II animals have decreased levels of vWF:Ag, with a disproportionate decrease in the level of high-molecular-weight multimers. The German shorthair pointer dog is a notable member in this category. The inheritance pattern is unknown. Type III animals have undetectable levels of vWF:Ag. The Scottish terrier (30%), Chesapeake Bay retrievers, and Shetland sheepdog (23%) are of this type. The inheritance pattern appears to be homozygous recessive in Scottish terriers and Chesapeake Bay retrievers and autosomal dominant trait with incomplete penetrance in Shetland sheepdogs. Von Willebrand disease has also been identified in rabbits, cats, horses, and swine. Ac-

quired causes of the disease in dogs are in dispute, but such causes do occur in humans.

Vascular Causes of Bleeding

Acquired

Injury to the endothelium, as occurs with Rocky Mountain spotted fever or heat stroke, may cause widespread coagulation. Acquired collagen disorders such as scurvy may be associated with bleeding because of the increased fragility of vessel walls. Localized inflammatory disease may be associated with hemorrhage. If recurrent localized hemorrhage is detected but a defect in either platelets or coagulation factors is not apparent, then a biopsy may be helpful in determining the cause of hemorrhage.

Hereditary

Hereditary collagen disorders, such as Ehlers-Danlos syndrome and Marfan syndrome, as well as acquired collagen disorders, such as scurvy and Cushing syndrome, have been associated with clinical bleeding. In part, bleeding results from increased vascular fragility caused by defective or decreased collagen, and in some cases, it is thought to be caused, again in part, by decreased platelet responsiveness to abnormal collagen.

Thrombosis

Thrombosis can be life-threatening, and it is a common ultimate cause of death in a wide variety of clinical diseases involving altered blood flow, endothelial injury, or hypercoagulable conditions. Clinical thrombosis is especially common in some specific clinical diseases.

Decreased circulating anticoagulant protein, notably AT-III, occurs in animals with nephrotic syndrome, because AT-III is a small-molecular-weight protein that is lost in the glomerular ultrafiltrate. Decreased levels of AT-III also occur in response to some drugs, such as asparaginase, a chemotherapeutic drug used in patients with lymphosarcoma. Increased concentrations of coagulation factors make blood hypercoagulable, and thrombosis may occur during late pregnancy after the administration of growth hormone implants or of some drugs, such as asparaginase. Cushing disease is associated with thrombosis, but the pathophysiology in dogs is unknown. Localized thrombosis can result from turbulent or misdirected blood flow, and generalized thrombosis can result from widespread vascular injury caused by chemicals, endotoxin, immunologic mechanisms, or infectious agents, such as infectious canine hepatitis virus or *Rickettsia rickettsii*.

CONCLUSION

Effective hemostasis is the product of coagulation factors, platelets, and vessels working in concert to cease the flow of blood from an injured vessel and allow healing and repair to occur, with re-establishment of blood flow to the tissues. Defects in any component of this delicate balance may result in excessive hemostasis (i.e., thrombosis) or inadequate hemostasis (i.e., bleeding). The challenge in each clinical case is to logically consider the possible causes and to fully evaluate them. Each clinical case should have at least an aPTT or ACT, a PT, a platelet count, and possibly, a bleeding time done to evaluate commonly encountered disturbances of hemostasis. Additional clinical evaluations are determined by the results of these tests and their relationship to the results of a thorough physical examination.

SUGGESTED READINGS

Bick RL. Coagulation abnormalities in malignancy: a review. Semin Thromb Hemost 1992;18:353–372.

Boudreaux MX. Platelets and coagulation: an update. Vet Clin North Am Small Anim Pract 1996;26:1065–1087.

Furie B, Furie BC. Molecular and cellular biology of blood coagulation. N Engl J Med 1992;326:800–806.

Jain N. Essentials of veterinary hematology. Philadelphia: Lea & Febiger, 1993.

Lassen ED, Swardson CJ. Hemostasis in the horse: normal functions and common abnormalities. Vet Clin North Am Equine Pract 1995; 11:351–389.

Loscalzo J, Schafer A. Thrombosis and hemorrhage. Cambridge, MA: Blackwell Scientific Publications, 1994.

Stamatoyannopoulos G, Nienhuis AW, Majerus PW, Varmus H, eds. The molecular basis of blood diseases. Philadelphia: WB Saunders, 1994:565–785.

Thomas JS. Von Willerband's disease in the dog and cat. Vet Clin North Am Small Anim Pract 1996;26:1089–1109.

Zwaal RFA. Coagulation and lipids. Boca Raton, FL: CRC Press, 1989.

APPENDIX 14.1

Minimum Laboratory Information Base to Evaluate a Patient with a Hemostatic Defect

1. Activated clotting time or activated partial thromboplastin time.
2. Prothrombin time.
3. Platelet count.
4. Bleeding time (possibly).

Other tests of hemostats are indicated by the results of these preliminary examinations.

Laboratory Methods in Clinical Practice

Bleeding Time

Method. Cause a reproducible wound (#11 BP blade, fixed to penetrate ⅛–¼ inch, or commercial product that creates a small wound 1 mm in depth) on a smooth, non-haired portion of the skin (e.g., gingiva, nasal planum, umbilicus, upturned lips held in place by a gauze tied around the muzzle, and so on). Next, gently remove beads of blood from wound margins, not touching the wound itself, with filter paper at 30-second intervals, and then record the time taken to stop bleeding.

Principle. Initial hemostasis reflects platelet function and numbers. May have rebleed phenomenon if fibrin clot does not adequately form after the initial cessation of bleeding, and this may be the result of coagulation factor deficiency.

Reference Range. 1–5 minutes

Note. The results of this test can be influenced by certain nonsteroidal anti-inflammatory drugs and by some sedatives or analgesics.

Activated Clotting Time (ACT)

Method. Draw 2 mL of venous blood into a prewarmed (37°C) Vacutainer tube (Becton-Dickinson, Franklin Lakes, NJ) containing sterile, diatomaceous earth. Begin timing with a stopwatch when blood first enters the tube. Invert the tube five times to mix, and then place it in 37°C heating block, removing it every 5 to 10 seconds after 1 minute of incubation to check for the first soft clot formation.

Principle. Contact activation proteins are fully activated when blood enters the tube. The time to clot formation depends on adequate mixing and activation, temperature, coagulation factor concentrations, and platelet numbers as well as function. Prolonged times suggest intrinsic or common pathway factor deficiencies. Platelet numbers must be very low to prolonged the ACT (<10,000 cells/mL). The ACT does not evaluate factor VII, and it generally does not evaluate platelets.

Reference Range

Dogs	79 ± 7.1 seconds
Horses	163 ±18 seconds
Cows	145 ±18 seconds

Note. Salicylates, anticoagulants, some antibiotics, and barbiturates can inhibit clot formation.

Activated Partial Thromboplastin Time (aPTT)

Method. Blood is collected from a vein nontraumatically into 3.8% sodium citrate anticoagulant in a blood:anticoagulant ratio of 9:1. Plasma is harvested by centrifugation and mixed with a platelet substitute, phospholipid (ether extract of brain); an activator such as kaolin, diatomaceous silica, or ellagic acid; and calcium. A pooled plasma sample is run as a control, samples are done in duplicate, and an average time is reported. Electrical impedance or optical end-point systems are used to detect fibrin clot formation. Factor XIII activity is not evaluated with this test, because only a loose, noncovalently linked clot is necessary for initiating an end point by optical, impedance, or manual methods.

Principle. Contact activator proteins are fully activated, and platelets are replaced by phospholipid. Normal time reflects adequate levels of intrinsic and common pathway factors.

Reference Range

Dogs	9–11 seconds
Cats	10–15 seconds
Horse	25–45 seconds

Note. Several types of contact activators are used commercially for the aPTT, and each activator has an associated normal reference range for a given species. The laboratory performing the test should provide a reference range for different species. Circulating anticoagulants (heparin, fibrinogen degradation products, autoantibodies) inhibit reaction. Mix equal volumes of normal plasma and patient plasma, and repeat the test. If the time corrects, there was a deficiency, not an anticoagulant, that caused the prolonged time. Nontraumatic venipuncture is very important, because release of tissue thromboplastin shortens most coagulation times. One or more factors must be decreased by 70 to 80% before significant prolongation occurs in the coagulation times (aPTT, ACT or PT) *(Fig. 14.19).*

Prothrombin time (PT)

Method. Blood is collected using the same method as that described for an aPTT, and plasma is harvested. Plasma is mixed with tissue thromboplastin (rabbit brain tissue thromboplastin) and calcium. The time to clot formation depends on the presence of factor VII and common pathway factors. Electrical impedance or optical end-point systems are used to detect fibrin clot formation. Factor XIII activity is not evaluated with this test, because only a loose, noncovalently linked clot is necessary for initiating an end point by optical, impedance, or manual methods.

Principle. Factor III is supplied with a platelet substitute, and normal time reflects adequate levels of factor VII and common pathway factors.

Reference Range

Dogs	6.4–7.4 seconds
Cats	7–11.5 seconds
Horses	9.5–11.5 seconds

Note. The aPTT and PT can be done in a local hospital, but plasma is best transported on ice. There should not be a long delay between collection and testing.

Fibrinogen Concentration

Method. Methods include heat precipitation (using a refractometer and heating plasma to 56°C–58°C for 3 minutes from blood collected with ethylenediaminetetraacetic acid [EDTA]), modified thrombin time, and immunologic methods. Heat precipitation is the least accurate when fibrinogen concentrations are low but the most accurate when fibrinogen is high. Modified thrombin time is most accurate if no dysfibrinogenemia is present. Immunologic methods do not require normal function of fibrinogen, which is the most abundant coagulation factor in plasma.

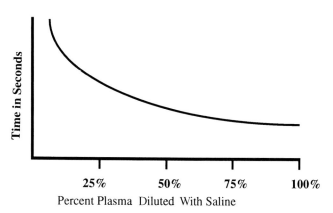

Figure 14.19 The approximate change in activated partial thromboplastin time (aPTT) or prothrombin time (PT) with serial dilutions of normal plasma using saline. A more than approximately 70% loss of plasma coagulation factor activity is associated with a marked change in coagulation time.

Reference Range

Dogs, sheep, and pigs	0.1–0.5 g/dL
Cats	0.05–0.3 g/dL
Cows	0.2–0.7 g/dL
Horses and goats	0.1–0.4 g/dL.

Note. Concentrations may be increased during inflammation or decreased when consumed during coagulation (e.g., disseminated intravascular coagulation).

Platelet Enumeration

Method. Methods include use of a hemocytometer and automated platelet enumeration by particle counters. Blood must be collected in EDTA using nontraumatic venipuncture, because trauma activates platelets and causes clumping. Feline platelets clump readily. If clumping is noted, then the platelet count is factitiously decreased. Platelets can be estimated when looking at a blood film. Less than three platelets per oil immersion field suggest the platelet count is 50,000 platelets/µL or less if platelet clumping is not noted in the feathered edge of the smear.

Reference Range

Dogs	200,000–500,000 platelets/µL
Cats	200,000–500,000 platelets/µL
Horses	100,000–600,000 platelets/µL
Cows	200,000–800,000 platelets/µL

Note. This test should include examination of bone marrow to evaluate platelet production and of blood film platelet morphology when evaluating circulating platelet numbers. Younger platelets are larger when viewed on peripheral blood films.

Fibrin(ogen) Degradation Products (FDPs)

Method. The most common method is to use the Thrombo Wellco Kit from Murex Diagnostics, Inc. (Norcross, GA). Immunoglobulin-coated latex beads that detect fragments D and E of fibrin or fibrinogen are mixed with diluted serum that has had an inhibitor of plasmin added. The beads agglutinate if sufficient D and E fragments are present. Results are reported as greater than 10 mg/mL or greater than 40 mg/mL. Other methods include FDP clumping of Staph A protein (Sigma Chemical Co., St. Louis, MO) and hemagglutination inhibition assay. This test is available in most laboratories and can be purchased by practitioners.

Principle. Activation of the contact activation system also activates plasmin. Fibrinogen and fibrin forming in a clot are broken down by plasmin, and the fragments circulate in the peripheral blood. Microvascular injury and repair are constantly occurring against a background of FDPs being produced (usually <10 mg/mL). Concentrations of FDPs increase with increased coagulation (as in disseminated intravascular coagulation).

Note. The FDPs inhibit thrombin and platelet function by competing with fibrinogen for binding sites, but they lack the structure to form cross-links or a fibrin meshwork.

Reference Range. Most animals have FDP levels of less than 10 mg/mL.

15

PRINCIPLES OF BLOOD TRANSFUSION AND CROSS-MATCHING

DIANE BROWN AND LINDA VAP

BLOOD GROUPS (BLOOD TYPES)

Blood groups or types are classifications made on the basis of species-specific antigens on the surface of erythrocytes. Erythrocyte antigens also may be present on platelets, on leukocytes, and in body tissues and fluids. Alloantibodies are naturally occurring antibodies against another blood type that are present in an animal's plasma even though that animal has not been exposed to those erythrocyte antigens. More commonly, antibodies against erythrocyte antigens are produced in response to exposure, either via blood transfusion or transplacentally. Blood groups in the common domestic species are described here.

Dog

The dog erythrocyte antigen groups or blood types are known as the DEA system. The dog has eight standard blood types: DEAs 1.1 and 1.2, and DEAs 3–8. The clinically important types are DEAs 1.1 and 1.2, which comprise approximately 60% of the canine population. In addition, DEA 7 may elicit an antibody response in dogs that lack it. Dogs with DEA 1.1 or 1.2 are called group A positive, whereas dogs with neither are called group A negative. Dogs do not have naturally occurring alloantibodies to DEA 1.1 or 1.2. In other words, dogs that are group A negative do not have naturally occurring antibodies against group A antigens, but antibodies can develop after exposure to group A–positive blood. The strongest antigen in the dog is DEA 1.1.

Cat

Three blood types are recognized in the feline AB blood group system. Type A is the most common and is estimated to be found in most (>95%) of domestic shorthair (DSH)/domestic longhair (DLH) cats in the United States. Type B occurs with varied frequency among certain breeds but, to date, has not been found in the Siamese, Burmese, Tonkinese, or Russian Blue breeds. A relatively high frequency (5%–25%) of type B has been reported in the Abyssinian, Birman, Himalayan, Scottish Fold, Somali, Maine Coon, Norwegian Forest, and Persian cat, whereas the highest frequency (25%–50%) has been reported in the British shorthair, Cornish Rex, and Devon Rex breeds. A higher percentage of DSH/DLH cats in the West Coast region of the United States, Europe, Japan, and Australia are reportedly type B. Type AB is extremely rare, however, and has been detected only among breeds in which type B also occurs. Type AB has been reported in DSH/DLH cats and in certain families of breeds among which type B blood also occurs, including the Abyssinian, Birman, British shorthair, Norwegian Forest, Somali, and Scottish fold, and Persian.

Cats have naturally occurring alloantibodies, with the exception of type AB cats, which have none. All type B cats have high serum concentrations of alloantibodies, which are strong hemagglutinins and hemolysins against type A erythrocytes. Type A cats have weak hemagglutinins and hemolysins. Newborn kittens have no alloantibodies because of their endotheliochorial placenta, but colostral transfer of immunoglobulin (Ig) G and, to a lesser extent, IgM occurs. Neonatal isoerythrolysis occurs in cats and is one cause of the fading kitten syndrome. Kittens at risk include those that are type A or AB and those that are born to type B queens. Because DSH/DLH cats have a low frequency of type B blood, less than 2% of random matings produce litters at risk for neonatal isoerythrolysis, whereas Birman and Devon Rex matings carry a risk of 15% and 25%, respectively, for producing neonatal isoerythrolysis.

Horse and Donkey

Seven blood groups/types (i.e., A, C, D, K, P, Q, U), which include 32 antigens, have been defined in the horse. Because of various antigenic combinations, approximately 400,000 equine blood types are possible, and no "universal donor" exists. Aa and Qa alloantigens are extremely immunogenic, and most cases of neonatal isoerythrolysis are associated with anti-Aa or -Qa antibodies. A donkey RBC antigen has been identified that has not been found in the horse; it is unique to the donkey and the mule. A mating between a donkey sire with this antigen and a horse mare may produce a foal at risk for neonatal isoerythrolysis.

Cow

Eleven blood groups have been identified in cattle (i.e., A, F, J, L, M, Z, R', B, C, S, T), but groups B and J have the greatest clinical relevance. The B group is extremely complex, thereby making closely matched transfusions very difficult. The J antigen is a lipid that is found in body fluid and adsorbed to erythrocytes; it is not a true erythrocyte antigen. Newborn calves do not have the J antigen but usually acquire it during the first six months of life. Indi-

viduals vary regarding the amount of J antigen that is present, and some cattle may have anti-J antibodies and develop transfusion reactions when receiving with J-positive blood. Vaccinations of blood origin (some anaplasmosis and babesiosis vaccines) may sensitize cows to erythrocyte antigens, which could result in neonatal isoerythrolysis in subsequent calves.

Sheep and Goat

Seven blood groups have been identified in sheep (i.e., A, B, C, D, M, R, X). The B system in these animals is analogous to the B system in cattle, and the R system is similar to the J system in cattle (i.e., antigens are soluble and passively adsorbed to erythrocytes). The blood groups of the goat (i.e., A, B, C, M, J) are very similar to those of sheep. Many of the reagents used for blood typing of sheep also have been used to type goats.

TRANSFUSION THERAPY

General Principles of and Indications for Blood Transfusion

In general, blood transfusions should not be administered to animals without blood typing and/or cross-matching the recipient and donor to decrease the likelihood of a transfusion reaction. In addition, the shortened survival of mismatched transfused cells results in ineffective therapy. Cross-matching and/or blood typing is particularly important in breeding females to avoid primary sensitization and risk of future offspring developing hemolytic disease. General guidelines and information related to transfusion medicine are summarized in *Table 15.1*; the reader is referred to the text for background and explanation. Blood typing for canine DEA 1.1 and for feline types A and B is feasible in the general veterinary practice. More extensive typing is available through universities and/or reference laboratories. Cross-matching, however, is a more practical procedure.

Blood transfusions are not without risk; therefore, they should be performed only when warranted. Clients should be questioned regarding any history of previous transfusion therapy, because a history of previous transfusion therapy warrants cross-matching. Whole-blood or blood-component therapy may be administered depending on availability and indication for transfusion. Blood-component therapy in domestic animals has been reviewed elsewhere, but the primary indication for blood transfusion is the treatment of severe anemia caused by hemorrhage, hemolysis, ineffective erythropoiesis, autoimmune hemolytic anemia, or neoplasia. Animals must be clinically evaluated on an individual basis. A rule of

TABLE 15.1 ANTIGENS AND PERTINENT FACTORS IN TRANSFUSION MEDICINE

Species	Major Immunogenic Antigens	Naturally Occurring Alloantibodies	Ideal Donor Type	First Tranfusion Risks and Recommendations	Compatible Transfused Cell Half-Life	Recommended Whole-Blood Dosage
Dog	DEA 1.1, 1.2 (Presence of either 1.1 or 1.2 also known as A positive)	Rare	DEA 1.1, 1.2 negative	Low without cross-match Use of ideal donor blood minimizes sensitization	21 days	20 mL/kg to increase HCT by 10 500-mL unit for large dogs
Cat	A most common B rare, except in certain breeds AB very rare	Common Anti-B, mild in type A cats Anti-A, strong in type B cats None in type AB cats	A in US for most breeds such as DSH/=DLH, Siamese No ideal donor for other breeds, especially Birman, British shorthair, Cornish, Devon Rex, Norwegian Forest, Somali, and Scottish Fold	For Siamese and most DSH/DLH: Low risk of tranfusion without typing or cross-match due to blood type A homogeneity Risk eliminated with blood typing or crossmatch Other Breeds: Risk increases considerably Use of type compatible or cross-matched blood is important due to B type incidence Type AB cats can safely receive A or B	29–39 days	20 mL/kg 60-mL syringe is a practical application vehicle
Horse	Complex system of 32 antigens in 7 blood groups	Occur Anti-Aa/Qa most important	None Aa/Qa negative are best starting choice	Should be cross-matched	2–6 days	Target of 20 mL/kg
	Donkey RBC antigen	Probably none		Donkey sire bred to horse mare, high risk for neonatal isoerythrolysis		
Cow	11 Blood groups B and J most important	Anti-J occasionally present in J-negative cattle	Not defined	Transfusions rarely performed in ruminants Cross-match recommended	2 days	Target of 20 mL/kg
Sheep and Goat	7 Blood groups Similar to cows B analogous to B and R analogous to J in cattle	Not characterized	Not defined	Transfusions rarely performed in ruminants Cross-match recommended	Unknown	Target of 20 mL/kg

DSH/DSL, domestic shorthair/domestic longhair; HCT, hematocrit.

199

thumb for the treatment of anemia is to transfuse when the hematocrit is less than 10% to 15%. Animals with acute-onset anemia, however, usually require transfusion before their hematocrit decreases to 15%, which contrasts with the situation in animals with chronic anemia. Additional indications for transfusion include hypovolemia, thrombocytopenia, clotting factor deficiency, and hypoproteinemia.

Donor Selection

Blood typing should be performed to select permanent blood donors. All donors should be healthy young adults that have never received a blood transfusion, undergo routine physical examinations as well as hematology and clinical chemistry evaluations, receive vaccinations, and are free of blood parasites and other infectious diseases. Female dog and cat donors should be nulliparous and spayed. Blood should be collected aseptically via jugular venipuncture. Donors should not be sedated with acepromazine, because it interferes with platelet function.

Dogs can donate between 13 and 17 mL of blood per kilogram of body weight every 3 to 4 weeks. Ideally, donors should be negative for antigens for DEAs 1.1, 1.2, 3, 5, and 7, greater than 25 kg, bled less than once per month to prevent iron deficiency, well nourished, and supplemented with oral iron. Donors should be negative for heartworm disease, babesiosis, brucellosis, ehrlichiosis, and Rocky Mountain spotted fever.

Donor cats can donate between 10 and 12 mL/kg. Healthy adult cats can donate 50 mL every 3 weeks. Donors should be type A, but depending on geography and breed prevalence, type B donors may be required. Donor cats should be negative for feline leukemia virus, feline immunodeficiency virus (FIV), feline infectious peritonitis, heartworm disease, and *Hemobartonella* sp.

Adult horses can safely donate approximately 6 to 8 L of blood. Whole blood can be taken every 2 to 4 weeks and plasma collected every week if the erythrocytes are returned to the donor. Donors should be negative for equine infectious anemia. Mares that have been pregnant or foaled and horses that have received blood or erythrocyte-contaminated plasma transfusions should be excluded as potential donors. A totally compatible blood transfusion is unlikely to be achieved in the horse. Thus, a donor that is genetically similar to the recipient is a natural choice, because erythrocyte alloantigen patterns generally are homologous within light horse breeds (e.g., Thoroughbreds). Aa and Qa alloantigens are extremely immunogenic; therefore, Aa- and Qa-negative donors that are free of plasma alloantibodies are the best choices as donors to recipients of unknown blood type.

Cattle can donate 8 to 14 mL/kg. Closely matched transfusions are very difficult in cattle.

Anticoagulants

Citrate-phosphate-dextrose-adenine (CPDA1) is the superior anticoagulant, because it maintains higher levels of 2,3-disphosphoglycerate (2,3-DPG) and adenosine triphosphate (ATP). Blood can be stored for 35 days in CPDA1. Acid-citrate-dextrose (ACD) allows storage of blood for 21 days. When using CPDA1 or ACD, use 1 mL of anticoagulant for every 7 mL of blood. Blood should be refrigerated in plastic blood bags. Heparin activates platelets and is not recommended for blood collection, but if heparin is used as the anticoagulant (625 U per 50 mL of blood), blood must be used immediately. Survival and functional usefulness of erythrocytes both decrease with increased storage temperature and storage because of glucose consumption and depletion of ATP and 2,3-DPG. To preserve platelets, blood should be collected into latex-free plastic bags or plastic syringes. Glass-bottle collection systems also are available for use; however, limitations include loss of platelets because of activation and inability to prepare components.

Administration

Blood should be filtered either before administration or as it is being given by using 170-μm pore, nonlatex filters if platelets are desired. To prevent hypothermia, blood should be warmed to not greater than 37°C before administration; higher temperatures cause lysis of erythrocytes and inactivation of clotting factors. Blood is administered intravenously through administration sets containing 0.9% saline. Lactated Ringer's solution, 5% dextrose in water, and hypotonic saline are contraindicated. Lactated Ringer's solution causes calcium chelation with citrate and subsequent clot formation. Dextrose-containing fluids cause swelling and lysis of erythrocytes, and hypotonic fluids lyse erythrocytes. Injection of undiluted citrate-containing anticoagulants may cause cardiac arrest.

Circulatory overload and heart failure can result from excessive and rapid injection of blood or plasma. Blood should be given intravenously at a rate not to exceed 10 mL/kg per hour; however, each patient must be assessed individually to establish an appropriate infusion rate. For example, hypovolemic patients may require an infusion rate of 20 mL/kg per hour, whereas patients with cardiac disease may require only 2 to 5 mL/kg per hour. If blood is administered too quickly, salivating, vomiting, and muscle fasciculations may occur. Transfusions should be completed within 4 hours to avoid contamination of warmed blood. The amount to be transfused is determined according to the patient's body weight, estimated blood volume, hematocrit of the recipient and of the donor, and the goal of therapy. A simple guideline is that 10 mL/kg of packed erythrocytes or 20 mL/kg of whole blood increases the hematocrit by 10% if the donor has a hematocrit of approximately 40%.

In dogs, the matched transfused erythrocyte half-life is approximately 21 days. In cats, the matched transfused erythrocyte half-life is approximately 34 days. The survival time of compatible transfused erythrocytes is only 2 to 6 days in horses and 2 days in cattle; therefore, blood transfusions should be reserved for life-threatening situations.

Preparations Used for Transfusions

Fresh whole blood is indicated for use in acute hemorrhage, anemia, coagulation disorders, and thrombocytopenia. Stored whole blood is indicated for use in anemia. Packed erythrocytes are recommended for anemic animals, particularly those with volume overload. These erythrocytes also may be washed with saline before administration to dilute any potentially harmful antibodies that may be present.

Uses for fresh-frozen or stored-frozen plasma include congenital or acquired deficiencies of coagulation factors and hypoproteinemia. Cryoprecipitated plasma is indicated for replacement of coagulation factors, but not for protein. Platelet-rich plasma is indicated for severe thrombocytopenia or thrombocytopathia.

Transfusion Reactions and Sequelae

Potential transfusion reactions may be acute or delayed. Acute intravascular hemolysis with hemoglobinemia and hemoglobinuria may be seen in animals receiving incompatible transfusions. Release of thromboplastic substances may lead to disseminated intravascular coagulopathy. Hypotension and shock secondary to the release of vasoactive substances, acute renal failure, and death also may occur. Delayed hemolysis is evidenced by a decrease in hematocrit between 2 days and 2 weeks after transfusion, and it occurs most commonly in previously transfused dogs with an antibody titer too low to detect by cross-matching. Usually, no hemoglobinemia or hemoglobinuria results; however, hyperbilirubinemia and bilirubinuria may result from extravascular hemolysis.

A first transfusion usually can be safely given to dogs without regard for donor blood type, because alloantibodies against the common canine erythrocyte antigens 1.1 and 1.2 do not exist. This may sensitize the recipient to immunogenic antigens such as 1.1, 1.2, 7, and others, however, and result in shortened survival times of the transfused cells on first transfusion and subsequent predisposition to severe transfusion reaction. The strongest antigen in dogs, DEA 1.1 elicits the most severe transfusion reaction.

In cats, AB-mismatched transfusions, whether initial or subsequent, may cause acute hemolytic incompatibility reactions. Because of alloantibodies, erythrocytes are destroyed immediately in cats; this contrasts with the situation in dogs, in which delayed transfusion reactions are more likely to occur. A type B transfusion to type A cat results in mild signs but also shortened erythrocyte survival, thus resulting in ineffective therapy. A type A transfusion to a type B cat results in an acute hemolytic transfusion reaction with massive intravascular hemolysis and serious clinical signs—even if it is the first transfusion. Type AB cats can safely receive type AB or A blood.

Neonatal isoerythrolysis is the destruction of erythrocytes in the circulation of offspring by alloantibodies of maternal origin that are absorbed from colostrum. Kittens at risk include those that are type A or AB and those that are born to type B queens. Nearly all cases in foals are caused by factor Aa in the A system and factor Qa in the Q system (acquired, not naturally occurring, alloantibodies). Signs usually develop 24 to 36 hours after suckling.

Complications that may be unrelated to erythrocyte antigen–antibody reactions include fever, allergic reactions, circulatory overload, citrate toxicosis, ammonia toxicosis, and infection. Fever is a common reaction to a blood transfusion, and it may occur in response to leukocyte or platelet antigens or to bacterial contamination of blood. Allergic reactions after transfusions are most commonly seen in the dog; sensitivity to plasma proteins generally is responsible. Circulatory overload is a potential sequela to whole-blood transfusion, particularly in patients with cardiovascular compromise. Citrate toxicity can result in acute decreases in the level of ionized serum calcium. Ammonia toxicity can occur with prolonged storage of blood, because the ammonia concentration increases over time. Patients with liver disease should be monitored closely for these latter two reactions. Infection is a potential risk of blood transfusion as a result of blood-borne parasites and viruses or contamination of stored blood. Proper health maintenance and screening of donors as well as proper handling and storage of blood help to minimize these risks.

CROSS-MATCHING BLOOD

General Principles

Cross-matching often is classified as either "major" or "minor" cross-matches. A major cross-match consists of adding patient serum to donor cells and following a specific protocol to determine the presence of agglutinating and/or hemolytic antibodies in the patient against the donor antigens. The presence of antibodies results in a positive in vitro reaction. A mild reaction may be seen 4 to 14 days after mismatched transfusions in patients that had no antibodies at the time of transfusion. A severe reaction occurs when blood is transfused to a patient in which antibodies are already present, whether naturally occurring or the result of a previous mismatched transfusion; moreover, isosensitization from transplacental immunization can result in high concentrations of antibodies. A cross-match should always be performed in dogs that have received previous transfusions.

A minor cross-match consists of adding donor serum to patient erythrocytes. If the donor has previously tested negative for antibodies, this step is unnecessary. Administration of antibodies in donor blood against patient erythrocytes may be avoided by transfusing packed or washed erythrocytes rather than whole blood.

An ethylenediaminetetraacetic acid (EDTA) tube and a clot tube from the recipient and each donor are preferred. If necessary, however, clotted samples may be used for the entire procedure. The EDTA plasma should not be used in place of serum, because this contributes to increased rouleaux formation and difficult interpretation of agglutination, particularly in the horse. Samples should be free of hemolysis and lipemia to aid in the interpretation of hemolytic reactions. The effects of hemolysis may be minimized by setting up a control tube with an equal number of drops of serum only to determine whether hemolysis is increased compared with the control. Specific procedures for cross-matching tests and blood typing are presented in Appendix 15.1.

ACKNOWLEDGMENT

The authors thank Dr. Kent Humber for his contributions to the large-animal sections of this chapter.

SUGGESTED READINGS

Bailey E, Conboy HS, McCarthy PF. Neonatal isoerythrolysis of foals: an update on testing. Proceedings of the Thirty-Third Annual Convention of the American Association of Equine Practitioners, New Orleans, Louisiana, November–December, 1987:341–353.

Bell K. The blood groups of domestic mammals. In: Agar NS, Board PG, eds. Red blood cells of domestic mammals. New York: Elsevier Science, 1983:133.

Giger U. The feline AB blood group system and incompatibility reactions. In: Kirk RW, ed. Current veterinary therapy XI. Philadelphia: WB Saunders, 1992:470–474.

Grigot-Wenk ME, Callan MB, Casal ML, et al. Blood type AB in the feline AB blood group system. Am J Vet Res 1996;57:1438–1442.

Hale AS. Canine blood groups and their importance in veterinary transfusion medicine. Vet Clin North Am Small Anim Pract. 1995;25:1323–1332.

Harrell K, Kristensen A, Parrow J. Canine transfusion reactions. Part I. causes and consequences. Compend Cont Educ 1997;19:181–190.

Harrell K, Kristensen A, Parrow J. Canine transfusion reactions. Part II. Prevention and treatment. Compend Cont Educ 1997;19:193–200.

Jain N. Hematologic techniques. In: Jain NC, ed. Schalm's veterinary hematology. Philadelphia: Lea & Febiger, 1986:71–74.

Jain NC. Immunohematology. In: Essentials of veterinary hematology. Philadelphia: Lea & Febiger, 1993:381–407.

Kristensen AT, Feldman BF. Blood banking and transfusion medicine. In: Ettinger SJ, Feldman EC, eds. Textbook of veterinary internal medicine. 4th ed. Philadelphia: WB Saunders, 1995:347–360.

McClure JJ, Parish SM. Diseases caused by allogeneic incompatibilities. In: Smith BP, ed. Large animal internal medicine. St. Louis: CV Mosby, 1990:1614–1625.

Stormont C, Suzuki Y, Rhode EA. Serology of horse blood groups. Cornell Vet 1964;54:439–452.

Traub-Dargatz JL, McClure JJ, Koch C, Schlipf JW. Neonatal isoerythrolysis in mule foals. J Am Vet Med Assoc 1995; 206:67–70.

Weiser MG. Principles of blood transfusion. In: Ettinger SJ, ed. Textbook of veterinary internal medicine. 3rd ed. Philadelphia: WB Saunders, 1989:2176–2180.

Williamson L. Blood and plasma therapy. In: Robinson NE, ed. Current therapy equine medicine III. Philadelphia: WB Saunders, 1992:517–520.

APPENDIX 15.1

Cross-Match Agglutination Test

The cross-match agglutination test is appropriate for dogs and cats, and it is used in conjunction with the lytic test for horses. The following procedure is modified from that described by Jain (see Suggested Readings):

1. Centrifuge clotted blood, and place serum into a prelabeled test tube.
2. Wash ethylenediaminetetraacetic acid (EDTA) anticoagulated erythrocytes by placing one or two drops of blood in a 12- × 75-mm, disposable glass test tube. Fill the tube with phosphate buffered saline (PBS). Mix, centrifuge for 1 minute at 3400 rpm, and then decant the supernatant. Repeat this procedure two additional times in most species and three additional times for horses.
3. After the final wash, make a 2% erythrocyte suspension of each specimen in PBS by adding 0.02 mL of packed, washed erythrocytes to 0.98 mL of PBS in a prelabeled test tube.
4. Place two drops of the recipient's serum and two drops of the donor's cell suspension in a 12- × 75-mm test tube and mix (i.e., major system). In a second tube, place two drops of the donor's serum and two drops of the recipient's erythrocyte suspension (i.e., minor system). To check for autoagglutination, set up controls

in the same manner by mixing the donor's erythrocytes with its own serum, and then follow the same procedure with the recipient's erythrocytes and serum.

5. Shake the rack of tubes, incubate for 30 minutes at room temperature, and then centrifuge for 1 minute at 3400 rpm.

6. Examine the supernatant for hemolysis. Shake the tubes gently by tapping with the finger to detect grossly visible agglutination of erythrocytes *(Figs. 15.1 and 15.2)*.

If no agglutination is observed, transfer a small amount to a glass slide and then examine under the low power of the microscope. Lower the condenser to increase the contrast. Erythrocytes are evenly dispersed *(Fig. 15.3)* if no agglutination is present. If present, agglutination appears as grape-like clusters of erythrocytes *(Fig. 15.4)*. *Rouleaux should not be confused with agglutination.* Rouleaux formation *(Fig. 15.5)* is common in horse blood, and it appears as stacks of coins.

Rouleaux and true agglutination may be further differentiated with the saline replacement procedure. First,

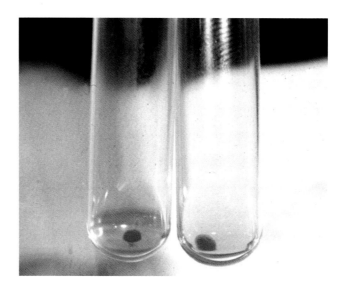

Figure 15.2 4+ Macroscopic agglutination. Note the tight button of cells. A reaction of this magnitude may be seen with a strong-reacting antibody, such as anti-A, which may be present in type B cats.

centrifuge the tube for 15 seconds, remove the serum by pipette and replace with two drops of PBS, mix, and then centrifuge at 3400 rpm for 15 seconds. Next, read for microscopic agglutination. Rouleaux should dissipate, whereas agglutination should remain.

Interpretation

Slight hemolysis in canine blood is nonspecific. Significant hemolysis and/or agglutination in one or both of the cross-matched tubes—but not in the controls—indicates an incompatibility and the need to select a new donor. In horses,

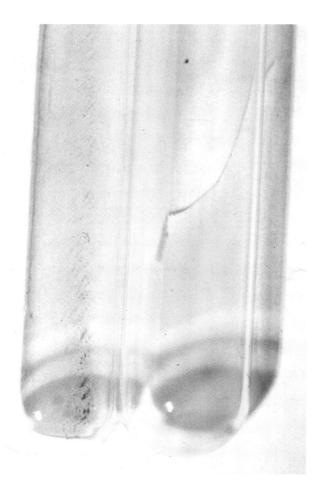

Figure 15.1 2+ Macroscopic agglutination *(left)* and negative control *(right)*.

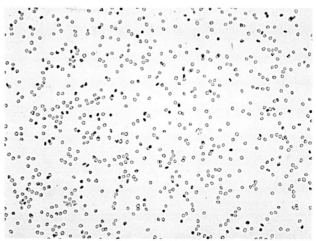

Figure 15.3 Negative microscopic agglutination. All the cells are evenly dispersed.

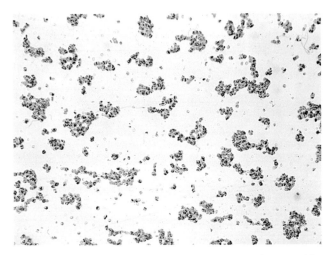

Figure 15.4 4+ Microscopic agglutination. Note the grape-like clusters. A microscopic reaction of this strength may be detectable macroscopically.

hemolysis in the agglutination test most likely indicates fragile or old cells rather than incompatibility. Therefore, hemolysis in horses should be ignored; however, if all cells are hemolyzed, then agglutination is impossible to detect. Positive control tubes indicate autoagglutination or contaminated reagents, thereby rendering positive cross-match tubes uninterpretable.

Cross-Match Hemolytic Test

The cross-match hemolytic test is required in cross-matching blood from sheep and cattle, because erythrocytes from these species tend not to agglutinate. Most equine isoantibodies act as hemolysins; thus, performing

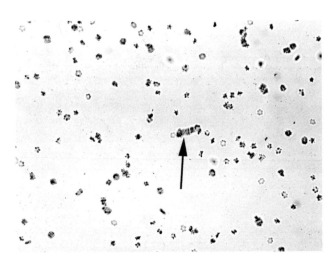

Figure 15.5 Rouleaux (coin-stacking phenomenon). This must not be confused with agglutination. It may indicate insufficient washing and commonly is seen with equine samples.

both the agglutination and hemolytic test in horses is prudent. In this test, fresh rabbit serum is used as the complement source. Because, however, all rabbits possess natural antibodies against horse erythrocytes, the antibodies must be removed before using the serum as a complement source.

Complement Absorption Procedure for Equine Cross-Match

Reagents

1. Lyophilized rabbit complement (Pel-Freez), store frozen.
2. $CaCL_2$-$MgCl_2$ solution, store refrigerated.
   a. $CaCL_2$, 14.7 g.
   b. $MgCl_2$, 20.35 g.
   c. Distilled H_2O, ≤1 L.
3. Na_2-EDTA solution.
   a. 74.4 g per 2 L of distilled H_2O.
   or
   b. Sequester-Sol (Baxter).
4. PBS (Sigma Diagnostics, catalog no. 1000-3), store refrigerated.
5. Normal horse erythrocytes. (Two lavender-top [EDTA], 10-mL tubes from one donor are adequate.)

Procedure of the University of California-Davis Veterinary Genetics Laboratory

1. Dilute each of three vials of thawed rabbit complement with 1 mL of distilled water.
2. Add 1 part EDTA (0.3 mL) to 10 parts (3 mL) complement.
3. Centrifuge the EDTA-anticoagulated whole blood, and remove the plasma. Wash two aliquots of horse erythrocytes three times with PBS. (Make enough for two absorptions.)
4. Add 1.1 mL of packed, washed horse erythrocytes to the complement solution. Incubate at room temperature for 30 minutes.
5. Harvest the complement solution, and repeat the absorption using fresh erythrocytes and incubating on ice instead of at room temperature for 30 minutes.
6. Centrifuge, collect absorbed rabbit complement (C′) into a flask on ice, and add 0.3 mL of $CaCL_2$-$MgCl_2$.
7. Aliquot the C′ in volumes of 0.5 mL in bullet tubes, and freeze at once. Label with the date and contents. Do not refreeze complement once thawed. (Do not store in a self-defrosting freezer, because the C′ thaws with each defrost cycle.)

Hemolytic Cross-Match Procedure

The following procedure is modified from that described by Jain:

1. Centrifuge the clotted samples, and place the serum into appropriately labeled tubes for the recipient and each donor.
2. Label the tubes for each cross-match and autocontrol. If the donor has not been previously screened for antibodies, a minor side cross-match also is performed using donor serum and recipient cells and following the procedure outlined below in steps 3–9.
3. Prepare 2% to 5% solutions of washed erythrocytes from the recipient and each donor as previously described, washing a total of four (instead of three) times.
4. Add two drops of serum to appropriately labeled tubes.
5. Add one drop of absorbed rabbit complement to the hemolytic phase cross-match and autocontrol tubes. Mix the tubes by gently shaking the rack. Complement is stored in the freezer. It must be thawed and used immediately; discard all unused portions.
6. Add one drop of the appropriate 2% to 5% washed erythrocyte suspension to the tubes.
7. Shake the rack to mix, and then place in a 37°C waterbath for 30 minutes.
8. Centrifuge the tubes at 3000 rpm (1000 g) for 15 seconds. Observe the supernatant in each tube for hemolysis; there is no need to check these tubes for agglutination.
9. Interpret and report the results.

The major cross-match is "incompatible" if the patient serum reacts with the donor's erythrocytes, and in this case, the donor blood should not be transfused. The minor cross-match is incompatible if the donor serum reacts with the recipient's erythrocytes. In this case, it should be reported as "minor-side incompatible" and only packed erythrocytes may be safely transfused.

A positive autocontrol indicates the presence of an autoantibody. It may induce uninterpretable results in the cross-match tubes.

Jaundice Foal Agglutination Test (Colostrum Cross-Match)

The jaundice foal agglutination test correlates highly with hemolytic blood group tests (performed by reference laboratories) at 1:16 dilutions. Lower dilutions have poorer correlations because of the viscosity of colostrum.

Materials

1. Centrifuge (300–600 g).
2. Test tube rack.
3. Disposable glass test tubes (12 × 75 mm).
4. Saline.
5. Colostrum (or serum) and EDTA whole blood from mare (erythrocytes teased from clotted blood may be used).

6. EDTA whole blood from foal (erythrocytes teased from clotted blood may be used).

Method

1. Label tubes for 1:2, 1:4, 1:8, 1:16, and 1:32 dilutions for the foal.
2. Add 1 mL of saline to all tubes.
3. Add 1 mL of colostrum to the tubes labeled as foal 1:2. Mix and remove 1 mL of the dilution and then add to the next consecutive tube. Repeat the procedure, discarding 1 mL from the 1:32 tube. Discard tube 8.
4. Add one drop of foal's whole blood to each tube and mix.
5. Centrifuge the tubes for 2 to 3 minutes at medium speed (300–600 g).
6. Invert the tubes and hold upside down, pouring out the liquid contents, and observe the status of the button of erythrocytes at the bottom of each tube. (It is easier to compare reactions if all four tubes are poured out at the same time.) Grade the agglutination as follows:

0	No agglutination	Cells flow easily down side of tube
1+	Weak agglutination	Cells in small clumps as they run down tube
2+	Strong agglutination	Cells in large clumps as they run down tube
3+	Complete agglutination	Cells remain tightly packed in a button

7. If no agglutination is present, report the test as being negative at all dilutions.
8. If agglutination is present, grade the reactions and continue with controls. (Controls may be set up along with the patient tubes during step one to save time.)

Controls

1. Foal auto control with 1 mL of saline and one drop of foal whole blood.
2. Mare colostrum/autocontrol, prepared by repeat steps 1 through 7 described earlier using colostrum and mare erythrocytes.

Interpretation

1. If all controls are negative, report the reactions of colostrum versus foal erythrocytes at all dilutions. A reaction at a dilution of 1:16 or greater is considered to be a high titer, and the colostrum should not be used.
2. A positive foal autocontrol indicates autoagglutination and the possibility that the foal has already nursed.
3. A positive mare colostrum/autocontrol indicates interference from the viscosity of the colostrum or a

technical problem. Reaction grades for the same dilu-tion should be compared between the mare auto-control and the foal cross-match tubes.

Typing Blood

Reagents and equipment described here are those used by the Colorado State University Veterinary Teaching Hospital.

Card Method

A simple, rapid method of blood typing cats and dogs is available in card form from **dms**laboratories (Flemington, NJ; 1-800-567-4367). One drop of buffered saline (pro-vided) is added to the reagent dried on the card, and one drop of EDTA-anticoagulated whole blood is added and mixed by rotating the card. The presence of macroscopic agglutination *(Fig. 15.6)* indicates which blood type is present. The entire procedure requires less than 5 minutes. The reagents, however, may deteriorate over time; there-fore, testing control samples with each patient sample is strongly recommended. Controls are included in the kit.

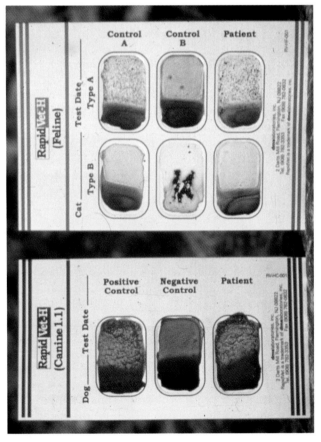

Figure 15.6   Canine and feline blood-typing cards. (Courtesy of **dms**laboratories.)

The feline card differentiates blood type A and B in cats. The canine card indicates the presence or absence of DEA 1.1 only. Therefore, the canine card should be used only as a screen for typing potential donors, because DEA 1.2 and 7 are not be detected. Donors typed as being A negative with the card should be further tested with DEA 1.2– and 7–specific antisera. The card is ade-quate for patient testing provided that all donors are known to be negative for DEA 1.1 and DEA 1.2.

Tube Method

The tube method is used to test dogs for blood types DEA 1.1 and 1.2 (DEA 1.1,2). Use of EDTA-anticoagu-lated whole blood is preferred, but clotted blood also can be used. The specimen should be fresh and free of he-molysis. Add four or five drops of blood from the EDTA tube or clotted blood to a 12- × 75-mm glass tube con-taining 0.9% PBS. Remove any clumps of cells with a wooden applicator stick if using a clotted sample. Centri-fuge at 3400 rpm (Sero-fuge II, Clay-Adams/Becton-Dickinson, Sparks, MD) for 1 minute, and then decant the PBS. Wash two more times by adding PBS, mixing, cen-trifuging, and decanting. After the last wash, add enough PBS to make an approximately 4% suspension of ery-throcytes. This suspension has the appearance of tomato juice, and it must have adequate erythrocytes to go through an additional set of washes at a later time.

Reagents required include DEA 1.1,2 antiserum (Mid-west Animal Blood Services, Stockbridge, MI; 517-851-8244). Store the antisera frozen in aliquots large enough to accommodate patient and control testing, but do not refreeze.

Procedure

1. For each sample to be tested, label two 12- × 75-mm, disposable glass tubes with the name or number. Label one tube "C" for Control and one tube "D" for DEA 1.1,2.
2. Add two drops of the 4% suspension of washed eryth-rocytes to each tube.
3. Add two drops of 0.9% PBS to the control tube.
4. Add two drops of DEA 1.1,2 antiserum to the DEA 1.1,2 tube.
5. Swirl the tubes to mix, and then incubate at 37°C for 15 minutes.
6. Centrifuge the tubes at 3400 rpm for 15 seconds (Sero-fuge II).

Read for hemolysis by observing the supernatant. Gently rock the tubes, and read for macroscopic and microscopic agglutination.

Interpretation.   Any blood that is positive for hemolysis and/or agglutination in the DEA 1.1,2 tube is type A positive—as long as the control tube is negative–and is *not* a universal blood donor. No further testing is necessary. A positive control tube suggests autoagglutination, which negates the interpretation of positive results in the DEA 1.1,2 tube. Any blood that is negative in both tubes for hemolysis and/or agglutination *must* be tested with Coombs' serum for incomplete antibodies using the same tubes (as described in the following section).

**Coombs Reaction to Detect
False-Negative Types**

The reagent required is Canine Coombs' Serum (VMRD, Pullman, WA), stored refrigerated.

Procedure

1. Wash the cells in both the "D" and "C" tubes three additional times with 0.9% PBS. Spin for 2 minutes at 34pp rpm (Serofuge II) for each wash to converse cells, and decant fluid between washes without removing any of the erythrocytes. After the third wash, invert the tubes and pour off as much of the fluid as possible to obtain a dry button. Insufficient washing results in a false-negative result.
2. Add one drop of Coombs reagent to each tube.
3. Swirl the tubes to mix, and then incubate at 37°C for 15 minutes.
4. Spin at 3400 rpm for 15 seconds.

Gently mix the tubes, and then read for macroscopic and microscopic agglutination. Hemolysis is not significant at this stage.

Interpretation

The samples showing no agglutination at this point are type A negative. The samples that agglutinate in the "D" tube at this point are type A positive. The "C" (i.e., control) tube should be negative. If this tube shows agglutination, then an autoantibody is present, and the blood type cannot be determined. Any positive Coombs' test result on the control tube using cells from a clot tube should be verified with an EDTA-anticoagulated sample. Calcium is bound by EDTA, which in turn prevents the activation of C_1 (i.e., complement) and, therefore, avoids interference by cold-reacting antibodies. A positive Coombs' test result in EDTA whole blood is clinically significant and suggests that the patient has autoantibodies.

Sample Preparation for Sending Blood-Typing Samples to Reference Laboratories

Large-animal blood typing requires acid-citrate-dextrose–anticoagulated blood for longer cell preservation. Usually, EDTA-anticoagulated whole blood is adequate for small-animal blood typing. Samples collected with an anticoagulant should be gently mixed, not shaken, immediately after collection. The EDTA-anticoagulated whole blood should be shipped cool (with, but not touching, a cold pack). All samples should be protected from temperature extremes and shipped by overnight delivery. The reference laboratory should be contacted to obtain more specific requirements regarding sample type, handling, and shipping. Most laboratories performing parental exclusion typing supply blood collection kits or mailers.

THREE

Hematology of Common

Nondomestic Mammals,

Birds, Reptiles, Fish,

and Amphibians

CHAPTER

16

MAMMALIAN HEMATOLOGY: LABORATORY ANIMALS AND MISCELLANEOUS SPECIES

BLOOD COLLECTION AND HANDLING

In general, the maximum amount of blood that can be safely collected during a single draw is 1% of the animal's body weight. For example, a 3.0-mL blood sample, although it rarely is needed, can be safely drawn from a healthy, 300-g rat, and a 0.15-mL blood sample can be safely drawn from an adult mouse. The blood volume will be restored within 24 hours of collection in most healthy mammals, but it may take 2 weeks for all the blood constituents to return to normal. If blood collection is required more frequently than every 2 weeks, a smaller sample size, such as 0.5% of the body weight, should be drawn each week. Blood that is collected from small mammals typically is placed in lithium heparin, because the blood sample volume is small. The heparinized blood then can be used for hematologic studies and clinical chemistries.

Blood samples often are difficult to obtain from small mammals. Such animals lack superficial vessels, and the deeper vessels may be covered with fat. In some cases,

chemical restraint may be necessary to safely handle mammals (e.g., primates) for blood collection. Training of some mammals, such as primates, for blood collection is desirable to prevent multiple anesthesias if frequent blood sampling is required. A number of collection sites are used to obtain blood from small mammals and are listed in *Table 16.1*.

In the clinical setting, the tail vein is the site of choice for blood collection from small mammalian patients with tails (e.g., mice and rats). Veins are located on either side of the tail in mice, and they can be dilated by placing the tail in warm water or under a heat lamp before collection. A tourniquet is placed at the base of the tail, and a 25-G needle is used to enter the lateral tail vein. Blood then is collected into a microcollection device, such as a microhematocrit tube or Microtainer (Becton-Dickinson, Rutherford, NJ), as it drips from the needle hub. Blood for hematology is collected into tubes containing an anticoagulant, such as ethylenediaminetetraacetic acid (EDTA) or heparin. Blood for clinical biochemistry analysis is collected into tubes containing heparin or no anticoagulant.

211

TABLE 16.1 BLOOD COLLECTION SITES IN LABORATORY ANIMALS AND MISCELLANEOUS SPECIES

	Retro-orbital	Tail Vein	Jugular Vein	Cranial Vena Cava	Lateral Saphenous Vein	Femoral Vein	Cephalic	Ear Vein	Cardio-centesis
Mice	X	X							X
Rats	X	X			X				X
Hamsters	X								X
Gerbils	X								X
Guinea pigs	X		X	X	X	X	X		X
Chinchillas	X		X	X	X	X	X		X
Rabbits			X		X		X	X	X
Ferrets		X	X	X	X		X		X
Primates					X	X	X		X
Minipigs		X	X	X	X		X	X	
Llamas			X		X			X	

212

A blood sample also can be obtained from the ventral tail artery of a rat that is placed in dorsal recumbency and under a general anesthetic. A 22-G (or smaller) needle attached to a 3-mL syringe with the plunger removed is used to collect the sample. The artery is located slightly off the ventral midline of the tail. The needle is inserted at a point one-third the length from the base of the tail using a 30° angle. Blood then fills the syringe because of pressure of the artery once the vessel has been penetrated. Pressure is applied to the collection site to control hemostasis after blood sampling.

Venipuncture of the tail artery also can be attempted in ferrets. The artery is approached along the ventral midline of the tail with a 22- or 21-G needle, which is directed toward the caudal vertebrae. The artery usually is 2 to 3 mm under the skin.

Blood may be collected from the lateral saphenous vein in small animals by applying a tourniquet above the stifle after clipping the hair. Shaving the hair off the lateral aspect of the tibia exposes the vein. The leg is extended, and a ⅝-inch, 25-G needle is used to cannulate the vein. Blood then is collected as it drips from the needle hub into a microcollection device. The lateral saphenous vein typically is small, however, and easily collapses, thereby making large sample volumes difficult to collect.

Blood collection from the retroorbital plexus commonly is performed in rodents and requires both technical skill and general anesthesia. A heparinized microhematocrit tube is placed in the medial canthus of the eye, and it is directed under the globe to the orbital venous plexus. With the rodent placed in lateral recumbency, the microhematocrit tube is rotated along its long axis while being advanced toward the venous plexus along the caudal one-half to two-thirds of the orbit. After blood collection, the area requires pressure for hemostasis.

Blood also can be collected from the ear of some animals (e.g. rabbits, miniature pigs, and llamas). Blood collection from the vessels in the ear of rabbits is performed by a simple drip method, vacuum ear bleeder, or a Vacutainer (Becton-Dickinson) method. Ear vessels can be dilated before collection by wrapping the ear in a warm towel or by applying a small amount of oil of wintergreen to the vessel to be punctured. The skin is cleaned with an alcohol wipe before venipuncture. A 25-G needle can be used to puncture the vessel, and the blood then is collected as it drips from the needle hub into a microcollection device. This procedure minimizes hematoma formation during sampling. In small rabbits, aspiration into a syringe or Vacutainer tube often results in collapse of the vessel. The vacuum ear bleeder method is performed by lacerating an ear vessel and then placing the ear inside a flask with a side arm, which is attached to a vacuum line and held firmly against the rabbit's head. This method generally is used for research rabbits, from which large sample volumes are needed.

Jugular venipuncture can be attempted in small mammals, although the jugular veins may be difficult to locate and positioning for the procedure can be stressful to the animal. Jugular venipuncture may require sedation or general anesthesia in some mammals (e.g., ferrets and rabbits). Blood collection in ferrets commonly is performed by jugular venipuncture; simply allowing the ferret to lick food during the procedure may be adequate to limit its movement without the need of anesthesia. After the neck has been shaved and extended, blood is collected from the jugular vein using a 22- to 25-G needle and a 3-mL syringe. The jugular vein of ferrets usually is more lateral than those of dogs and cats, and when the head and neck are extended, it generally runs between the thoracic inlet and the angle of the mandible. Often, the vein cannot be visualized, especially in large males.

Blood collection from the jugular vein of miniature pigs often requires sedation to prevent excessive struggling. The pig is held in dorsal recumbency with the snout extended forward and the forelimbs held caudally to stretch the skin on the neck. A 20- to 22-G, 1.5-inch needle is inserted perpendicularly to the skin and into the jugular furrow. Because the jugular vein is protected by a large amount of fat in the ventral neck area, sampling blood can be difficult with this technique.

Jugular venipuncture can be accomplished in llamas even though the vein cannot be seen. The lower site for jugular venipuncture in the llama is located medial to the ventral projections of the transverse process of the fifth or sixth cervical vertebrae, which can be palpated. The upper site for jugular venipuncture is located just dorsal to the tendon of the sternomandibularis muscle, along a line extending from the ventral border of the mandible.

Blood frequently is collected from the cranial vena cava in small mammals, but this approach may produce bleeding into the thoracic cavity. Venipuncture of the cranial vena cava commonly is performed in ferrets (actually, jugular venipuncture is commonly performed using this approach). The ferret is held in dorsal recumbency with the forelimbs held along its sides and the head and neck extended. A 23-G (or smaller) needle attached to a 3-mL syringe is inserted into the thoracic cavity between the first rib and the manubrium, and it then is advanced caudally at a 45° angle to the body and directed toward the opposite rear limb. The plunger is pulled back as the needle is slowly advanced or withdrawn, thereby allowing blood to enter the syringe.

The cranial vena cava is the most commonly used site for blood collection from miniature pigs. A 19- or 20-G, 1.5-inch needle is used to collect blood from pigs weighing less than 50 pounds; a 3.5-inch spinal needle often is necessary for pigs weighing more than 50 pounds. The needle is inserted in the angle made by the manubrium and the first rib, and it is directed toward the opposite scapular spine. Negative pressure then is applied to the syringe as the needle is advanced. When blood enters the syringe, the needle is held in place until the collection is complete.

Cardiocentesis also can be used to collect blood from small mammals, but this method should be reserved for terminal procedures because of the risk for death during the procedure. Cardiocentesis requires general anesthesia, because the heart often moves away from the needle during the procedure. The small mammal is placed in dorsal recumbency, and the heart is located by palpation. The needle is inserted slightly to the left of and under the manubrium and then is advanced toward the heart, which is stabilized by a thumb and forefinger.

GENERAL HEMATOLOGIC FEATURES OF LABORATORY AND LESS COMMON DOMESTIC MAMMALS

The hematology of laboratory and less common domestic mammals is similar to that of the more common domestic mammals. Obtaining meaningful reference values can be difficult, however, because of variations associated with blood collection, environmental factors, and laboratory procedures. Blood collection often causes stress or requires chemical restraint. The hemogram can vary with age, environmental conditions, diet, and gender. In addition, laboratory procedures and sample handling are not standardized, thereby creating variability between data sets. *Tables 16.2 and 16.3* provide guidelines or suggested reference ranges for erythrocyte and leukocyte parameters, respectively, in laboratory and uncommon domestic mammals.

The erythrocytes of mammals are small compared with the nucleated erythrocytes of other vertebrates. Mammalian erythrocytes are biconcave discs, except in the camelids (e.g., camels, alpacas, and llamas), which have elliptical erythrocytes. The small, nonnucleated, biconcave shape minimizes the hemoglobin-to-surface distance during gas exchange and increases the cell plasticity to improve movement through the blood vessels, thereby increasing the delivery of oxygen to tissues. The hemoglobin content and packed cell volume (PCV) remain relatively constant among mammals, but the total erythrocyte count and mean cell size vary. As a result, an inverse relationship between cell size and number exists.

The granulocytes of nondomestic mammals vary in appearance, but they can be classified as being neutrophils or heterophils, eosinophils, and basophils. The heterophils of rabbits and some rodents previously were called pseudoeosinophils, because their granules do not stain neutral with Romanowsky stains but instead are distinctly eosinophilic. Neutrophils of mice often have nonlobed nuclei, and those of normal primates have lobes that are separated by fine filaments. Cytochemical and ultrastruc-

tural features of cells also differ between species. For example, the neutrophils of ruminants, rhesus monkeys (*Macaca mulatta*), and hamsters lack lysozyme activity, and alkaline phosphatase activity is less in the neutrophils of rhesus monkeys and mice than is typically found in dogs and cats. Neutrophils of mammals are phagocytic; one of their primary functions is to destroy microorganisms. The circulating neutrophil concentration increases with inflammation, especially that associated with invading microorganisms (e.g., bacteria).

The granules of eosinophils become intensely eosinophilic with maturation because of the basic protein content. The ultrastructure of the granules in mammalian eosinophils reveals a distinct, crystalline shape that varies with the species. For example, a trapezoidal pattern is found in the eosinophils of primates, guinea pigs, and rodents, and a needle-shaped pattern is found in those of rabbits. Mammalian eosinophils have phagocytic activity similar to that of neutrophils, but they are less effective. Eosinophilias are associated with metazoan infections (especially those involving helminth larvae), allergic inflammation (especially those associated with mast cell and basophil degranulation), and antigen–antibody complexes. Therefore, eosinophilia suggests one of these processes.

Mammalian basophils have characteristic cytoplasmic granules that are strongly basophilic in Romanowsky-stained blood films. Unlike the basophils of lower vertebrates, those of mammals tend to have lobed nuclei. The ultrastructural appearance of the granules varies with the species. For example, a coiled, threaded pattern is observed in the basophil granules from primates and rabbits, and a homogenous pattern is observed in those from rodents. Basophils participate in both allergic and delayed hypersensitivity reactions.

Mammalian monocytes generally are the largest leukocytes in peripheral blood films, and their appearance is similar in all species. The monocyte nucleus varies in shape, but the moderately abundant cytoplasm typically is light blue-gray. When visible, very fine granules appear to be azurophilic in Romanowsky-stained preparations. Monocytes engulf and degrade microorganisms, abnormal cells, and cell debris. Monocytes also regulate immune responses and myelopoiesis.

The appearance of mammalian lymphocytes varies depending on the species, lymphocyte type, and degree of activation. Mammalian lymphocytes vary in size, color of the cytoplasm (light to dark blue), and degree of nuclear chromatin condensation.

In general, the leukocyte morphology of nondomestic mammals provides a reliable indication of disease. The presence of immature cells, toxic neutrophils, and Döhle bodies are more reliable criteria for infectious diseases than are the total leukocyte and differential counts, given the amount of information known regarding various strains and breeds.

TABLE 16.2 ERYTHROCYTE PARAMETERS FOR LABORATORY ANIMALS AND MISCELLANEOUS SPECIES[a]

	PCV (%)	RBC (× 10⁶ cells/µL)	Hb (g/dl)	MCV (fL)	MCHC (%)	MCH (pg)	Reticulocytes (%)
Mice[b]	40.4 32.8–48.0	8.3 6.5–10.1	13.1 10.1–16.1	49.1 42.3–55.9	32.3 29.5–35.1	15.9 13.7–18.1	4.7 0–11.3
Rats[b]	46.1 2.5 41.1–51.1	7.8 6.6–9.0	14.8 13.2–16.4	59.0 6.4 52.6–65.4	32.4 30.2–34.6	18.9 16.5–21.3	2.2 0–4.6
Guinea pigs[b]	42.1 35.9–48.3	5.1 4.1–6.1	12.9 10.5–15.3	83.0 75.0–91.0	30.6 28.2–33.0	—	2.3 0–6.1
Hamsters[b]	52.5 47.9–57.1	7.5 2.7–12.3	16.8 13.4–19.2	71.2 64.8–77.6	—	—	—
Chinchilla[b]	38.3 25.0–52.0	6.6 5.2–9.9	11.7 8.8–15.4	58.0 —	—	—	—
Rabbits[b]	42.0 36.6–47.4	6.0 5.2–6.8	13.3 11.5–15.1	70.4 64.6–76.2	31.7 29.5–33.9	22.3 21.1–24.5	3.7 1.1–6.3
Ferrets[c]	49.2 42–55	8.11 6.8–9.8	16.2 14.8–17.4	47.1 42.6–51.0	32.0 30.3–34.9	15.0 13.7–16.0	5.3 2–14
Rhesus monkeys[b]	42.1 37.7–46.5	5.4 4.6–6.2	12.2 11.0–13.4	78.6 69.0–88.2	28.9 26.3–31.5	22.8 19.4–26.2	—
Squirrel monkeys[d]	42.0 33.6–50.4	7.5 5.9–9.1	14.1 11.1–17.1	57.0 47.2–66.8	—	—	—
Chimpanzee[d]	41.4 36.0–46.8	5.6 4.6–6.6	13.5 11.5–15.5	74.3 65.3–83.3	—	24.2 21.6–26.8	—
Minipigs[e]	44.6 36.4–52.8	7.0 5.6–8.8	14.9 12.5–17.3	64.4 57.0–71.8	33.2 31.6–34.8	21.4 18.8–24.0	—
Llamas[b]	35.0 25.0–45.0	13.7 10.1–17.3	15.2 11.3–19.0	25.8 22.0–29.5	42.6 38.9–46.2	11.1 9.6–12.6	1.2 0–2.4
White-tailed deer[f]	— 55.0–61.0	— 17.0–20.0	— 17.0–21.0	—	—	—	—
Mule deer[f]	46.7 45.5–47.9	8.8 8.4–9.2	16.4 15.8–17.0	—	—	—	—

Hb, hemoglobin; MCH, mean cell hemoglobin; MCHC, mean cell hemoglobin concentration; MCV, mean cell volume; PCV, packed cell volume; RBC, red blood cells.
[a] Values are presented as means and reference ranges.
[b] Data from Jain NC. Essentials of veterinary hematology. Philadelphia; Lea & Febiger, 1993:54–71.
[c] Data from Fox JG. Normal clinical and biologic parameters. In: Fox JG, ed. Biology and diseases of the ferret. Philadelphia; Lea & Febiger, 1988;159–173.
[d] Data from Loeb W. Primate clinical pathology. In: Fowler ME, ed. Zoo and Wild Animal Medicine. 2nd ed. Philadelphia; WB Saunders, 1986;705–710.
[e] Data from Radin MJ, Weiser MG, Fettman MJ. Hematologic and serum biochemical values for Yucatan miniature swine. Lab Anim Sci 1986;36:425–427.
[f] Data from Kitchen H. Hematological values and blood chemistries for a variety of Artiodactylids. In: Fowler ME, ed. Zoo and Wild Animal Medicine. 2nd ed. Philadelphia; WB Saunders, 1986;1003–1017.

TABLE 16.3 LEUKOCYTE PARAMETERS OF LABORATORY ANIMALS AND MISCELLANEOUS SPECIES[a]

	White Blood Cells	Units	Neutrophils — Bands	Neutrophils — Mature	Lymphocytes	Monocytes	Differential — Eosinophils	Basophils	Platelets
Mice[b]	6.33 (2.61–10.05)	(×10³ cells/μL)	0 (0–0.02)	1.20 (0.4–2.0)	4.86 (1.27–8.44)	0.14 (0–0.29)	0.08 (0–0.17)	0 (0–0.02)	1.16 (×10⁶ cells/μL) (0.78–1.54)
Rats[b]	9.98 (7.30–12.66)	(×10³ cells/μL)	0 (0–0.02)	2.48 (1.25–3.71)	7.07 (5.07–9.07)	0.25 (0.05–0.44)	0.17 (0.04–0.30)	0 (0–0.03)	1.04 (×10⁶ cells/μL) (0.84–1.24)
Guinea pigs[b]	11.11 (8.22–14.0)	(×10³ cells/μL)	0 (0–0.01)	2.50 (1.35–3.65)	8.01 (5.47–10.55)	0.31 (0.06–0.56)	0.27 (0–0.69)	0 (0–0.02)	0.55 (×10⁶ cells/μL) (0.39–0.71)
Hamsters[b]	7.62 (6.32–7.92)	(%)	—	29.9 ± 8.0	73.5 ± 9.4	2.5 ± 0.8	1.1 ± 0.02	0	—
Chinchilla[b]	8.0 (2.2–45.1)	(%)	—	44.6 (10.0–78.0)	53.6 (19.0–98.0)	1.2 (0.0–5.0)	0.5 (0.0–9.0)	0.4 (0.0–11.0)	—
Rabbits[b]	8.18 (6.30–10.06)	(×10³ cells/μL)	0	2.35 (1.49–3.21)	5.18 (3.36–7.00)	0.25 (0.05–0.45)	0.08 (0.01–0.15)	0.21 (0.06–0.36)	0.43 (×10⁶ cells/μL) (0.25–0.61)
Ferrets[c]	10.5 (4–18)	(%)	—	59.5 (43–84)	33.4 (12–50)	4.4 (2–8)	2.6 (0–5)	0.2 (0–1)	545 (×10³ cells/μL) (310–910)
Rhesus monkeys[b]	10.95 (8.08–13.82)	(%)	<1	41.4 ± 11.4	55.7 ± 11.5	<1	2.7 ± 1.8	<1	—
Squirrel monkeys[d]	8.0 (5.1–10.9)	(%)	<1	51.1 ± 15.1	41.0 ± 14.4	3.0 ± 2.7	5.2 ± 6.5	<1	—
Chimpanzee[d]	12.5 (7.4–17.6)	(%)	<1	52.0 ± 14.6	43.0 ± 14.0	1.1 ± 1.2	2.6 ± 3.2	0.2 ± 0.5	349 (×10³ cells/μL) (216–482)
Minipigs[e]	12.6 (6.6–18.6)	(%)	0.2 (0.0–1.2)	41.9 (17.5–66.3)	45.6 (19.2–72.0)	7.5 (1.1–13.9)	4.1 (0.0–10.0)	0.5 (0.0–2.5)	440 (×10³ cells/μL) (201–679)
Llamas[b]	15.7 (8.0–23.3)	(×10³ cells/μL)	0.06 (0.0–0.13)	9.53 (4.18–14.87)	4.3 (0.96–7.64)	0.67 (0.0–1.34)	2.95 (0.07–5.83)	0.15 (0.0–0.30)	—
White-tailed deer[f]	2.25 (1.5–3.0)	(%)	—	32.5 (30.0–35.0)	62.5 (55.0–70.0)	2.0	8.5 (2.0–15.0)	1.0 (0.0–2.0)	—
Mule deer[f]	3.0 (2.9–3.1)	(%)	—	40.6 (39.4–41.8)	43.4 (42.3–44.5)	6.2 (5.7–6.7)	8.3 (7.7–8.9)	0.4 (0.3–0.5)	—

[a] Values are presented as means and reference ranges.
[b] Data from Jain NC. Essentials of veterinary hematology. Philadelphia; Lea & Febiger, 1993:54–71.
[c] Data from Fox JG. Normal clinical and biologic parameters. In: Fox JG, ed. Biology and diseases of the ferret. Philadelphia; Lea & Febiger, 1988;159–173.
[d] Data from Loeb W. Primate clinical and clinical pathology. In: Fowler ME, ed. Zoo and Wild Animal Medicine. 2nd ed. Philadelphia; WB Saunders, 1986;705–710.
[e] Data from Radin MJ, Weiser MG, Fettman MJ. Hematologic and serum biochemical values for Yucatan miniature swine. Lab Anim Sci 1986;36:425–427.
[f] Data from Kitchen H. Hematological values and blood chemistries for a variety of Artiodactylids. In: Fowler ME, ed. Zoo and Wild Animal Medicine. 2nd ed. Philadelphia; WB Saunders, 1986;1003–1017.

HEMATOLOGIC FEATURES OF RODENTS

Mice and Rats

Hematologic parameters of mice and rats are influenced by a variety of factors, including site of sample collection, age, gender, strain, anesthesia, method of restraint, and stress. In rats, blood collected from the heart yields a significantly lower erythrocyte and leukocyte concentration, hemoglobin concentration, and hematocrit compared with samples taken from the retroorbital sinus and tail. A distinct circadian rhythm affects the peripheral leukocyte concentrations, with an increase in the circulating leukocyte concentration occurring during the light phase and a decrease occurring during the dark phase. A distinct decrease in the total leukocyte concentration, associated with a decrease in the lymphocyte concentration, occurs in mice after the stress, such as occurs during transportation. Thus, establishing reference hematologic values for mice and rats is difficult because of many strains and variations in blood collection methods, sample handling techniques, and environmental conditions. Published reference ranges for several strains of rats and mice are available, however, and the reader should refer to the suggested readings list at the end of this chapter and to Table 16.2.

The erythrocyte half-life in a small rodent is from 45 to 68 days, which is relatively short compared with that in larger mammals. Polychromasia is commonly observed on blood films from small rodents, and adults normally have a greater degree of reticulocytosis, with means that average between 2% to 7% *(Fig. 16.1)*. Erythrocyte concentrations in females tend to be less than those of males.

Howell-Jolly bodies are found in small numbers of erythrocytes among normal rats and mice. The rouleaux formation of erythrocytes rarely is seen, however, even with inflammatory disease.

Granulocytes of mice and rats often have nuclei without distinct lobes, and they typically have a horseshoe, sausage, or ring (doughnut) shape *(Fig. 16.2)*. The ring shape may result from a gradually increasing hole that develops in the nucleus during maturation of the granulocyte. Nuclear segmentation occurs as the ring breaks during maturation and then begins to form constrictions.

Neutrophils usually have a colorless cytoplasm, but they may contain a few dust-like, red granules, thus appearing to be diffusely pink with Romanowsky stains *(Fig. 16.3)*. Eosinophils usually are larger than neutrophils and have a ring- or U-shaped nucleus, a basophilic cytoplasm, and numerous small, round eosinophilic cytoplasmic granules that may be arranged in small clumps *(Fig. 16.4)*. Basophils are present in small numbers and contain numerous basophilic granules *(Fig. 16.5)*. Basophils should be differentiated from the mast cells that may appear in peripheral blood, especially when cardiocentesis is performed. The size of lymphocytes ranges from that of erythrocytes to that of neutrophils. The cytoplasm of lymphocytes stains light blue, and azurophilic cytoplasmic granules occasionally are found in large lymphocytes *(Fig. 16.6)*.

The leukocyte concentrations of mice and rats demonstrate a distinct diurnal variation and also vary markedly between strains. An age-dependent variation exists in the neutrophil:lymphocyte (N:L) ratio, with the lymphocyte concentration decreasing and the neutrophil concentration increasing as rodents age.

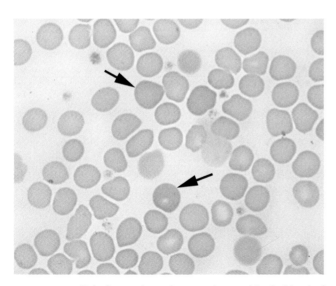

Figure 16.1 Polychromatic erythrocytes (arrows) in the blood of a rat. Wright-Giemsa stain, 500×.

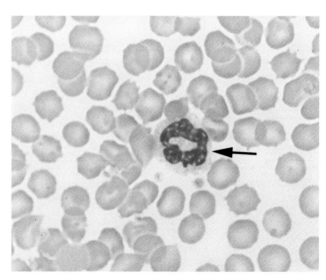

Figure 16.2 A neutrophil (arrow) with a nucleus forming a ring in the blood of a rat. Wright-Giemsa stain, 500×.

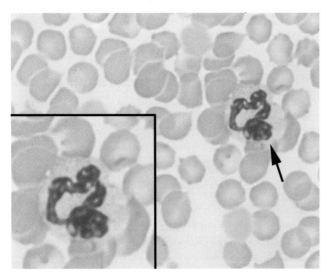

Figure 16.3   A neutrophil (arrow) with fine, pink cytoplasmic granules in the blood of a rat. Wright-Giemsa stain, 500×.

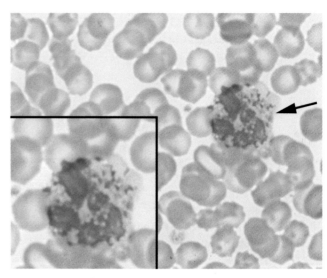

Figure 16.5   A basophil (arrow) in the blood of a rat. Wright-Giemsa stain, 500×.

Platelet concentrations in rodents tend to be high compared with those in larger domestic mammals. Platelet concentrations of greater than 1×10^6 cells/µL are common.

Guinea Pigs

Guinea pigs have larger erythrocytes than other rodents, and polychromasia and macrocytosis characterize the regenerative responses to anemia. The neutrophils of guinea pigs contain granules that stain eosinophilic and that often are referred to as being heterophils or pseudoeosinophils *(Fig. 16.7)*. Although they stain differently than the neutro-

phils of domestic mammals with Romanowsky stains, the neutrophils of guinea pigs are equivalent in function. The granules of guinea pig eosinophils are larger than those of neutrophils, and they are round to rod-shaped, thereby making eosinophils easy to differentiate from neutrophils *(Fig. 16.8)*. The granules of basophils are reddish-purple to black. Large lymphocytes of guinea pigs often contain a single, large cytoplasmic inclusion referred to as a Kurloff body *(Fig. 16.9)*. The finely granular and occasionally vacuolated Kurloff bodies stain homogeneously red with Romanowsky stains and positive with toluidine blue and periodic acid-Schiff. They occur in low numbers

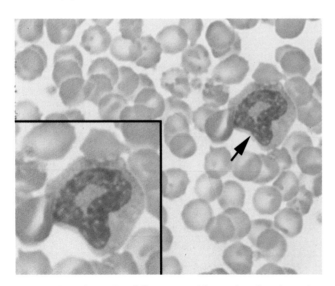

Figure 16.4   An eosinophil (arrow) with a nucleus forming a ring in the blood of a rat. Wright-Giemsa stain, 500×.

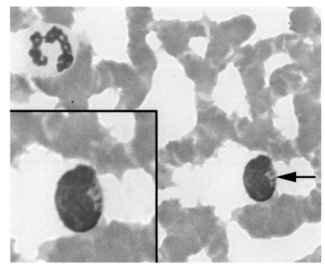

Figure 16.6   A lymphocyte with azurophilic granules (arrow). Wright-Giemsa stain, 500×.

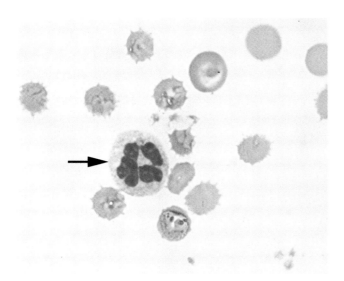

Figure 16.7   A neutrophil (arrow) in the blood of a guinea pig. Wright-Giemsa stain, 500×.

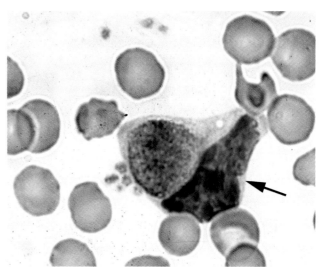

Figure 16.9   A lymphocyte (arrow) containing a Kurloff body in the blood of a guinea pig. Wright-Giemsa stain, 500×.

among immature male guinea pigs, thereby suggesting that they are influenced by sex hormones.

Other Rodents

The hematologic features of hamsters, gerbils, and chinchillas resemble those of mice and rats. As with rats and mice, polychromasia is a normal finding in blood films from hamsters and gerbils, and Howell-Jolly bodies are common. The neutrophils of chinchillas typically are hyposegmented and resemble those of dogs with the Pelger-Huët anomaly.

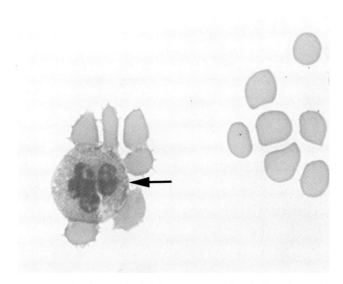

Figure 16.8   An eosinophil (arrow) in the blood of a guinea pig. Wright-Giemsa stain, 500×.

HEMATOLOGIC FEATURES OF RABBITS

The rabbit erythrocyte is a biconcave disk. As with rodents, polychromatic erythrocytes and reticulocytes are common in the blood films of normal rabbits. Polychromasia commonly is observed in 2% to 4% of the erythrocyte population in normal rabbits, and nucleated erythrocytes and Howell-Jolly bodies occasionally are observed. The estimated half-life of rabbit erythrocytes is between 57 and 67 days. As with most other mammalian species, a regenerative response to anemia in rabbits is characterized by increased anisocytosis, polychromasia, nucleated erythrocytes, and Howell-Jolly bodies. Anemia commonly is associated with a variety of diseases in rabbits. Infectious diseases often produce increased numbers of nucleated erythrocytes.

The rabbit neutrophil has a polymorphic nucleus that stains light blue to purple with Romanowsky stains. The cytoplasm of rabbit neutrophils typically stains diffusely pink with Romanowsky stains because of the fusion of many small, acidophilic granules (i.e., primary granules) *(Fig. 16.10)*. These cells often are referred to as pseudo-eosinophils or heterophils in the literature because of the larger eosinophilic cytoplasmic granules (i.e., secondary granules) that stain dark pink to red with Romanowsky stains. Rabbit neutrophils are ultrastructurally, functionally, and biochemically equivalent to those of other domestic mammals and humans. An occasional neutrophil with characteristics of the Pelger-Huët anomaly (i.e., hyposegmented) may be observed in the blood films from normal rabbits. Rabbit neutrophils are easily distinguished from eosinophils, which have large eosinophilic granules.

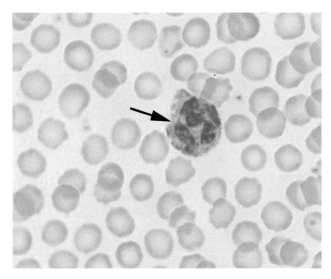

Figure 16.10 A neutrophil (heterophil; arrow) in the blood of a rabbit. Wright-Giemsa stain, 500×.

The eosinophils of rabbits are larger than the neutrophils. The large cytoplasmic granules of rabbit eosinophils are more numerous than those of neutrophils. Eosinophil granules are poorly defined and stain intensely pink to a dull pink-orange with Romanowsky stains, thereby creating a tinctorial quality that differs from that of the neutrophil granules. The nucleus of the eosinophil is bilobed to U-shaped *(Fig. 16.11)*.

Rabbits typically have more basophils than other species. Commonly, 5% of leukocytes are basophils, but this number can be as high as 30% in rabbits with no apparent abnormalities.

Rabbit lymphocytes are morphologically similar to those of other domestic mammals and humans. Most

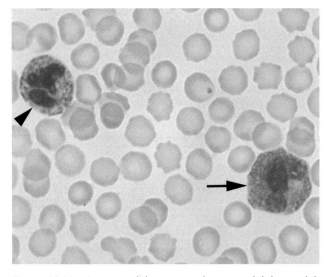

Figure 16.11 An eosinophil (arrow) and a neutrophil (heterophil; arrowhead) in the blood of a rabbit. Wright-Giemsa stain, 500×.

lymphocytes are small, but large lymphocytes, comparable in size to neutrophils, also may be present. Azurophilic granules often are present in the cytoplasm of the large lymphocytes.

Rabbit monocytes are similar to those in other domestic mammals. The nucleus varies from lobulated to bean-shaped, and the cytoplasm stains blue and may contain a few vacuoles.

The normal leukocyte concentration of rabbits typically is reported to range between 6000 and 10,000 cells/μL. Lymphocytes tend to be the predominant leukocyte; however, variations occur with age, methods of restraint, and methods of blood collection, all of which may alter the N:L ratio. A bimodal increase in the leukocyte concentration is seen with increasing age, with the highest lymphocyte concentration occurring at 3 months and then slowly declining and the highest neutrophil concentration occurring among older animals. Therefore, rabbits that are 12 months of age or younger have lower N:L ratios (30%:65%) than do rabbits 13 to 26 months of age, which typically have equal numbers of neutrophils and lymphocytes. A stress response associated with restraint during blood collection can result in a 15% to 30% decrease in the total leukocyte concentration. A mature neutrophilia and lymphopenia characterize glucocorticoid-mediated changes in the leukogram.

Rabbits generally do not develop leukocytosis with bacterial infections, but they do develop an increased absolute neutrophil concentration and a decreased absolute lymphocyte concentration. This reversal of the N:L ratio also is associated with increased serum cortisol concentrations. The neutrophil morphology (e.g., the presence of toxicity) may aid in distinguishing an infectious cause from corticosteroid excess. Therefore, the N:L ratio and absolute neutrophil and lymphocyte concentrations appear to be more reliable indicators of inflammatory disorders than total leukocyte concentrations.

HEMATOLOGIC FEATURES OF FERRETS

The hematology of ferrets resembles that of domestic carnivores. Ferrets commonly are anesthetized for blood collection. However, use of inhalant anesthetics, such as isoflurane, enflurane, and halothane, result in significant and rapid decreases in the red blood cell count, hematocrit, and hemoglobin concentration. In fact, the hemoglobin concentration can decrease by as much as 33% with use of these inhalant anesthetics. Splenic sequestration and anesthetic-induced hypotension are possible causes for this response in ferrets. The red blood cell count, hematocrit, and hemoglobin concentration return to normal within 45 minutes of recovery from the anesthetic. Use of manual restraint or an injectable anesthetic (e.g., ketamine) is required to avoid this effect in the erythron.

The hemogram of domestic ferrets (*Mustela putorius*) is influenced by both gender and age. Young hobs (i.e., male ferrets) have a lower red-blood-cell concentration, hematocrit, and hemoglobin concentration than adult hobs and young jills (i.e., female ferrets). Jills experience a decrease in the hematocrit with age.

Common causes of nonregenerative anemia in domestic ferrets include malignant neoplasia (e.g., lymphoma), systemic infections, and hyperestrogenism in intact females. Gastrointestinal ulcers are a common cause of blood loss anemia.

The morphology of ferret leukocytes is similar to that of dogs. In normal ferrets, the neutrophil concentrations are higher than the lymphocyte concentrations. Ferrets experience an increase in the neutrophil concentration and a decrease in the lymphocyte concentration with increasing age. The total leukocyte count of healthy ferrets can be as low as 3000 cells/µL. Ferrets cannot develop a marked leukocytosis with inflammatory disease. Concentrations of greater than 20,000 cells/µL are unusual, and a left shift appears to be rare.

HEMATOLOGIC FEATURES OF PRIMATES

The mature erythrocytes of primates are biconcave discs of approximately 7.5 µm in diameter, but the red cell parameters of primates vary with age and sex. Neonates have a higher total erythrocyte concentration, hemoglobin concentration, and PCV compared with adults. The erythron rapidly decreases as animals become subadults, but then increases after puberty. Adult male primates have a higher erythrocyte concentration, hemoglobin concentration, and PCV compared with adult female primates. The reticulocyte concentration of most normal primates is less than 2.0%. Small numbers of Howell-Jolly bodies may be seen in the blood films from primates. Erythrocyte rouleaux formation occurs with inflammatory disease.

Excitement and exertion associated with capture and restraint produce splenic contraction and a corresponding increase in the PCV. Use of an anesthetic (e.g., ketamine) reduces this effect.

Neutrophils of some primates, such as orangutans (*Pongo pygmaeus*), have very small eosinophilic granules, whereas those of others, such as chimpanzees (*Pan* sp.), have very small basophilic granules. Lymphocytosis, which is associated with restraint-related epinephrine release, can be prevented with use of ketamine anesthesia. Occasional binucleate lymphocytes are found in the blood of normal primates.

Leukocyte concentrations as great as 15,000 cells/µL are more typical of nonexcited primates; however, concentrations as great as 30,000 cells/µL can occur with ex-

citement. An increased number of immature neutrophils (i.e., bands) is indicative of inflammation. Most species demonstrate toxic neutrophils with inflammation, and some species, such as rhesus monkeys (*Macaca mulatta*) and orangutans commonly exhibit neutrophil toxicity in the form of Döhle bodies. A marked, transient leukocytosis with lymphocytosis occurs in primates in response to antigenic challenges (e.g., adenovirus infection). Leukemias associated with high concentrations of large lymphocytes often have viral causes, such as *Herpesvirus saimiri* and RNA oncornavirus infections.

Blood parasites, including microfilaria and trypanosomes, commonly are present in wild-caught primates, especially New World monkeys. These parasites have a low virulence, however, and generally are considered to be an incidental finding. *Plasmodium* gametocytes and schizonts often appear as incidental findings in the erythrocytes of asymptomatic wild-caught primates. Gametocytes of *Hepatocystis*, which is a mildly pathogenic parasite, may be seen in the blood films of some African monkeys.

HEMATOLOGY OF MINIPIGS

The hemograms of minipigs (e.g., pot-bellied pigs) do not vary significantly from those of domestic pigs. Therefore, hematologic studies of minipigs are interpreted in the same way as those of domestic pigs. Erythrocyte spiculation, which is characterized by sharp, pointed projections from the cells, is common in the blood films of normal minipigs *(Fig. 16.12)*.

The neutrophils of pigs have irregularly stained nuclei with irregular margins, and they often are coiled and lack

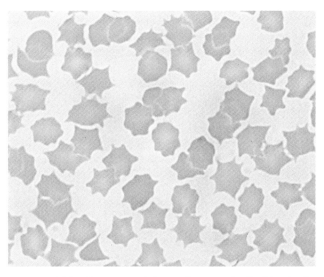

Figure 16.12 Crenation of the erythrocytes in the blood of a minipig. Wright-Giemsa stain, 500×.

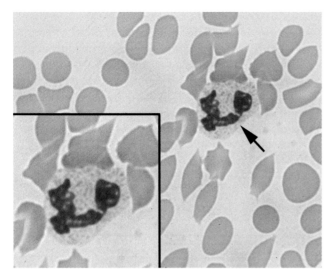

Figure 16.13 A neutrophil (arrow) with fine cytoplasmic granules in the blood of a minipig. Wright-Giemsa stain, 500×.

complete lobation. The cytoplasm of porcine neutrophils contains small, pink granules with Romanowsky stains *(Fig. 16.13)*. Porcine eosinophils have round to oval, orange cytoplasmic granules. The nucleus often appears to be a band *(Fig. 16.14)*. Normal minipigs have total leukocyte concentrations as great as 22,000 cells/μL because of the excitement leukocytosis associated with handling for blood collection. The lymphocyte concentration is greater than the neutrophil concentration in healthy pigs. Physiologic leukocytosis results from a transient neutrophilia and lymphocytosis. Minipigs, like other animals with low

N:L ratios, mount a lower leukocyte response than animals with high N:L ratios and inflammatory diseases, and they may show only a reversal of the N:L ratio with mild inflammatory diseases. Marked neutrophilia is associated with more severe inflammatory diseases.

HEMATOLOGY OF LLAMAS

The erythrocytes of camelids, including camels, alpaca, and llamas, are elliptical, thin, and flat *(Fig. 16.15)*. Llamas are adapted to life at high altitudes, and their erythrocyte function allows them to survive low atmospheric oxygen tension without developing polycythemia and associated high blood viscosity. The elliptical shape of the erythrocytes may allow for easier passage through the capillaries, and the thin shape allows for rapid gas exchange. Healthy llamas have a small mean cell volume, ranging between 20 and 30 fL, and a relatively high mean cell hemoglobin concentration, ranging between 40 and 45 g/dL. Camelid erythrocytes are more resistant to hemolysis in hypotonic saline than those of other mammals. Llamas have high erythrocyte concentrations, but the small size of the erythrocytes result in relatively low PCVs. Llama erythrocytes are too small for the threshold range of the automated, multichannel instruments commonly used for obtaining total erythrocyte concentrations; therefore, use of threshold modifications or manual techniques are required. The hemoglobin of llamas has an oxygen–hemoglobin dissociation curve that is shifted to the left compared with those of other mammals, thereby

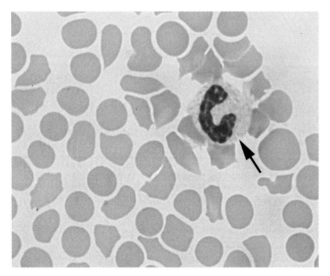

Figure 16.14 A band cell (arrow) in the blood of a minipig. Wright-Giemsa stain, 500×.

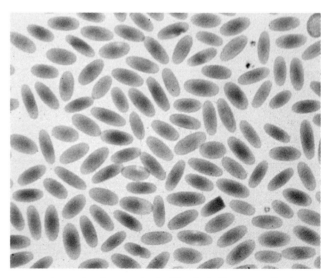

Figure 16.15 Erythrocytes in the blood of a llama. Wright-Giemsa stain, 500×.

allowing for high saturation of hemoglobin with oxygen at low atmospheric oxygen tension. The PCVs and hemoglobin concentrations of adult male llamas are greater than those of adult female and juvenile llamas. Erythrocytes become flattened and ellipsoid during the final stages of maturation, and reticulocytes and nucleated erythrocytes are round. Erythrocyte rouleaux formation does not occur in camelids, even those with inflammatory diseases.

Anemia in llamas is indicated by a PCV of less than 24%. The presence of reticulocytes and nucleated erythrocytes is indicative of a regenerative response. Iron deficiency anemia in llamas is characterized by microcytosis, hypochromasia, decreased hemoglobin concentration and mean cell hemoglobin concentration, hypoferremia, and decreased transferrin saturation. The red-cell morphologic features include marked poikilocytosis, anisocytosis, asymmetric distribution of hemoglobin (interpreted as hypochromia), folded erythrocytes, and dacryocytes *(Fig. 16.16)*. Erythrocyte volume distribution histograms are more sensitive than mean cell volumes in the detection of microcytosis. Hypochromic erythrocytes often have an eccentric, irregular distribution of hemoglobin. Folding of erythrocytes may be associated with a change in the thickness: diameter ratio as a result of iron deficiency. Hypochromasia with marked anisocytosis also can be associated with copper deficiency in camelids.

Neutrophils are the predominant leukocyte in normal blood films. Absolute lymphocyte concentrations are greater and eosinophil concentrations are less in juvenile compared with adult llamas. Neutrophilia (>25,000 cells/μL), increased plasma fibrinogen (>400 mg/dL), and a non-

regenerative anemia are indicative of inflammatory disease, and the presence of immature neutrophils is supportive of inflammatory disease. A stress leukogram is indicated by neutrophilia and lymphopenia. A physiologic leukocytosis associated with excitement is common in llamas. A neutropenia (<4000 cells/μL) with a left shift, toxic neutrophils, and lymphopenia is suggestive of overwhelming septicemia and endotoxemia.

HEMATOLOGY OF DEER

Erythrocytes in most species of normal deer exhibit in vitro sickling. The erythrocytes circulate as round cells, but sickling occurs during preparation of blood films after blood collection. Sickling occurs when the cells are exposed to oxygen and also appears to be affected by pH. Nearly all erythrocytes sickle at a pH of 7.4. Sickling can be prevented, however, by acidifying the blood. Sickled cells appear as crescent, holly leaf, match stick, and burr shapes, depending on the hemoglobin variant *(Fig. 16.17)*. Deer blood contains several hemoglobin types that polymerize or crystallize in the oxygenated state, thereby leading to sickle cell formation.

Excitement and stress during restraint result in high erythrocyte and leukocyte counts. Male deer have higher PCVs and erythrocyte counts compared with female deer. Erythrocytes in deer exhibit a high degree of rouleaux formation with inflammatory disease.

Lymphocytes are the predominant leukocyte in normal deer. During the rutting period, male deer have higher neutrophil concentrations compared with female deer.

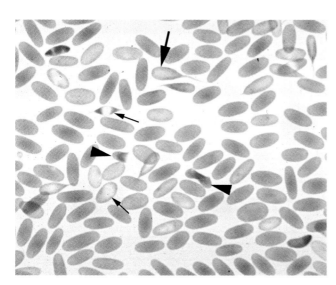

Figure 16.16   Folded erythrocytes (arrowheads), hypochromic erythrocytes (thin arrows), and dacryocytes (large arrow) in the blood of a llama with iron deficiency anemia, 500×.

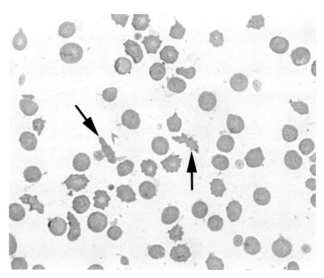

Figure 16.17   Sickling of erythrocytes (arrows) in the blood of a deer, 500×.

SUGGESTED READINGS

Rodents

Bean-Knudsen DE, Wagner JE. Effect of shipping stress on clinico-pathologic indicators in F344/N rats. Am J Vet Res 1987;48: 306–308.

Drozdowicz CK, Bowman TA, Webb ML, Lang CM. Effect of in-house transport on murine plasma corticosterone concentration and blood lymphocyte populations. Am J Vet Res 1990;51:1841–1846.

Leonard R, Ruben Z. Hematology reference values for peripheral blood of laboratory rats. Lab Anim Sci 1986;36:277–281.

Ringer DH, Dabich L. Hematology and clinical biochemistry. In: Baker HJ, Lindsey JR, Weisbroth SH, eds. The laboratory rat. Volume 1: biology and disease. New York: Academic Press, 1979:105–121.

Suber RL, Kodell RL. The effect of three phlebotomy techniques on hematological and clinical chemical evaluation in Sprague-Dawley rats. Vet Clin Pathol 1985;14:23–30.

Wright JR, et al. Hematological characteristics of the BB Winstar rat. Vet Clin Pathol 1983;12:9–13.

Rabbits

McLaughlin RM, Fish RE. Clinical biochemistry and hematology. In: Manning PJ, Ringler DH, Newcomer CE, eds. The biology of the laboratory rabbit. New York: Academic Press, 1974:111–127.

Ferrets

Fox JG. Normal clinical and biologic parameters. In: Fox JG, ed. Biology and diseases of the ferret. Philadelphia: Lea & Febiger, 1988: 159–173.

Kawasaki TA. Normal parameters and laboratory interpretation of disease states in the domestic ferret. Semin Avian Exotic Pet Med 1994;3:40–47.

Lee EJ, Moore WE, Fryer HC, et al. Haematological and serum chemistry profiles of ferrets (*Mustela putorius furo*). Lab Anim 1982; 16:133–137.

Marini RP, Jackson LR, Esteves MI, et al. Effect of isoflurane on hematologic variables in ferrets. Am J Vet Res 1984;55:1479–1483.

Primates

Bennett JS, Gossett KA, McCarthy MP, et al. Effects of ketamine hydro-chloride on serum biochemical and hematologic variables in Rhesus monkeys (*Macaca mulatta*). Vet Clin Pathol 1992;21:15–18.

Huser H-J. Atlas of comparative primate hematology. New York: Academic Press, 1970.

Minipigs

Parsons AH, Wells RE. Hematologic values of the Yucatan miniature pig. Vet Clin Pathol 1989;18:90–92.

Radin MJ, Weiser MG, Fettman MJ. Hematologic and serum biochemical values for Yucatan miniature swine. Lab Anim Sci 1986; 36:425–427.

Llamas

Andreasen CB, Gerros TC, Lassen ED. Evaluation of bone marrow cytology and stainable iron content in healthy adult llamas. Vet Clin Pathol 1994;23:38–42.

Fowler ME. Medicine and surgery of South American camelids. Ames, IA: Iowa State University Press, 1991.

Fowler ME, Zinkl JG. Reference ranges for hematologic and serum biochemical values in llamas (*Lama glama*). Am J Vet Res 1989; 50:2049–2053.

Garry F. Clinical pathology of llamas. Vet Clin North Am Food Anim Pract 1989;5:55–70.

Jain NC, Keeton KS. Morphology of camel and llama erythrocytes as viewed with scanning electron microscope. Br Vet J 1974;130: 288–291.

Lewis JH. Comparative hematology—studies on camelidae. Comp Biochem Physiol (A) 1976;55:367–371.

McLaughlin BG, Evans CN, McLaughlin PS, et al. An *Eperythrozoon*-like parasite in llamas. J Am Vet Med Assoc 1990;197:1170–1175.

Morin DE, Garry FB, Weiser MG. Hematologic responses in llamas with experimentally-induced iron deficiency anemia. Vet Clin Pathol 1993;22:81–86.

Morin DE, Garry FB, Weiser MG, et al. Hematologic features of iron deficiency anemia in llamas. Vet Pathol 1992;29:400–404.

Reagan WJ, Gary F, Thrall MA, et al. The clinicopathological, light, and scanning electron microscopic features of eperythrozoonosis in four naturally infected llamas. Vet Pathol 1990;27:426–431.

Smith BB, Reed PJ, Pearson EG, et al. Erythrocyte dyscrasia, anemia, and hypothyroidism in chronically underweight llamas. J Am Vet Med Assoc 1991;198:81–88.

Van Houten D, Weiser MG, Johnson LW, et al. Reference hematologic values and morphologic features of blood cells in healthy adult llamas. Am J Vet Res 1992;53:1773–1775.

Weiser MG, Fettman MJ, Van Houten D, et al. Characterization of erythrocytic indices and serum iron values in healthy llamas. Am J Vet Res 1992;53:1776–1779.

Deer

Chapple RS, English AW, Mulley RC, et al. Haematology and serum biochemistry of captive unsedated Chital deer (*Axis axis*) in Australia. J Wildl Dis 1991;27:396–406.

Seal US, Erickson AW. Hematology, blood chemistry and protein polymorphisms in the white-tailed deer (*Odocoileus virginianus*). Comp Biochem Physiol 1969;30:695–713.

General

Hawkey CM. Comparative mammalian haematology. London: William Heinemann Medical Books, 1975.

Hawkey CM, Dennett TB, Peirce MA. Color atlas of comparative veterinary hematology. London: Wolfe Medical Publications, 1989.

Jain NC. Essentials of veterinary hematology. Philadelphia: Lea & Febiger, 1993.

Parmley RT. Mammals. In: Rowley AF, Ratcliffe NA, eds. Vertebrate blood cells. Cambridge, UK: Cambridge University Press, 1988: 337–424.

Schalm OW, Jain NC, Carrol EJ. Veterinary hematology. 3rd ed. Philadelphia: Lea & Febiger, 1975.

Weiser MG. Comparison of two automated multi-channel blood cell counting systems for analysis of blood of common domestic animals. Vet Clin Pathol 1983;12:25–32.

Weiser MG. Modification and evaluation of an automated blood cell counter for blood analysis in veterinary hematology. J Am Vet Med Assoc 1987;190:411–415.

C H A P T E R

17

HEMATOLOGY OF BIRDS

Clinical avian hematology is relatively new to veterinary medicine. Before 1980, avian hematology was used primarily as a research tool in the poultry industry. The first comprehensive description of hemic cytology was by Lucas and Jamroz in 1961 (1). Their atlas described the various cells in the peripheral blood and hemic tissue of poultry, and it formed the basis of avian hematology. In 1980, the Association of Avian Veterinarians was formed by veterinarians experiencing an increased number of pet birds (primarily psittacine birds) being presented to their clinical practices. Since then, the number of birds seen in veterinary practices has increased significantly. Avian hematology is approached in a manner similar to that of human and mammalian hematology, but a few differences require modification of the hematologic procedures. Major differences include the presence of nucleated erythrocytes, thrombocytes, and heterophil granulocytes in the peripheral blood of birds.

This chapter discusses the basics of clinical avian hematology. Topics include blood collection techniques, laboratory methods, evaluation of peripheral blood cells, and identification of common blood parasites.

COLLECTION AND HANDLING OF BLOOD SAMPLES

The amount of blood that can be safely removed from a bird depends on its body size and health status. A blood

volume representing 1% or less of body weight usually can be withdrawn from healthy birds without detrimental effects. For example, a healthy, 80-g cockatiel (*Nymphicus hollandicus*) can easily tolerate removal of a 0.8 mL blood sample. The sample size taken from severely ill birds, however, must be reduced. For routine hematologic evaluations in birds, a sample size of 0.2 mL usually is adequate. A variety of collection methods have been used to obtain blood from birds, and the method chosen depends on the size of the bird, peculiarities of the species, preference of the collector, volume of blood needed, and physical condition of the patient.

Venous blood provides the best sample for hematologic studies. Blood collected from capillary beds (i.e., clipping of a toenail) usually results in abnormal cell distributions and contains both cells and other substances not found in venous blood, such as tissue fluid, macrophages, and cellular debris. Veins commonly used for venipuncture include the jugular, cutaneous ulnar (wing or brachial), and medial metatarsal (caudal tibial). Blood can be collected using a needle and syringe when performing venipuncture on the jugular or other large veins. A short (≤1 inch), 25- to 22-G needle attached to a 3- to 6-mL syringe commonly is used for jugular venipuncture. A needle with an extension tube, such as a butterfly catheter (Abbott Hospitals, North Chicago, IL) aids in stabilization of the needle during sample collection. Blood also can be collected after venipuncture by allowing it to flow through the needle and drip into a microcollection device. Collecting blood by allowing it to flow through the needle, rather than by aspirating it into a syringe, minimizes hematoma formation. A variety of these devices (Microtainer tubes, Becton-Dickinson, Rutherford, NJ) are available. Microcollection tubes containing ethylenediaminetetraacetic acid [EDTA] are available for hematologic studies, but they also are available as plain tubes, with or without a serum separator, and as tubes containing heparin (lithium heparin is preferred) for studies of blood chemistry.

Jugular venipuncture most commonly is used for collecting blood from birds, because most small birds do not have other veins that are large enough for venipuncture (2–6). Jugular venipuncture involves lightly wetting the feathers with alcohol to expose the featherless tract (apterla) of skin that overlies the jugular furrow. The right jugular vein is the vein of choice for this procedure, because it either is the only jugular vein present or is the larger of the two jugular veins. Jugular venipuncture is performed by using an appropriate-sized needle and providing proper restraint, with the bird's head and neck extended to allow the jugular vein to fall into the jugular furrow *(Figs. 17.1 and 17.2)*. Jugular venipuncture provides a rapid collection time and the ability to easily collect adequate amounts of blood, even in small birds. The tendency for hematoma formation can be minimized with proper attention to technique and hemostasis.

Another common procedure for blood collection in medium to large birds is venipuncture of the cutaneous ulnar (brachial) vein. This vein crosses the ventral surface of the humeroradioulnar joint (elbow), and it is easily visualized by wetting the area lightly with alcohol. Using an appropriate-sized needle, blood can be collected after

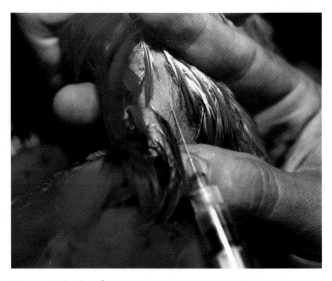

Figure 17.2   Jugular venipuncture in a macaw (*Ara maczo*).

cannulation of this vein either by aspiration into a syringe or by allowing it to drip from the needle hub into a microcollection tube *(Figs. 17.3 through 17.5)*.

Blood also can be collected by aspiration or the drip technique from the medial metatarsal (caudal tibial) vein, which is located on the caudomedial aspect of the tibiotarsus just above the tarsal joint. Because this vein is protected by the surrounding muscles of the leg, hematoma formation is minimal *(Figs. 17.6 through 17.8)*.

Clipping the toenail and lancet wounding are two other methods of blood collection, but these should be reserved for very small birds or for when attempts at venipuncture have failed. After alcohol cleansing, the toenail

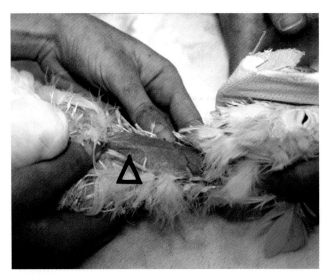

Figure 17.1   Location of the right jugular vein in a cockatoo (*Cacatua moluccensis*).

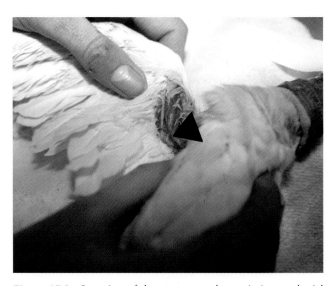

Figure 17.3   Location of the cutaneous ulnar vein in a cockatiel (*Nymphicus hollandicus*).

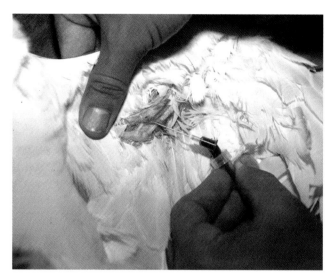

Figure 17.4 Cannulation of the cutaneous ulnar vein of a cockatoo (*Cacatua moluccensis*) using the drip method for blood collection.

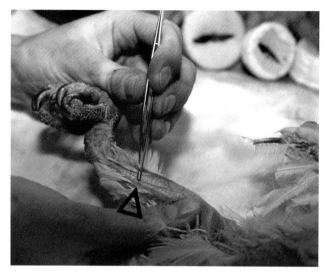

Figure 17.6 Location of the medial metatarsal vein in a cockatoo (*Cacatua moluccensis*).

is clipped until blood flows freely for collection into a microcollection tube. After blood collection from the cut nail, hemostasis is accomplished by applying a hemostatic agent such as silver nitrate or ferrous subsulfate. Blood collection by this technique yields a poor sample for hematologic studies, however, because the blood is from the capillary bed and usually contains microclots, which interfere with cell counts. Capillary blood also frequently is contaminated with tissue fluid that affects hematologic data. Toenail clipping may result in temporary lameness because of nail damage. An alternative to nail clipping for blood collection from small birds is to collect blood

after lancet wounding of vascular structures, such as the cutaneous ulnar vein, medial metatarsal vein, and external thoracic vein. After alcohol cleansing of the skin overlying the vein, the vessel is punctured through the skin using a lancet (i.e., needle), and the blood is allowed to drip into a microcollection tube.

Large volumes of blood can be collected from birds by cardiac puncture or occipital venous sinus puncture (2,7–10). These procedures are potentially dangerous, however, and should be reserved for birds that are used for research or are to be euthanized. Cardiac puncture can be performed using either an anterior or a lateral approach. The heart is approached anteriorly by inserting

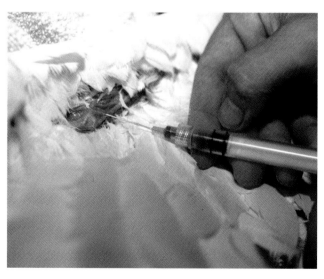

Figure 17.5 Aspiration of blood from the cutaneous ulnar vein in a cockatoo (*Cacatua moluccensis*).

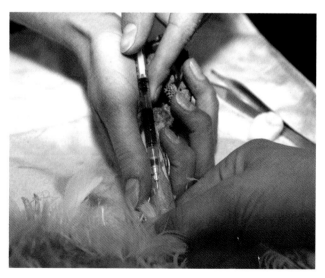

Figure 17.7 Aspiration of blood from the medial metatarsal vein in a cockatoo (*Cacatua moluccensis*).

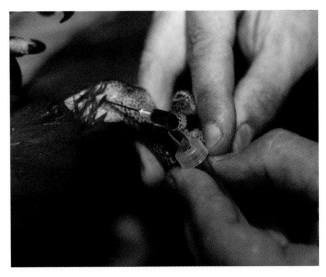

Figure 17.8   Cannulation of the medial metatarsal vein in a macaw using the drip method for blood collection (*Ara maczo*).

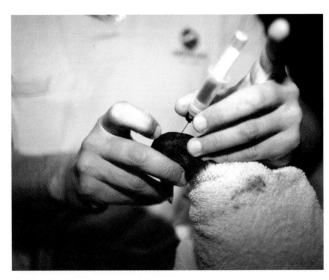

Figure 17.9   Blood collection from the dorsal occipital venous sinus in a puffin (*Fratercula cirrhata*).

a needle along the ventral floor of the thoracic inlet with the bird in dorsal recumbency. Care should be taken to avoid the ingluvies (crop) in some avian species. The needle is inserted near the "V" that is formed by the furcula, and it is directed toward the bird's dorsum and caudal toward the heart. Once the heart is penetrated, the vibration can be felt to ensure proper needle placement, and blood is then aspirated. In galliforme birds, the heart can be approached laterally by inserting the needle in the fourth intercostal space near the sternum (keel) with the bird held in lateral recumbency. This approach, however, may vary with the species.

Blood collection from the occipital venous sinus requires use of evacuated glass tubes with appropriate needles and needle holders. The occipital venous sinus is located at the junction of the dorsal base of the skull and the first cervical vertebra, and it can be located by palpation while holding the bird's head firmly flexed and positioned in a straight line with the cervical vertebrae. A needle is inserted through the skin at a 30° to 40° angle to the vertebrae. As soon as the needle penetrates the skin, the rubber stopper of the evacuated tube is perforated gently and the needle advanced until the sinus is reached *(Fig. 17.9)*. Penetration of the sinus results in a rapid flow of blood into the tube. Blood collection by either puncture of the heart or the occipital venous sinus requires proper restraint and technique to avoid permanent damage to the heart or brainstem—and even possible death of the patient.

Blood samples collected without use of an anticoagulant require immediate processing. Dilutions for cell counting and preparation for blood films must be quickly performed with such samples. Because of the urgency for

rapid processing of nonanticoagulated blood, most avian blood samples are collected into tubes containing an anticoagulant. Ethylenediaminetetraacetic acid, heparin, and sodium citrate are commonly used, and each has both advantages and disadvantages. The anticoagulant of choice for avian hematology is EDTA, because it allows for proper staining of cells and does not tend to clump leukocytes (2–4). Hematologic testing, however, should be performed soon after blood collection to avoid artifacts, such as increased cell smudging, which is created by prolonged exposure to any anticoagulant. Excessive liquid anticoagulants dilute the blood sample, thereby resulting in artifactually decreased hematocrit and total cell concentrations, and excessive dry anticoagulants may cause shrinkage of red blood cells, thus affecting the hematocrit. Blood from certain avian groups, such as crows and jays, may show incomplete anticoagulation or partial hemolysis when collected in EDTA (3,4). Heparin has the advantage of providing anticoagulated blood for hematology and plasma for evaluations of blood chemistry. Heparinized blood, however, may result in improper staining of cells, thereby resulting in erroneous leukocyte counts and poor cellular morphology in stained blood films (2–4). Heparin also causes clumping of leukocytes and thrombocytes and resultant, inaccurate cell counts. A 3.8% sodium citrate solution, used in a ratio of one part citrate solution to nine parts blood, is the anticoagulant of choice for coagulation studies; however, it should not be used for other hematologic evaluations.

Blood films can be made using a variety of techniques. The standard two-slide wedge or push-slide method that is commonly used for preparing human and mammalian blood films also can provide adequate blood films for avian hematology (2,11,12). This method usually provides good cellular distribution and adequate monolayer fields for proper slide evaluation. Use of precleaned, bevel-edged microscope slides is advised to minimize cell damage during preparation of blood films. To minimize cell damage, a drop of commercially available, purified bovine albumin can be applied to a glass microscope slide, which with by an equal amount of blood placed on top of the albumin before making the blood film. The albumin should not be allowed to dry before making the blood film. Alternately, blood films can be prepared by using a slide and coverslip or by using two coverslips. With proper attention to technique, these methods minimize cellular disruption while maintaining good cellular distribution with monolayered areas for examination (13,14). The coverslip is pulled across a drop of blood that has been placed on a glass microscope slide or coverslip. A disadvantage of the coverslip method, however, is the inability to use an automatic stainer.

Wright, Wright-Giemsa, Wright-Leishman, and May Grünwald-Giemsa stains have been used for staining air-dried, avian blood films for hematologic examination. Quick stains or modified Wright stains (Diff-Quik, American Scientific Products, Division of American Hospital Supply Corporation, McGraw Park, IL; Hemacolor, Miles Laboratories, Elkhart, IN) also can be used to stain avian blood films. Use of automatic slide stainers (Hema-Tek, Ames Division of Miles Laboratories, Elkhart, IN; Harleco Midas II, EM Diagnostic Systems,Gibbstown, NJ) simplifies the staining procedure and provides a means for consistency and high-quality staining of blood films. Automatic stainers remove much of the staining variation that occurs with hand-staining methods.

ERYTHROCYTES

Morphology

Evaluation of avian erythrocyte morphology involves observation of the cells in a monolayer ×1000 field in which approximately half the erythrocytes are touching one another (15). In general, such fields represent approximately 200 erythrocytes in most species of birds. Monolayer fields may be difficult to achieve, however, in severely anemic birds (i.e., films are too thin) or in poorly prepared blood films (i.e., films made too thick or thin). Avian erythrocytes should be evaluated on the basis of size, shape, color, nucleus, and presence of cellular inclusions (15,16,17). A semiquantitative scale can be used to estimate the number of abnormal erythrocytes based on the average number per monolayer ×1000 field *(Table 17.1)*.

Mature avian erythrocytes generally are larger than mammalian erythrocytes but smaller than reptilian eryth-

TABLE 17.1 SEMIQUANTITATIVE MICROSCOPIC EVALUATION OF AVIAN ERYTHROCYTE MORPHOLOGY[a]

	1+	2+	3+	4+
Anisocytosis	5–10	11–20	21–30	>30
Polychromasia	2–10	11–14	15–30	>30
Hypochromasia	1–2	3–5	6–10	>10
Poikilocytosis	5–10	11–20	21–50	>50
Erythroplastids	1–2	3–5	6–10	>10

[a] Based on the average number of abnormal cells per ×1000 monolayer field.

rocytes. Avian erythrocytes vary in size depending on the species, but they generally range between 10.7×6.1 μm to $15.8 \times 10.2 \times$ μm (18). Mature avian erythrocytes are elliptical and have an elliptical, centrally positioned nucleus. Nuclear chromatin is uniformly clumped and becomes increasingly condensed with age. In Wright-stained blood films, the nucleus stains purple, whereas the cytoplasm stains orange-pink with a uniform texture *(Fig. 17.10)*.

Changes in the size of avian erythrocytes include microcytosis, macrocytosis, and anisocytosis. A significant change in the mean size of the erythrocyte is reflected in the mean corpuscular volume (MCV). The presence of macrocytes or microcytes also should be noted during assessment of the blood film. The degree of variation in the size of erythrocytes (anisocytosis) can be scored from 1+ to 4+ based on the number of variable-sized erythrocytes in a monolayer field (15) (Table 17.1). Erythrocyte

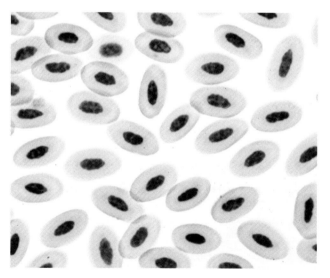

Figure 17.10 Normal erythrocytes in the blood film of a duck *(Glaucionette clangula)*. Modified Wright-Giemsa stain, 500×.

subpopulations have been reported in ducks, in which larger erythrocytes (MCV, 308 fL/cell) most likely represent those most recently released from the hematopoietic tissue and smaller cells (MCV, 128 fL/cell) most likely represent the older, aging cells (19).

Variations in erythrocyte color include polychromasia and hypochromasia. Polychromatophilic erythrocytes occur in low numbers (usually <5% of erythrocytes] in the peripheral blood of most normal birds. The degree of polychromasia can be graded according to the guideline presented in Table 17.1. The cytoplasm of polychromatophilic erythrocytes is weakly basophilic, and the nucleus is less condensed than in mature erythrocytes (Fig. 17.11) Polychromatophilic erythrocytes are similar in size to mature erythrocytes, and they appear as reticulocytes when stained with vital stains such as new methylene blue.

Reticulocytes are the penultimate cell in the erythrocyte maturation series, and their presence in the peripheral blood of normal birds suggests that the final stages of red-cell maturation occur in circulating blood. Determination of the reticulocyte concentration can be made by staining erythrocytes with a vital stain such as new methylene blue. Reticulocytes have a distinct ring of aggregated reticular material that encircles the nucleus (Fig. 17.12). As the cells mature, the amount of aggregated reticular material decreases and becomes more dispersed throughout the cytoplasm. With further maturation, the reticular material becomes nonaggregated, thereby resembling the "punctate" reticulocytes of felids. Most mature avian erythrocytes contain a varying amount of aggregate or punctate reticulum. Reticulocytes that reflect the current erythrocyte regenerative response, however,

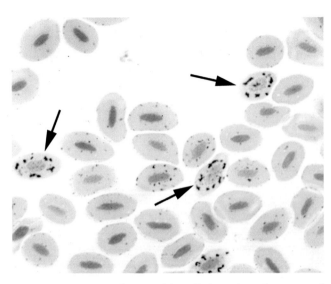

Figure 17.12 Reticulocyte with a distinct ring of aggregated reticulum encircling the red-cell nucleus in the blood film of an eagle (*Aquila chrysaetus*). Brilliant cresyl blue, 500×.

are those with a distinct ring of aggregated reticulum that encircles the red-cell nucleus (2,4).

Hypochromatic erythrocytes are abnormally pale in color compared with mature erythrocytes, and they have an area of cytoplasmic pallor that is greater than half the cytoplasmic volume (Fig. 17.13). They also may have cytoplasmic vacuoles and round, pyknotic nuclei. A significant hypochromasia is reflected as a decrease in the mean corpuscular hemoglobin concentration (MCHC) and mean corpuscular hemoglobin (MCH) values. The degree of hypochromasia can be estimated using the scale presented in Table 17.2.

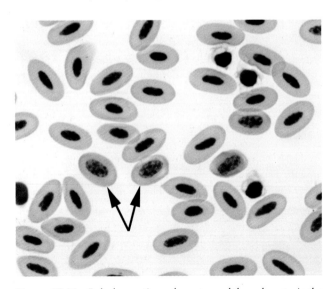

Figure 17.11 Polychromatic erythrocytes and thrombocytes in the blood film of an owl (*Strix vaira*). Modified Wright-Giemsa stain, 500×.

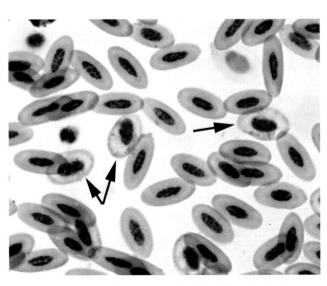

Figure 17.13 Hypochromasia in the blood film of a duck (*Netta rufina*). Modified Wright-Giemsa stain, 500×.

TABLE 17.2 NATT-HERRICK SOLUTION AND STAIN[a]	
Sodium chloride (NaCl)	3.88 g
Sodium sulfate (NaSO₄)	2.50 g
Sodium phosphate (Na₂HPO₄)	1.74 g
Potassium phosphate (KH₂PO₄)	0.25 g
Formalin (37%)	7.50 mL
Methyl violet	0.10 g

[a] Bring to 1000 mL with distilled water and then filter through Whatman #10 medium-filter paper.

In most species of birds, the shape of erythrocytes is relatively uniform. The degree of poikilocytosis can be estimated using the scale outlined in Table 17.1.

Atypical erythrocytes occasionally are present in the peripheral blood of normal birds, and such erythrocytes may represent artifacts associated with preparation of the blood film. Careful examination of erythrocyte morphology may reveal significant clues in the detection of disorders affecting avian erythrocytes. As mentioned, the degree of polychromasia and reticulocytosis and the presence of immature erythrocytes in the peripheral blood aid in the assessment of red-blood-cell regeneration. The presence of many hypochromatic erythrocytes (i.e., 2+ hypochromasia or greater) indicates an erythrocyte disorder such as iron deficiency.

Atypical erythrocytes may vary in both size and shape. A slight variation in the size of erythrocytes (1+ anisocytosis) is considered to be normal for birds. A greater degree of anisocytosis, however, usually is observed in birds with a regenerative anemia and is associated with polychromasia. Likewise, minor deviations from the normal shape of avian erythrocytes (1+ poikilocytosis) is considered to be normal in the peripheral blood of birds, but marked poikilocytosis may indicate erythrocytic dysgenesis. Round erythrocytes with oval nuclei occasionally are found in the blood films of anemic birds and suggest a dysmaturation of the cell cytoplasm and nucleus, which may be a result of accelerated erythropoiesis.

The nucleus may vary in its cellular location and contain indentions, protrusions, or constrictions. Anucleated erythrocytes (erythroplastids) or cytoplasmic fragments occasionally are found in normal avian blood films *(Fig. 17.14)*. The nucleus may contain chromophobic streaking, which suggests chromatolysis, or achromic bands, which indicate nuclear fracture with displacement of the fragments (1). Mitotic activity associated with erythrocytes in blood films suggests a marked regenerative response or erythrocytic dyscrasia *(Fig. 17.15)*. Perinuclear rings are common artifacts of improper slide preparation

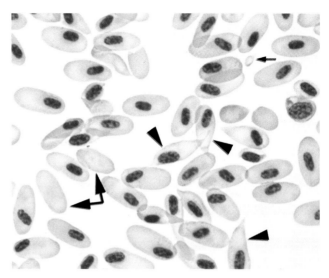

Figure 17.14 Erythroplastids (large arrows), erythrocyte fragments (small arrow), and dactylocytes (arrow head) in a blood film with marked anisocytosis and poikilocytosis from a lovebird (*Agapornis roseicollis*). Modified Wright-Giemsa stain, 500×.

(e.g., exposure to solvent or formalin fumes, or allowing the slide to dry too slowly), and they represent nuclear shrinkage. Clear, irregular, refractile spaces in the cytoplasm occur when blood films are allowed to dry too slowly. This artifact, which is a form of erythrocyte crenation, should not be confused with avian blood parasites, such as gametocytes of *Hemoproteus* and *Plasmodium* (2). Disruption or smudging of avian erythrocytes is the most common artifact of slide preparation. Severely ruptured cells result in the presence of purple, amorphous nuclear material in the blood film.

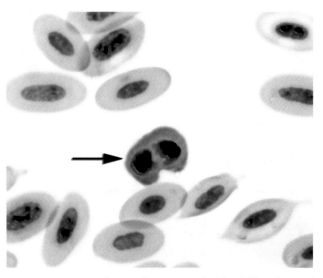

Figure 17.15 Dividing erythrocytes in the blood film of an owl (*Nyctea scandiaca*). Modified Wright-Giemsa stain, 500×.

Binucleate erythrocytes rarely occur in the blood films of normal birds. Large numbers of binucleated erythrocytes plus other features of red-blood-cell dyscrasia, however, suggest neoplastic, viral, or genetic disease (20).

Punctate basophilia is characterized by punctate aggregations of small, irregular, basophilic-staining granules throughout the cytoplasm of erythrocytes in Wright-stained smears. As in mammalian hematology, punctate basophilia is most likely associated with degenerative changes in ribosomal ribonucleic acid and is indicative of a response to anemia or, rarely, lead poisoning. Basophilic stippling can be affected by preparation and staining of the blood film. Using fresh blood without an anticoagulant or rapid drying of blood films made from EDTA-anticoagulated blood provides the best films for demonstrating basophilic stippling (21). Such stippling is less apparent when alcohol fixation of blood is used. Heinz bodies rarely are reported in birds and are the result of hemoglobin denaturation (oxidized hemoglobin) (22). Heinz bodies appear as round to irregularly shaped, pale-blue, cytoplasmic inclusions with new methylene blue stain; as round to irregular inclusions of densely stained hemoglobin with Wright stain; or as refractile inclusions in unstained erythrocytes. Agglutination of erythrocytes in blood films also is a rare, abnormal finding.

Laboratory Evaluation

Laboratory evaluation of avian erythrocytes involves the same routine procedures as that used in mammalian hematology, but with a few modifications. The standard manual technique for using microhematocrit capillary tubes and centrifugation (12,000 g for 5 min) can be used to obtain a PCV (i.e., hematocrit). Hemoglobin concentration is determined by the cyanmethemoglobin method with one modification: the free nuclei from lysed erythrocytes must be removed by centrifugation of the cyanmethemoglobin reagent–blood mixture before obtaining the optical density value to avoid overestimation of the hemoglobin concentration.

The total erythrocyte concentration in birds can be determined using the same automated or manual methods as those used for determinating total erythrocyte counts in mammalian blood. Automated cell counters (Coulter counter, Coulter Corporation, Miami, FL) provide a rapid, reliable method for obtaining total red-blood-cell concentrations. Two manual methods for obtaining total red-blood-cell count in birds are the erythrocyte Unopette (Becton-Dickinson) method used in mammalian hematology and the Natt-Herrick method, which involves preparation of Natt-Herrick solution to be used as a stain and diluent (23) (Table 17.2). A 1:200 dilution of the blood is made using the Natt and Herrick solution and red-blood-cell diluting pipettes. After mixing, the diluted

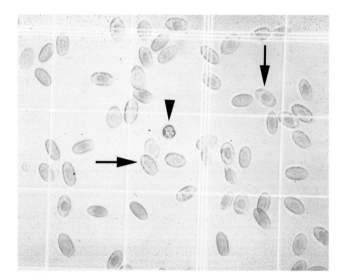

Figure 17.16   Appearance of erythrocytes (arrows) and a leukocytes (arrow head) in a hemocytometer using the erythrocyte Unopette method, 250×.

blood is discharged into a hemacytometer counting chamber, and the cells are allowed to settle for 5 minutes, to the ruled surface, before counting. Erythrocytes located in the four corner and the central squares of the hemacytometer chamber are counted when using either of the manual methods *(Figs. 17.16 and 17.17).* The number obtained then is multiplied by 10,000 to calculate the total red-blood-cell count per cubic millimeter (mm³) of blood.

The MCV, MCH, and MCHC also can be calculated for avian hematology using the same formulas as those used for mammals.

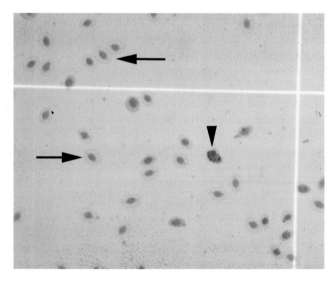

Figure 17.17   Appearance of erythrocytes (arrows) and a granulocyte (arrow head) in a hemocytometer using Natt and Herrick method, 250×.

Normal Erythrocyte Physiology

The total erythrocyte concentration and PCV of birds are influenced by age, sex, hormonal influences, hypoxia, environmental factors, and disease (19). In general, the total erythrocyte count and PCV increase with age and are higher in male than female birds. Estrogen depresses erythropoiesis, whereas androgens and thyroxin stimulate erythropoiesis (19). Birds, like mammals, respond to blood loss and blood destruction by increasing erythropoietin production, which stimulates erythropoiesis. Avian erythropoietin, which is a glycoprotein produced by the kidney, acts directly on the bone marrow to increase erythrocyte production. Avian erythropoietin does not stimulate mammalian erythropoiesis, however, and mammalian erythropoietin has no effect on avian hematopoiesis (19).

Avian hemoglobin has four iron-containing heme subunits, as with mammalian hemoglobin, but the protein moieties (i.e., globulins) are different (19). In avian erythrocytes, the phosphate compounds influencing the affinity of hemoglobin for oxygen also differ from those in mammals. The hemoglobin of mature birds contains myoinositol pentophosphate, not the 2,3-diphosglycerate as in mammals (24). Inositol pentophosphate causes hemoglobin to have a lower affinity for oxygen, and it shifts the oxygen dissociation curve to the right of the mammalian curve. Therefore, avian tissues can extract oxygen more readily from hemoglobin than mammalian tissues can.

Responses in Disease

The PCV is the quickest and most practical method for evaluating the red-cell mass of birds. As in mammals, the PCV in birds is affected by the number and size of the erythrocytes as well as by changes in the plasma volume that do not affect the actual cell concentrations. These include increased plasma volume (hemodilution), decreased plasma volume (hemoconcentration), improper blood sampling (hemodilution), and epinephrine administration and hypothermia, which may result in hemoconcentration. The normal PCV for many species of birds ranges between 35% and 55%. Therefore, a PCV of less than 35% suggests anemia, and a PCV of greater than 55% suggests dehydration or erythrocytosis (polycythemia). The latter condition can be differentiated by the total serum protein: increased total protein indicates dehydration, whereas normal or low total protein indicates erythrocytosis.

Typically, polychromatic erythrocytes make up 5% or less of the erythrocyte population in blood films from normal birds. The degree of erythrocyte polychromasia and reticulocytosis indicates the degree of erythrogenesis. Anemic birds with greater than 10% polychromasia (3+ and 4+ polychromasia) are exhibiting an appropriate regen-

erative response to their anemia. Those with a smaller response, however, are not. The number of reticulocytes also indicates a bird's current response to anemia. Therefore, the reticulocyte count can be used in conjunction with assessment of the degree of polychromasia to determine the bird's current erythropoietic response.

Other evidence of active erythropoiesis is the presence of binucleate, immature erythrocytes and an increased number of normal, immature erythrocytes in the peripheral blood. Immature erythrocytes (i.e., rubricytes) in peripheral blood films in addition to increased polychromasia indicates a marked erythrocyte response *(Fig. 17.18)*. In cases of nonanemic birds, however, these cells indicate abnormal erythropoiesis. Immature erythrocytes also may suggest early release from the hematopoietic tissue after anoxic insult or toxicity (i.e., lead poisoning).

The causes of anemia in birds include blood loss [hemorrhagic anemia], increased red cell destruction [hemolytic anemia], and decreased red cell production [depression anemia]. The most common causes of hemorrhagic anemia in birds include traumatic injury, blood-sucking parasites, coagulopathies, and hemorrhagic lesions of internal organs, such as ulcerated neoplasms, gastric ulcerations, and rupture of the liver or spleen. Heavy infestation with blood-sucking ectoparasites such as ticks or mites (i.e., *Dermanyssus* mites) or with gastrointestinal parasites such as coccidia can lead to severe blood loss anemia in birds. Coagulopathies that result in blood loss anemia usually are acquired and often are associated with toxicities such as aflatoxicosis or coumarin poisoning or severe liver disease such as papovavirus infections (25–28). Birds can tolerate acute blood loss better than

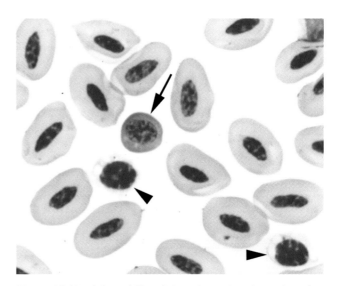

Figure 17.18 A basophilic rubricyte (arrow) and two thrombocytes (arrow heads) in a blood film of an eagle (*Aquila chrysaetus*). Modified Wright-Giemsa stain, 500×.

mammals, and diving and flying birds are more resistant to blood loss than nondiving birds such as galliformes. The mobilization and restoration of fluid during the first 90 minutes after bleeding in chickens is approximately 13% to 17% of the initial blood volume per hour, which is twice that of dogs (19).

Hemolytic anemia can result from parasitemias, septicemia, and toxicities. Most avian blood parasites have the potential to cause anemia in the host; however, the two parasites that most frequently are associated with hemolytic anemia are *Plasmodium* and *Aegyptianella*. Salmonellosis or spirochetosis commonly cause bacterial septicemia that results in severe hemolytic anemia (29). Toxicoses that lead to increased erythrocyte destruction include aflatoxins, certain plant chemicals (i.e., mustards), and petroleum products (30–32). Ingestion of petroleum products may produce a Heinz body anemia. Hemolytic anemia occurs in marine birds associated with oil pollution and is characterized by low red-cell indices and numerous immature erythrocytes (33). Although rare, immune-mediated anemia may result in hemolysis, with red-cell agglutination being present in the blood film (4). Hemolytic anemias typically are characterized by a marked regenerative response (34). Although hemochromatosis usually does not affect the hemogram, one report in a psittacine with hemochromatosis indicated a severe anemia with a marked regenerative response (4+ polychromasia and immature erythrocytes as early as prorubricytes) (35). The hemochromatosis may have altered the maturation of erythrocytes as a result of defective iron uptake.

A nonregenerative, normocytic, normochromic anemia indicates decreased erythropoiesis (depression anemia), which can develop rapidly in birds with inflammatory diseases, especially those involving infectious agents. Birds appear to develop anemias from a lack of erythropoiesis more quickly than mammals, perhaps because of the relatively short erythrocyte half-life in birds compared with that in mammals (36,37). Although the avian erythrocyte life span varies with the species, it is generally shorter than those in mammals. For example, the erythrocyte life span is 28 to 35 days in chickens, 42 days in pigs, 35 to 45 days in pigeons, and 33 to 35 days in quails (37). The degree of polychromasia or reticulocytosis is poor to absent in birds with depression anemias. Disorders frequently associated with depression anemia in birds include tuberculosis, aspergillosis, chlamydiosis, chronic hepatic or renal disease, hypothyroidism, neoplasia, and other chronic inflammatory diseases (27,38).

Hypochromasia can be seen with iron deficiency, chronic inflammatory diseases, and lead toxicosis (4,39). Chronic lead toxicosis also may be associated with an inappropriate release of normal-appearing, immature erythrocytes into the peripheral blood of nonanemic birds *(Fig. 17.19)*. In this condition, the blood film reveals small,

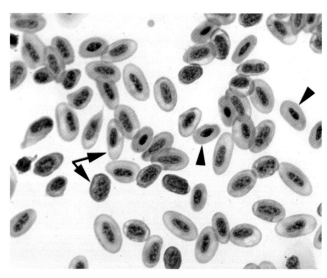

Figure 17.19 Marked numbers of immature erythrocytes in a blood film of a duck (*Anas platyrhynchos*) with a normal packed cells volume (42%). This duck has lead poisoning. Wright stain, 250×.

senescent, mature erythrocytes with pyknotic nuclei and immature erythrocytes (usually rubricytes) without the presence of normal, mature erythrocytes. This hematologic response resembles the inappropriate release of nucleated erythrocytes in the blood of nonanemic dogs affected by chronic lead poisoning. Basophilic stippling in the cytoplasm of erythrocytes may be seen with lead poisoning in birds, but this is rare. Stippled basophilia more commonly is associated with erythrocyte regeneration and hypochromic anemia. Hypochromasia also is associated with nutritional deficiencies, especially iron deficiency anemia. Hypochromatic erythrocytes frequently appear in the blood films from birds with chronic inflammatory diseases, presumably related to iron sequestration as part of the bird's defense against infectious agents. In such cases, hypochromatic cells often are observed in blood films before the red-cell indices (MCHC and MCH) suggest hypochromasia *(Fig. 17.20)*.

A macrocytic, normochromic anemia occurs in birds with food restriction or folic acid deficiency (40). Folic acid deficiency causes defective DNA synthesis, thereby causing nuclear maturation to be out of step with hemoglobinization of the cytoplasm (41). Food restriction anemia also is associated with leukopenia, thrombocytopenia, abnormal erythrocyte shapes (marked poikilocytosis), and hypersegmentation of granulocytes (40).

Erythrocytosis (polycythemia) rarely is reported in birds (42). The conditions that are associated with polycythemia in mammals most likely cause polycythemia in birds as well. A primary erythrocytosis is a myeloproliferative disorder resulting in an absolute erythrocytosis.

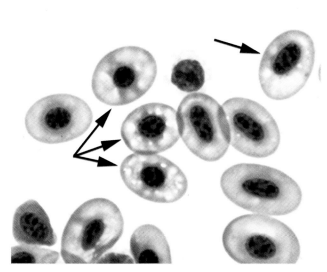

Figure 17.20 Hypochromatic erythrocytes in the blood film of a domestic goose (*Anser anser*) with a marked inflammatory leukogram. Wright stain, 500×.

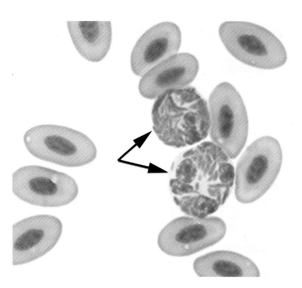

Figure 17.21 Normal heterophils in the blood film of an eagle (*Aquila chrysaetus*). Modified Wright-Giemsa stain, 500×.

Most reported cases of an absolute erythrocytosis (PCV, usually >70%) in birds are secondary and associated with chronic pulmonary disease. Cardiac insufficiency, however, also may result in an erythrocytosis. An increase in erythropoietin associated with renal disease is another causative consideration for this disorder. A relative erythrocytosis associated with dehydration is responsible for most avian cases with an erythrocytosis.

The presence of numerous immature erythrocytes (especially rubriblasts) and abnormal-appearing immature erythrocytes in the peripheral blood of birds indicates erythrocytic neoplasia. Erythroblastosis in poultry with avian leukosis complex is an example of this condition.

LEUKOCYTES

Morphology

Leukopoiesis in normal birds appears to be similar to that in mammals, in that leukocytes are released into the peripheral circulation only when they are mature. Leukocytes in avian blood include lymphocytes, monocytes, and granulocytes. The granulocytes are classified as heterophils, eosinophils, and basophils. Heterophils are the most abundant granulocyte in most birds. The cytoplasm of normal, mature heterophils appears colorless and contains eosinophilic granules (dark orange to brown-red) with Romanowsky stains *(Fig. 17.21)*. The cytoplasmic granules typically are elongate (rod or spiculated shaped), but they may appear oval to round in some species. Heterophil granules frequently have a distinct central body that

appears to be refractile. The granules may be affected by the staining process and appear atypical (i.e., poorly stained, partially dissolved, or fused). The nucleus of mature heterophils is lobed (usually two to three lobes) with coarse, clumped chromatin that stains purple. The nucleus often is partially hidden by the cytoplasmic granules.

Avian heterophils are functionally equivalent to mammalian neutrophils. They actively participate in inflammatory lesions, and they are phagocytic (43,44). The cytoplasmic granules of heterophils contain lysozyme and proteins needed for bactericidal activity, although some avian species, such as chickens, have heterophils that lack peroxidase activity (45–48). Heterophils phagocytize microorganisms and destroy them by oxygen-dependent and -independent mechanisms. Although chicken heterophils lack the alkaline phosphatase, catalase, and myeloperoxidase needed for oxygen-dependent killing of microorganisms, they do consume oxygen and produce oxygen radicals and hydrogen peroxide, but to a lesser extent than in mammalian neutrophils (49). Therefore, avian heterophils rely more heavily on oxygen-independent mechanisms, lysozyme, and cationic proteins (i.e., acid hydrolases and cathepsin) to destroy microorganisms (49).

Ultrastructural studies of avian heterophils reveal primary, secondary, and tertiary granules (50). Primary granules are the most numerous, and they appear as electron-dense, fusiform rods (1.5×0.5 μ) with a circular central body. Secondary granules (diameter, 0.5 μ) are less dense and contain eccentric inclusions composed of loose, filamentous material. Tertiary granules (0.1 μm) have a dense core that is separated from a membranous envelope of an electron-luscent area. Based on the results of biochemical evaluations of chicken heterophils, myeloperoxidase and alkaline phosphatase also are absent (47,48). Chicken heterophil granules do not stain with alkaline phosphatase, peroxidase, Sudan black B, acid phosphatase, naphthol AS-D chloroacetate esterase methods, or periodic acid-Schiff (51). Small and medium granules may be seen ultrastructurally in avian heterophils, and these probably represent maturation stages of the cytoplasmic granules (50).

Abnormal appearing heterophils in blood films include both immature and toxic heterophils. Immature heterophils have increased cytoplasmic basophilia, non-segmented nuclei, and immature cytoplasmic granules compared with normal, mature heterophils *(Fig. 17.22)*. Immature heterophils most frequently encountered in the blood are myelocytes and metamyelocytes. Heterophil myelocytes are larger than mature heterophils, and they have blue cytoplasm as well as secondary, rod-shaped granules, which occupy less than half the cytoplasmic volume, and a round to oval, nonsegmented nucleus. Heterophil metamyelocytes resemble myelocytes, except that the nucleus is indented and the rod-shaped granules occupy more than half the cytoplasmic volume. Band heterophils resemble mature heterophils, except that the nucleus is not lobed. It often is difficult to recognize a band cell, because the nucleus is hidden by the cytoplasmic granules. Therefore, a true assessment regarding the concentration of band cells in avian blood films requires use of a nuclear stain, such as hematoxylin, which stains only the nucleus and not the cytoplasmic granules.

In response to severe systemic illness, avian heterophils exhibit toxic changes similar to those in mammalian neutrophils (2,11,12). Toxic changes in avian heterophils are subjectively quantified as to the number of toxic cells and

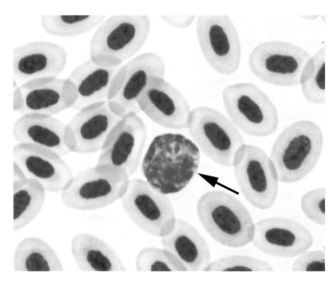

Figure 17.23   Mildly toxic (1+) heterophils in the blood film of a robin (*Turdus migratorius*). Wright stain, 500×.

the severity of toxicity, as in mammalian hematology (15). Toxic heterophils have increased cytoplasmic basophilia, vacuolization, abnormal granulation (degranulation, granules that appear deeply basophilic, and granules that appear to coalesce into large, round granules), and degeneration of the cell nucleus *(Figs. 17.23 through 17.26)*. The degree of heterophil toxicity can be rated subjectively on a scale of 1+ to 4+. A 1+ degree of toxicity is assigned when heterophils exhibit increased cytoplasmic basophilia. A 2+ degree of toxicity is assigned when heterophils have deeper cytoplasmic basophilia and partial degranulation. A 3+ degree of toxicity is assigned when heterophils

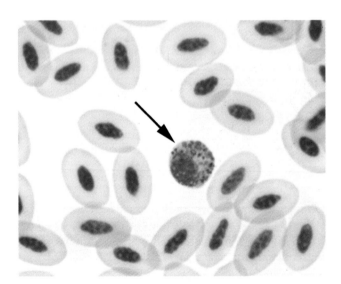

Figure 17.22   A toxic heterophil myelocyte in the blood film of a parrot (*Amazona viridigenalis*). Wright stain, 500×.

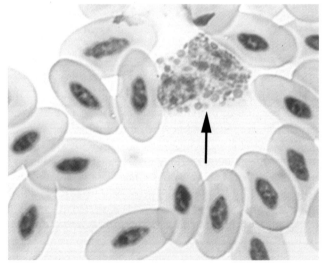

Figure 17.24   A heterophil with marked toxicity (3+) in the blood film of an ostrich (*Struthio camelus*). Wright stain, 500×.

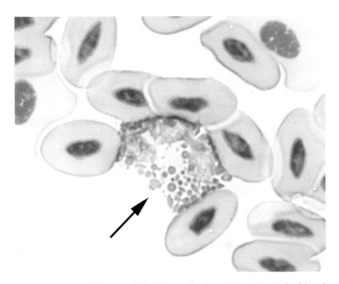

Figure 17.25 A heterophil with marked toxicity (4+) in the blood film of an ostrich (*Struthio camelus*). Wright stain, 500×.

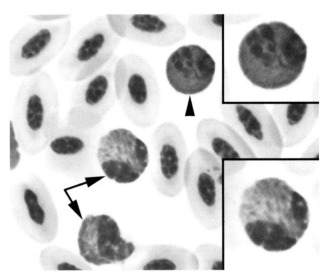

Figure 17.27 Heterophils (arrows) and an eosinophil (arrow head) in the blood film of an owl (*Bubo virginianus*). Modified Wright-Giemsa stain, 500×.

exhibit deep cytoplasmic basophilia, moderate degranulation, abnormal granules, and cytoplasmic vacuolization, and a 4+ degree of toxicity is assigned when heterophils exhibit deep cytoplasmic basophilia, moderate to marked degranulation with abnormal granules, cytoplasmic vacuolization, and karyorrhexis or karyolysis. The number of toxic heterophils are graded as few (5–10%), moderate (11–30%), and marked (>30%).

Most avian eosinophils are the same size as heterophils but have round, strongly eosinophilic cytoplasmic granules, although the granules in some species are oval to elongate. In general, eosinophil granules stain more in-

tensely that heterophil granules *(Figs. 17.27 and 17.28)*. The cytoplasmic granules of eosinophils lack the central, refractile body seen in many avian heterophils. The cytoplasm of eosinophils stains clear blue, in contrast to the colorless cytoplasm of normal, mature heterophils. The nuclei of eosinophils are lobed and usually stain darker than heterophil nuclei. The cytoplasmic granules of eosinophils frequently are affected by Romanowsky stains. The granules may appear to be large, swollen, and round, and they also may appear colorless or to stain pale blue *(Fig. 17.29)*. Eosinophils vary in appearance species of birds (4,52).

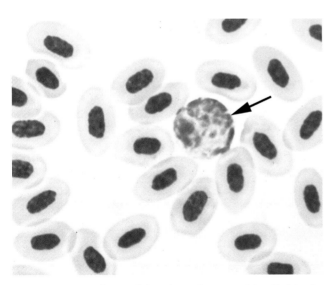

Figure 17.26 A heterophil with moderate toxicity (2+) in the blood film of a robin (*Turdus migratorius*). Wright stain, 500×.

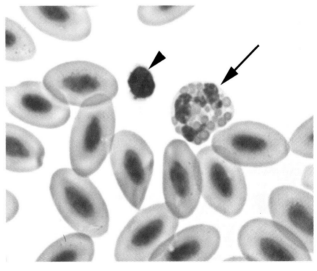

Figure 17.28 An eosinophil (arrow) and a thrombocyte (arrow head) in the blood film of a flamingo (*Phoenicopterus ruber*). Wright stain, 500×.

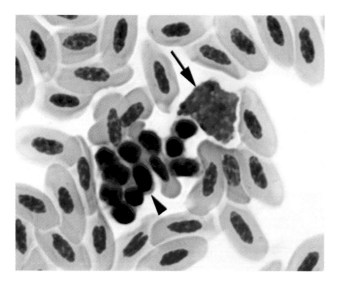

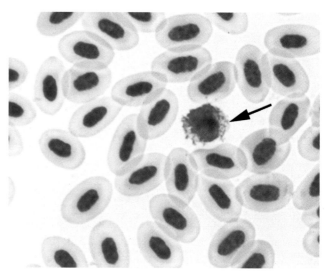

Figure 17.29 An eosinophil with blue-staining granules and clumped thrombocytes in the blood film of a parrot (*Psitticus erithacus*). Wright stain, 500×.

Figure 17.30. A basophil in the blood film from a robin (*Turdus migratorius*). Wright stain, 500×.

The ultrastructure of avian eosinophils reveals large, spherical, primary granules and mature, rod-shaped, specific granules. In some birds, the specific granules possess a crystalline core (50). The larger primary granules most likely are precursors to the smaller, specific granules. Similar to mammalian eosinophils, specific granules possess a high concentration of arginine and enzymes, such as peroxidase, acid phosphatase, and arylsulfatase (50). Cytochemical staining of chicken eosinophils indicate a positive reactivity for peroxidase, acid phosphatase, and Sudan black B (51). Therefore, these reactions can be used to distinguish eosinophils from heterophils.

Avian basophils contain deeply metachromic granules that often obscure the nucleus. The nucleus usually is nonlobed, thereby causing avian basophils to resemble mammalian mast cells (*Figs. 17.30 and 17.31*). The cytoplasmic granules of basophils frequently are affected by alcohol-solubilized stains, and they may partially dissolve or coalesce and appear abnormal in blood films stained with Romanowsky stains. Avian basophils frequently are found in the peripheral blood, in contrast to mammalian basophils, which rarely are found in the blood films of normal animals. The function of avian basophils is not known. However, it is presumed to be similar to that of mammalian basophils and mast cells, because their cytoplasmic granules contain histamine (50,53). They also participate in acute inflammatory and type IV hypersensitivity reactions (54,55).

Avian lymphocytes resemble mammalian lymphocytes. Typically, they are round cells that often show cytoplasmic irregularity when they mold around adjacent erythrocytes in the blood film (*Figs. 17.32 through 17.34*). Lym-

phocytes have a round, occasionally slightly indented, centrally or slightly eccentrically positioned nucleus. The nuclear chromatin is heavily clumped or reticulated in mature lymphocytes, and the cytoplasm typically is scant, except in large lymphocytes, thereby giving lymphocytes their high nucleus:cytoplasm (N:C) ratio. Large lymphocytes of birds resemble those found in bovine blood films. Large lymphocytes can be confused with monocytes, however, because of their size, cytoplasmic volume, and pale-staining nuclei. The lymphocyte cytoplasm usually appears to be homogenous and weakly basophilic (pale blue), and it lacks both vacuoles and granules. Cyto-

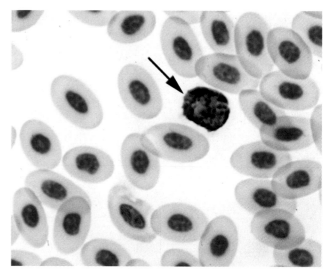

Figure 17.31 A basophil in the blood film from a chicken (*Gallus gallus formadomestica*). Modified Wright-Giemsa stain, 500×.

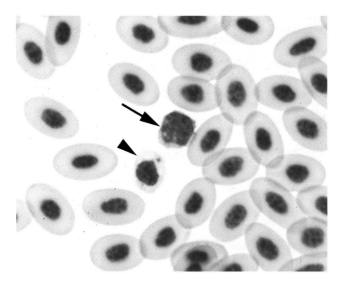

Figure 17.32 A small lymphocyte (arrow) and thrombocyte (arrow head) in the blood film of a chicken (*Gallus gallus formadomestica*). Wright stain, 500×.

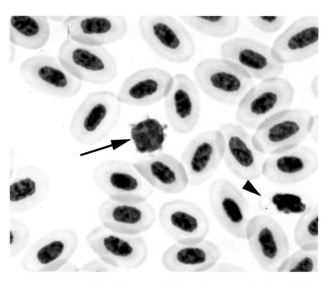

Figure 17.34 A lymphocyte and thrombocyte in the blood film of a robin (*Turdus migratorius*) Wright stain, 500×.

plasmic features are important when differentiating small lymphocytes from thrombocytes. The latter have clear, colorless cytoplasm that often appears to be vacuolated, with a few distinct specific granules. Occasionally, cells in the blood films of birds have features of both thrombocytes and lymphocytes. These intermediate cells have small, round to oval nuclei with coarsely clumped chromatin and moderately abundant, blue-tinged cytoplasm that lacks both vacuoles and granules. Cytochemical properties indicate these cells to be lymphocytes (56). Occasionally, lymphocytes may contain distinct azurophilic granules or irregular cytoplasmic projections.

Abnormal lymphocytes are classified as either reactive or blast-transformed lymphocytes. Reactive lymphocytes are small to medium lymphocytes with heavily clumped nuclear chromatin and deeply basophilic cytoplasm. Lymphocytes develop into reactive lymphocytes when antigenically stimulated. Blast-transformed lymphocytes are large lymphocytes with dispersed, smooth nuclear chromatin, which may contain nucleoli *(Figs. 17.35 and 17.36)*. They have basophilic cytoplasm that may exhibit a prominent, clear, perinuclear halo or Golgi zone. These lymphocytes have anaplastic features and may be neoplastic, but they also may result from immunologic stimulation (15).

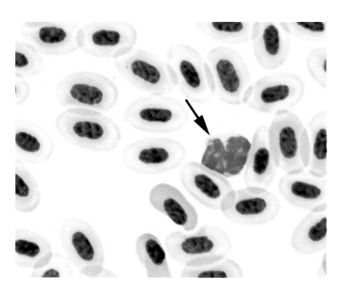

Figure 17.33 A lymphocyte with a cleft nucleus in the blood film of a robin (*Turdus migratorius*). Wright stain, 500×.

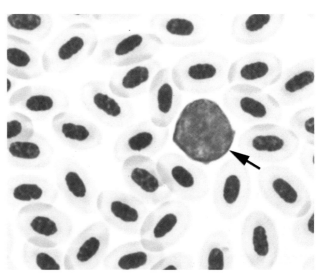

Figure 17.35 A reactive lymphocyte in the blood film of a parrot (*Amazona aestiva*). Wright stain, 500×.

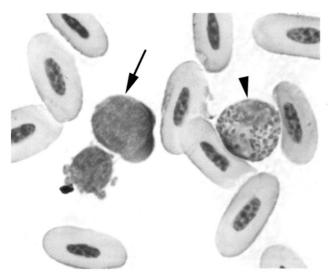

Figure 17.36 A reactive lymphocyte (arrow); small, mature lymphocyte; and heterophil (arrow head) in the blood film of a penguin (*Spheniscus demersus*). Wright stain, 500×.

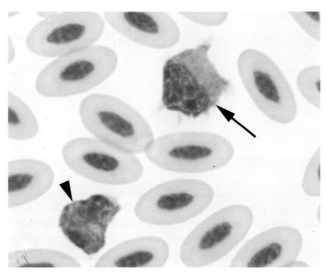

Figure 17.38 A monocyte (arrow) and a heterophil (arrow head) in the blood film of a cockatoo (*Cacatua moluccensis*). Wright stain, 500×.

Plasma cells also can be found in the peripheral blood of birds. These are large B lymphocytes with eccentrically positioned mature nuclei; abundant, deeply basophilic cytoplasm; and a distinct Golgi zone. Lymphocytes that contain prominent azurophilic granules are also considered to be reactive.

Avian monocytes typically are the largest leukocyte, and they resemble their mammalian counterpart, varying in shape from round to ameboid. Monocytes have abundant, blue-gray cytoplasm that may appear to be slightly opaque, and they contain vacuoles or fine, dust-like eosinophilic granules *(Figs. 17.37 and 17.38)*. Avian monocytes frequently exhibit two distinct zones in the cytoplasm: a light-staining perinuclear area, and a darker-staining area. The monocyte nucleus can vary in shape and is relatively pale, with less chromatin clumping compared with lymphocyte nuclei. The ultrastructure of avian monocytes and macrophages reveals a cytoplasmic membrane that is composed of blebs or filaments, a prominent Golgi apparatus, many ribosomes, and a variable number of pinocytic vesicles and lysosomes (50). Monocytes exhibit phagocytic activity and migrate into tissues to become macrophages (57). They possess biologically active chemicals that are involved in inflammation and destruction of invading organisms. Monocytes also have an important immunologic role in antigen processing (50).

Laboratory Evaluation

The presence of nucleated erythrocytes and thrombocytes in avian blood precludes use of the routine methods used to count leukocytes in mammalian blood. Automated methods for counting white blood cells in mammalian blood produce erroneous results when applied to avian blood, because all the cells in the peripheral blood of birds are nucleated. Also, the size of the erythrocytes is similar to the size of many of the leukocytes; thrombocytes and small lymphocytes also are similar in size. Therefore, direct and semidirect, manual methods for obtaining total leukocyte concentrations in birds have been developed. A commonly used semidirect method involves the staining of avian heterophils and eosinophils with phloxine B as the diluent. Phloxine B commonly is used as a specific stain for eosinophils in mammalian blood. The procedure is simplified by using the Eosinophil Unopette 5877 system (Becton-Dickinson), which was developed for determining total eosinophil concentrations in mammalian blood (58).

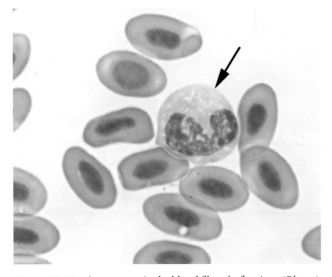

Figure 17.37 A monocyte in the blood film of a flamingo (*Phoenicopterus ruber*). Modified Wright-Giemsa stain, 500×.

The blood is diluted 1 : 32 with the phloxine B solution in the Unopette vial using the 25-µL pipette that is provided. After a Neubauer-ruled hemacytometer chamber has been properly loaded with the blood–phloxine mixture and allowed to stand in a humid chamber for a minimum of 5 minutes, the eosin-stained heterophils and eosinophils are counted in both sides of the chamber (18 large squares) *(Fig. 17.39)*. The hemacytometer should be loaded immediately after proper mixing of the blood and phloxine diluent, because red blood cells also may stain after prolonged exposure. The total heterophil and eosinophil concentration per cubic millimeter of blood (heterophils + eosinophils/mm³) is calculated using the formula for obtaining a total eosinophil count in mammalian blood:

$$\text{Heterophils} + \text{Eosinophils}/\text{mm}^3 = \frac{\text{Cells counted} \times 10 \times 32}{18}$$

The total leukocyte concentration (TWBC/mm³) is calculated after completing a leukocyte differential using the following formula:

$$\text{TWBC}/\text{mm}^3 = \frac{\left(\text{Heterophils} + \text{Eosinophils}/\text{mm}^3\right) \times 100}{\%\,\text{Heterophils and eosinophils}}$$

The TWBC/mm³ can be obtained using one calculation with the following formula:

$$\text{TWBC}/\text{mm}^3 = \frac{\text{Eosin-stained cells} \times 1.111 \times 16 \times 100}{\%\,\text{Heterophils and eosinophils}}$$

where the number of eosin-stained cells are counted in both sides of the hemacytometer (18 large squares).

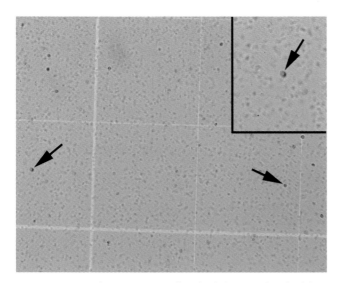

Figure 17.39 The appearance of acidophils stained with phloxine dye in a hemocytometer chamber, 100×.

A direct method for obtaining total leukocyte concentrations in avian blood is to make a 1 : 200 dilution with Natt-Herrick solution (Table 17.2) using a standard red blood cell–diluting pipette or by adding 20 µL of blood to 4 mL of the Natt-Herrick solution (Fig. 17.17). The total leukocyte concentration is obtained by counting all the leukocytes (dark-blue cells) in the nine large squares in the ruled area of the hemacytometer chamber using the following formula:

$$\text{TWBC}/\text{mm}^3 = (\text{Total cells in nine large squares} + 10\%) \times 200$$

The advantage to this method is that a total erythrocyte and thrombocyte count also can be obtained using the same charged hemacytometer. A disadvantage is that differentiating thrombocytes from small lymphocytes often is difficult, thus creating errors in the counts. Staining for 60 minutes in the Natt-Herrick solution, however, improves the differentiation between small lymphocytes and thrombocytes (59).

A second method for obtaining a direct total leukocyte count in birds is to dilute the anticoagulated blood 1 : 100 with 0.01% toluidine blue in phosphate-buffered saline before charging a Neubauer-ruled hemocytometer (60,61). Cells that are equal to or larger than the width of the erythrocytes are counted in the nine large squares of the hemacytometer. The total leukocyte count is calculated using the standard formula:

$$\text{TWBC}/\text{mm}^3 = \frac{\text{No. of cells} \times 10 \times 100}{9}$$

Or, to simplify the math,

$$\text{TWBC}/\text{mm}^3 = (\text{Number of cells} + 10\%) \times 100$$

Toluidine blue stains leukocytes blue, erythrocytes pale orange, and thrombocytes pale blue. Counting cells that are equal to or larger than the width of erythrocytes should rule out thrombocytes, which tend to be smaller in width than erythrocytes. Small lymphocytes tend to be equal to or larger than the width of erythrocytes. Immature erythrocytes are distinguished from small lymphocytes by their round to irregular shape; their round, centrally positioned nucleus with dark, irregularly clumped chromatin; and their moderate volume of basophilic hyalin cytoplasm. A corrected total leukocyte concentration can be obtained when a large number of immature erythrocytes are present by using the following formula:

$$\text{Corrected WBC}/\text{mm}^3 = \frac{\text{TWBC} \times 100}{100 + \text{No. of immature RBCs per 100 leukocytes}}$$

With counting methods requiring use of a hemocytometer, the difference between the counts obtained from each chamber should not exceed 10% to ensure accuracy between the two sides. If the difference does exceed 10%, the procedure should be repeated. The semidirect method using the phloxine stain is easier to perform and is more precise for hemocytometer counting than the Natt and Herrick method (62). To our knowledge, no comparisons have been made for the toluidine blue method; however, the results should be similar to those with the Natt and Herrick method. Because the semidirect method using phloxine B stain for determination of total leukocyte counts in birds depends on the leukocyte differential, especially the number of heterophils and eosinophils, it becomes less accurate as the level of mononuclear leukocytes exceeds that of the granulocytes.

Crude estimation of the cell numbers from blood films is an inappropriate method for obtaining a total leukocyte count in birds. Estimated leukocyte counts should be used only when quantitative counts (i.e., phloxine B, Natt and Herrick, or toluidine blue methods) are unavailable or as a means of detecting submission or laboratory error (e.g., if the number of leukocytes observed in a blood film appears to be less than that reported from a quantitative count) (15).

Crude estimation of the leukocyte concentration in a well-prepared blood film is made by obtaining the average number of leukocytes in five monolayer ×1000 (oil-immersion) fields and using the following formula:

$$\text{Estimated WBC/mm}^3 = \frac{\text{Average no. of WBC}}{1000}$$

The number 1000 is the average number of erythrocytes in five monolayer ×1000 fields, and 3,500,000 is the approximate number of erythrocytes per cubic millimeter in birds with normal PCVs. If the PCV is outside the normal range of 35% to 55%, then the estimated count should be corrected for the PCV using the following formula:

$$\text{Corrected Estimated WBC/mm}^3 = \frac{\text{Estimated WBC} \times \text{Observed PCV}}{\text{Normal PCV (45\%)}}$$

Less experienced observers may wish to obtain an estimated total leukocyte count by determining the average number of leukocytes per field in ten monolayer ×40 (high-dry) fields and then multiplying by 2000 (63).

Accurate interpretation of leukocyte counts, especially when determined by the semidirect method, depends on the accurate identification and differentiation of leukocytes in the blood film.

Responses in Disease

Avian leukograms often vary widely between normal birds of the same species. Because birds often become excited when handled, the blood collection process usually results in a physiologic leukocytosis, and this physiologic response increases the concentration of heterophils and lymphocytes in the peripheral blood. Normal total leukocyte reference intervals obtained from birds generally are broader than those obtained from domestic mammals. Thus, avian leukogram values must differ greatly from the normal reference intervals to have diagnostic significance.

The general causes of a leukocytosis in birds include inflammation, which may be associated with infectious or noninfectious causes, toxicities, hemorrhage into a body cavity, rapidly growing neoplasms, and leukemia. A leukocyte differential aids in the assessment of a leukocytosis. Because leukocytosis often is caused by inflammation, a heterophilia usually is present as well. The magnitude of the heterophilia depends on both the cause and the severity of the inflammation: the greater the degree of heterophilia, the greater the severity of the inflammation. A leukocytosis and heterophilia can be associated with inflammation in response to localized or systemic infections caused by a spectrum of infectious agents (i.e., bacteria, fungi, chlamydia, viruses, and parasites) and noninfectious causes (i.e., traumatic injury or toxicities). A marked leukocytosis and heterophilia often are associated with diseases produced by common avian pathogens, such as *Chlamydia*, *Mycobacterium*, and *Aspergillus*. A slight to moderate leukocytosis in birds also can occur with excess endogenous or exogenous glucocorticoids (stress leukogram). A corticosteroid-induced leukocytosis reveals a slight to moderate, mature heterophilia and lymphopenia. The heterophil:lymphocyte (H:L) ratio can be used as an index of stress in birds. The magnitude of leukocytosis and heterophilia during disease or corticosteroid excess varies with the H:L ratio, with greater responses being seen in species with normal H:L ratios of 3.0:1 versus those with ratios of 0.5:1. The H:L ratio can be used as an index of stress in birds. Initially, species that normally have high numbers of circulating lymphocytes (e.g., anseriformes) may show a leukopenia but, later (i.e., up to 12 hours) demonstrate typical leukocytosis, heterophilia, and lymphopenia (64–66). Species that normally have greater numbers of circulating heterophils (e.g., galliformes) show a less dramatic change in the stress leukogram.

Immature heterophils rarely are present in the peripheral blood of normal birds. When they do occur, however, their presence usually results from excessive peripheral utilization of mature heterophils, with depletion of the mature storage pool in the hematopoietic tissue that indicates a severe inflammatory response, especially when associated with a leukopenia (67). Marked increases in the concentration of immature heterophils also may result from granulocytic leukemia, which is a rare condition in birds.

Toxic heterophils are associated with severe, systemic illness such as septicemia, viremia, chlamydiosis, mycotic infections, and severe tissue necrosis. The degree of heterophil toxicity usually indicates the severity of the bird's condition, and a marked number of 4+ toxic heterophils indicates a grave prognosis.

Leukopenia is associated with either consumption of peripheral leukocytes or decreased production. Heteropenia results from decreased survival of mature heterophils or from decreased or ineffective production. Leukopenias associated with heteropenias can occur with severe bacterial infections or certain viral diseases (e.g., Pacheco's parrot disease) (68,69) Leukopenia and heteropenia with the presence of immature heterophils suggest exhaustion of the mature heterophil storage pool because of excessive peripheral demand for heterophils, as seen with severe inflammation. A degenerative response is reflected by a leukopenia, heteropenia, immature heterophils, and toxic heterophils. Degenerative responses and depletion are differentiated by the presence of toxic heterophils or by following the decreasing leukocyte count with serial leukograms. Bone marrow evaluation also may be helpful. In general, a degenerative response in the leukogram of a bird indicates a poor prognosis for survival. As discussed, leukopenia and lymphopenia can occur as an early, corticosteroid-induced leukogram response in some species of birds (64). Leukopenias and lymphopenia also may suggest a viral cause, although such causes have been poorly documented in birds.

Lymphocytosis may occur with antigenic stimulation. An occasional reactive lymphocyte may be found in blood films from normal birds; however, many reactive lymphocytes suggest antigenic stimulation associated with infectious disease (Figs. 17.35 and 17.36). Lymphocytosis also can occur with lymphocytic leukemia (e.g., avian leukosis). In some cases of lymphocytic leukemia, immature lymphocytes may be present in the blood film. A marked lymphocytosis in which most lymphocytes appear as small, mature lymphocytes with scalloped cytoplasmic margins also has been associated with lymphoid neoplasia (2,70,71).

Lymphopenia can occur with glucocorticosteroid excess, which may be more pronounced in some avian species than others. Immunosuppressive drugs also may cause lymphopenia.

Monocytosis often is associated with infectious diseases caused by organisms that typically cause granulomatous inflammation, such as *Mycobacterium* and *Chlamydia*, and fungi, such as *Aspergillus*. Chronic bacterial granulomas and massive tissue necrosis also may result

in monocytosis. A monocytosis has been seen in certain nutritional deficiencies, such as zinc deficiency, as well (72).

Because the exact functions of avian eosinophils are not known, interpreting the cause of peripheral eosinophilia is difficult in birds. Although this avian granulocyte was given the name "eosinophil," avian eosinophils may behave differently than mammalian eosinophils. Studies have shown that avian eosinophils may participate in delayed (type IV) hypersensitivity reactions, a participation that does not occur with mammalian eosinophils (73). Experiments using parasite antigens have failed to induce peripheral eosinophilias, although eosinophilias associated with gastrointestinal nematode infestations have been reported (74). Despite limited knowledge regarding the function of avian eosinophils, peripheral eosinophilia in birds can be loosely interpreted as being a response to internal or external parasitism or exposure to foreign antigens (i.e., hypersensitivity response).

Eosinopenia may be difficult to document in birds. If present, it is expected to be associated with a stress response or with administration of glucocorticosteroids.

Basophilia is rare in birds. Because avian basophils produce, store, and release histamine, they may have a function similar to that of mammalian basophils (75). Therefore, avian basophils may participate in immediate hypersensitivity reactions, release mediators for thrombocyte activation, cause smooth muscle contractions, initiate edema, and affect coagulation. Basophils appear to participate in the initial phase of acute inflammation in birds; however, this usually is not reflected as a basophilia on the leukogram (76,77) Peripheral basophilia may suggest early inflammation or an immediate hypersensitivity reaction in birds. A stress-related basophilia occurs in chickens subjected to food restriction, but this response may be age or duration dependent (40,78).

THROMBOCYTES AND HEMOSTASIS

Morphology

Thrombocytes are nucleated cells that are found in the peripheral blood of birds. They tend to be round to oval cells with a round to oval nucleus that contains densely clumped chromatin. The nucleus is more rounded than an erythrocyte nucleus, and cells have a high N:C ratio. Normal, mature thrombocytes have a colorless to pale-gray cytoplasm, which often has a reticulated appearance. The appearance of the cytoplasm is an important feature in differentiating thrombocytes from small, mature lymphocytes (Figs. 17.32, 17.34, and *17.40*). Cytoplasmic vacuolation can occur in activated or phagocytic thrombocytes. Thrombocytes frequently contain one or more distinct eosinophilic (specific) granules, which usually are

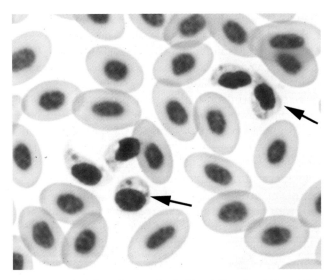

Figure 17.40 Thrombocytes in the blood film of a chicken (*Gallus gallus formadomestica*). Modified Wright-Giemsa stain, 500×.

located in one area of the cytoplasm. Thrombocytes participate in the hemostatic process and, like mammalian platelets, tend to clump in blood films. Activated thrombocytes occurring in aggregates may have indistinct cellular outlines or cytoplasmic pseudopodia.

Ultrastructurally, the cytoplasm resembles that of mammalian platelets (55). The granules that frequently are seen in thrombocytes at light microscopy appear as aggregates of many small granules at electron microscopy. The specific granules contain primarily 5′-hydroxytryptamine, and they are an unlikely source of thromboplastin (37). Thrombocytes aggregated in clumps show degranulation of specific granules, cellular degeneration, and nuclear pyknosis. Avian thrombocytes contain a large amount of serotonin, and some studies suggest that they are capable of phagocytosis and may participate in removing foreign materials from the blood (79).

Laboratory Evaluation

The thrombocyte concentration of most avian species studied ranges between 20,000 and 30,000 cells/mm³, or 10 to 15 thrombocytes per 1000 erythrocytes (2,55). The actual thrombocyte concentration is difficult to determine, because thrombocytes tend to clump. Therefore, their concentration often is reported as either normal, increased, or decreased, based on estimates made from peripheral blood films. Approximately one to five thrombocytes can be seen in a monolayer ×1000 (oil-immersion) field in a blood film from a normal bird, unless the thrombocytes clump excessively during preparation. Thrombocytopenia is suggested by thrombocyte numbers less than one per monolayer ×1000 field, and thrombocytosis is suggested by

numbers greater than five in an average monolayer ×1000 field. A thrombocyte concentration can be obtained with the same hemacytometer used for obtaining total leukocyte and erythrocyte counts with the Natt and Herrick method. The number of thrombocytes counted in the central large square on both sides of the Neubauer-ruled hemocytometer is multiplied by 1000 to obtain the number of thrombocytes per microliter of blood. An estimated thrombocyte count can be obtained from the blood film using the same formula as that for estimation of the total leukocyte count:

Estimated thrombocytes/µL =

$$\frac{\text{Average number of thrombocytes in 5 fields (×1000)} \times 3{,}500{,}000}{1000}$$

Again, if the PCV is outside the normal range of 35% to 55%, then the estimated thrombocyte count should be adjusted for the PCV as follows:

Corrected thrombocyte count/µL = Estimated thrombocyte count × Observed PCV/Normal PCV (45%)

Responses in Disease

Avian thrombocytes are derived from mononuclear precursors in the bone marrow. Immature thrombocytes occasionally are present in the peripheral blood of birds. They are larger, round to oval cells, with round to oval nuclei and basophilic cytoplasm compared with mature thrombocytes *(Fig. 17.41)*. The mid and late immature thrombocytes most commonly are seen when immature cells are present (see the discussion of avian

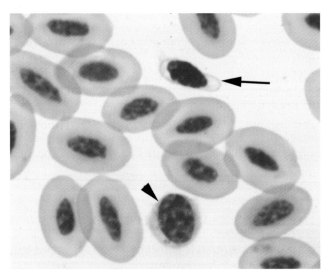

Figure 17.41 A mature thrombocyte (arrow) and a late immature thrombocyte (arrow head) in the blood film of an eagle (*Aquila chrysaetus*). Modified Wright-Giemsa stain, 500×.

hematopoiesis). The presence of immature thrombocytes usually indicates a regenerative response to excessive utilization of thrombocytes. Young birds tend to have relatively higher numbers of circulating thrombocytes than adult birds (50).

Thrombocytopenia results from either decreased bone marrow production or excessive peripheral utilization or destruction. A decreased thrombocyte concentration often is associated with severe septicemia and, possibly, diffuse intravascular coagulation.

The initial hemostatic plug of birds is formed through the adhesion and aggregation of thrombocytes, and the secondary hemostatic plug develops through the coagulation cascade after injury to a blood vessel wall. Most clotting factors involved in avian blood coagulation are similar to those in mammals. Although evidence suggests an intrinsic clotting mechanism in some avian species, coagulation of avian blood appears to depend on the extrinsic clotting system, which involves the release of tissue thromboplastin (i.e., factor III) (18). The extrinsic and common pathways can be evaluated using a one-step prothrombin time test. Avian brain thromboplastin is required for avian prothrombin time testing, because commercially available rabbit-brain thromboplastin and other mammalian sources give unreliable results in birds. The normal prothrombin time for most birds is 13 seconds or less (80). Studies suggest that the source of thromboplastin should be from the brain of the same species of bird as the patient for accurate prothrombin time determinations (18,80).

Whole blood (capillary) clotting times in birds usually are less than 5 minutes; however, normal values appear to range between 2 and 10 minutes (18). The whole-blood clotting time is more variable than the prothrombin time.

COMMON AVIAN BLOOD PARASITES

Protozoan parasites, especially *Hemoproteus*, *Plasmodium*, *Leukocytozoon*, and microfilaria of filarial nematodes, commonly are found in avian blood films. Their identification usually can be made using the stains commonly used for evaluating blood cells. Films made from fresh blood, without addition of an anticoagulant, provide samples with fewer artifacts affecting the parasite.

Hemoproteus

Protozoan blood parasites of the genus *Hemoproteus* are common in many species of wild birds. The only forms of the parasite in the peripheral blood of birds are gametocytes, which range in size from small, developing, ring forms to the elongate, crescent-shaped, mature gametocyte that partially encircles the erythrocyte nucleus to

form the characteristic "halter shape" (81) *(Fig. 17.42)*. The mature gametocyte typically occupies greater than half the cytoplasmic volume of the host erythrocyte, and it causes minimal displacement of the host cell nucleus: the nucleus is never pushed to the cell margin. *Hemoproteus* gametocytes contain refractile, yellow to brown pigment granules that represent iron pigment deposited as a result of hemoglobin utilization. Macrogametocytes stain dark blue with Romanowsky stains and have iron pigment dispersed throughout the cytoplasm of the parasite, whereas microgametocytes stain pale blue to pink and have iron pigment aggregated into a spherical mass. Occasionally, extraerythrocytic macrogametes and microgametes can be found in blood films, especially those made from blood collected several hours before the film was actually prepared *(Fig. 17.43)*. Extraerythrocytic macrogametes are round and resemble those within erythrocytes. Microgametes are small, spindle-shaped structures scattered throughout the blood film. Usually, these forms are found in the midgut of the insect host after a blood meal.

Blood-sucking insect vectors, such as hippoboscid flies and midges of the genus *Culicoides*, transmit *Hemoproteus*. The insect host ingests gametocytes when it feeds, and the parasites then undergo a series of developmental stages to become sporozoites within the salivary gland. Sporozoites are injected into the new avian host when the insect feeds. The sporozoites enter the bird's vascular endothelial cells in various tissues (primarily the lung, liver, bone marrow, and spleen) and then undergo schizogony. *Hemoproteus* schizonts occasionally are found in cytologic or histologic samples of infected tissue, and they appear as large, round cysts containing numerous multinucleated bodies or cytomeres. Each cytomere produces

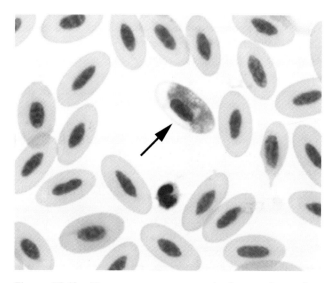

Figure 17.42 *Hemoproteus* gametocyte in the cytoplasm of an erythrocyte of a cockatoo (*Cacatua moluccensis*). Wright stain, 500×.

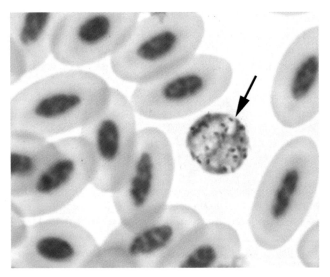

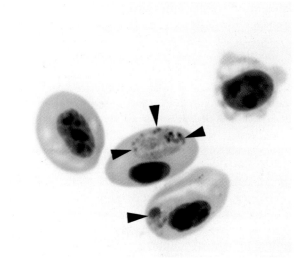

Figure 17.43 Extracellular macrogametocyte of *Hemoproteus* in the blood film of an owl (*Bubo virginianus*). Wright stain, 500×.

Figure 17.44 *Plasmodium* gametocytes in the erythrocyte cytoplasm from a skua (*Catharacta skua*). Wright stain, 500×.

numerous merozoites that escape into the bloodstream when the endothelial cell and cytomeres rupture. Merozoites enter erythrocytes to become gametocytes, which then are ingested by insect hosts to complete the cycle.

The pathogenicity of *Hemoproteus* generally is low, and parasitized birds rarely show evidence of disease. Clinical disease, however, can occur in certain avian species, such as pigeons and quail, nestlings, and in birds suffering from other diseases that, perhaps, result in immunodeficiencies. The clinical signs include hemolytic anemia, anorexia, and depression. Hepatomegaly and splenomegaly may be observed at postmortem evaluation.

The degree of parasitemia associated with *Hemoproteus* can be used as an index to assess the recovery of birds, especially raptors, from traumatic injuries or diseases. For example, an injured raptor may present with marked *Hemoproteus* parasitemia; with greater than 15% of the erythrocytes being affected. As the bird recovers from its injuries, however, the parasitemia decreases dramatically. Presumably, this represents an improved immune status of the bird.

Plasmodium

Parasites of the genus *Plasmodium* can be pathogenic and responsible for malaria, which affects certain species of birds (e.g., canaries, penguins, ducks, pigeons, raptors, and domestic poultry). Many avian species appear to be asymptomatic carriers of the parasite, however, and do not develop the clinical disease. Outbreaks of avian malaria occur sporadically in endemic areas, especially during seasons associated with increased mosquito populations. Clinical signs associated with avian malaria include

anemia, anorexia, depression, and acute death. The hemogram often reveals hemolytic anemia, leukocytosis, and lymphocytosis. Hemoglobinuria or biliverdinuria also may occur. Splenomegaly and hepatomegaly often are seen on postmortem examination.

Detection of *Plasmodium* is based on presence of the organism in blood films. Unlike *Hemoproteus*, stages other than the gametocyte, such as schizonts and trophozoites, can be found within erythrocytes, thrombocytes, and leukocytes *(Figs. 17.44 through 17.46)*. Certain *Plasmodium* sp. have round to irregular gametocytes that cause

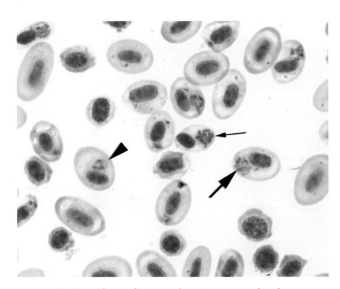

Figure 17.45 *Plasmodium* trophozoites (arrow head), gametocytes (large arrow), and schizonts (small arrow) in the cytoplasm of erythrocytes from a skua (*Catharacta skua*). Wright stain, 500×.

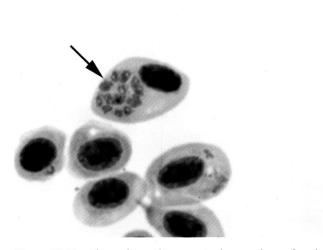

Figure 17.46 *Plasmodium* schizogony in the cytoplasm of erythrocytes from a skua (*Catharacta skua*). Wright stain, 500×.

marked displacement of the host-cell nucleus, whereas other species have elongate gametocytes that do not displace the host-cell nucleus. Like those of *Hemoproteus*, *Plasmodium* gametocytes contain refractile, yellow to brown, iron pigment granules, which tend to be scattered, and macrogametocytes stain deeper blue than microgametocytes. *Plasmodium* trophozoites are small, round to oval, ameboid forms containing a large vacuole that pushes the parasite nucleus to one edge, thereby giving the trophozoite a "signet-ring" appearance. Schizonts are round to oval inclusions that contain several deeply staining merozoites; the number of merozoites is used to determine the *Plasmodium* species. Schizonts with developing merozoites exhibit clusters of merozoites that appear to be fused, which is in contrast to mature merozoites, which appear to be distinct bodies and separate from each other. Identification of the *Plasmodium* species depends on the location and appearance of the schizonts and gametocytes (81).

The life cycle of *Plasmodium* is similar to that of *Hemoproteus*, except that culicine mosquitoes act as intermediate hosts and schizogony occurs in the red blood and endothelial cells of various organs (81). The key features used to differentiate *Plasmodium* from *Hemoproteus* are the presence of schizogony in the peripheral blood, parasite stages within thrombocytes and leukocytes, and gametocytes causing marked displacement of the erythrocyte nucleus.

Leukocytozoon

Leukocytozoon, which is a protozoan parasite commonly found in the blood of wild birds, is identified by

large, dark-staining macrogametocytes or light-staining microgametocytes. The large gametocytes grossly distort the infected host cell, thereby elongating and distending the cell and making the identification of the cell difficult *(Fig. 17.47)*. Some parasitologists believe that immature erythrocytes rather than leukocytes, as suggested by the name of the parasite, serve as the host cell for *Leukocytozoon* (81). As with *Hemoproteus*, only the gametocytes of *Leukocytozoon* occur in the peripheral blood. Parasitized cells appear to have two nuclei: a dark-staining, host-cell nucleus that lies along the cell membrane; and a pale pink–staining, parasite nucleus that lies adjacent to the host-cell nucleus. *Leukocytozoon* gametocytes do not contain the refractile pigment granules seen in the gametocytes of *Hemoproteus* and *Plasmodium*.

Leukocytozoon is transmitted by black flies (Simuliidae), which act as intermediate hosts and inject sporozoites into the blood of susceptible avian species. The sporozoites invade the endothelial and parenchymal cells of various tissues such as the liver, heart, and kidney, in which schizogony occurs. Schizonts mature and then rupture to release merozoites that infect erythrocytes and, possibly, leukocytes. Merozoites become gametocytes in the peripheral blood or are ingested by macrophages to become megaloschizonts in tissues such as the liver, lung, and kidney. Megaloschizonts also release merozoites that develop into gametocytes.

The pathogenicity of *Leukocytozoon* usually is low; however, certain species can be highly pathogenic for some birds, such as young waterfowl and turkeys. The clinical signs associated with this parasite include anemia, anorexia, and depression (82–85). Clinical laboratory evaluation may reveal a hemolytic anemia, leukocytosis, and

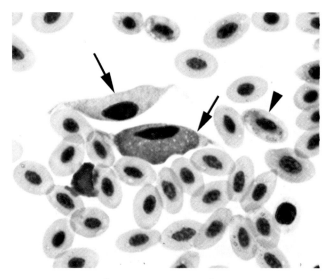

Figure 17.47 *Leukocytozoon* macro- and microgametocytes (arrows) in the blood film of a hawk (*Buteo jamaicensis*). A *Hemoproteus* gametocyte (arrow head) is also present. Wright stain, 500×.

elevated serum enzymes such as aspartate aminotransferase or alanine aminotransferase, thereby suggesting hepatocellular necrosis. Postmortem findings may include splenomegaly and hepatomegaly with hepatic necrosis.

Microfilaria

Microfilaria of filarial nematodes commonly are found in the peripheral blood of many species of birds *(Fig. 17.48)*. The adult filarial nematodes usually are not seen unless they occur in peripheral locations, such as in the fluid of distended joints. Adult filarial nematodes may occur anywhere within the body of birds, but they most frequently are seen in the air sacs, subcutaneously, or in the body cavities. Most of these parasites are considered to be nonpathogenic and cause little harm to their host.

Other, Less Common Avian Blood Parasites

Other parasites that are seen less frequently in the peripheral blood of birds include *Atoxoplasma*, *Aegyptianella*, *Trypanosoma*, and *Borrelia*. *Atoxoplasma* is a coccidian parasite that often is found in passerine birds, which can be highly pathogenic, especially to canaries (86,87). It is transmitted directly via oocysts in the feces. Atoxoplasmosis is diagnosed on the basis of demonstrating characteristic sporozoites within the lymphocytes on peripheral blood films or cytologic imprints of the liver, spleen, or lung. The sporozoites appear as pale, eosinophilic, round to oval, intracytoplasmic inclusions within lymphocytes, monocytes, or macrophages in Romanowsky-stained preparations *(Fig. 17.49)*. The sporozoites indent the host lymphocyte nucleus, thereby resulting in a char-

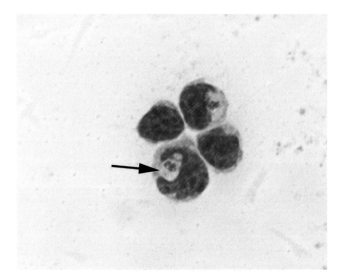

Figure 17.49 An *Atoxoplasma* inclusion in a lymphocyte from a buffy coat film of a thrush (*Garrulax chinensis*). Wright stain, 500×.

acteristic crescent shape (88). Sporozoites of *Atoxoplasma* lack pigment granules, but detection of *Atoxoplasma* in the peripheral blood can be improved by using a preparation of a buffy-coat film to concentrate the leukocytes for examination.

Aegyptianella is a minute parasite of avian erythrocytes that lacks pigment granules. It is a piroplasma that can affect several avian species, usually those originating in tropical or subtropical climates. *Aegyptianella pullorum* occurs in chickens, geese, ducks, and turkeys. The organism is detected by demonstrating the developing forms within erythrocytes in blood films *(Fig. 17.50)*. Three

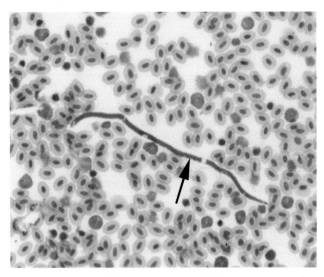

Figure 17.48 A microfilaria in the blood film of a cockatoo (*Cacatua moluccensis*). Wright stain, 250×.

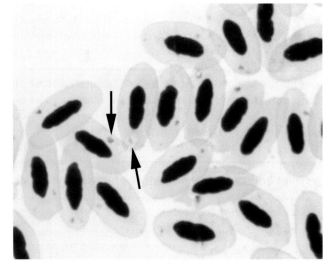

Figure 17.50 *Aegyptianella* inclusions within the erythrocytes of a parrot (*Amazona finschi*). Wright stain, 500×.

forms can occur (81). One form, the initial body, is a small, anaplasma-like structure that is less than 1 μm in diameter and appears as a round, basophilic, intracytoplasmic inclusion. A second form is a round- to piriform-shaped inclusion with pale-blue cytoplasm and a chromatin body at one pole resembling those of *Babesia*. The third form is a larger (2–4 μm), round to elliptical inclusion. *Aegyptianella* can be pathogenic, resulting in anemia, anorexia, and diarrhea. Postmortem findings include splenomegaly, hepatomegaly, and hepatic as well as renal degeneration.

Trypanosomes (*Trypanosoma*) occasionally are found in the peripheral blood of wild birds, especially passerines, galliformes, waterfowl, and pigeons. They are transmitted by biting insects such as mosquitoes, hippoboscid flies, and blackflies or mites. Avian trypanosomes resemble those found in mammals. They have an undulating membrane; a slender, tapering posterior end; and a short, anteriorly directed flagellum. Trypanosomes usually are considered to be an incidental finding.

Borrelia anserina is the causative agent of avian spirochetosis, which can affect several species of birds, especially galliformes and waterfowl. It is transmitted by arthropod vectors such as ticks and mites. *Borrelia* is a loosely spiraled spirochete that tapers into fine filaments and is found free in the plasma. During the acute stages of the disease, the organism is spiral shaped; however, as the disease progresses and the bird nears death, the organism may appear abnormal or clumped and often is difficult to find. In acute avian spirochetosis, affected birds are depressed, anemic, and weak. Postmortem findings include splenomegaly and hepatomegaly. Birds recovering from the disease exhibit a regenerative anemia.

AVIAN HEMATOPOIESIS

Bone Marrow

The bone marrow is the primary site for erythropoiesis, granulopoiesis, and thrombopoiesis during late embryonic development and post-hatched birds (55,89) In some adult birds, such as chickens, the hematopoietic activity of the bone marrow primarily is associated with erythropoiesis and, possibly, thrombopoiesis, with only a small reserve of granulopoiesis compared to that of mammalian bone marrow (90). Therefore, compared with mammals, granulopoiesis in mature birds is more diffuse and is found in a variety of tissues. During embryonic development, granulocyte stem cells colonize to create foci of granulopoiesis in the spleen, kidney, lungs, thymus, gonad, pancreas, and other tissues, including the bone marrow (1,91, 92). The bone marrow also provides an environment for lymphocyte maturation. Because it is the most readily available source of hematopoietic tissue in birds, the bone marrow is used to evaluate disorders of blood cells. Cytologic evaluation of the bone marrow is indicated in avian patients with nonregenerative anemia, heteropenia, and other unexplained alterations involving the cellular elements in circulating blood.

Bone Marrow Collection

Marrow samples for cytologic evaluation can be successfully obtained in most avian species via bone marrow aspiration. The best source of bone marrow for most birds is the proximal tibiotarsus, because the procedure at this location is relatively simple (2,93). Marrow may be collected from the sternum (keel), however, and from most of the long bones, except the pneumatic bones. A general anesthetic usually is not required, but a local anesthetic can be used with caution in large birds. The type of biopsy needle used for aspiration depends on the size of the bird, location of the biopsy site, and preference of the cytologist. Biopsy needles commonly used for bone marrow collection in both domestic mammals and humans (Jamshidi bone marrow biopsy–aspiration needles and disposable Jamshidi Illinois-Sternal/Iliac aspiration needles, Kormed Corp., Minneapolis, MN) can be used for marrow collection in birds. The pediatric sizes are preferred, however, because of the relatively small bone size in most birds compared with mammals. Spinal needles containing a stylet can be used for marrow collection in very small birds.

The procedure for collecting bone marrow from the proximal tibiotarsus begins with application of a skin disinfectant, as for any surgical procedure. The medial or cranial aspect of the proximal tibiotarsus just below the femoral-tibiotarsal joint is a suitable location for aspiration, because only a minimal amount of soft tissue overlies the bone in this area. After application of a local anesthetic, a small incision is made using a scalpel blade to facilitate passage of the needle through the skin. The needle with stylet is placed against the bone *(Fig. 17.51)*, and using gentle pressure and rotary movements, the needle then is advanced into the marrow cavity. A perpendicular approach to the bone should be used. The hand not being used to manipulate the needle is used to stabilize the tibiotarsus. Once the needle is positioned into the marrow cavity, the stylet is removed, and a 6- to 12-mL syringe is attached *(Fig. 17.52)*. Marrow is aspirated into the lumen of the needle by applying negative pressure to the syringe using the syringe plunger *(Fig. 17.53)*. Excessive or prolonged negative pressure should be avoided to minimize blood contamination of the marrow sample. Unlike collection of bone marrow from most mammals, avian marrow should not appear in the syringe (except in very large birds) because of the small marrow volume in most birds.

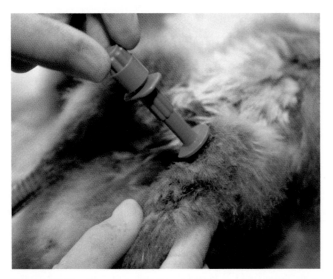

Figure 17.51   Placement of a Jamshidi Illinois-Sternal/Iliac aspiration needle (Kormed Corp, Minneapolis, MN) in the proximal tibiotarsus of a flamingo chick (*Phoenicopterus ruber*).

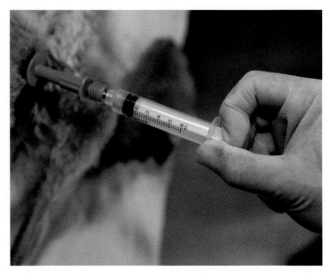

Figure 17.53   Aspiration of a bone marrow sample.

Therefore, the marrow sample is found in the lumen of the biopsy needle.

When aspiration is completed, the needle and syringe are removed from the tibiotarsus while making sure that negative pressure is not being applied to the syringe. The needle is removed from the syringe, and the syringe is filled with air to force the marrow from the lumen onto a glass microscope slide. A second glass microscope slide is placed atop of the marrow sample, and the marrow is allowed to spread between the two slides as they are pulled apart. Bone marrow samples also can be obtained from the keel (sternum) of some birds, such as galliformes; the biopsy needle is introduced into the widest part of the

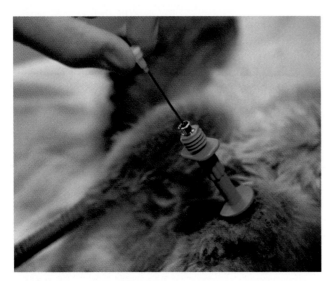

Figure 17.52   Removal of the stylet from a bone marrow aspiration needle.

sternal ridge in the manner as described for the proximal tibiotarsus.

Marrow core biopsies for histologic evaluation can be obtained from birds using a technique similar to that of marrow aspiration. Once the biopsy needle is introduced into the bone marrow space, the stylet is removed, and the needle is advanced deeper into the marrow cavity, toward the opposite cortex. Once the opposite cortex has been reached, the needle is twisted and redirected slightly to detach the marrow plug within the lumen of the needle. Gentle vacuum may be applied to the syringe to aid in holding the marrow plug in the needle as the needle is withdrawn from the marrow cavity. The marrow core sample is removed by reinsertion of the stylet (usually beginning at the tip of the needle) to push the sample out of the needle. Imprint films can be made from the core sample for cytologic evaluation before the sample is placed in 10% neutral-buffered formalin. A sample holder often is required to maintain the marrow core while it is being fixed in the formalin solution.

Examination of Avian Bone Marrow

Bone marrow slides are stained with the same Romanowsky stains used for blood films. Interpretation of avian bone marrow begins with scanning of the marrow film using the ×10 microscope objective to evaluate both the number and the distribution of cells. Because an actual cell count of a bone marrow sample cannot be obtained, the cellularity is estimated by evaluating the ratio of fat and cells in marrow particles and is compared with the cellularity of normal bone marrow. The degree of cellularity is estimated as poor, normal, or high.

The distribution of cells can be estimated as well. Myeloid, erythroid, and thrombocytic elements may appear to be normal, hypoplastic (decreased), or hyperplastic (increased). A more objective approach is to perform an actual differential count based on 1000 cells or more, but this is more time-consuming and may not provide more information.

In addition to estimating the degree of cellularity and evaluating the distribution of cell types in the marrow sample, the cytologist also should estimate the myeloid:erythroid ratio. Any changes involving the maturation sequence of each cell line should be noted as well. The cell lines include erythrocytes, granulocytes (heterophils, eosinophils, and basophils), monocytes, and thrombocytes. Other cells that occasionally are found include lymphocytes, plasma cells, osteoblasts, and osteoclasts. The presence of abnormal cells also should be noted.

An accurate interpretation of the bone marrow response can be made only in conjunction with knowledge regarding the current peripheral blood cellular response. Therefore, a hemogram made from a blood sample collected at the same time as the bone marrow sample should be evaluated.

Erythropoiesis

Avian erythropoiesis occurs within the lumen of the vascular sinusoids in the bone marrow (37,50,55,89). These sinuses are lined by elongated endothelial cells that are associated with the most immature cells of the erythroid series. The more mature cells are located in the lumen of the sinuses. The vascular sinuses communicate with a central vein.

Avian erythropoietin, which is a glycoprotein that differs structurally from mammalian erythropoietin, is necessary for the multiplication and differentiation of precursor stem cells committed to the erythroid series (37, 94). Erythropoietin can be obtained from the blood of anemic birds, and the site of its production is considered to be the kidney.

The stages of maturation in normal avian erythropoiesis appear to be similar to those of mammals. The terminology used for the different stages of erythrocyte maturation, however, varies in the literature (1,2,4,55). In general, seven stages are recognizable in red-blood-cell development based on findings with Romanowsky stains. These include rubriblasts (proerythroblasts), prorubricytes (basophilic erythroblasts), basophilic rubricytes (early polychromatic erythroblasts), early polychromatic rubricytes (late polychromatic erythroblasts), late polychromatic rubricytes (orthochromic erythroblasts), polychromatic erythrocytes, and mature erythrocytes. As erythroid cells mature, the nuclear size decreases, the chromatin becomes increasingly condensed, the nuclear

shape changes from round to ellipsoid, the amount of cytoplasm increases, the hemoglobin concentration increases (resulting in increasing eosinophilia), and the cell shape changes from round to ellipsoid. Unlike mammalian erythrocytes, avian erythrocytes normally retain their nucleus.

Rubriblasts

Rubriblasts are large, round, deeply basophilic cells with a large, round, central nucleus that results in a high N:C ratio *(Fig. 17.54)*. The nuclear chromatin typically is coarsely granular, and large, prominent nucleoli or nucleolar rings are present. The cytoplasm is deeply basophilic, with clear spaces most likely representing mitochondria.

Prorubricyte

The prorubricyte resembles the rubriblast, but it lacks the prominent nucleoli. The N:C ratio is high, and the large nucleus usually is surrounded by a narrow rim of blue cytoplasm. The cytoplasm is predominantly basophilic but may contain spots of reddish material, suggesting the beginning of hemoglobin development. The cytoplasm lacks the mitochondrial spaces of the rubriblast.

Rubricyte

Rubricytes are round cells that are smaller than rubriblasts and prorubricytes. They can be divided into three stages, based primarily on the appearance of the cytoplasm. The basophilic rubricyte is the earliest rubricyte

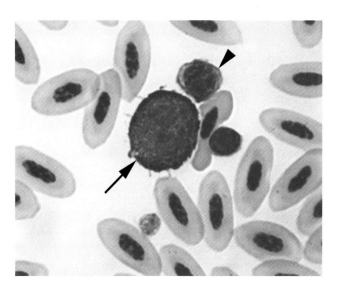

Figure 17.54 A rubriblast (arrow) and late polychromatic rubricyte (arrow head) from the bone marrow of a parrot (*Psittacus erithacus*). Wright stain, 500×.

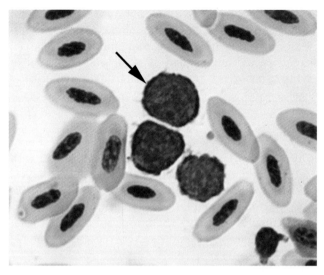

Figure 17.55   Three basophilic rubricytes and a lymphocyte from the bone marrow of a parrot (*Psittacus erithacus*). Wright stain, 500×.

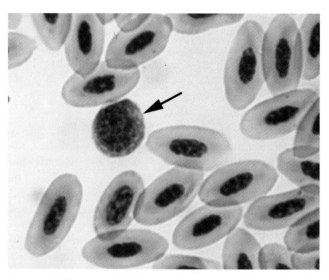

Figure 17.57   An early polychromatic rubricyte from the bone marrow of a parrot (*Psittacus erithacus*). Wright stain, 500×.

stage and is characterized by a homogenous, basophilic cytoplasm and a round nucleus with clumped chromatin *(Figs. 17.55 and 17.56)*. The next stage, the early polychromatophilic rubricyte, is smaller than the basophilic rubricyte and has a gray (basophilic to slightly eosinophilic) cytoplasm because of increased hemoglobin production (Figs. 17.56 and *17.57)*. The nucleus of early polychromatophilic rubricytes contains clumped chromatin and is small in relation to the amount of cytoplasm. The final rubricyte stage, the late polychromatophilic rubricyte, is ellipsoid and has more eosinophilic (eosinophilic gray to weakly eosinophilic) cytoplasm than earlier stages

(Fig. 17.58). The nucleus of late polychromatophilic rubricytes varies from round to slightly ellipsoid, with irregularly clumped chromatin.

Polychromatophilic Erythrocytes and Mature Erythrocytes

Cells in the final stages of erythropoiesis are the polychromatophilic erythrocyte and the mature erythrocyte. These cells are found in the peripheral blood of normal birds and were described earlier. The mature erythrocyte has a flattened, ellipsoid shape. The nuclear chromatin is condensed and transcriptionally inactive.

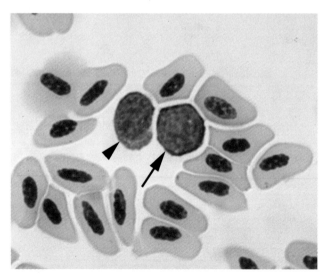

Figure 17.56   A basophilic rubricyte (arrow) and late polychromatic rubricyte (arrow head) from the bone marrow of a parrot (*Psittacus erithacus*). Wright stain, 500×.

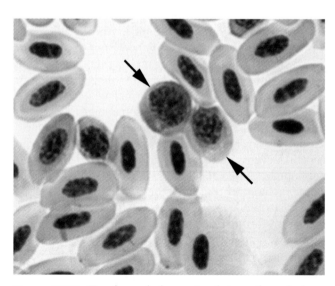

Figure 17.58   Two late polychromatic rubricytes from the bone marrow of a parrot (*Psittacus erithacus*). Wright stain, 500×.

Granulopoiesis

Avian granulocytes appear to develop in a manner similar to those of mammals. The maturation stages have been described based on their morphologic appearance, primarily in chicken bone marrow. Thus, the study of avian hematopoiesis lags behind research in mammalian hematopoiesis, in which morphologic criteria are only part of the overall evaluation. Avian granulocytes show a progressive decrease in size and cytoplasmic basophilia as they mature, which is similar to the granulocytes of mammals. Specific cytoplasmic granules appear during the later stages of development and then progressively increase in number, until a full complement is reached in the cytoplasm of the mature granulocyte. The nuclei of granulocytes initially are round and progress toward segmentation, except for basophils, which do not segment, and the nuclear chromatin becomes increasingly condensed with maturity. The developmental stages of avian granulocytes include, in order of maturation, myeloblasts (granuloblasts), progranulocytes (promyelocytes), myelocytes, metamyelocytes, band cells, and mature granulocytes.

Myeloblasts

Avian myeloblasts are large, round cells with a high N:C ratio *(Fig. 17.59)*. The cytoplasm stains a lighter blue than that of rubriblasts. Myeloblast nuclei typically are round, with delicate reticular (fine) chromatin and prominent nucleoli. Myeloblasts do not contain specific cytoplasmic granules and, possibly, represent a stage that is common to all granulocytes. Myeloblasts frequently are associated with other developing granulocytes, especially on imprints of bone marrow core biopsy specimens.

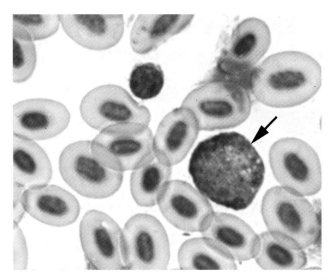

Figure 17.60 An early progranulocyte from the bone marrow of a parrot (*Psittacus erithacus*). Wright stain, 500×.

Progranulocytes

Avian progranulocytes are large cells with light blue cytoplasm and slightly eccentric nuclei *(Figs. 17.60 and 17.61)*. The N:C ratio is smaller than that of myeloblasts because of an increase in cytoplasm. The nuclear chromatin often has a delicate reticular pattern. Nucleoli are absent, and nuclear margins may be indistinct. Progranulocytes contain primary (immature) granules that vary in appearance among the types of granulocytes. Heterophil progranulocytes contain primary granules that vary in color and shape. They often appear as orange spheres (primary granules) and rings or as deeply basophilic spheres and rings.

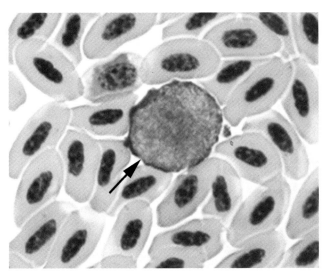

Figure 17.59 A myeloblast from the bone marrow of a parrot (*Psittacus erithacus*). Wright stain, 500×.

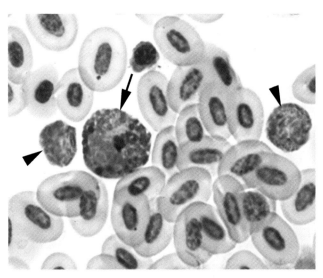

Figure 17.61 A late progranulocyte (arrow) and two heterophils (arrow heads) from the bone marrow of a parrot (*Psittacus erithacus*). Wright stain, 500×.

Eosinophil progranulocytes contain only brightly staining, orange, primary granules, and they appear to lack the dark magenta granules and rings found in heterophil progranulocytes. Basophil progranulocytes contain basophilic granules that appear to be smaller than the specific basophilic granules and the immature granules of the heterophil series. Fewer ring forms are seen in basophil progranulocytes.

Myelocytes

Myelocytes are smaller than myeloblasts and progranulocytes, and they contain the secondary or specific granules of the mature granulocytes, thereby making identification of this cell somewhat simple *(Figs. 17.62 and 17.63)*. The round to oval nuclei of myelocytes appear to be more condensed than the nuclei of myeloblasts and progranulocytes. Heterophil myelocytes typically are round cells, with a light blue cytoplasm that contains a mixture of rod-shaped specific granules and primary granules and rings. The eosinophilic, rod-shaped specific granules occupy less than half the cytoplasmic volume. Eosinophil myelocytes lack the deeply basophilic granules and rings that occasionally are found in early heterophil myelocytes. Basophil myelocytes contain basophilic specific granules that occupy less than half the cytoplasmic volume. The specific basophil granules have a slightly eosinophilic tinge, compared with the deep violet of the smaller primary granules that also may be present.

Metamyelocytes

Metamyelocytes are slightly smaller than myelocytes, have slightly indented nuclei, and possess specific cytoplasmic granules that occupy greater than half the cytoplasmic

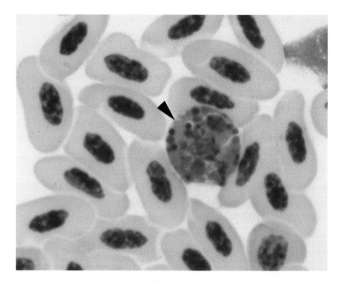

Figure 17.63   An eosinophil myelocyte with primary granules from the bone marrow of a parrot (*Psittacus erithacus*) that has blue granules in the eosinophils. Wright stain, 500×.

volume *(Figs. 17.64 and 17.65)*. Heterophil and basophil metamyelocytes have fewer primary granules than myelocytes and progranulocytes.

Band Cells and Mature Granulocytes

Band cells resemble mature granulocytes, except that the nucleus appears as a curved or coiled band rather than segmented. Identifying band cells often is difficult, because the exact shape of the nucleus is obscured by specific cytoplasmic granules. A specific nuclear stain such as hematoxylin usually is required to determine the concentra-

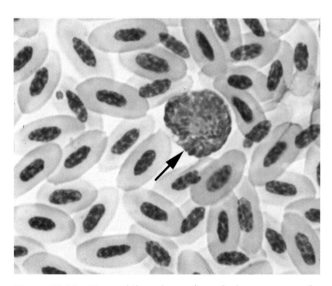

Figure 17.62   Heterophil myelocyte from the bone marrow of a parrot (*Psittacus erithacus*). Wright stain, 500×.

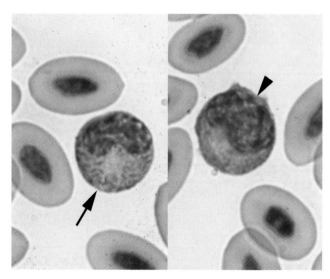

Figure 17.64   Toxic heterophil metamyelocyte (arrow) and myelocyte (arrow head) from the peripheral blood of a duck (*Anas platyrhynchos*). Wright stain, 500×.

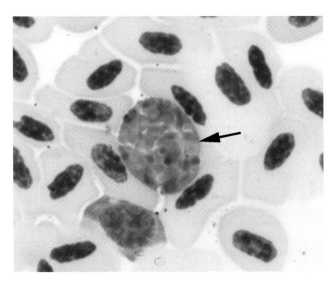

Figure 17.65 An eosinophil metamyelocyte from a parrot (*Psittacus erithacus*) with blue granules in the eosinophils. Wright stain, 500×.

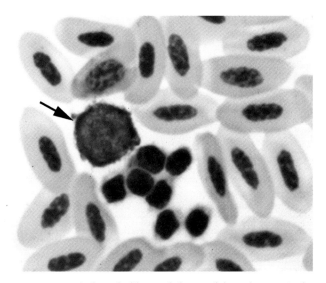

Figure 17.66 A thromboblast and cluster of thrombocytes in the bone marrow from a parrot (*Psittacus erithacus*). Wright stain, 500×.

tion of band cells. Because mature basophils lack a segmented nucleus, the band stage of basophils is not apparent. Mature granulocytes generally are the most abundant cell of each granulocytic cell line in the bone marrow of normal birds and were described earlier.

Thrombocytes

Avian thrombocytes appear to derive from a distinct line of mononuclear cells in the bone marrow, unlike mammalian platelets, which are cytoplasmic fragments of large, multinucleated megakaryocytes. The thrombocyte series consists of thromboblasts, immature thrombocytes, and mature thrombocytes. Thromboblasts resemble rubriblasts, but they tend to be smaller, with round nuclei having fine to punctate nuclear chromatin and one or more nucleoli *(Fig. 17.66)*. The cytoplasm is scant, stains deeply basophilic, and may contain clear spaces. They tend to be round to oval, with cytoplasmic blebs.

Immature thrombocytes are divided into three groups—early, mid, and late immature thrombocytes—based on their degree of maturity. Early immature thrombocytes are intermediate in size between thromboblasts and more mature stages *(Fig. 17.67)*. They tend to be round to oval and have more abundant cytoplasm than thromboblasts. The cytoplasm is basophilic and may contain vacuoles. The nuclear chromatin is aggregated into irregular clumps. Mid immature thrombocytes are slightly elongate or irregular, with pale blue cytoplasm *(Fig. 17.68)*. Cytoplasmic specific granules and vacuoles occasionally are seen at this stage of development. The nucleus contains heavy chromatin clumping. Late immature thrombocytes are oval and slightly smaller than the mid immature stage (Figs. 17.67 and 17.68). The cytoplasm stains pale blue,

with vaguely defined, clear areas. Specific granules frequently are seen at one pole of the cell. The nucleus is oval and has densely packed chromatin. The mature thrombocyte is the definitive cell in the thrombocyte series and was described earlier.

Other Cells in Avian Bone Marrow

Monocytes and Macrophages

Monocytopoiesis is poorly defined in birds. Granulocytic precursor cells may be similar to—or even the same as—monocytic precursor cells (55). Monocytes originating in hematopoietic tissues become the monocytes and macro-

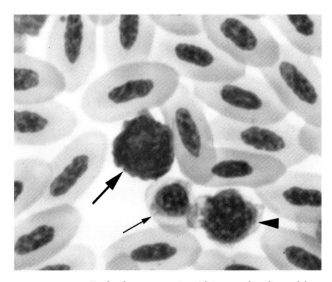

Figure 17.67 Early (large arrow), mid (arrow head), and late (small arrow) immature thrombocytes in the bone marrow of a parrot (*Psittacus erithacus*). Wright stain, 500×.

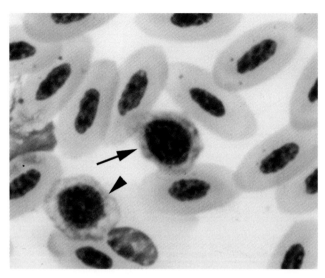

Figure 17.68 A mid (arrow) and late immature (arrow head) thrombocyte in the bone marrow of a parrot (*Psittacus erithacus*). Wright stain, 500×.

phages found in blood and body tissues, respectively. A variety of tissues, notably bone marrow, embryonic yolk sac, and spleen, can produce macrophage colonies (55). Mature monocytes are described in the discussion of leukocytes. Macrophages within the bone marrow usually contain iron pigment within the cytoplasm, because they are involved with iron metabolism during hemoglobin synthesis and catabolism. Iron may appear as gray to black granulation or as golden, crystalline material.

Lymphocytes

Aggregates of lymphocytes are found within the bone marrow of birds, although major sites of lymphopoiesis in adult birds are located in the spleen, liver, intestines, and cecal tonsils (50). Avian lymphocytes can be classified as B lymphocytes (providing humoral immunity) or T lymphocytes (responsible for cell mediated immunity), but these two cell types usually cannot be differentiated based on morphology alone. B lymphocytes differentiate in the bursa of Fabricius, and T-lymphocytes differentiate in the thymus.

Immature avian lymphocytes are larger than mature lymphocytes, and they are classified as either lymphoblasts or prolymphocytes based on morphology. Lymphoblasts have large nuclei, with fine chromatin, and they contain one or more prominent nucleoli. The cytoplasm is relatively abundant and deeply basophilic. Prolymphocytes resemble lymphoblasts, but their nuclear chromatin is coarser and nucleoli are not present. Mature lymphocytes have coarse chromatin that typically is clumped. Cytoplasm is scant and stains light blue.

Osteoblasts

Avian osteoblasts are large cells found in the bone marrow that resemble those of mammals. They have abundant, foamy, basophilic cytoplasm, with a distinct, clear Golgi apparatus. The nucleus is round to oval and eccentrically located in the cell, contains reticular to coarsely granular chromatin, and possesses one or more distinct nucleoli. Osteoblasts are polygonal to fusiform, and they may have indistinct cytoplasmic margins.

Osteoclasts

Osteoclasts are large, multinucleated, giant cells with an ameboid shape. The cytoplasm is weakly basophilic and vacuolated, and red cytoplasmic granules may be present. Nuclei are round to oval and often contain prominent nucleoli.

Hematopoietic Tissues Other than Bone Marrow

Bursa of Fabricius

Based on research using domestic chicken and quail embryos, lymphoid cells first appear in the developing bursa of the 13- to 15-day embryo (50). Granulopoiesis also occurs in the developing bursa of the 12- to 13-day chicken embryo, but it disappears either at or just before hatching. The bursa reaches its maximum growth around 4 weeks after hatching then gradually undergoes involution during a 2- to 3-month period.

During development, the bursa contains numerous deeply basophilic, lymphoid precursor cells (50). Lymphoid precursors reach a maximum number in the 13- to 25-day embryo and then decline as lymphoid differentiation progresses. Lymphoid precursors may originate from an external source, such as the yolk sac or bone marrow. Seeding of the bursa with lymphoid precursor cells appears to occur in the 7- to 14-day embryo, depending on the species. Thus, the sole source of B lymphocytes in the adult bird is the self-regenerating aggregates of B lymphocytes that originated in the bursa and then spread to the spleen, liver, intestines, and cecal tonsils.

Thymus

The thymus is organized into a cortex consisting of densely packed lymphoid cells and a medulla. Lymphoid precursors originating from the yolk sac or bone marrow begin to colonize the thymus during the first 4 to 8 days of development, depending on the species (50). The influx of lymphoid precursors appears to last from 24 to 36 hours and then ends abruptly. The invasion of the thymus by precursors is followed by a 4- to 5-day refractory period before another influx occurs. This cyclic colonization of the thymus by lymphoid stem cells consists of two to three colonization periods, which may extend into the post-hatchling period, depending on the species. This contrasts with colonization of the bursa, which occurs during a distinct, single episode in the embryo before hatching. T lymphocytes acquire their T antigen during a 24-hour period of development around the time of the second wave of colonization, between days 12 to 15 of embryonic life. T lymphocytes originating in the thymus spread to the spleen, liver, intestines, and cecal tonsils, and they are the predominate lymphoid cell of the spleen and peripheral blood of hatched birds.

Spleen

T and B lymphocytes appear at different locations in the white pulp of the spleen (50). The central arteries of the white pulp are surrounded by a periarteriolar lymphoid sheath, which is comprised of densely packed T lymphocytes. Capillaries branching at right angles from the central arteries are surrounded by periellipsoid lymphoid tissue consisting of B lymphocytes. B lymphocytes also are found at the germinal centers located within the periarteriolar lymphoid sheath. During embryonic development, the spleen participates in erythropoiesis and granulocytopoiesis. Granulopoiesis becomes more predominant as the embryo matures. At hatching, however, the granulocytes begin to disappear, and by 3 days, they are replaced by lymphocytes.

REFERENCES

1. Lucas AJ, Jamroz C. Atlas of avian hematology. USDA monograph 25. Washington, DC: U.S. Department of Agriculture, 1961.
2. Campbell TW. Avian hematology and cytology. Ames, IA: Iowa State University Press, 1988.
3. Dein FJ. Hematology. In: Harrison GJ, Harrison LR, eds. Clinical avian medicine and surgery. Philadelphia: WB Saunders, 1986: 174–191.
4. Hawkey CM, Dennett TB. Color atlas of comparative veterinary hematology. London: Wolfe Medical Publications, 1989.
5. Law GRJ. Blood samples from the jugular vein of turkeys. Poult Sci 1960;39:1450–1452.
6. Stevens RWC, Ridgeway GJ. A technique for bleeding chickens from the jugular vein. Poult Sci 1966;45:204–205.
7. Andrews FX. Simplified heart puncture in poultry diagnosis. J Am Vet Med Assoc 1950;16:38–39.
8. MacArthur FN. An improved method of obtaining blood from the chicken heart. Poult Sci 1944;23:542–544.
9. Utter JM, LeFebure EA, Greenlaw JJ. A technique for sampling blood from small passerines. Auk 1970;88:169–171.
10. Vullaume A. A new technique for taking blood samples from ducks and geese. Avian Pathol 1983;12:389–391.
11. Coles EH. Veterinary clinical pathology. 4th ed. Philadelphia: WB Saunders, 1986:53–54.
12. Schalm OW, Jain NC, Carroll EJ. Veterinary hematology. 3rd ed. Philadelphia: Lea & Febiger, 1975:21.
13. Davidson I, Henry JB. Todd-Sanford clinical diagnosis by laboratory methods. 15th ed. Philadelphia: WB Saunders, 1974.
14. Dein FJ. Laboratory manual of avian hematology. East Northport, NY: Association of Avian Veterinarians, 1984.
15. Weiss DJ. Uniform evaluation and semiquantitative reporting of hematologic data in veterinary laboratories. Vet Clin Pathol 1984; 13:27–31.
16. Rebar AH, Lewis HB, DeNicola DB, et al. Red cell fragmentation in the dog: an editorial review. Vet Pathol 1981;18:415–426.
17. Bessis M: Blood smears reinterpreted. Berlin: Springer-Verlag, 1977.
18. Sturkie PD, Griminger P. Body fluids: blood. In: Sturkie PD, ed. Avian physiology. 4th ed. New York: Springer-Verlag, 1986: 102–129.
19. Herbert R, Nanney J. Spano JS, Pedersoli WM, Krista LM. Erythrocyte distribution in ducks. Am J Vet Res 1989;50:958–960.
20. Romagnano A, et al. Binucleate erythrocytes and erythrocytic dysplasia in a cockatiel. Proc Assoc Avian Vet 1994:83–86.
21. George JW, Duncan JR. Effect of sample preparation on basophilic stippling in bovine blood smears. Vet Clin Pathol 1981;10:37–39.
22. Maxwell MH. The production of a "Heinz body" anaemia in the domestic fowl after oral ingestion of dimethyl disulphate: a haematological and ultrastructural study. Res Vet Sci 1981;30:233–238.
23. Natt MP, Herrick CA. A new blood diluent for counting erythrocytes and leucocytes of the chicken. Poult Sci 1952;31:735–738.
24. Coates ML. Hemoglobin function in the vertebrates: an evolutionary model. J Mol Evol 1975;6:285–307.
25. Gaskin JM. Psittacine viral diseases: a perspective. J Zool Wildl Med 1989;20:249–264.
26. Jacobson ER, Hines SA, Quesenberry K, et al. Epornitic of papova-like virus-associated disease in a psittacine nursery. J Am Vet Med Assoc 1984;185:1337–1341.
27. Lothrop C, et al. Miscellaneous diseases. In: Harrison GJ, Harrison LR, eds. Clinical avian medicine and surgery. Philadelphia: WB Saunders, 1988:525–536.
28. Wainright PO, Pritchard NG, Fletcher OJ, Davis RB, Clubb S. Identification of viruses from Amazon parrots with a hemorrhagic syndrome and a chronic respiratory disease. First International Conference on Zoological and Avian Medicine, 1987:15–19.
29. Assoku R, Pehale W, Buxton A. An immunological basis for the anemia of acute Salmonella gallinarium infection of chickens. Clin Exp Immunol 1970;7:865–874.
30. Fry DM, Addiego L. Hemolytic anemia complicates the clearing of oiled seabirds. Wildl J 1987;10:3–6.
31. Leighton FA, Peakall DB, Butler RG. Heinz body hemolytic anemia from ingestion of crude oil: primary toxic effect in marine birds. Science 1983;220:871–873.
32. White J. Protocol for the rehabilitation of oil-affected waterbirds. Proc Assoc Avian Vet 1990;153–163.
33. Yamato O, Goto I, Meade Y. Hemolytic anemia in wild seaducks caused by marine oil pollution. J Wildl Dis 1996;32:381–384.
34. Christie G. Hematological and biochemical findings in an experimentally produced hemolytic anemia in eight-week-old brown leghorn cockerels. Br Vet J 1979;135:279–285.
35. Rupiper DJ, Read DH. Hemochromatosis in a Hawk-head parrot (Deroptyus accipitrinus). J Avian Med Surg 1996;10:24–27.
36. Campbell TW, Dein FJ. Avian hematology: the basics. Vet Clin North Am Small Anim Pract 1984;14:223–248.
37. Sturkie PD. Blood: physical characteristics, formed elements, hemoglobin, and coagulation. In: Sturkie PD, ed. Avian physiology. New York: Springer-Verlag, 1976:53–75.
38. Newell SM, McMillan MC, Moore FM. Diagnosis and treatment of lymphocytic leukemia and malignant lymphoma in a Pekin duck (Anas platyrhynchas domesticus). JAAV 1991;5:83–86.
39. Lloyd M. Heavy metal ingestion: medical management and gastroscopic foreign body removal. JAAV 1992;6:25–26.
40. Maxwell MH, Robertson GW, Anderson IA, Dick LA, Lynch M. Haematology and histology of seven-week-old broilers after early food restriction. Res Vet Sci 1991;50:290–297.

41. Jain NC. Essentials of veterinary hematology. Philadelphia: Lea & Febiger, 1993:211–213.
42. Taylor M. Polycythemia in the Blue and Gold macaw—a case report of three cases. Proceedings of the First International Conference on Zoological and Avian Medicine, 1987:95–104.
43. Topp RC, Carlson HC. Studies on avian heterophils. II: histochemistry. Avian Dis 1972;16:369–373.
44. Topp RC, Carlson HC. Studies on avian heterophils. III: phagocytic properties. Avian Dis 1972;16:374–380.
45. Daimon T, Caxton-Martins A. Electron microscopic and enzyme cytochemical studies on granules of mature chicken granular leucocytes. J Anat 1977;123:553–562.
46. Hodges RD. Normal avian (poultry) haematology. In: Archer RK, Jeffcott LB, eds. Comparative clinical haematology. London: Blackwell Scientific Publications, 1977:483–517.
47. Brune K, Spitznagel JK. Peroxidaseless chicken leukocytes: isolation and characterization of anti-bacterial granules. J Infect Dis 1973;127:84–94.
48. Pinneall R, Spitznagel JK. Chicken neutrophils: oxidative metabolism in phagocytic cells devoid of myeloperoxidase. Proc Natl Acad Sci U S A 1975;72:5012–5015.
49. Dri P, Bisiacchi B, Cramer R, Bellavite P, de Nicola G, Patriama P. Oxidative metabolism of chicken polymorphonuclear leucocytes during phagocytosis. Mol Cell Biochem 1978;22:159–166.
50. Dieterien-Lievre F: Birds. In: Rawley AF, Ratcliffe NA, eds. Vertebrate blood cells. Cambridge, UK: Cambridge University Press, 1988:257–336.
51. Andreasen CB, Latimer KS. Cytochemical staining characteristics of chicken heterophils and eosinophils. Vet Clin Pathol 1990;19:51–54.
52. Lind PJ, et al. Morphology of the eosinophil in raptors. JAAV 1990;4:33–38.
53. Hodges RD. The histology of the fowl. London: Academic Press, 1974.
54. Carlson HC, Allen JR. The acute inflammatory reaction in chicken skin: blood cellular response. Avian Dis 1969;14:817–833.
55. Fox AJ, Solomon JB. Chicken non-lymphoid leukocytes. In: Rose LN, Payne LN, Freeman MB, eds. Avian immunology. Edinburgh, Poultry Science, 1981:135–166.
56. Swayne DE, Stockman SL, Johnson GS. Cytochemical properties of chicken blood cells resembling both thrombocytes and lymphocytes. Vet Clin Pathol 1986;15:17–24.
57. Harmon BG, Blisson JR. Disassociation of bacterial and fungistatic activities from the oxidative burst of avian macrophages. Am J Vet Res 1993;51:71–75.
58. Costello RT. A Unopette for eosinophil counts. Am J Clin Pathol 1970;54:249–250.
59. Robertson GW, Maxwell MH. Modified staining techniques for avian blood cells. Br Poult Sci 1990;31:881–886.
60. Zinkle JG. Avian hematology. In: Jain CJ, ed. Schalm's veterinary hematology. Philadelphia: Lea & Febiger, 1986:261–262.
61. Joseph V, Wagner D, Stouli J, Palagi L. Toluidine blue stain for avian WBC count. JAAV 1989;3:191–229.
62. Dein FJ, Wilson BA, Fischer MT. Avian leucocyte counting using the hemocytometer. J Zool Wildl Med 1994;25:432–437.
63. Lane R. Basic techniques in pet avian clinical pathology. Vet Clin North Am Small Anim Pract 1991;21:1157–1179.
64. Davidson TF, Flack IH. Changes in the peripheral blood leucocyte populations following an injection of corticotropin in the immature chicken. Res Vet Sci 1981;30:79–82.
65. Bhattacharyya TK, Sarkar AK. Avian leucocytic responses induced by stress and corticoid inhibitors. Ind J Exp Biol 1968;6:26–28.
66. Gross WB, Siegel HS. Evaluation of the heterophil/lymphocyte ratio as a measure of stress in chickens. Avian Dis 1983;27:972–979.
67. Tangredi BP. Heterophilia and left shift with fatal diseases in four psittacine birds. J Zool Anim Med 1981;12:13–16.
68. Rosskopf WJ, Woerpel RW, Howard EB, Holshus HJ. Chronic endocrine disorder associated with inclusion body hepatitis in a Sulfur-crested Cockatoo. J Am Vet Med Assoc 1981;179:1273–1276.
69. Olson C. Avian hematology. In: Biester HE, Swarte LH, eds. Diseases of poultry. 5th ed. Ames, IA: Iowa State University Press, 1965:100–119.
70. Campbell TW. Lymphoid leukosis in an Amazon parrot—a case report. Proc Assoc Avian Vet 1984;229–234.
71. Purchase GH, Burmester BD. Leukosis/sarcoma group. In: Hofstad MS, ed. Diseases of poultry. Ames, IA: Iowa State University Press, 1978:418–468.
72. Wight PA, et al. Monocytosis in experimental zinc deficiency of domestic birds. Avian Pathol 1980;9:61–66.
73. Maxwell MH, Burns RB. Experimental stimulation of eosinophil stimulation and of eosinophil production in the domestic fowl. Res Vet Sci 1986;41:114–123.
74. Maxwell MH. Attempted induction of an avian eosinophilia using various agents. Res Vet Sci 1980;29:293–297.
75. Chad N, Eyre P. Immunological release of histamine and SRS in domestic fowl. Can J Comp Med 1978;42:519–524.
76. Montali RJ. Comparative pathology of inflammation in the higher vertebrates (reptiles, birds, and mammals). J Comp Pathol 1988;99:1–26.
77. Carlson HC, Hacking MA. Distribution of mast cells in chicken, turkey, pheasant, and quail and their differentiation from basophils. Avian Dis 1972;16:574–577.
78. Maxwell MH, Robertson GW, Spence S, McCorquodale CC. Comparison of haematological values in restricted and ad libitum-fed domestic fowls. II. White blood cells and thrombocytes. Br Poult Sci 1990;31:399–405.
79. Grecchi R, Saliba AM, Mariano M. Morphological changes, surface receptors and phagocytic potential of fowl mononuclear phagocytes and thrombocytes in vivo and in vitro. J Pathol 1980;130:23–31.
80. Campbell TW, Coles EH. Avian clinical pathology. In: Coles EH, ed. Veterinary clinical pathology. 4th ed. Philadelphia: WB Saunders, 1986:279–301.
81. Soulsby EJL. Helminths, arthropods, and protozoa of domesticated animals. 7th ed. Philadelphia: Lea and Febiger, 1982.
82. Fite RW. Diagnosis and control of Leucocytozoonosis in canaries. Proceedings of the First International Conference of Zoological and Avian Medicine, 1987:33–35.
83. Dresser SS. Schizogony and gametogony of Leucocytozoon simondi and associated reactions in the avian host. J Protozool 1967;14:224–254.
84. Miller RE, Trampel DW, Desser SL, Boever WJ. Leucocytozoon simondi infection in European and American eiders. J Am Vet Med Assoc 1983;183:1241–1244.
85. Siccardi FJ, Rutherford HO, Derieux WT. Pathology and prevention of Leucocytozoon smithi infection of turkeys. J Am Vet Med Assoc 1971;158:1902.
86. Dorrestine GM, Vand de Hage MN, Zwart P. Diseases of passerines, especially canaries and finches. Proc Assoc Avian Vet 1985;53–70.
87. Flammer K. Clinical aspects of atoxoplasmosis in canaries. Proceedings of the First International Conference of Zoological and Avian Medicine, 1987:33–35.
88. Levine ND. The genus Atoxoplasma (Protozoa, Apicomplexa). J Parasitol 1982;68:719–723.
89. Campbell F. Fine structure of the bone marrow of the chicken and pigeon. J Morphol 1967;123:405–440.
90. Glick B, Rose C. Cellular composition of the bone marrow in the chicken. I. Identification of cells. Anat Rec 1976:185:235–246.
91. Jones AW. Granulopoiesis in the embryonic chick lung: a histologic study. Poult Sci 1973;52:1600–1603.
92. Del Cacho E, Gallego M, Bascuas JA. Granulopoiesis in the pineal gland of chickens. Am J Vet Res 1991;52:449–452.
93. Van der Heyden N. Bone marrow aspiration technique in birds. Proc Assoc Avian Vet 1986:53–60.
94. Rosse WF, Waldmann TA. Factors controlling erythropoiesis in birds. Blood 1961;27:654–661.

CHAPTER

18

HEMATOLOGY OF REPTILES

Evaluation of the hemogram and blood film is part of the laboratory evaluation of reptilian patients. Hematology is used to detect conditions such as anemia, inflammatory diseases, parasitemias, hematopoietic disorders, and hemostatic alterations. Hematologic evaluation involves examination of the erythrocytes, leukocytes, and thrombocytes in the peripheral blood.

COLLECTION AND HANDLING OF BLOOD SAMPLES

Blood samples for hematologic and blood biochemical studies can be collected from reptiles using a variety of methods, with the choice depending on the peculiarities of the species, volume of blood needed, size of the reptile, physical condition of the patient, and preference of the collector. A few venipuncture sites are available for blood sampling from some reptiles. (1,2,3); however, because the lymphatic vessels often accompany blood vessels in reptiles, a mixture of blood and lymph frequently occurs with venipuncture of the peripheral vessels (4,5). The mixing of lymphatic fluid with the blood sample is variable, and it dilutes the cellular components of the blood, thereby resulting in a lower packed cell volume (PCV), hemoglobin concentration (Hb), total erythrocyte count (TRBC), and leukocyte count (4). Therefore, the collection site chosen for a blood sample influences the hematologic values.

Jugular venipuncture can be used to collect blood from reptiles, especially chelonians (turtles and tortoises) *(Fig. 18.1)*. An advantage of jugular venipuncture is that it minimizes the chances for the hemodilution of the sample with lymphatic fluid; however, jugular venipuncture may require chemical restraint. With the head and neck extended, the jugular vein is approached as it lies just under the skin in a line between the angle of the mandible and the thoracic inlet. The right jugular vein may be larger than the left in some species (6).

The dorsal coccygeal (dorsal postoccipital or occipital) vein or venous plexus (sinus) is a common location for obtaining blood samples in reptiles, especially tortoises, turtles, and crocodilians, but samples from this location commonly are diluted with a variable amount of lymphatic fluid, which can be seen as a clear liquid entering the syringe. The dorsal coccygeal venous plexus is reached by inserting the hypodermic needle along the dorsal aspect of the neck, just off the midline and lateral to the cervical vertebrae. In some species, the venous plexus is located on the right side of the neck. To collect blood from sea turtles using this technique, a 20-G, 1.0- to 1.5-inch needle is inserted in an area located one-third of the distance from the dorsal midline to the lateral aspect of the neck and one-third of the distance from the head to the carapace (7) *(Fig. 18.2)*. Blood is collected either into a syringe or an evacuated tube. This method also may be used for other chelonians, such as tortoises and freshwater, semiaquatic turtles. The dorsal coccygeal vein or

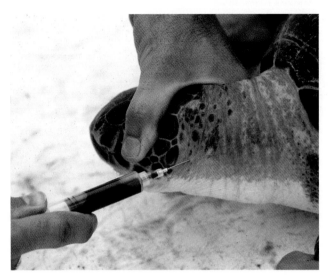

Figure 18.1 Blood collection by jugular venipuncture in a turtle (*Chelonia mydas*).

sinus is approached just behind the nuchal crest or occipital along the dorsal midline in crocodilians.

Cardiocentesis commonly is performed for blood collection from reptiles, especially snakes. The heart of a snake is located by observing the heartbeats, which move the ventral scutes overlying the heart, or by palpation. Because the heart will move caudally and cranially, it should be stabilized at the apex and base using a thumb and forefinger during sample collection (2). A needle (i.e., a thin-wall, 22- or 23-G needle attached to a 3–6-mL syringe) is inserted under the scute—not through the scale—and then advanced into the heart. Usually, the attached syringe fills slowly as the heart pulsates *(Fig. 18.3)*. The

heart of small lizards can be located by transillumination of the thoracic cavity. Cardiocentesis may be harmful in lizards, however, and it is not commonly used for blood collection in this group of reptiles. Cardiocentesis of chelonians is performed by passing a needle through the plastron along the midline at the junction of the humeral and pectoral scutes. In small chelonians, a hole is drilled through the plastron using an 18- to 20-G needle, whereas a sterile drill bit may be required for larger chelonians. After the procedure, the hole drilled through the plastron should be sealed with an epoxy. If multiple samples are required, a larger hole can be drilled into the plastron over the heart and then plugged with a rubber stopper from a blood collection tube, which is sealed into position with epoxy (8). This provides an access port to the heart for blood collection.

The ventral coccygeal vein (ventral caudal or tail vein) also is a common site for blood collection in reptiles, especially lizards, snakes, and crocodilians. This vein lies just ventral to the caudal vertebrae. To collect blood from the ventral coccygeal vein, a 22- to 23-G, 1-inch needle is inserted under a ventral scale or the ventral midline and then is directed toward the vertebrae *(Fig. 18.4)*. Slight negative pressure should be applied to the syringe as the needle is being advanced. Often, a vertebra is encountered before blood enters the needle, and in such cases, the needle is withdrawn slowly until blood flows into the syringe. Lizards and crocodilians can be bled from the tail in this manner by extending the tail over the edge of a table and approaching the site from underneath. This method of restraint is better tolerated by most reptiles compared with holding them in dorsal recumbency. Lizards also can be restrained in a vertical position by allowing them to cling to a cage door, thereby permitting access to the ventral

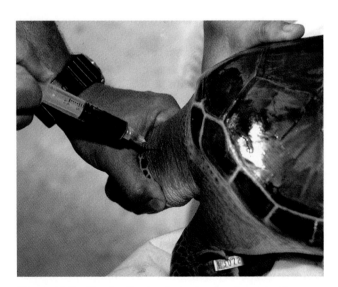

Figure 18.2 Blood collection from the dorsal coccygeal venous sinus of a turtle (*Chelonia mydas*).

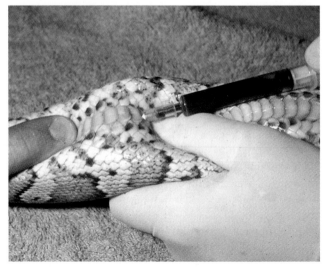

Figure 18.3 Blood collection by cardiocentesis of a snake.

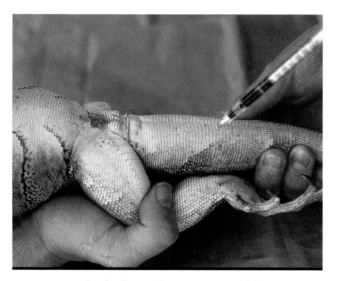

Figure 18.4 Blood collection by venipuncture of the ventral coccygeal vein of a lizard (*Iguana iguana*) using the ventral approach.

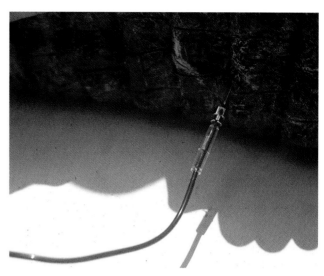

Figure 18.6 Blood collection from the ventral coccygeal vein of an alligator (*Alligator mississippiensis*) using the lateral approach.

tail. In addition, a lateral approach can be used in lizards and crocodilians by inserting the needle along the lateral aspect of the tail in an area where a natural groove or line occurs *(Figs. 18.5 and 18.6)* The needle tip should be placed just beneath the caudal vertebra and into the vein.

Other, less commonly used procedures for collecting blood from reptiles include sampling from the brachial vein or artery, palatine-pterygoid vein, ventral abdominal vein, and toenails. Blood collection from the brachial vein or artery is a blind approach, but it may be attempted in chelonians or lizards. Samples obtained using this method, however, frequently are diluted with lymph. Blood can

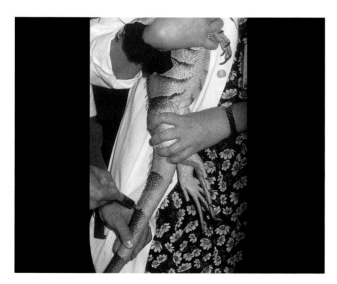

Figure 18.5 Blood collection by venipuncture of the ventral coccygeal vein of a lizard (*Iguana iguana*) using the lateral approach.

be collected from the palatine-pterygoid veins in the oral cavity of medium and large snakes, but this method requires either a cooperative patient or general anesthesia. In addition, these veins are fragile and easily lacerated. Blood can be collected by aspiration into a syringe or by allowing the blood to flow from the needle hub into a microcollection tube. Lizards have large ventral abdominal veins that lie just under the skin on the ventral midline, and although this vein is easily located, it also is easily lacerated. Thus, hemostasis after venipuncture can be a problem. To minimize bleeding, the vein can be cannulated with a needle and blood collected from the needle hub into a microcollection tube. Lastly, although blood from a capillary bed provides a poor sample for hematologic studies, blood from a clipped toenail may be the only collection procedure available in very small reptiles (i.e., <30 g). After cleaning of the toenail, the nail is clipped using nail trimmers, and blood is collected into a microcollection tube. A styptic powder or solution is used to aid clotting.

The blood volume of reptiles is estimated to range between 5% and 8% of the body weight, and most species tolerate withdrawal of as much as 10% of the blood volume (or 1% of body weight) without detrimental effects (2). Only 0.2 to 0.3 mL of blood is required for routine hematologic studies; most reptiles tolerate this loss.

Blood should be collected into an anticoagulant for hematologic evaluations. Although ethylenediaminetetraacetic acid generally is the anticoagulant of choice for hematologic studies, blood from reptiles, especially chelonians, often undergoes hemolysis in its presence. Therefore, use of an alternative anticoagulant, such as lithium heparin, is necessary. Heparin creates a blue tinge to blood films and may cause clumping of leukocytes and thrombocytes, thereby creating difficulties in obtaining accurate cell counts. To minimize these effects of heparin, the blood sample should be processed soon after collection, and slides should be made as soon as possible. A blood film made from a drop of blood that contains no anticoagulant and is taken from the needle immediately after collection can be used to avoid interference with anticoagulants during staining.

REPTILIAN ERYTHROCYTES

Morphology

Mature erythrocytes in reptiles generally are larger than those in birds and mammals. Reptilian erythrocytes are ellipsoidal cells with centrally positioned, oval to round nuclei, dense purple chromatin, and often, irregular margins *(Fig. 18.7)*. The cytoplasm stains uniformly orange-pink with Romanowsky stains such as Wright stain. Polychromatophilic erythrocytes have nuclear chromatin that is less dense and cytoplasm that is more basophilic than in mature erythrocytes. Immature erythrocytes occasionally are seen in the peripheral blood of reptiles, especially very young animals or those undergoing ecdysis. Immature erythrocytes are round to irregular cells with large, round nuclei and basophilic cytoplasm *(Fig. 18.8)*. The nucleus lacks the dense chromatin clumping of the mature cell. Immature erythrocytes often appear to be smaller than mature erythrocytes, probably for the same reasons as those described for avian hematology (see Chapter 17). Mitotic activity associated with erythrocytes is common in the peripheral blood of reptiles *(Fig. 18.9)*.

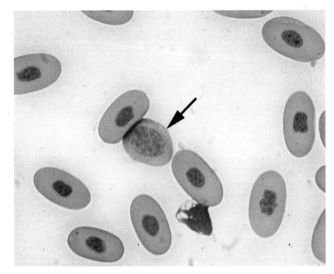

Figure 18.8 An immature erythrocyte (early polychromatic rubricyte) in the peripheral blood of a snake (*Corallus canina*). Modified Wright-Giemsa stain, 500×.

Reticulocytes are detected by staining cells with a vital stain such as new methylene blue. Reptilian reticulocytes, like avian reticulocytes, have a distinct ring of aggregated reticulum that encircles the red-cell nucleus. These cells best correspond to the polychromatophilic erythrocytes found in Romanowsky-stained blood films, and they probably are the cells that were recently released from erythropoietic tissues *(Fig. 18.10)*. Basophilic stippling commonly occurs in reticulocytes with Romanowsky stains.

Round to irregular basophilic inclusions frequently are seen in the cytoplasm of erythrocytes in the peripheral blood films from many species of reptiles *(Fig. 18.11)*.

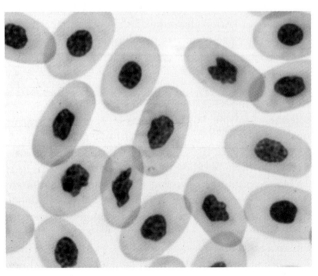

Figure 18.7 Normal erythrocytes in the blood film of a snake (*Python molurus bivittatus*). Modified Wright-Giemsa stain, 500×.

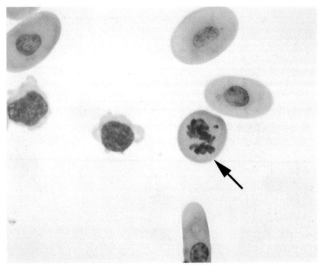

Figure 18.9 An erythrocyte exhibiting mitotic activity in the peripheral blood of a snake (*Boa constrictor*). Modified Wright-Giemsa stain, 500×.

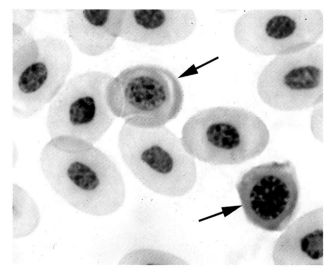

Figure 18.10 Polychromatic erythrocytes in the blood film of a lizard (*Iguana iguana*). Modified Wright-Giemsa stain, 500×.

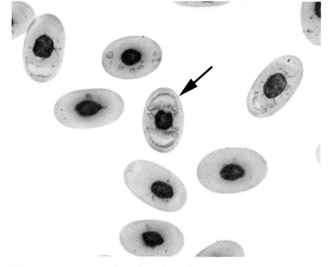

Figure 18.12 Irregular refractile artifacts are commonly found in the cytoplasm of reptilian erythrocytes. Modified Wright-Giemsa stain, 500×.

These inclusions most likely represent an artifact of slide preparation, because blood films made repeatedly from the same sample often reveal varying degrees of these inclusions. Electron-microscopic images suggest that these inclusions are degenerate organelles (9). Other artifacts found in the erythrocyte cytoplasm include vacuoles and refractile clear areas *(Fig. 18.12)*. These can be minimized with careful preparation of blood films.

Laboratory Evaluation

Laboratory evaluation of the reptilian erythron involves determination of the PCV, TRBC, and Hb of blood. The

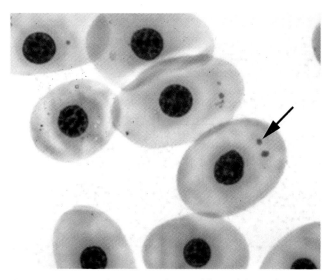

Figure 18.11 Erythrocytes with round basophilic inclusions in the blood film of a turtle (*Macroclemys temminckii*). Modified Wright-Giemsa stain, 500×.

PCV is obtained by microhematocrit centrifugation. A PCV also can be calculated by electronic cell counters that are accurately adjusted for each species according to differences in erythrocyte sizes. Microhematocrit centrifugation, however, is the most practical method for obtaining PCVs of reptilian blood.

A TRBC can be determined by a manual hemocytometer counting method or by an electronic cell counter. Two manual methods that commonly are used to obtain a TRBC in reptilian blood involve either an erythrocyte Unopette system (Becton-Dickinson, Rutherford, NJ) or Natt-Herrick solution (see Chapter 17). The erythrocyte Unopette system is the easier method, because the 1:200 dilution of the whole, anticoagulated blood is made using the diluent, pipette, and mixing vial provided with the kit. In contrast, the Natt and Herrick method requires preparation of the diluent/stain solution and use of a red blood cell–diluting pipette. Blood is drawn to the 0.5 mark on the red blood cell–diluting pipette, and Natt-Herrick solution then is drawn to the 101 mark to prepare the 1:200 dilution. With both methods, the diluted blood is discharged onto the hemocytometer counting chamber and allowed to settle for a minimum of 5 minutes before counting. The total number of erythrocytes in the four corner and central squares of the central, large square of the Neubauer-ruled counting chamber is obtained using ×40 (i.e., high-dry) magnification *(Fig. 18.13)*. The TRBC is calculated by multiplying the number of erythrocytes that are counted by 10,000.

The Hb is determined by the same technique as that described for avian hematology (see Chapter 17). The cyan-methemoglobin method or automated procedures, such as use of the Hemoglobinometer (Coulter Electronics, Hialeah, FL), can determine the Hb of reptilian blood.

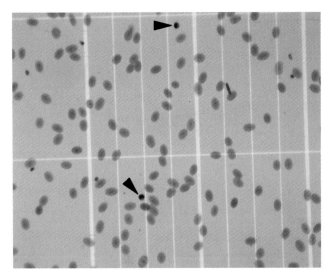

Figure 18.13 Appearance of erythrocytes and dark-staining leukocytes (arrow heads) in the Neubauer-ruled hemocytometer using Natt-Herrick solution, 100×.

The cyanmethemoglobin reagent–blood mixture requires centrifugation to remove the free nuclei from the lysed erythrocytes before measuring the optical density to obtain an accurate Hb value.

Responses in Disease

Reptiles have lower TRBCs compared with those of mammals and birds (10), and the TRBC appears to have an inverse relationship with the size of the erythrocytes (10). Lizards tend to have smaller erythrocytes than other reptiles; therefore, they have higher TRBCs (10,11) Snakes have lower TRBC values than lizards but greater values than chelonians. The TRBC, Hb, and PCV values vary with a number of factors, including the environment (TRBC values are highest before and lowest immediately after hibernation), nutritional status; and gender (males tend to have higher TRBCs than females) (10–14).

The normal PCV of most reptiles ranges between 20% and 40% (12,15,16). Therefore, a PCV of less than 20% suggests anemia, a PCV of greater than 40% suggests either hemoconcentration or erythrocytosis (polycythemia).

The causes of anemia in reptiles are similar to those described for birds and mammals. Anemia can be classified as hemorrhagic (i.e., blood loss), hemolytic (i.e., increased red-cell destruction), or depression anemia (i.e., decreased red-cell production). Hemorrhagic anemias usually result from traumatic injuries or blood-sucking parasites; however, other causes, such as a coagulopathy or an ulcerative lesion, should be considered as well. Hemolytic anemia can result from septicemia, parasitemia, or toxemia. Depression anemia usually is associated with

chronic inflammatory diseases, especially those associated with an infectious agent. Other causes that should be considered for depression anemia in reptiles include chronic renal or hepatic disease, neoplasia, chemicals, and possibly, hypothyroidism.

The degree of polychromasia or reticulocytosis in the blood films of normal reptiles generally is low, and it represents less than 1% of the erythrocyte population. This may be associated with the long erythrocyte life span (600–800 days in some species) and, therefore, with the slow turnover rate of reptilian erythrocytes compared with those of birds and mammals (10,12). The relatively low metabolic rate of reptiles also may be a factor. Young reptiles tend to have a greater degree of polychromasia than adults.

Slight anisocytosis and poikilocytosis is considered to be normal for most reptilian erythrocytes. Moderate to marked anisocytosis and poikilocytosis are associated with erythrocytic regenerative responses and, less commonly, with erythrocyte disorders. An increased polychromasia and number of immature erythrocytes is seen in reptiles responding to anemic conditions. Young reptiles or those undergoing ecdysis also may exhibit an increased polychromasia and immature erythrocyte concentration. Erythrocytes exhibiting binucleation, abnormal nuclear shapes (anisokaryosis), or mitotic activity can be associated with marked regenerative responses *(Fig. 18.14)*. These nuclear findings, however, also may occur in reptiles awakening from hibernation or in association with severe inflammatory disease, malnutrition, and starvation (17). Basophilic stippling usually suggests a regenerative response, but it may also be seen in patients with lead toxicosis. Hypochromatic erythrocytes are associated with iron deficiency or chronic inflam-

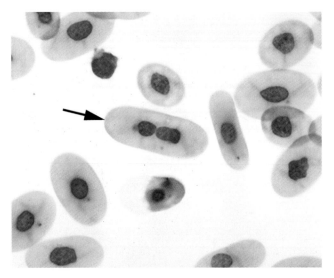

Figure 18.14 A binucleated erythrocyte in the peripheral blood of a snake (*Boa constrictor*). Modified Wright-Giemsa stain, 500×.

matory disease (presumably in association with iron sequestration).

REPTILIAN LEUKOCYTES

Morphology

The granulocytes of reptiles can be classified into two groups, acidophils and basophils, based on their appearance in blood films prepared with Romanowsky stains. The acidophils are further divided into heterophils and eosinophils. Reptilian heterophils generally are round cells with eosinophilic (bright orange), fusiform cytoplasmic granules *(Figs. 18.15 through 18.18)* The cytoplasm of normal heterophils is colorless. The mature heterophil nucleus typically is round to oval and is eccentrically positioned in the cell, with densely clumped nuclear chromatin. Some species of lizards have heterophils with lobed nuclei (14). Heterophils range between 10 and 23 μm in size but vary between species and individual blood samples (14).

The cytoplasmic granules of reptilian heterophils usually are peroxidase negative, except in a few species of snakes and lizards (9,10,18–20). In addition, reptilian heterophils do not stain for alkaline phosphatase (9). Therefore, reptilian heterophils are functionally equivalent to mammalian neutrophils, but they most likely behave like avian heterophils, in that they rely more heavily on oxygen-independent mechanisms to destroy phagocytized microorganisms.

Eosinophils in most reptilian blood films are large, round cells with spherical, eosinophilic cytoplasmic granules *(Figs. 18.18 and 18.19)*. The granules of some species

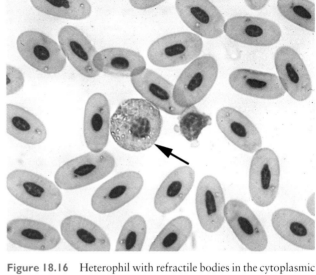

Figure 18.16   Heterophil with refractile bodies in the cytoplasmic granules of a snake (*Python molurus bivittatus*). Modified Wright-Giemsa stain, 500×.

of reptiles, such as iguanas, stain blue with Romanowsky stains. The cytoplasmic granules of eosinophils also stain positive for peroxidase in some species of reptiles, thereby allowing easy differentiation between eosinophils and heterophils (9). Like heterophils, eosinophils vary in size with the species. For example, snakes have the largest eosinophils, whereas lizards have the smallest (14). The nucleus typically is central in its cellular position and is variable in shape, ranging from slightly elongated to lobed.

Basophils usually are small, round cells that contain basophilic, metachromatic cytoplasmic granules, which often obscure the nucleus *(Fig. 18.20)*. When visible, the

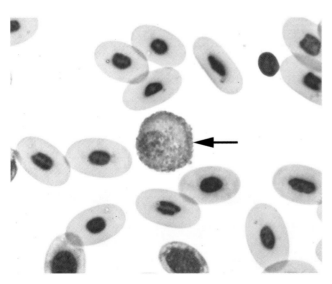

Figure 18.15   A heterophil in the blood film of a snake (*Python molurus bivittatus*). Modified Wright-Giemsa stain, 500×.

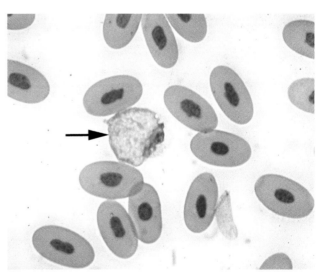

Figure 18.17   Heterophil with partially dissolved granules in the blood film of a snake (*Corallus canina*). Modified Wright-Giemsa stain, 500×.

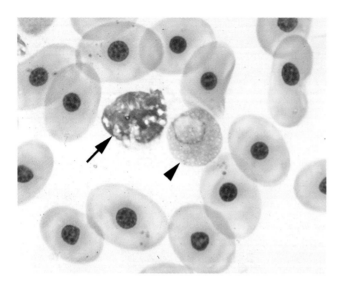

Figure 18.18   A heterophil (arrow) with fusiform cytoplasmic granules and an eosinophil (arrow head) with round cytoplasmic granules in the blood film of a turtle (*Macroclemys temminckii*). Modified Wright-Giemsa stain, 500×.

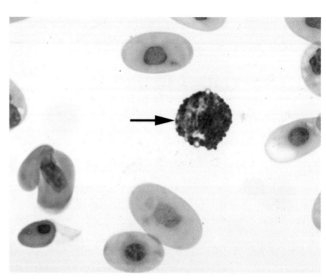

Figure 18.20   A basophil in the blood film of a snake (*Boa constrictor*). Modified Wright-Giemsa stain, 500×.

cell nucleus is slightly eccentric in position and nonlobed. Basophil granules frequently are affected by water-based stains, which cause them to partially dissolve. Therefore, alcohol fixation and use of Romanowsky stains provide the best staining results for reptilian basophils. Like acidophils, basophils vary in size according to the species, but they generally range between 7 and 20 μm (14). Lizards tend to have small basophils, whereas turtles and crocodiles have large basophils (14).

Reptilian lymphocytes resemble those of birds and mammals. They vary in size from small (5–10 μm) to large (15 μm) (10,14). Lymphocytes are round cells that exhibit irregularity when they mold around adjacent cells in the blood film or fold at their cytoplasmic margin *(Fig. 18.21)*. They have a round or slightly indented nucleus that is centrally or slightly eccentrically positioned in the cell; nuclear chromatin is heavily clumped in mature lymphocytes. Typically, lymphocytes have a large nucleus:cytoplasm ratio. The typical small, mature lymphocyte has scant slightly basophilic (pale blue) cytoplasm. Large lymphocytes have more cytoplasmic volume compared with small lymphocytes, and the nucleus

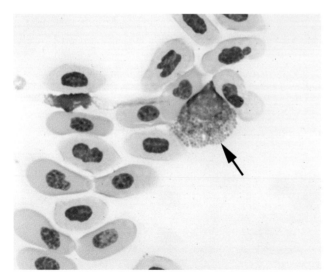

Figure 18.19   An eosinophil with blue cytoplasmic granules in the blood film of a lizard (*Iguana iguana*). Modified Wright-Giemsa stain, 500×.

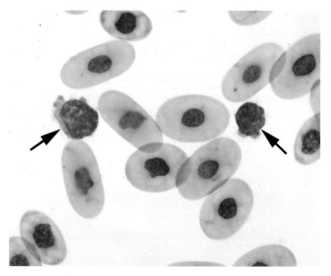

Figure 18.21   Small mature lymphocytes in the blood film of a snake (*Boa constrictor*). Modified Wright-Giemsa stain, 500×.

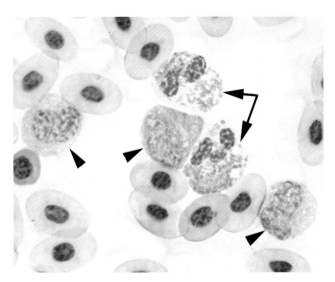

Figure 18.22 Three monocytes (arrow heads) and two heterophils (arrows) in the blood film of a lizard (*Iguana iguana*). Modified Wright-Giemsa stain, 500×.

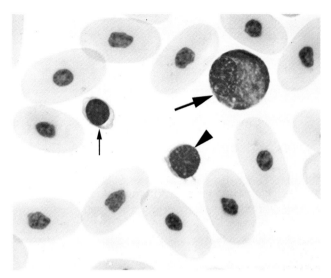

Figure 18.23 An azurophilic monocyte (large arrow), lymphocyte (arrow head), and thrombocyte (small arrow) in the blood film of a snake (*Boa constrictor*). Modified Wright-Giemsa stain, 500×.

often is pale staining. The cytoplasm of a normal lymphocyte appears to be homogenous and lacks both vacuoles and granules.

Monocytes generally are the largest leukocytes in the peripheral blood of reptiles, and they resemble those of birds and mammals *(Fig. 18.22)*. They vary in shape from round to ameboid. The nucleus also is variable in shape, ranging between round to oval to lobed. The nuclear chromatin of monocytes is less condensed and stains relatively pale compared with the nuclei of lymphocytes. The abundant cytoplasm of monocytes stains blue-gray, may appear to be slightly opaque, and may contain vacuoles or fine, dust-like eosinophilic or azurophilic granules. Although monocytes that have an azurophilic appearance to the cytoplasm often are referred to as azurophils in the literature, their cytochemical and ultrastructural characteristics are similar to those of monocytes: therefore, they should be reported as monocytes rather than as a separate cell type (10,17,19) *(Figs. 18.23 and 18.24)*. The term *azurophilic monocyte* can be used for these cells.

Laboratory Evaluation

Evaluation of the reptilian leukogram involves determination of a total and a differential leukocyte count and examination of the leukocyte morphology on a stained blood film. Manual counting methods are used to obtain total leukocyte concentrations in reptiles for the same reasons they are used in avian hematology: the presence of nucleated erythrocytes and thrombocytes in the blood of reptiles precludes the use of electronic cell-counting procedures. Two manual methods commonly used to obtain a total leukocyte count in reptilian blood are the

Natt and Herrick method and the phloxine B method (see Chapter 17) (Fig. 18.13). In species of reptiles that normally have higher numbers of circulating lymphocytes than of heterophils, the Natt and Herrick method is preferred, because the accuracy of the phloxine B method relies on large numbers of heterophils and eosinophils.

Responses in Disease

The percentage of heterophils in the leukocyte differential of normal reptiles varies with the species. Heterophils

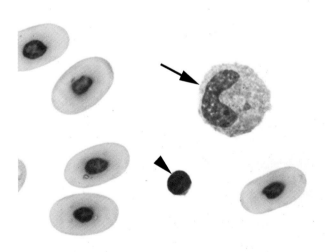

Figure 18.24 An azurophilic monocyte (arrow) and lymphocyte (arrow head) in the blood film of a tortoise (*Gopherus polyphemus*). Modified Wright-Giemsa stain, 500×.

can represent as much as 40% of the leukocytes in some normal reptilian species (10,11,15,21–24). The heterophil concentration in reptiles also is influenced by seasonal factors. For example, the heterophil concentration is highest during the summer months and is lowest during hibernation (11). Because the primary function of heterophils is phagocytosis, significant increases in the heterophil count of reptiles usually are associated with inflammatory disease, especially microbial and parasitic infections or tissue injury. Noninflammatory conditions that may result in heterophilia include stress (i.e., glucocorticosteroid excess), neoplasia, and heterophilic leukemia.

Heterophils may appear to be abnormal in reptiles suffering from a variety of diseases. For example, heterophils may exhibit varying degrees of toxicity with inflammatory diseases, especially those involving infectious agents such as bacteria. Toxic heterophils exhibit increased cytoplasmic basophilia, abnormal granulation (i.e., dark blue to purple granules or granules with abnormal shapes and staining), and cytoplasmic vacuolation *(Figs. 18.25 through 18.29)*. Degranulated heterophils may be associated with artifacts of blood-film preparation or represent toxic changes. Nuclear lobation in species that normally do not lobate their heterophil nuclei also is an abnormal finding and suggests severe inflammation.

The number of circulating eosinophils in normal reptiles is variable. In general, lizards tend to have low numbers of eosinophils compared with some species of turtles, which can have as much as 20% eosinophils (10,11, 15,21–24). Like heterophils, the number of eosinophils present in the peripheral blood is influenced by environmental factors, such as seasonal changes. The number of eosinophils generally is lower during the summer months

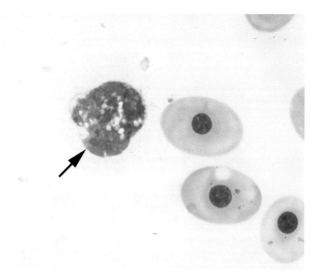

Figure 18.26   A moderately toxic (2+) heterophil in the blood film of a turtle (*Macroclemys temminckii*). Modified Wright-Giemsa stain, 500×.

and highest during hibernation in some species (11). Eosinophilia may be associated with parasitic infections and stimulation of the immune system (25).

The percentage of basophils in the differential leukocyte count of normal reptiles can range from 0% to 40% (10,11,15,21–24). Seasonal variation in the basophil concentration is minimal, unlike that in the acidophil concentration, which varies with the season (14). Some species of reptiles normally have high numbers of circulating basophils. For example, some species of turtles typically have circulating basophil numbers that represent as much

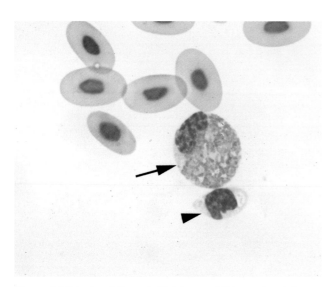

Figure 18.25   A mildly toxic (1+) heterophil (arrow) and thrombocyte (arrow head) in the blood film of a snake (*Python molurus bivittatus*). Modified Wright-Giemsa stain, 500×.

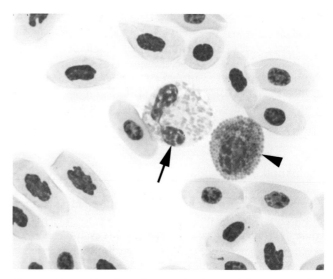

Figure 18.27   A moderately toxic (2+) heterophil (arrow) and an eosinophil (arrow head) in the blood film of a lizard (*Iguana iguana*). Modified Wright-Giemsa stain, 500×.

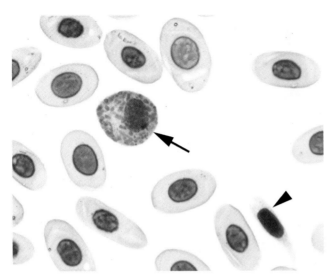

Figure 18.28 A heterophil showing marked toxicity (3+) and a thrombocyte in the blood film of a tortoise (*Gopherus agassizii*). Modified Wright-Giemsa stain, 500×.

as 40% of the leukocyte differential, although the reason for this is unknown (26,27).

Based on the results of cytochemical and ultrastructural studies, reptilian basophils most likely function in a manner similar to that of mammalian basophils. They appear to process surface immunoglobulins and to release histamine on degranulation (10,26,27). Basophilias have been associated with parasitic and viral infections (10).

The lymphocyte concentration in reptilian blood also varies and can represent more than 80% of the normal leukocyte differential in some species (10). Lymphocyte

numbers are influenced by several environmental and physiologic factors. Like heterophils and eosinophils, lymphocytes also are influenced by seasonal change; lymphocyte counts tend to be lowest during the winter months and highest during the summer months (10,11,23). Temperate reptiles have decreased numbers—or even absent—lymphocytes during hibernation, after which the lymphocyte concentration increases (28–31). Tropical reptiles also demonstrate decreased numbers of circulating lymphocytes during the winter months despite their lack of hibernation (10). Lymphocyte numbers also are affected by gender, with the female members of some species having significantly higher lymphocyte concentrations than males of the same species (10,11).

Reptilian lymphocytes function in a manner similar to those of birds and mammals. They have the same major classes of lymphocytes, B and T lymphocytes, that are involved with a variety of immunologic functions. Unlike those in birds and mammals, however, the immunologic responses of ectothermic reptiles are influenced greatly by the environment. For example, low temperatures may suppress—or even inhibit—the immune response in reptiles.

Lymphopenia often is associated with malnutrition or is secondary to a number of diseases because of stress and immunosuppression. Lymphocytosis occurs during wound healing, inflammatory disease, parasitic infection (e.g., anasakiasis and spirorchidiasis), and viral infections. Lymphocytosis also occurs during ecdysis (16). The presence of reactive lymphocytes and, less commonly, of plasma cells suggests stimulation of the immune system *(Fig. 18.30)*. These cells resemble those of birds and mammals. Reactive lymphocytes have more abundant,

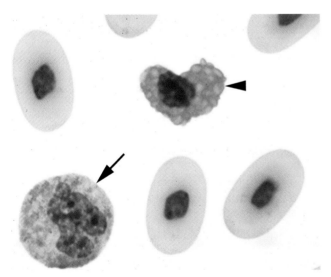

Figure 18.29 A heterophil with marked toxicity (3+) and an eosinophil in the blood film of a tortoise (*Gopherus polyphemus*). Modified Wright-Giemsa stain, 500×.

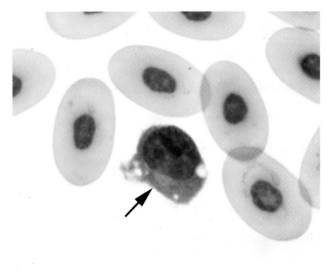

Figure 18.30 A reactive lymphocyte (plasma cell) in the blood film of a tortoise (*Gopherus polyphemus*). Modified Wright-Giemsa stain, 500×.

deeply basophilic cytoplasm compared with normal lymphocytes, and their nuclear chromatin may appear to be less condensed. Plasma cells have abundant, intensely basophilic cytoplasm that contains a distinct Golgi zone and an eccentrically positioned nucleus.

Monocytes generally occur in low numbers in the blood films of normal reptiles, ranging between 0% and 10% of the leukocyte differential (10,11,15,21–24,32,33). Snakes typically have monocytes with an azurophilic appearance to the cytoplasm, which frequently is referred to as azurophils in the literature (17) (Figs. 18.23 and 18.24). The monocyte concentration changes little with seasonal variation (11). Monocytosis suggests inflammatory diseases, especially granulomatous inflammation.

Although considered to be rare, several cases of leukemia have been reported in reptiles (34–38). The myeloproliferative diseases of reptiles can be classified in the same manner as those in mammals. Special cytochemical studies may be required to identify the abnormal cells.

THROMBOCYTES AND HEMOSTASIS

Morphology

Thrombocytes of reptiles appear as elliptical to fusiform, nucleated cells *(Fig. 18.31)*. The centrally positioned nucleus has dense nuclear chromatin that stains purple, whereas the cytoplasm typically is colorless and may contain a few azurophilic granules. Activated thrombocytes are common and appear as clusters of cells with irregular cytoplasmic margins and vacuoles. Thrombocytes appear to be devoid of cytoplasm when aggregated.

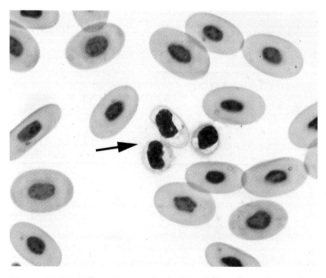

Figure 18.31   Thrombocytes in the blood film of a snake (*Python molurus bivittatus*). Modified Wright-Giemsa stain, 500×.

Laboratory Evaluation

The actual thrombocyte concentration may be difficult to determine, because thrombocytes tend to clump both in vitro and when exposed to heparin, which is a commonly used anticoagulant in reptilian hematology. The thrombocyte concentration can be measured using the Natt and Herrick method for obtained erythrocyte and leukocyte counts. After preparing the 1:200 dilution of the blood with Natt-Herrick solution and charging a Neubauer-ruled hemocytometer, the number of thrombocytes in the entire central ruled area (i.e., the central, large square) are counted on both sides of the hemocytometer. The number of thrombocytes per microliter of blood is obtained by multiplying that number by 1000. A subjective thrombocyte concentration can be determined based on the number of thrombocytes that appear in a stained blood film, and it can be reported as either reduced, normal, or increased. Thrombocytes typically occur in numbers that range between 25 and 350 thrombocytes per 100 leukocytes in the blood film of normal reptiles (10).

Responses to Disease

Reptilian thrombocytes have a significant role in thrombus formation, and they function similarly to avian thrombocytes and mammalian platelets. The ultrastructural features of activated reptilian thrombocytes include pseudopodia with fine, granular material and many fibrin-like filaments radiating both between and around the cells (10,28). Immature thrombocytes of reptiles resemble the immature thrombocytes of birds and, when present in blood films, represent a regenerative response. Thrombocytopenias of reptiles most likely result from excessive peripheral utilization of thrombocytes or decreased thrombocyte production. Thrombocytes with polymorphic nuclei are considered to be abnormal, and they may be associated with severe inflammatory disease (17).

CONSIDERATIONS IN THE INTERPRETATION OF THE REPTILIAN HEMOGRAM

When evaluating the hematologic responses of reptiles, external factors such as environmental conditions that may enhance or inhibit the animal's response to disease should not be overlooked. The cellular responses in the blood of reptiles are less predictable than those in the blood of endothermic mammals and birds whose cellular microenvironments are more stable. A number of intrinsic factors, such as age and gender, also affect the hematologic data from reptiles. In addition, a number of sample-handling factors, such as the site of blood collection, type of anticoagulant used, method of cell counting, and type of stain used, add to the variability of reptilian hemogram values. All these factors complicate the establishment of normal reference values in reptiles. Therefore, total and differential leukocyte counts must differ greatly (i.e., twofold or greater increase or decrease) from normal reference values to be considered significant.

Hematology is most valuable as a tool for assessing the response of reptilian patients to disease or therapy. A favorable response in the leukogram is a shift from a leukocytosis or leukopenia to a normal leukocyte concentration. A normal heterophil, eosinophil, or monocyte count after a heterophilia, eosinophilia, or monocytosis, respectively, usually indicates improved patient status. Disappearance of toxic heterophils, reactive lymphocytes, and plasma cells from the blood film indicates improvement and a favorable response to therapy. Anemic reptiles exhibiting an erythrocytic regenerative response have a better prognosis compared with those exhibiting little or no response. Similarly, a normal thrombocyte concentration after a thrombocytopenia indicates a favorable response. Therefore, hematology can be a valuable tool in the assessment of reptilian patients.

BLOOD PARASITES

Blood parasites are common in reptiles. Their presence usually is considered to be an incidental finding; however, some have the potential of causing disease, such as hemolytic anemia.

Common hemoprotozoa include the hemogregarines, trypanosomes, and *Plasmodium*. Less commonly encountered hemoprotozoans include *Leishmania*, *Saurocytozoon*, *Hemoproteus*, and *Schellackia*, and the piroplasmids. Microfilaria also commonly are found in the peripheral blood films of reptiles.

Hemogregarines

Hemogregarines are the most common group of sporozoan hemoparasites affecting reptiles, especially snakes. The three genera of hemogregarines that are common in reptiles are *Hemogregarina*, *Hepatozoon*, and *Karyolysus* (39). The hemogregarines are not easily differentiated based on the appearance of their gametocytes within the cytoplasm of erythrocytes or tissue schizonts (39,40). The hemogregarines found in snakes usually belong to the genus *Hepatozoon* and those of freshwater, semiaquatic turtles usually to the genus *Hemogregarina*; *Karyolysus* typically occurs in Old World lizards and, possibly, tree snakes (39–42). No cases of hemogregariniasis have been reported in sea turtles, and the parasites are rare in tor-

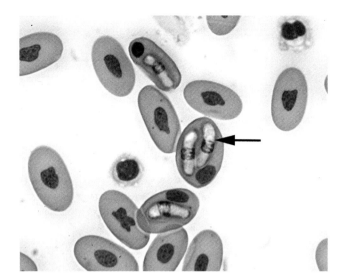

Figure 18.32 A hemogregarine, most likely *Hepatozoon*, in the blood film of a snake (*Corallus canina*). Modified Wright-Giemsa stain, 500×.

toises (40). Accurate classification of the hemogregarines into their appropriate genus cannot be accomplished based on their appearance in the blood film alone. Therefore, the general term *hemogregarine* is used when reporting their presence in blood films during hematologic examinations.

Hemogregarines are identified by the presence of intracytoplasmic gametocytes in erythrocytes. *(Figs. 18.32 and 18.33)* The sausage-shaped gametocytes lack the refractile pigment granules found in the gametocytes of *Plasmodium* and *Hemoproteus*, and they distort the host cell

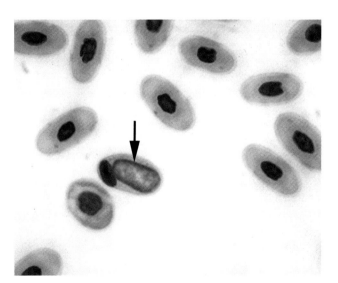

Figure 18.33 An erythrocytic inclusion resembling that of a hemogregarine in the blood film of a tortoise (*Geochelone emys*). Modified Wright-Giemsa stain, 500×.

by creating a bulge in the cytoplasm. Typically, only one gametocyte is found per erythrocyte; however, in heavy infections, two gametocytes may be found in one cell.

Hemogregarines have a life cycle that involves sexual reproduction (sporogony) in an invertebrate host and asexual multiplication (merogony) in a reptilian host. The parasite infects the reptilian host when the sporozoites are transmitted from the invertebrate host as it feeds on the blood of the reptile or is ingested by the reptile (40). Several biting, invertebrate hosts (i.e., mites, ticks, mosquitoes, flies, and bugs) can transmit the parasite to terrestrial reptiles, whereas leeches appear to be the primary intermediate host for the hemogregarines of aquatic reptiles (39). Reptilian hemogregarines are well adapted to their natural host and do not cause clinical disease; however, because they are relatively nonhost-specific, they can cause significant clinical disease in unnatural or aberrant host species (43,44). Such infections result in severe inflammatory lesions associated with schizonts in a variety of organs (43–46).

Trypanosomes

The trypanosomes found in reptiles resemble those found in mammals and birds. They are large, extracellular, flagellate protozoa with a blade-like shape, a single flagellum, and a prominent, undulating membrane *(Fig. 18.34)*. For transmission, they require a blood-sucking invertebrate host, such as biting flies for terrestrial reptiles or leeches for aquatic reptiles (40,42). Trypanosomes have been found in all orders of reptiles, have a worldwide distribution, rarely cause clinical disease, and often are associated with lifelong infections.

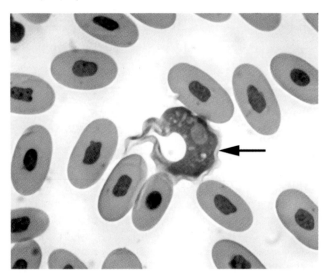

Figure 18.34 A trypanosome in the blood film of a snake (*Corallus canina*). Modified Wright-Giemsa stain, 500×.

Plasmodium

More than 60 species of *Plasmodium* have been described in reptiles; most have been identified in lizards and a few in snakes (39,47). *Plasmodium* in reptiles resemble those found in birds (see Chapter 17). The gametocytes have refractile pigment granules that aid in differentiation between *Plasmodium* and hemogregarines. Also, unlike hemogregarines, *Plasmodium* schizogony (packets of merozoites) can occur in blood cells. The trophozoites are small, signet-ring structures in the cytoplasm of erythrocytes. The life cycle of *Plasmodium* involves a sporogony stage in an insect host (e.g., mosquito) and schizogony and gametogony in a reptile host. Infections with *Plasmodium* can result in a severe hemolytic anemia.

Leishmania

Leishmania rarely are seen in blood films of reptiles. The organism is related to trypanosomes, and it primarily infects lizards (40). When present, the organism (i.e., amastigote or leishmanial stage) appears as a round to oval inclusion of 2 to 4 μm with blue cytoplasm and an oval, red nucleus in the cytoplasm of thrombocytes or mononuclear leukocytes. Leishmaniasis is primarily identified using culture techniques (48).

Saurocytozoon

Saurocytozoon produce large, round gametocytes that lack pigment granules in the cytoplasm of leukocytes in peripheral blood films. Only the gametocyte stage is found in the peripheral blood, and schizogony occurs in the tissues. The organism resembles *Leukocytozoon* of birds, because it grossly distorts the host cell that it parasitizes (see Chapter 17). As indicated by its name, this is a parasite of lizards and, most likely, is transmitted by mosquitoes (40).

Lainsonia and Schellackia

Lainsonia and *Schellackia* are coccidian parasites of lizards and snakes. They produce schizonts that can be found in the intestinal epithelium and sporozoites that can be found in the peripheral blood (40). The sporozoites are intracytoplasmic inclusions that are seen in erythrocytes and mononuclear leukocytes, primarily lymphocytes that resemble those of *Atoxoplasma* in birds (see Chapter 17). The parasite is identified by the round to oval, pale-staining, nonpigmented inclusions that deform the host-cell nucleus into a crescent shape. *Schellackia* and *Lainsonia* are transmitted by mites or, possibly, by ingestion of oocysts from feces.

Piroplasmids

The piroplasmids of reptiles include *Babesia*, *Aegyptianella* (*Tunetella*), and *Sauroplasma* or *Serpentoplasma*. They have been reported in chelonians, lizards, and snakes (40), and they appear as small, nonpigmented inclusions in the cytoplasm of erythrocytes. The inclusions are small, round to piriform, nonpigmented, and signet ring–like vacuoles measuring from 1 to 2 μm in diameter *(Fig. 18.35)*. Piroplasmids commonly found in the peripheral blood erythrocytes of lizards are referred to as *Sauroplasma*, whereas the same organisms in the blood of snakes are called *Serpentoplasma*. The piroplasmids are transmitted by biting insects or arthropods. They reproduce by either schizogony or binary fission.

Pirohemocyton

Pirhemocytonoisis is characterized by the presence of intraerythrocytic inclusions in lizards. The inclusions appear as red, punctate to oval bodies that may be associated with vacuoles (albuminoid vacuoles) and irregular, pale-staining areas in the cytoplasm of erythrocytes in Giemsa-stained blood films (49) *(Fig. 18.36)*. Similar inclusions have been reported in snakes and turtles (39). These intra-erythrocytic inclusions of reptiles were previously considered to be a piroplasm, referred to as Pirhemocyton, until ultrastructural studies revealed the presence of a virus consistent with members of the Iridoviridae (49). One report of pirhemocytonosis in snakes was suggestive of an oncornavirus based on the results of ultrastructural

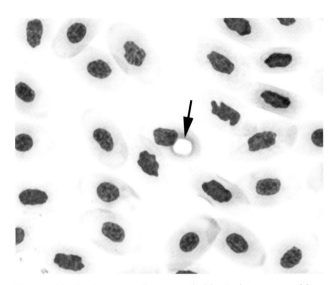

Figure 18.36 A rectangular, vacuole-like inclusion resembling that of pirohemocyton in the cytoplasm of an erythrocyte in the blood film of a lizard (*Iguana iguana*). Modified Wright-Giemsa stain, 500×.

studies (50). As the infection develops, the inclusions increase in size, measuring between 0.5 and 1.5 μm (49). A single inclusion per erythrocyte is typical; however, two inclusions per cell may occur on occasion. Natural infections with the lizard erythrocytic virus appear to be nonfatal, even with high viremias (i.e., >85% of the erythrocytes are infected) that result in the appearance of spindle-shaped or thin, elongate erythrocytes (49).

Hemoproteus

Hemoproteus (*Haemocystidium*) has been reported in lizards, turtles, and snakes (40,47). They resemble the *Hemoproteus* found in birds; only the gametocytes with refractile pigment granules are found in the peripheral blood films (see Chapter 17). The parasite can cause dehemoglobinization of the infected erythrocyte (47).

Microfilaria

Microfilaremia in reptiles typically is not associated with clinical signs of illness or changes in the hemogram or blood biochemical profile. The reptile typically survives for years with these parasites, and microfilaria are detected as an incidental finding on examination of routine Romanowsky-stained blood films. Microfilaria are produced by adult female filarid nematodes, which can live in various locations in the body of a reptile. Microfilaria are ingested by a suitable blood-sucking arthropod (i.e., tick or mite) or insect (i.e., mosquito), in which they develop

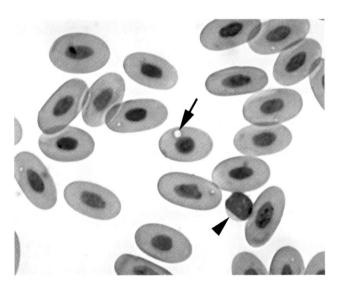

Figure 18.35 An erythrocytic cytoplasmic *Serpentoplasma* inclusion (arrow) in the blood film of a snake (*Corallus canina*). A small lymphocyte is also present (arrow head) Modified Wright-Giemsa stain, 500×.

into the infective, third-stage larval form. The life cycle is complete when the infective form enters a new reptilian host during intermediate-host feeding.

HEMATOPOIESIS

The bone marrow appears to be the primary site for erythropoiesis, granulopoiesis, and thrombopoiesis in adult reptiles. The bone marrow of some reptiles, especially turtles and tortoises, is not gelatinous, and hematopoietic cells may be difficult to sample for study. A saline-soak technique can be used for turtles in which a 2-mm thickness of bone is allowed to soak for 18 to 24 hours at 4°C, then agitated for 30 minutes, and the solution centrifuged to obtain the hematopoietic cells (51).

Erythropoiesis in the bone marrow occurs within the vascular space of the reticular stroma (9). Foci of extramedullary erythropoiesis, in the liver and spleen, are common. The maturation stages of reptilian erythrocytes appear to be similar to those of birds and mammals. In general, seven recognizable stages are involved in erythrocyte development: rubriblasts, prorubricytes, basophilic rubricytes, early polychromatic rubricytes, late polychromatic rubricytes, polychromatic erythrocytes, and mature erythrocytes. The morphologic features of these cells are similar to those described in birds (see Chapter 17).

As the reptilian erythrocytes mature, the cells become larger and the cytoplasm increasingly eosinophilic because of increased hemoglobin synthesis. A clear, size-related progression in erythrocyte development may not be evident in some species, but the shape of the cell changes from spherical to a flattened ellipsoid with maturation. The erythrocyte nucleus also decreases in size, with its shape changing from round to ellipsoid, and the nuclear chromatin becomes increasingly condensed as the cell matures. Sudan black B stain can be used as an erythrocyte marker that stains the cytoplasm of erythrocyte precursors and mature erythrocytes dark gray to black (51).

Developing granulocytes are morphologically similar to mammalian granulocytes and are associated with the extravascular spaces of the bone marrow reticular stroma (9). The maturing granulocytes migrate through the endothelial cells of the sinusoids to enter the bloodstream. The maturation stages of the granulocytes of reptiles also resemble those of birds (see Chapter 17) *(Fig. 18.37)*. As the granulocyte matures, the cell decreases in size, and the cytoplasm becomes less basophilic. Specific, characteristic granules appear in the myelocyte and metamyelocyte stages of development, and these increase in number with maturation. The nuclear chromatin becomes increasingly condensed with maturity, and in those species that lobate their nuclei, the nucleus changes from round to segmented. Mature and immature heterophils from

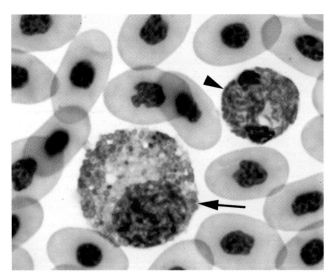

Figure 18.37   A progranulocyte (arrow) and a mature heterophil (arrow head) from a lizard (*Iguana iguana*). Modified Wright-Giemsa stain, 500×.

some species stain positive with chloroacetate esterase, α-naphthyl butyrate esterase, α-naphthyl acetate esterase, and leukocyte alkaline phosphatase chemical stains (10, 51,52,53). The cytoplasmic granules of the eosinophils of some reptiles typically are large, round, and pink with Romanowsky stains and golden brown with Benzedrine peroxidase, which helps in the differentiation of eosinophil precursors from heterophil precursors (10,51,52,53).

Thrombopoiesis in reptiles is similar to that in birds (see Chapter 17). The elliptical, mature thrombocytes are derived from round precursor cells. As thrombocytes develop, they become smaller and the cytoplasm less basophilic. The shape of the cell nucleus changes from round to oval with maturity. During the later stages of development, the nuclear chromatin becomes densely packed, and specific cytoplasmic granules may appear. It often is difficult to differentiate thrombocytes from lymphocytes in hematopoietic specimens. Special chemical stains may be used to differentiate the two in some species, in which thrombocytes stain positive with periodic acid-Schiff, acid phosphatase, and α-naphthyl butyrate esterase and lymphocytes do not (10,51,53).

The thymus is the first lymphoid organ to develop in reptiles. The lymphocytes derive from bloodborne stem cells, which most likely originate from the yolk sac (9). The origin of the immunoglobulin-producing cells (i.e., B lymphocytes) is unknown, because a reptilian equivalent to the avian bursa of Fabricius has not been found. During the early stages of splenic development, large numbers of granulocytes are present, indicating granulopoiesis. With later development, however, they disappear, and the spleen becomes primarily involved with lymphopoiesis (9). Lymphopoiesis of reptiles resembles that of mammals and birds. Reptilian lymphoblasts, prolymphocytes, and mature lymphocytes appear to be identical to those found in birds and mammals, and they can be found in lympho-poietic tissues such as the spleen.

REFERENCES

1. Samour HJ, Risley D, March T, et al. Blood sampling techniques in reptiles. Vet Rec 1984;114:472–476.
2. Jacobson ER. Blood collection techniques in reptiles: laboratory investigations. In: Fowler ME, ed. Zoo and wild animal medicine: current therapy 3. Philadelphia: WB Saunders, 1993:144–152.
3. Owens DW, Ruiz GJ. New methods of obtaining blood and cerebrospinal fluid from marine turtles. Herpetologica 1980;36:17–20.
4. Gottdenker NL, Jacobson ER. Effect of venipuncture sites on hematologic and clinical biochemical values in desert tortoises (*Gopherus agassizii*). Am J Vet Res 1995;56:19–21.
5. Crawshaw GJ. Comparison of plasma biochemical values in blood and blood-lymph mixtures from red-eared sliders, *Trachemys scripta elegans*. Bull Assoc Rept Amphib Vet 1996;6:7–9.
6. Jenkins JR. Diagnostic and clinical techniques. In: Mader DR, ed. Reptile medicine and surgery. Philadelphia: WB Saunders, 1996:264–276.
7. Campbell TW. Sea turtle rehabilitation. In: Mader DR, ed. Reptile medicine and surgery. Philadelphia: WB Saunders, 1996:427–436.
8. Wimsatt J. Personal communication, Feb. 16, 1999.
9. Alleman AR, Jacobson ER, Raskin RE. Morphologic and cytochemical characteristics of blood cells from the desert tortoise (*Gopherus agassizii*). Am J Vet Res 1992;53:1645–1651.
10. Sypik J, Borysenko M. Reptiles. In: Rowley AF, Ratcliffe NA, eds. Vertebrate blood cells. Cambridge, UK: Cambridge University Press, 1988:211–256.
11. Duguy R. Numbers of blood cells and their variations. In: Gans C, Parsons TC, eds. Biology of the reptilia. New York: Academic Press, 1970;3:93–109.
12. Frye FL. Hematology as applied to clinical reptile medicine. In: Frye FL. Biomedical and surgical aspects of captive reptile husbandry. 2nd ed. Malabar, FL: Krieger Publishing, 1991;1:209–277.
13. Mussachia XJ, Sievers ML. Effects of induced cold torpor on blood of *Chrysemys picta*. Am J Physiol 1956;187:99–102.
14. Saint Girons MC. Morphology of the circulating blood cell. In: Gans C, Parsons TC, eds. Biology of the reptilia. New York: Academic Press, 1970;3:73–91.
15. Marks SK, Citino SB. Hematology and seurm chemistry of the radiated tortoise (*Testudo radiata*). J Zool Wildl Med 1990;21:342–344.
16. Wallach JD, Boever WJ. Diseases of exotic animals, medical and surgical management. Philadelphia: WB Saunders, 1983:983–987.
17. Hawkey CM, Dennett TB. Color atlas of comparative veterinary hematology. London: Wolfe Medical Publications, 1989:6–147.
18. Mateo MR, Roberts ED, Enright FM. Morphological, cytochemical, and functional studies of peripheral blood cells in young healthy American alligators (*Alligator mississippiensis*). Am J Vet Res 1984;45:1046–1053.
19. Montali RK. Comparative pathology of inflammation in higher vertebrates (reptiles, birds, and mammals). J Comp Pathol 1988;99:1–26.
20. Caxton-Martins AE, Nganwuchu AM. A cytochemical study of the blood of the rainbow lizard (*Agama agama*). J Anat 1978;125:477–480.
21. Taylor K, Kaplan HM. Light microscopy of the blood cells of *Pseudemyd* turtles. Herpetologica 1961;17:186–192.
22. Wood FE, Ebanks GK. Blood cytology and hematology of the green sea turtle, *Chelonia mydas*. Herpetologica 1984;40:331–336.
23. Jacobson ER, Gaskin JM, Brown MB, et al. Chronic upper respiratory tract disease of free-ranging desert tortoises, *Xerobates agassizii*. J Wildl Dis 1990;27:296–316.
24. Wright KM, Skeba S. Hematology and plasma chemistries of captive prehensile-tailed skinks (*Corucia zebrata*). J Zool Wildl Med 1992;23:429–432.
25. Mead KF, Borysenko M. Surface immunoglobulins on granular and agranular leukocytes in the thymus and spleen of the snapping turtle, *Chelydra serpentina*. Dev Comp Immunol 1984;8:109–120.
26. Mead KF, Borysenko M, Findlay SR. Naturally abundant basophils in the snapping turtle, *Chelydra serpentina*, possess cytophilic surface antibodies with reaginic function. J Immunol 1983;130:384–340.
27. Sypek JP, Borysenko M, Findlay SR. Anti-immunoglobulin induced histamine release from naturally abundant basophils in the snapping turtle, *Chelydra serpentina*. Dev Comp Immunol 1984;8:358–366.
28. Wright RK, Cooper EL. Temperature effects on ectothermic immune responses. Dev Comp Immunol 1981;5(Suppl 1):117–122.
29. Hussein MF, et al. Effect of seasonal variation on the immune system of the lizard, *Scinus scinus*. J Exp Zool 1979;209:91–96.
30. Hussein MF, et al. Lymphoid tissue of the snake, *Spalerosophis diadema*, in the different seasons. Dev Comp Immunol 1979;3:77–88.
31. Hussein MF, Badir N, El Ridi R, Akef M. Differential effect of seasonal variation on lymphoid tissue of the lizard, *Chalecides ocellatus*. Dev Comp Immunol 1978;2:297–310.
32. Taylor KW, Kaplan HM, Hirano T. Electron microscope study of turtle blood cells. Cytologia 1963;28:248–256.
33. Otis VS. Hemocytological and serum chemistry parameters of the African puff adder, *Bitis arietans*. Herpetologica 1973;29:110–116.
34. Goldberg SR, Holshuh HJ. A case of leukemia in the desert spiny lizard (*Sceloporus magister*). J Wildl Dis 1991;27:521–525.
35. Langenberg JA, et al. Hematopoietic and lymphoreticular tumors in zoo animals. Lab Invest 1983;48:48A.
36. Frey FL, Carney J. Acute lymphocytic leukemia in a boa constrictor. J Am Vet Med Assoc 1973;163:653–654.
37. Frey FL, Carney J. Myeloproliferative disease in a turtle. J Am Vet Med Assoc 1972;161:595–599.
38. Desser SS, Weller I. Ultrastructural observations on the granular leucocytes of the tuatara, *Sphenodon punctatus* (Gray). Tissue Cell 1979;11:703–715.
39. Telford SR. Haemoparasites of reptiles. In: Hoff GL, Frye FL, Jacobson ER, eds. Diseases of amphibians and reptiles. New York: Plenum, 1984:385–517.
40. Keymer IF. Protozoa. In: Cooper JE, Jackson OF, eds. Diseases of reptilia. San Diego: Academic Press, 1981;1:233–290.
41. Lowichik A, Yeager RG. Ecological aspects of snake hemogregarine infections from two habitats in southern Louisiana. J Parasitol 1987;73:1109–1115.
42. Frye FL. Hemoparasites. In: Frye FL, ed. Biomedical and surgical aspects of captive reptile husbandry. 2nd ed. Melbourne, FL: Krieger Publishing, 1991;1:209–277.
43. Wozniak EJ, Telford SR, McLaughlin GL. Employment of the polymerase chain reaction in the molecular differentiation of reptilian hemogregarines and its application to preventative zoological medicine. J Zool Wildl Med 1994;25:538–549.
44. Wozniak EJ, Telford SR. The fate of possibly two Hepatozoon species naturally infecting Florida black racers and watersnakes in potential mosquito and soft tick vectors: histological evidence of pathogenicity in unnatural host species. Int J Parasitol 1991;21:511–516.
45. Griner LA: Pathology of zoo animals. San Diego: Zoological Society of San Diego, 1983.
46. Wozniak EJ, McLaughlin GL, Telford SR. Description of the vertebrate stages of a hemogregarine species naturally infecting Mojave Desert sidewinder rattlesnakes (*Crotalus cerastes cerastes*). J Zool Wildl Med 1994;25:103–110.

47. Jacobson E. Parasitic diseases of reptiles. In: Fowler ME, ed. Zoo and wild animal medicine. 2nd ed. Philadelphia: WB Saunders, 1986:162–181.

48. Campbell TW. Hemoparasites. In: Mader DR, ed. Reptile medicine and surgery. Philadelphia: WB Saunders, 1996:379–381.

49. Telford SR, Jacobson ER. Lizard erythrocytic virus in East African chameleons. J Wildl Dis 1993;29:57–63.

50. Daly JJ, Mayhue M, Menna JH, Calhoun CH. Viruslike particles associated with Pirhemocyton inclusion bodies in the erythrocytes of a water snake, *Nerodia erythrogster flavigaster*. J Parasitol 1980;66:82–87.

51. Garner MM, Homer BL, Jacobson ER, et al. Staining and morphologic features of bone marrow hematopoietic cells in desert tortoised (*Gopherus agassizii*). Am J Vet Res 1996;57:1608–1615.

52. Cannon MS. The morphology and cytochemistry of the blood leukocytes of Kemp's ridley sea turtles (*Lepidochelys kempi*). Can J Zool 1992;70:1336–1340.

53. Bounous DI, Dotson TK, Brooks RL, et al. Cytochemical staining and ultrastructural characteristics of peripheral blood leukocytes from the yellow rat snake (*Elaphe obsoleta quadrivitatta*). Comp Haematol Int 1996;6:86–91.

CHAPTER

19

HEMATOLOGY OF FISH

Hematologic evaluation of fish is not routinely used in establishing the diagnosis of fish diseases, but it can be useful in the detection of diseases affecting the cellular components of blood. Certain diseases of fish result in anemia, leukopenia, leukocytosis, thrombocytopenia, and other abnormal changes of the blood cells. Evaluation of the hemogram also may be useful in following the progress of the disease or the response to therapy.

COLLECTION AND HANDLING OF BLOOD SAMPLES

Blood for diagnostic sampling can be collected safely from fish that are greater than 3 inches (8 cm) in length (1). The collection procedure itself should be accomplished in less than 30 seconds, however, because fish that are held out of water for longer periods suffer from respiratory distress and electrolyte imbalance. Blood for hematologic evaluation should be collected in either heparin or ethylenediaminetetraacetic acid (EDTA) as an anticoagulant. Disadvantages of heparin include the tendency for leukocytes and thrombocytes to clump and the creation of a blue tinge to blood films with Romanowsky stains. In addition, if the blood sample contains a small clot, heparin may not prevent coagulation once it has started. Disadvantages of EDTA include the hemolysis of erythrocytes in some fish species. Hemolysis also can occur with the use of tricaine sedation or anesthesia, but cooling the

blood sample to 25°C and rapidly preparing the film can minimize the hemolysis associated with tricaine (1).

Blood can be collected from fish via the caudal vertebral vein or artery. Venipuncture of these vessels can be accomplished with or without sedation or anesthesia, and the caudal vertebral vein or artery can be approached either ventrally or laterally. The ventral approach involves insertion of the needle under a scale along the ventral midline near the base of the caudal peduncle (Fig. 19.1). The needle is then directed toward the vertebral bodies. After reaching the vertebral bodies, the needle is withdrawn slightly, both ventrally and laterally, while negative pressure is applied to the syringe. Once the vessels have been entered, blood will begin to enter the syringe. The needle may need to be rotated slightly to properly position the needle hub in the vessel to facilitate collection of the blood.

A lateral approach to the caudal vertebral vessels is performed by inserting the needle a few millimeters below the lateral line near the base of the caudal peduncle (Fig. 19.2). The needle is then directed toward the midline and under the vertebral bodies, and blood is aspirated into the syringe as described for the ventral approach.

Blood can be collected from the heart or bulbous arteriosus using a ventral approach. The needle is inserted slightly caudal to the apex of the V-shaped notch formed by the gill covers (opercula) and isthmus, and it is then advanced toward the heart while a slight vacuum is applied to the syringe. Blood will enter the syringe once the

277

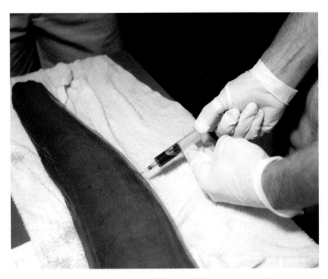

Figure 19.1   Venipuncture of the caudal vein in an eel (*Gymnothorax funebria*) using the ventral approach.

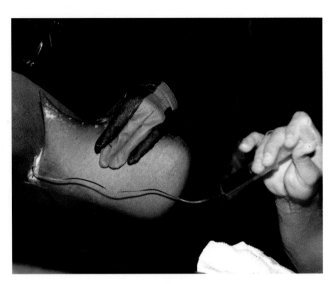

Figure 19.3   Blood collection from a shark (*Negaprion brevirostris*) using the blood vessel under the dorsal fin.

heart is penetrated. An anterolateral approach through an opened gill opercular cover also can be used to reach the heart. In this approach, the needle is directed caudally, from a point one-third of the distance between the ventral limit of the cavity (gill chamber) and medial to the bony support of the caudal wall of the opercular cavity. The needle is then advanced toward the heart using a slight vacuum. Cardiocentesis carries a greater risk of damage to the fish than use of the caudal vertebral vessels for blood collection.

Blood can be collected from large sharks using the vein that courses caudal and slightly ventral to the dorsal fins.

With the shark restrained in ventral recumbency or in a sling with its back exposed, a needle is inserted through the soft skin just under the caudal aspect of a dorsal fin as it is lifted dorsally *(Fig. 19.3)*. The needle is then directed under the dorsal fin but is kept to the back and slightly off the midline. Use of a needle with an extension tube is often helpful for keeping the needle in position should the shark move during the procedure. Advantage of this method compared with venipuncture of the caudal vertebral vessels in large sharks include ease of access to the vessel and restraint of large sharks when using the dorsal fin approach.

ERYTHROCYTES OF FISH

Morphology

Normal, mature erythrocytes of fish are oval to ellipsoidal, have abundant pale eosinophilic cytoplasm, and include a centrally positioned, oval to ellipsoidal nucleus in Romanowsky-stained blood films *(Fig. 19.4)*. The long axis of the nucleus is parallel to that of the cell, except in a few species with round erythrocyte nuclei. The nuclei of fish erythrocytes can be large, occupying as much as one-fourth (or more) of the cell volume. The nuclear chromatin is densely clumped and stains dark purple. The cytoplasm typically is homogeneous, but it may contain variable amounts of rarefied or pale-staining areas or vacuoles associated with the degeneration of organelles (2).

Both the size and number of erythrocytes vary between species of fish and, depending on the physiologic conditions, even within a single species (3). For example, the erythrocytes of fish belonging to the class Chondrichthyes

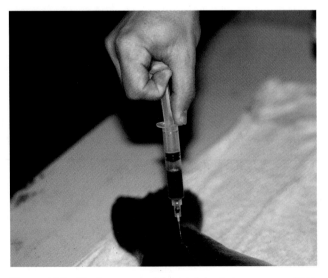

Figure 19.2   Venipuncture of the caudal vein in a grouper (*Epinephelus sp.*) using the lateral approach.

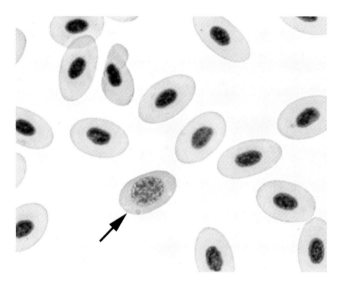

Figure 19.4 Normal mature erythrocytes and a polychromatic erythrocyte (arrow) in the blood of a bony fish (*Gymnothrorax funebris*). Wright's stain, 500×.

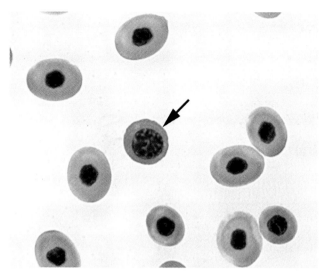

Figure 19.6 An immature erythrocyte (arrow) in the blood of a cartilaginous fish (*Pristis pectinata*). Wright's stain, 500×.

(sharks and rays) generally are larger than those of the class Osteichthyes (bony fish) (4) *(Fig. 19.5)*. Mature erythrocytes of some fish are biconvex, with a central swelling that corresponds to the position of the nucleus, whereas those of other species are flattened and biconcave (3).

Slight to moderate anisocytosis and polychromasia are normal in many species of fish. Polychromatic erythrocytes have a pale blue cytoplasm compared with that of mature erythrocytes. They also may appear to be more rounded and to have a less condensed nuclear chromatin.

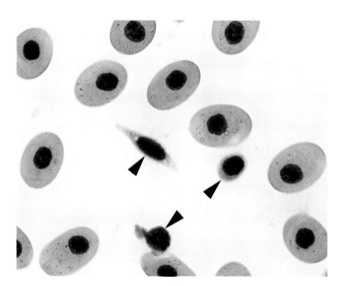

Figure 19.5 Mature erythrocytes and thrombocytes (arrowheads) in the blood of a cartilaginous fish (*Pristis pectinata*). Wright's stain, 500×.

Because erythropoiesis occurs in the peripheral blood of normal fish, immature erythrocytes may be found in blood films (2,4,5). Immature erythrocytes have larger, less condensed nuclei and less cytoplasm than mature erythrocytes *(Fig. 19.6)*. Immature erythrocytes (i.e., rubriblasts, prorubricytes, and rubricytes) are round cells with centrally positioned, round nuclei. Depending on the stage of development, the cytoplasmic volume varies in both the amount and intensity of basophilic staining with Romanowsky stains. Erythroid cells in mitosis also may be present in the peripheral blood films from normal fish.

Ultrastructurally, mature fish erythrocytes have a finely granular cytoplasm with no inclusions, whereas immature erythrocytes have a cytoplasm with mitochondria, Golgi complex, and small vacuoles (6).

Laboratory Evaluation

Determination of packed cell volume (PCV) is the most commonly used method for evaluating the red cell mass of fish. The microhematocrit method is used for obtaining a PCV of fish blood.

Although a variety of methods have been used to determine the hemoglobin concentration in fish blood, the cyanmethemoglobin method provides the most consistent results (7). As with avian and reptilian hemoglobin determinations, this procedure requires centrifugation of the blood–cyanmethemoglobin reagent mixture to remove the free erythrocyte nuclei before measurement of optical density.

A total erythrocyte count (TRBC) in fish can be determined by a manual counting method using a hemocytometer or by an electronic cell counter. Three manual

TABLE 19.1   MODIFIED DACIE'S FLUID FOR OBTAINING TOTAL CELL COUNTS IN FISH BLOOD[a]

40% Formaldehyde	10 mL
Trisodium citrate	31.3 g
Brilliant cresyl blue	1.0 gm
Distilled water	1 L

[a] Filter Dacie's fluid before use.

methods that can be used to obtain TRBCs in fish blood use the erythrocyte Unopette system (Becton-Dickinson, Rutherford, NJ), Natt-Herrick solution (see Chapter 17), or modified Dacie's solution (8, 9) *(Table 19.1)*. The erythrocyte Unopette method is the easiest of the three, because the 1:200 dilution of whole anticoagulated blood is made using the diluent, pipette, and mixing vial provided with the kit. The Natt-Herrick and modified Dacie's staining methods require preparation of the diluent/stain solution and use of the red blood cell–diluting pipette. Blood is drawn to the 0.5 mark on the pipette, and either Natt-Herrick or modified Dacie's stain is drawn to the 101 mark to prepare the 1:200 dilution. The diluted blood is then discharged onto the hemocytometer counting chamber and is allowed to settle for a minimum of 5 minutes before counting. With these stains, the oval erythrocytes show a small, dark blue nucleus that is surrounded by a colorless to faint pink cytoplasm. The total number of erythrocytes in the four corner and central squares in the central, large square of a Neubauer-ruled hemocytometer chamber is obtained using ×40 (high dry) magnification. The TRBC is calculated by multiplying the numbers of erythrocytes by 10,000.

The red blood cell indices (i.e., mean erythrocyte volume [MCV], mean corpuscular hemoglobin concentration [MCHC], and mean cell hemoglobin) can be calculated using standard formulas. However, the direct, electronic measurement of MCV appears to be more sensitive for detecting changes in the erythrocyte size in fish and is more reproducible than the calculated MCV (10).

Responses in Disease

The standard practices for collecting, handling, and analyzing blood from mammals and birds can be misleading when applied to fish. Emersion and handling of fish for venipuncture or cardiocentesis can have a marked effect on the hemogram, significantly increasing the hematocrit by as much as 25% (11,12). The magnitude of this effect relates directly to the handling and analytic time. Handling of fish for as little as 20 seconds results in the release of catecholamines, which tend to cause hemocon-

centration and swelling of the erythrocytes. Therefore, the hematocrit increases, but the hemoglobin concentration remains the same, thereby resulting in a decreased MCHC (11,12). The increase in blood catecholamines causes ion exchanges (Na^+/H^+ and Cl^-/HCO^-) across the erythrocyte membrane; thus, as Na^+ and Cl^- enter the cell, water follows osmotically, causing the cell to swell (12). Cannulation methods have been developed for use in research fish to minimize these effects; however, these methods are impractical for use in clinical studies (12).

In general, the PCV of fish is lower than that of mammals and birds (13). Hematocrits vary both between and within fish species, and they appear to correlate with the normal activity of the fish, with less active fish having lower hematocrits than active, fast-swimming fish (4,14). Hematocrits also vary during the life cycle of fish. For example, during prespawning conditions, Atlantic salmon (*Salmo salar*) have high hematocrits compared with those during spawning (4). Age, sex, water temperature, photoperiod, and seasonal variation also may influence the PCV of fish (15–19). In fact, the PCV in some species of male fish are large enough to require two reference intervals (17).

Cartilaginous fish (sharks and rays) and bony fish appear to have different gas transport systems, which affect their erythrocyte parameters. Bony fish exhibit a high cardiac workload and blood pressure, which are associated with a higher PCV and smaller erythrocytes (14). Sharks and rays, however, exhibit relatively modest cardiac workload, higher cardiac output, higher blood volumes, and increased flow rates, which are associated with lower concentrations of larger cells (14).

In general, fish with PCVs of greater than 45% usually are considered to be dehydrated, particularly when this finding is supported by increased serum osmolality or total protein. Anemic fish have low PCVs (<20%); however, for some species, such as the Port Jackson shark (*Heterodontus portusjacksoni*), normal PCVs may be as low as 20% (13).

Fish with regenerative anemia often have an increased concentration of polychromatic and immature erythrocytes in their blood films. Anemic fish that exhibit little or no polychromasia have nonresponsive anemia. A microcytic normochromic anemia has been associated with environmental stresses, such as increased population densities (19,20). A microcytic hypochromic anemia with marked poikilocytosis has been reported in trout (*Salmo gairdneri*) that were fed diets containing yeast, thereby resulting in oxidative damage to erythrocytes (21). Anemias associated with erythrocytes having pyknotic nuclei, erythroplastids (i.e., erythrocytes without nuclei), and red-blood-cell fragmentation have been associated with conditions that interfere with the splenic removal of senescent red blood cells from the peripheral circulation (22). Abnormal erythrocyte nuclei (i.e., amitosis, segmentation, and fragmentation) as well as formation of erythroplastids may relate to nutritional disorders, such as deficiency of folic acid or vitamin E and toxicosis from rancid oils and environmental pollutants (3,23).

Because the immature erythrocytes of fish are smaller than the mature erythrocytes, microcytosis often is associated with marked hemorrhagic or hemolytic anemias, in which the regenerating, immature erythrocytes represent the majority of the peripheral blood erythrocytes (24). Hemorrhagic anemias of fish are associated with trauma, blood-sucking parasites, vitamin K deficiency, and septicemia (bacteria or viral). For example, enteric red mouth disease (yersiniosis) of fish produces a hemorrhagic septicemia and a hemogram that is characterized by leukocytosis, low PCV, and reticulocytosis (1). Hemolytic anemias of fish may be associated with toxins (bacterial or environmental), viral infections (erythrocytic necrosis virus), certain nutritional deficiencies, and hemoparasites (24). Nitrite poisoning (e.g., brown blood disease, new tank syndrome) of fish results in severe hemolytic anemia. Nitrite is readily absorbed from the gills and enters into the blood, where it then oxidizes hemoglobin to methemoglobin, which in turn gradually changes the blood from red to brown in color. A hemolytic anemia then results as splenic macrophages remove the affected erythrocytes from the circulation (22).

Several nutritional deficiencies have been produced experimentally in fish. For example, folic acid deficiencies result in normochromic macrocytic anemias, and vitamin B_{12} deficiencies result in hypochromic anemias (24). Folate deficiency has been suggested as being a cause of the chronic hemolytic anemia that occurs in channel catfish (*Ictalurus punctatus*) (25).

FISH LEUKOCYTES

Leukocytes (especially the granulocytes) exhibit a wide variation in appearance among fish species. This has led to controversy and confusion when applying the nomenclature and classification of piscine leukocytes on the basis of such descriptions from avian and mammalian Romanowsky-stained blood films. Evaluation of the cellular ultrastructure, differential cytochemical staining, immunofluorescence, and function testing of fish leukocytes, however, has helped to alleviate some of this controversy in some species.

Leukocytes of Commonly Studied Bony Fish

Channel Catfish

Ultrastructural and cytochemical studies have identified heterophils, basophils, lymphocytes, and monocytes in the peripheral blood of channel catfish (4,26–28).

These results support the classification of these cells in Romanowsky-stained blood films.

Goldfish

On the basis of electron microscopy, leukocytes found in the peripheral blood of goldfish (*Carassius auratus*) can be classified as lymphocytes, monocytes, heterophils, eosinophils, and rarely, basophils (29). On the basis of cytochemical reaction, goldfish leukocytes can be classified as lymphocytes, heterophils, monocytes, and an atypical, segmented granulocyte (26).

Salmonids (Trout and Salmon)

On the basis of cytochemical staining, salmonids appear to have three types of leukocytes: lymphocytes, neutrophils, and monocytes.

Bass

Striped bass (*Morone saxatulis*) leukocytes are classified as lymphocytes, neutrophils, and monocytes.

Sturgeon

Four types of leukocytes—lymphocytes, monocytes, neutrophils, and eosinophils—have been described in white sturgeon (26).

Summary

Cytochemical studies of piscine leukocytes appear to support the use of mammalian leukocyte terminology as a classification scheme. In general, neutrophils or heterophils, lymphocytes, and monocytes commonly are reported in the peripheral blood films of fish belonging to the class Osteichthyes (teleost or bony fish). Myeloperoxidase stain is used to differentiate neutrophils from true heterophils, because neutrophils stain positive and heterophils stain negative (30–33). Eosinophils and basophils are rare in the peripheral blood of bony fish (34,35).

Leukocytes of Sharks and Rays

The peripheral blood of fish belonging to the class Chondrichthyes (cartilaginous fish, such as sharks and rays) contain leukocytes that can be classified as granulocytes, lymphocytes, or monocytes. The granulocytes exhibit marked variation in both numbers and types between species, and the granulocyte classification scheme is based on the results of ultrastructural and cytochemical studies performed in blood samples from the lesser spotted dogfish (*Scliorrhinus canicula*), which has been used as a model for cartilaginous fish (4). The granulocytes are classified as either G_1 (type I), G_2 (type II), or G_3 (type III). Basophils also can be found in the peripheral blood of cartilaginous fish.

Morphology

Neutrophils of Bony Fish

The neutrophils of bony fish tend to be round to slightly oval cells with eccentric nuclei *(Fig. 19.7)*. The nucleus of mature neutrophils vary in shape, being round, oval, indented (metamyelocyte type), elongated (band cell type), or segmented, and usually with two to three lobes. Nonsegmented nuclei are the most common in the granulocytes of bony fish. The nuclear chromatin is coarsely clumped, and it stains deeply basophilic in Romanowsky-stained blood films. The neutrophils of bony fish have abundant colorless, grayish, or slightly acidophilic-staining cytoplasm; small cytoplasmic granules also may be present. The staining of the granules varies, however, and depends on the species or the maturity of the cell. The small, cytoplasmic granules of the neutrophils vary from gray to pale blue or red. Interspecies differences in the cytochemical reactions of bony fish neutrophils are observed; however, in general, they resemble the neutrophils of mammals. Piscine neutrophils that exhibit distinct, rod-shaped cytoplasmic granules on Romanowsky stains often are classified in the literature as heterophils. Some species, such as goldfish and carp (*Cyprinus carpio*), have granulocytes with distinct and slightly acidophilic cytoplasmic granules, colorless cytoplasm, and eccentric, partially lobed nuclei on Romanowsky stains. These cells often are clas-

sified as heterophils rather than neutrophils, although they do have cytochemical properties similar to those of neutrophils in other fish. They measure approximately 10 μm in diameter. These heterophils are peroxidase and Sudan black B positive when the granules are immature, but they are peroxidase negative in mature granules (4). An atypical, segmented granulocyte that does not appear to be analogous to any leukocyte of mammals or birds has been found in blood films from goldfish (26). Neutrophils from channel catfish and certain species of eel also contain prominent eosinophilic, rod-shaped cytoplasmic granules resembling those of avian heterophils on the basis of Romanowsky stains. The granules of these cells are strongly peroxidase positive (4). Similar cells have been found in a number of other bony fish as well. In salmonids, such as rainbow trout (*Onchorhynchus mykiss*) and coho salmon (*Onchorhynchus kisutch*), these neutrophils are the predominant granulocyte, as in most bony fish. Piscine neutrophils often reveal artifacts of blood film preparation, causing the cells to appear large and with swollen, pale nuclear chromatin (karyolysis).

Eosinophils of Bony Fish

Eosinophils rarely are reported in the blood films from bony fish, and some investigators doubt whether they exist at all in some species (34,36). When present, however, they appear as intermediate to large granulocytes, with distinct eosinophilic granules and pale blue cytoplasm. The nucleus varies from round (more common) to segmented. They can be distinguished from heterophils on the basis of cytochemistry and ultrastructural findings, although the absence of crystalloids (used as a fingerprint for mammalian eosinophils) often is the rule with piscine eosinophils (34). Eosinophils have been reported in goldfish, white sturgeon, and channel catfish (6,26,29,37). Piscine eosinophils tend to be round, with round to rod-shaped eosinophilic-stained cytoplasmic granules (with Romanowsky stain) *(Fig. 19.8)*. The granules of piscine eosinophils often are less distinct compared with those of birds and mammals. These granules also have a tinctorial quality that differs from those of heterophils with distinct eosinophilic granules.

The eosinophils of carp are approximately 7.5 μm in diameter, and they have an eccentric nucleus that is indented, sausage-shaped, or bilobate as well as eosinophilic, cytoplasmic granules that are larger than those of the heterophils (4).

Basophils of Bony Fish

Basophils are rare in the peripheral blood of bony fish and have been reported only in a few species (34,35). Baso-

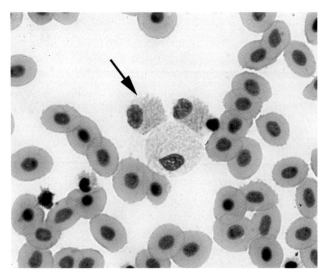

Figure 19.7   Three neutrophils (arrow) in the blood of a bony fish (*Artromotus ocellatus*). Wright's stain, 500×.

283

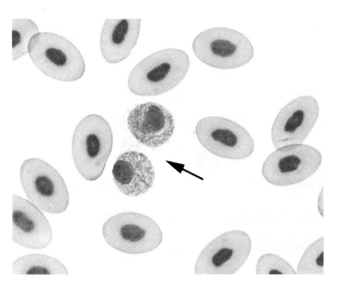

Figure 19.8 Two eosinophils (arrow) with distinct cytoplasmic granules in the blood of a bony fish *Gymnothrorax funebris*). Wright's stain, 500×.

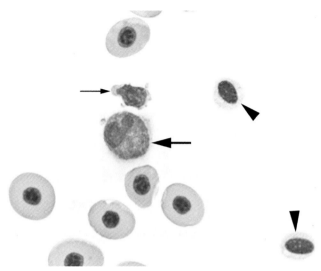

Figure 19.10 A G₁ granulocyte (arrow), lymphocyte (thin arrow), and thrombocytes (arrowhead) in the blood of a cartilaginous fish (*Pristis pectinata*). Wright's stain, 500×.

phils are identified as round cells that have round, basophilic cytoplasmic granules that often obscure the cell nucleus *(Fig. 19.9)*. The nucleus is large, eccentric, and round. The nuclear chromatin is homogeneous. The basophils of carp measure between 10 and 20 μm (4). When present, basophils occur in low numbers.

Granulocytes of Sharks and Rays

In cartilaginous fish, G₁ (type I) granulocytes typically have an eccentric, irregular, nonlobed nucleus; colorless cytoplasm; and round to oval, eosinophilic cytoplasmic

granules *(Fig. 19.10)*. The nucleus may be lobed in some species. These cells resemble avian heterophils, and they often are the most common form of the granulocytes. The G₂ (type II) granulocytes have a lobed nucleus and a colorless cytoplasm that lacks distinct granules *(Fig. 19.11)*. These cells resemble mammalian neutrophils. The G₃ (type III) granulocytes are characterized by a lobed nucleus (in some species), pale blue cytoplasm, and strongly eosinophilic, round to rod-shaped cytoplasmic granules *(Fig. 19.12)*. The cytoplasmic granules in the G₃ granulocytes have tinctorial qualities that differ from those of the G₁ granulocytes in the same blood film *(Fig. 19.13)*.

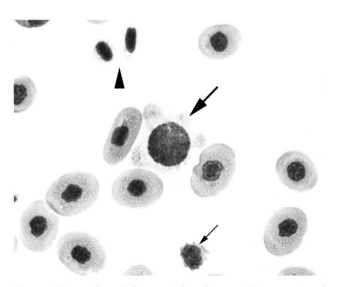

Figure 19.9 A basophil (arrow), lymphocyte (thin arrow), and thrombocyte (arrowhead) in the blood of a cartilaginous fish (*Pristis pectinata*). Wright's stain, 500×.

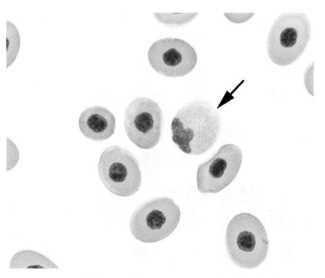

Figure 19.11 A G₂ granulocyte (arrow) in the blood of a cartilaginous fish (*Pristis pectinata*). Wright's stain, 500×.

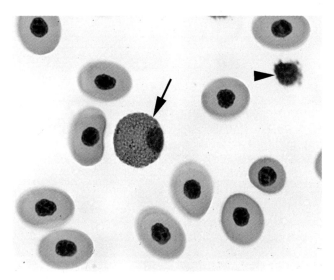

Figure 19.12   A G₃ granulocyte (arrow) and small lymphocyte (arrowhead) in the blood of a cartilaginous fish (*Pristis pectinata*). Wright's stain, 500×.

The G₃ granulocytes of cartilaginous fish resemble avian eosinophils.

The granulocytes of sharks and rays tend to stain negatively for peroxidase, β-glucuronidase, and Sudan black B but positive for acid phosphatase, aryl sulfatase, and acid naphthyl AS-D chloroacetate esterase (4). The eosinophilic granulocytes (G₁ and G₃) of the elasmobranchs share few morphologic and cytochemical characteristics with mammalian eosinophils. The function and interrelationships of the granulocytes in cartilaginous fish are not

known; however, they appear to be separate cell types rather than intermediate stages of one cell type (4). Not all species of cartilaginous fish exhibit all the granulocytes described for the lesser spotted dogfish (*Scyliorhinus canicula*). For example, only G₁ and G₃ granulocytes have been found in the rays *Raja clavata* and *Raja microcellata* (4). Basophils occasionally are found in peripheral blood films of some species of cartilaginous fish.

Lymphocytes of Fish (Bony and Cartilaginous)

Lymphocytes frequently are the most abundant leukocyte in peripheral blood films of fish, and they resemble their counterparts in avian and mammalian blood films *(Fig. 19.14)*. They typically measure between 5 and 8 μm in diameter. Lymphocytes tend to be round, but they may mold around adjacent cells in the blood film. They have a high nucleus:cytoplasm ratio, with coarsely clumped, deeply basophilic nuclear chromatin. The scant cytoplasm of small mature lymphocytes stains a homogenous pale blue. An occasional lymphocyte possesses azurophilic cytoplasmic granules. Reactive lymphocytes in blood films from fish resemble those of birds and mammals, with abundant, deeply basophilic cytoplasm and an occasional, distinct Golgi complex *(Fig. 19.15)*. Plasma cells also may be seen in small numbers on the peripheral blood films of many species of fish.

Monocytes of Fish (Bony and Cartilaginous)

Monocytes occasionally are reported in the blood films of most species of fish, and they resemble monocytes of birds

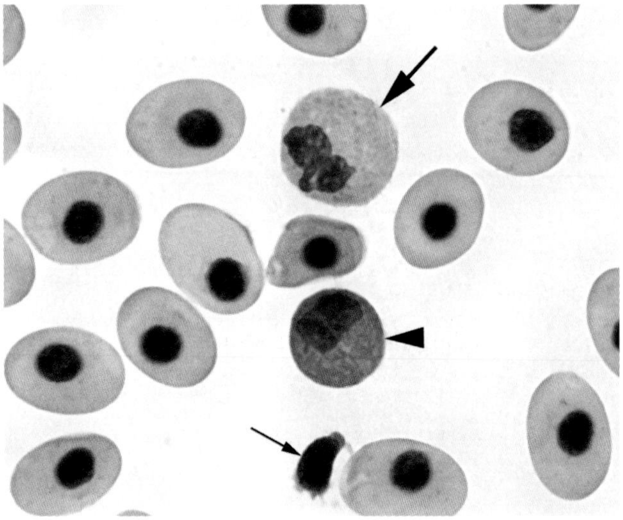

Figure 19.13   A G₁ (arrow) and a G₃ (arrowhead) granulocyte and lymphocyte (thin arrow) in the blood of a cartilaginous fish (*Negaprion brevirostris*). Wright's stain, 500×.

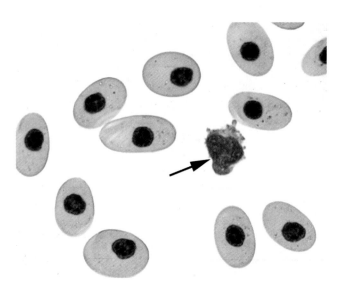

Figure 19.14   A lymphocyte (arrow) in the blood of a cartilaginous fish (*Negaprion brevirostris*). Wright's stain, 500×.

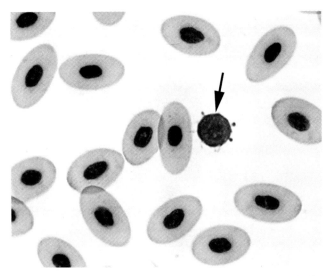

Figure 19.15   A reactive lymphocyte (arrow) in the blood of a bony fish (*Gymnothrorax funebris*). Wright's stain, 500×.

and mammals. They are large, mononuclear leukocytes, with abundant blue-gray to blue agranular cytoplasm, which may contain vacuoles *(Fig. 19.16)*. The cytoplasmic margins may be indistinct or ragged because of the presence of pseudopodia. The nucleus varies in shape (kidney-shaped to bilobate) and generally occupies less than 50% of the cytoplasmic volume. The nuclear chromatin of monocytes generally is more granular and less clumped compared with that of lymphocyte nuclei. Results of ultrastructural studies indicate that monocytes in all species of fish are similar to those in other vertebrates. The term

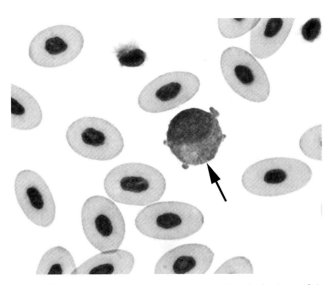

Figure 19.16   A monocyte (arrow) in the blood of a bony fish (*Gymnothrorax funebris*). Wright's stain, 500×.

monocyte/macrophage frequently is used to classify piscine monocytes, because cells resembling transformational forms between monocytes and macrophages often are found in peripheral blood films. The term *monocyte*, however, is reserved for those found in peripheral blood, and the term *macrophage* is reserved for those found elsewhere. Fish monocytes can be differentiated from immature granulocytes and lymphocytes by the positive, nonspecific esterase reaction in monocytes.

Laboratory Evaluation

The same problems associated with obtaining total leukocyte counts in birds and reptiles also apply in fish. Because fish have nucleated erythrocytes and thrombocytes, manual counting methods are used. Direct leukocyte counting methods using a Neubauer-ruled hemocytometer and a variety of staining and diluting solutions have been used (8,9,38,39). Natt and Herrick's method commonly is used, and the procedure is the same as that described for obtaining total leukocyte counts in avian and reptilian blood (see Chapters 17 and 18). The leukocytes appear blue and stain darker than erythrocytes stained with Natt-Herrick. It may be difficult to distinguish small, mature lymphocytes from thrombocytes if the counts are made using a ×10 objective; cells are more accurately identified at higher magnifications. Staining for 60 minutes in Natt-Herrick's solution also may improve the differentiation between small lymphocytes and thrombocytes. Advantages of the Natt and Herrick procedure include the ability to obtain a total erythrocyte, leukocyte, and thrombocyte count using the same charged hemocytometer. In addition, the technique can be applied to blood samples obtained from all lower vertebrates.

A leukocyte differential is obtained from a Romanowsky-stained blood film. Applying a drop of albumin to the slide during preparation of the blood film often is advantageous to minimize smudging of the cells. Quickly drying the blood film using a hair dryer also may help to alleviate cellular artifacts associated with blood film preparation (1).

Responses in Disease

Piscine neutrophils and heterophils participate in inflammatory responses. They are not always phagocytic, however, and little is known regarding their function, including their methods of intracellular killing and digestion of phagocytized organisms. Because the function of fish granulocytes is not known, viewing them as being homologous to the granulocytes of higher vertebrates is appropriate. Therefore, interpretation of the changes may not be in granulocyte concentrations of peripheral blood can be difficult. Broad generalizations can be made, however, until the results of further studies indicate the specific functions and responses of these cells to disease. For example, an increased concentration of fish neutrophils or heterophils often is associated with inflammatory diseases, especially those involving infectious agents (28). A relative neutrophilia or heterophilia often is associated with lymphopenias, which can be interpreted as a stress response in fish (5).

Eosinophils are found in low concentrations (0%–3% of the leukocyte differential) in the peripheral blood of normal fish. Piscine eosinophils participate in inflammatory responses along with neutrophils (heterophils) and macrophages, and they appear to have a limited phagocytic capability (4). Piscine eosinophils apparently are involved in the control of infections with metazoan parasites, and they participate in the immune responses to antigenic stimulation (5). Therefore, an increased eosinophil concentration in the peripheral blood of fish suggests an inflammatory response associated with parasitic infections or antigenic stimulation.

The functions of the granulocytes of cartilaginous fish are not known; however, they appear to participate in inflammatory responses. Because the granulocytes account for 20% to 30% of the leukocytes in sharks and rays, the normal granulocyte:lymphocyte ratio typically is low (<0.5). An increase in the granulocyte concentration is indicative of an inflammatory response. A decrease in the lymphocyte concentration results from conditions that reduce the number of circulating lymphocytes, such as stress responses. Both increases in the granulocyte concentrations and decreases in the lymphocyte concentrations of sharks can be associated with bacterial septicemias. The leukogram of cartilaginous fish can be used to follow the progress of these fish during the course of the disease or in response to therapy. For example, an initial increase in the granulocyte concentration or decrease in the lymphocyte concentration that has returned to normal indicates a favorable response to therapy and prognosis.

Piscine monocytes are actively phagocytic cells, and they participate in acute inflammatory responses in fish (4). Monocytes occur in low numbers (<5% of the leukocyte differential) in the peripheral blood of normal fish. Therefore, a monocytosis is suggestive of an inflammatory response in fish that is, perhaps, associated with an infectious agent.

Lymphocytes are the most commonly observed leukocytes in the peripheral blood of most normal fish, in which they typically represent greater than 60% (and as much as 85% in some species) of the leukocyte differential. Lymphocytes play a major role in the humoral and cell-mediated immunity of fish. Therefore, lymphocytosis is suggestive of immunogenic stimulation, whereas lymphopenia is suggestive of immunosuppressive conditions, such

as stress or excess exogenous glucocorticosteroids (40). Bacterial septicemias commonly affect fish and result in marked leukopenias and lymphopenias (41).

THROMBOCYTES AND HEMOSTASIS

The blood of fish clots in response to injury, as it does in other vertebrates. The speed and effectiveness in fish, however, are variable. Clotting is much more rapid in bony fish compared with sharks and rays. Sharks and rays appear to rely primarily on the extrinsic pathways of coagulation; the addition of skin, high calcium solutions, sea water, or other extrinsic factors enhances clotting (4). Clot formation in bony fish usually occurs within 5 minutes, whereas clotting in samples taken from sharks and rays can take 20 minutes or longer.

Morphology

Fish thrombocytes are smaller than erythrocytes, vary in shape, and can be round, elongate, or spindle-shaped. In addition, the shape may vary with the stage of maturity or the degree of reactivity. The oval and elongated forms tend to be nonreactive, mature thrombocytes (Fig. 19.17). Immature thrombocytes are round in some species, whereas spindle-shaped thrombocytes appear to be reactive forms and often are found in clumps. The cytoplasm of the piscine thrombocyte is colorless to faint blue; the nucleus is condensed and follows the shape of the cell. Fish thrombocytes also may contain a variable amount of eosinophilic cytoplasmic granules (Fig. 19.18).

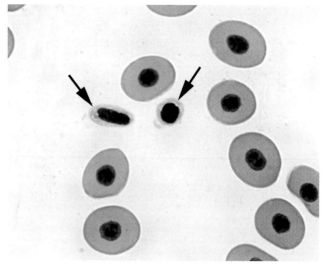

Figure 19.17   Thrombocytes (arrow) in the blood of a cartilaginous fish (*Pristis pectinata*). Wright's stain, 500×.

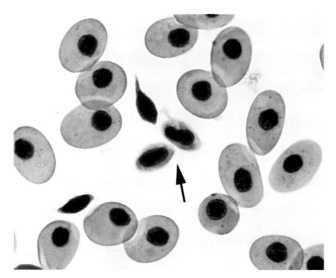

Figure 19.18   Thrombocytes (arrow) with eosinophilic cytoplasmic granules in the blood of a cartilaginous fish (*Negaprion brevirostris*). Wright's stain, 500×.

Like those in birds and reptiles, thrombocytes in fish often are confused with small, mature lymphocytes. Lymphocytes, however, have slightly more abundant, mildly basophilic cytoplasm compared with thrombocytes. The nucleus of the lymphocyte also usually is larger and less condensed compared with that of the thrombocyte. Fish thrombocytes usually stain weakly positive with periodic acid-Schiff and positive for acid phosphatase (26).

Laboratory Evaluation

The total thrombocyte count can be obtained via the same hemocytometer charged with diluting solutions (i.e., Natt-Herrick solution) used to obtain a total erythrocyte and leukocyte count. The thrombocytes resemble erythrocytes in the hemocytometer, but they are much smaller and appear to be round to oval, with a greater nucleus:cytoplasm ratio compared to erythrocytes. All squares in the central, large square of a Neubauer hemocytometer are counted on both sides. The average number of thrombocytes in one large hemocytometer square is calculated and then multiplied by 2000 to obtain the total thrombocyte count per microliter. Because thrombocytes tend to clump, however, accurate counts may be difficult to achieve.

Responses in Disease

During the clotting process in fish, fibrinopeptides are formed after the cleavage of fibrinogen, which is under the control of thrombin. These fibrinopeptides differ from those produced by mammals; however, the basic structure of fibrin in fish, though much larger than its mammalian counterpart, is the same as that in mammals. Fish thrombocyte aggregation differs from mammalian platelet aggregation. For example, fish thrombocytes convert arachidonic acid to prostaglandins with little, if any, thromboxane formation, whereas thromboxane is a potent inducer of platelet aggregation in mammals (4). Thrombocyte aggregation in sharks is temperature reversible, which is a feature not seen with mammalian platelet aggregation (4). Shark thrombocyte aggregation also is independent of thrombin and adenosine diphosphate. Therefore, both the control and the outcome of thrombocyte aggregation in fish may not be the same as mammals.

Glucocorticoid excess in fish tends to decrease the thrombocyte concentration and increase the clotting time (13). Prolonged clotting times also occur with vitamin K deficiency; dietary requirements for vitamin K have been determined for salmonids and channel catfish (5).

BLOOD PARASITES

Hemogregarina sp.

Hemogregarina sp. affecting fish resemble those described in the blood films of reptiles, and they are identified by characteristic gametocytes in the cytoplasm of erythrocytes (see Chapter 18). The gametocytes lack refractile pigment granules and may create a bulge in the cytoplasmic membrane. Little is known regarding the life cycle of fish hemogregarines, but they most likely require a blood-feeding, intermediate host, such as leeches, copepods, and isopods. Therefore, they more frequently are found in wild-caught fish. Often, the *Hemogregarina* sp. gametocytes in the peripheral blood of fish are considered to be an incidental finding; however, some species can cause anemia, leukocytosis with a marked left shift, and large granulomas in internal organs (1,42).

Trypanosomes

Trypanosomes occasionally may be found in blood films of fish, especially wild-caught, cold-water species. They can occur in high concentration (1,000,000 organisms/µL) and are especially prevalent in the imprints of kidney tissue (4). Infections with trypanosomes can result in fatal anemias. Leeches act as the intermediate host for the trypanosomes, and the infective trypomastigotes develop and then enter the fish host when the leech takes a blood meal. Trypanosomes are identified by their slender and serpentine shape, single anterior flagellum, prominent and undulating membrane, nucleus, and kinetoplast. On wet-mount preparations, the trypanosomes exhibit rapid, wriggling movements but have no forward motion.

Trypanoplasms

Trypanoplasms are hemoparasites that resemble trypanosomes morphologically, except that they are more pleomorphic (a slender, serpentine shape is most common), have two flagella (one directed anteriorly and one posteriorly), and kinetosomes. Their life cycle is similar to that of the trypanosomes. A prepatent period occurs after infection, and then parasitemia (i.e., cryptobiasis) results in either death of the fish or disappearance of the trypanoplasmas from the blood (4). *Trypanoplasma borreli* causes a severe anemia in cyprinids (i.e. Koi, goldfish, and carp), and the disease is referred to as sleeping sickness (4). Anemia, exophthalmia, ascites, and splenomegaly occur in freshwater salmonids (i.e. trout) with *T. salmositica*; *T. bullocki* infects marine fish, especially flatfish species along the western Atlantic and Gulf of Mexico (4). On wet-mount preparations, trypanoplasms exhibit flowing, ameboid motility, which aids in their identification (4).

Piroplasmids

Babesiosoma, Haemohormidium, Haematractidium, and *Mesnilium* are genera of piroplasmids that have been described in fish. As with the hemogregarines, little is known regarding their life cycle, which most likely requires a blood-feeding, intermediate host. Piroplasmids are identified by their intracytoplasmic inclusions in circulating erythrocytes, which can vary from small, ring-like forms to anaplasma-like inclusions. Piroplasmids may cause hemolytic anemia in fish.

Microsporidians

Enterocytozoon salmonis is an intranuclear microsporidium that primarily infects hematopoietic cells of salmonids. The infected cells exhibit intranuclear inclusions. This organism was once considered to be the causative agent of plasmacytoid leukemia of Chinook salmon (*Onchorhynchus tshawytscha*). The presence of high reverse-transcriptase activity in the affected tissues from these fish, however, suggests that an oncogenic retrovirus may be the causative agent for that disease (43).

Viral Inclusions

Intracytoplasmic inclusions occur in the erythrocytes of fish with viral erythrocytic necrosis (i.e., piscine erythrocytic necrosis), erythrocytic inclusion body syndrome, and coho anemia. Viral erythrocytic necrosis occurs in a variety of marine fish, including salmon, cod, and herring. The disease is characterized by marked poikilocytosis, a single intracytoplasmic inclusion (0.3–4.0 μm) within the erythrocytes, and karyolysis of the red-blood-cell nuclei (1). Erythrocytic inclusion body syndrome of young salmonids is characterized by progressive, severe anemia, which is caused by a viral agent that creates 0.8- to 3.0-μm intracytoplasmic inclusions within the erythrocytes (1). A Leishman-Giemsa stain provides the best results for demonstrating the inclusions. An anemia that occurs in seawater-reared coho salmon (*Oncorhynchus kisutch*) results from 0.1- to 2.0 -μm intracytoplasmic inclusions, which often are rod-shaped within the erythrocytes (1).

HEMATOPOIESIS

Cartilaginous fish (Chondrichthyes) lack bone marrow and lymph nodes, but they do have a lymphoid thymus, spleen, and other lymphomyeloid tissues. Significant hematopoietic activity occurs in the sinusoids of the red pulp area of the spleen, where erythrocytes, thrombocytes, and lymphocytes develop (4). Little evidence, however, suggests that granulopoiesis occurs in the spleen of these fish. Development of erythrocytes in these fish appears to occur in the same manner as that in mammals. The peripheral blood may be an important component of erythropoiesis, because several stages of erythrocyte development can be found in the routine blood films from cartilaginous fish. The epigonal organ, which is associated with the gonad, and Leydig's organ, which is situated in the submucosa of the alimentary tract, are the major sites for granulopoiesis in cartilaginous fish (4). Myeloblasts, progranulocytes, myelocytes, metamyelocytes, and mature granulocytes have been described in these unique lymphomyeloid tissue.

The principle lymphomyeloid tissues of bony fish (Osteichthyes) are the thymus, spleen, and kidney. The thymus, which is the first lymphoid organ to develop, seeds the spleen and kidney with lymphocytes. The kidney is a major blood-forming organ in bony fish; the pronephric (anterior or head) and opisthonephric (main or trunk) kidneys are the sites of hematopoiesis in these fish. The opisthonephric kidney also functions as an excretory organ. Therefore, the kidney (primarily the pronephros) is the principal site for the differentiation and development of erythrocytes, granulocytes, lymphocytes, monocytes, and possibly, thrombocytes in most bony fish (4). The typical stages of granulocyte development have been identified for each type of granulocyte in the kidney of bony fish. The spleen of teleost fish is similar to that of elasmobranchs, but it typically has a secondary role in hematopoiesis, except in some species in which it is the only hematopoietic organ (4).

REFERENCES

1. Noga EJ. Fish disease, diagnosis and treatment. St. Louis: Mosby, 1996.
2. Stokes EE, Firkin BG. Studies of the peripheral blood of the Port Jackson shark (*Heterodontus portusjacksoni*) with particular reference to the thrombocyte. Br J Haematol 1971;20:427–435.

3. Hibiya T, ed. An atlas of fish histology: normal and pathological features. Tokyo: Kodansha, 1985.
4. Rowley AF, et al. Fish. In: Rowley AF, Ratcliffe NA, eds. Vertebrate blood cells. Cambridge: Cambridge University Press, 1988:19–127.
5. Stoskopf MK. Fish medicine. Philadelphia: WB Saunders, 1993.
6. Hyder SL, Cayer ML, Pettey CL. Cell types in peripheral blood of the nurse shark: an approach to structure and function. Tissue Cell 1983;15:437–455.
7. Larsen HN, Snieszko SF. Comparison of various methods of determination of hemoglobin in trout blood. Prog Fish Cult 1961;23:8–17.
8. Natt MP, Herrick CA. A new blood diluent for counting the erythrocytes and leukocytes of the chicken. Poult Sci 1952;31:735–738.
9. Dacie JV, Lewis K. Practical hematology. 4th ed. London: Churchill Livingstone, 1968.
10. Haley PJ, Weiser MG. Erythrocyte volume distribution in rainbow trout. Am J Vet Res 1985;46:2210–2211.
11. Heming TA. Clinical studies of fish blood: importance of sample collection and measurement techniques. Am J Vet Res 1989;50:93–97.
12. Railo E, Nikinmaa M, Soivio A. Effects of sampling of blood parameters in the rainbow trout, *Salmo gairdneri* Richardson. J Fish Biol 1985;26:725–732.
13. Campbell TW. Tropical fish medicine. Fish cytology and hematology. Vet Clin North Am Small Anim Pract 1988;18:347–364.
14. Danilo WF, Eble GJ, Kassner G, Capriario FX, Dafre AL, Ohira M. Comparative hematology in marine fish. Comp Biochem Physiol 1992;102A:311–321.
15. Kamra SK. Effect of starvation and refeeding on some liver and blood constituents of Atlantic cod. J Fish Res Board Can 1966;23:975–982.
16. Haws GT, Goodnight CJ. Some aspects of the hematology of two species of catfish in relation to their habitats. Physiol Zool 1962;35:8017.
17. Sano T. Hematological studies of the culture fishes in Japan. J Tokyo Univ Fish 1960;46:68–87.
18. Summerfelt RC. Measurement of some hematological characteristics of goldfish. Prog Fish Cult 1967;29(10):13–20.
19. Burton CB, Murray SA. Effects of density on goldfish blood—I. Hematology. Comp Biochem Physiol 1979;62A:555–558.
20. Murray SA, Burton CB: Effects of density on goldfish blood—II. Cell morphology. Comp Biochem Physiol 1979;62A:559–562.
21. Sanchez-Muiz FJ, de la Higuera M, Varela G. Alterations of erythrocytes of the rainbow trout *Salmo gairdneri* by the use of *Hansenula anomola* yeast as sole protein source. Comp Biochem Physiol 1982;72A:693–696.
22. Ellis AE. Bizarre forms of erythrocytes in a specimen of plaice, *Pleuronectes platessa* L. J Fish Dis 1984;7:411–414.
23. Eiras JC. Erythrocyte degeneration in the European eel, *Anguilla anguilla*. Bull Eur Assoc Fish Pathol 1983;3:8–10.
24. Ferguson HW. Systemic pathology of fish. Ames, IA: Iowa State University Press, 1989.
25. Plumb JA, Liu PR, Butterworth CE. Folate-degrading bacteria in channel catfish feeds. J Appl Aguacult 1991;1:33–43.
26. Zinkl JG, Cox WT, Kono CS. Morphology and cytochemistry in leucocytes and thrombocytes of six species of fish. Comp Haematol Int 1991;1:187–195.
27. Cannon MS, et al. An ultrastructural study of the leukocytes of the channel catfish, *Ictalurus punctatus*. J Morphol 1980;164:1–23.
28. Ellsaesser CF, et al. Analysis of channel catfish peripheral blood leukocytes by bright field microscopy and flow cytometry. Trans Am Fish Soc 1985;114:279–285.
29. Weinreb EL. Studies on the fine structure of teleost blood cells in peripheral blood. Anat Rec 1963;147:219–238.
30. Andreasen CB, Latimer KS. Cytochemical staining characteristics of chicken heterophils and eosinophils. Vet Clin Pathol 1990;19:51–54.
31. Jain NC. Schalm's veterinary hematology. 4th ed. Philadelphia: Lea & Febiger, 1986:275–281.
32. Jain NC, et al. A comparison of cytochemical techniques to demonstrate peroxidase activity in canine leukocytes. Vet Clin Pathol 1988;17:87–89.
33. Montali RJ. Comparative pathology of inflammation in higher vertebrates (reptiles, birds, and mammals). J Comp Pathol 1988;99:1–26.
34. Ellis AE. The leukocytes of fish: a review. J Fish Biol 1977;11:453–491.
35. Saunders DC. Differential blood cell counts of 121 species of marine fishes of Puerto Rico. Trans Am Microsc Soc 1966;85:427–499.
36. Catton WT. Blood cell formation of certain teleost fishes. Blood 1951;6:39–60.
37. Williams RW, Warren MC. Some observations on the stained blood cellular elements of channel catfish, *Ictalurus punctatus*. J Fish Biol, 1976;9:491–496.
38. Blaxhall PC, Daisley KW. Routine hematological methods for use with fish blood. J Fish Biol 1973;5:771–781.
39. Shaw AE. A direct method for counting the leukocytes, thrombocytes, and erythrocytes of bird blood. J Pathol Bacteriol 1930;32:833–835.
40. McLeay DJ. Effects of cortisol and dexamethasone on the pituitary-interrenal axis and abundance of white blood cell types in juvenile coho salmon, *Oncorhynchus kisutch*. Gen Comp Endocrinol 1973;21:441–450.
41. Brenden RA, Huizinga HW. Pathophysiology of experimental *Aeromonas hydrophila* infection in goldfish, *Carassius auratus* (L.). J Fish Dis 1986;9:163–167.
42. Ferguson HW, Roberts RJ. Myeloid leucosis associated with sporozoan infection in cultured turbot (*Scophthalmus maximus* L.). J Comp Pathol 1975;85:317–326.
43. Newbound GC. Production of monoclonal antibodies specific for antigens derived from tissue of chinook salmon (*Oncorhynchus tshawytscha*) affected with plasmacytoid leukemia. Am J Vet Res 1993;54:1426–1431.

CHAPTER

20

HEMATOLOGY OF AMPHIBIANS

Compared with other vertebrates seen in veterinary practices, amphibians are unique, because their normal life cycle includes a metamorphosis from a larval to an adult form. Amphibians have adapted to aquatic, terrestrial, fossorial, and alpine environments, and their normal hematologic parameters vary accordingly. Amphibians, especially frogs of the Ranidae family, are often used in research, but hematologic evaluation of amphibians is not routinely used in establishing the diagnosis of amphibian diseases. In fact, establishing reference values and the hematologic interpretation can be challenging because of the various extrinsic and intrinsic factors that influence these results. Extrinsic factors, such as environmental temperature, photoperiod, water-quality parameters, diet, and population density, should be noted whenever reference values are reported. Adaptation to a specific environment also influences the hematologic parameters. Important intrinsic factors include gender and age; larval and adult stages should be considered as separate entities, each with their own reference range.

COLLECTION AND HANDLING OF BLOOD

Blood can be collected from frogs and toads by venipuncture of the ventral abdominal or lingual vein or by cardiocentesis. Adequate restraint for blood collection may require sedation or anesthesia, such as submersion of the amphibian in a 0.05% solution of tricaine methanesul-

phonate. Care must be taken to avoid breaking the fragile mandibular bones while holding the mouth open to collect blood from the lingual vein. Excess saliva is swabbed from below the tongue, after which a large vein of the lingual venous plexus on the ventral aspect of the tongue is punctured with a 25-G needle. Blood is then allowed to flow into a microcollection or hematocrit tube. Venipuncture of the ventral abdominal vein of larger frogs and toads is accomplished by insertion of a 25-G needle through the ventral midline in a craniodorsal direction, midway between the sternum and the pelvis *(Fig. 20.1)*. Blood is collected either by the drip method or by aspiration into a small syringe. Because lymphatic vessels accompany blood vessels in amphibians, a mixture of blood and lymph frequently occurs with venipuncture of the ventral abdominal vein. This mixing of lymphatic fluid with the blood sample is variable, but it will dilute the cellular components of the blood, thereby resulting in lower packed cell volume (PCV), hemoglobin concentration, and erythrocyte and leukocyte concentrations. Cardiocentesis is performed by placing the frog or toad in dorsal recumbency and locating the heart either by visualizing the pulsing heart or by use of a Doppler scan. Once the heart is located, a 25-G needle is inserted into the ventricle, and blood is aspirated into a syringe.

Blood collection from salamanders and newts can be accomplished by venipuncture of the ventral abdominal vein or by cardiocentesis, in the same manner as that described for frogs and toads. In addition, venipuncture of the ventral coccygeal vein can be performed by insertion

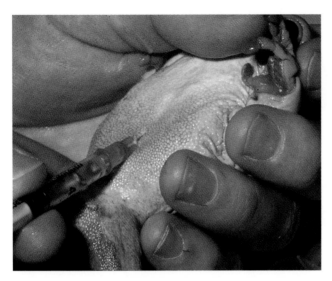

Figure 20.1   Blood collection from a tree frog (*Litoria caerulea*) using the ventral abdominal vein.

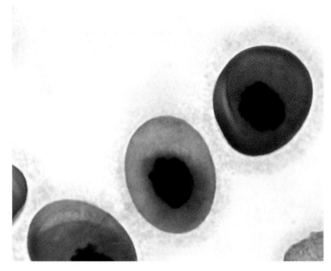

Figure 20.2   Erythrocytes in the blood of a salamander (*Ambystoma tigrinum*). Wright's stain, 500×.

of a 25-G needle to a point just below the coccygeal vertebrae, after which blood is aspirated into a syringe. This technique should be avoided, however, in salamanders and newts with tail autotomy (i.e., a natural ability to lose their tail), because the tails may break off during the procedure. Collection of blood after tail amputation has been used in research, but it should not be used in clinical practice.

Blood for hematologic studies in amphibians should be collected using lithium heparin as an anticoagulant. Ethylenediaminetetraacetic acid usually causes hemolysis of amphibian blood and, therefore, should be avoided. Syringes may be pretreated with lithium heparin, or blood can be allowed to drip from the needle hub into a microcollection tube containing lithium heparin.

ERYTHROCYTES OF AMPHIBIANS

Morphology

Erythrocytes of amphibians are nucleated, elliptic discs *(Fig. 20.2)*. The cells usually have a distinct nuclear bulge, and the nuclear margins often are irregular. Amphibian erythrocytes are large compared with those of other vertebrates. The mean size of a variety of frog and toad erythrocytes is 22 × 14 μm. The cytoplasm of frog and toad erythrocytes is homogenous and packed with hemoglobin. Ultrastructural analysis reveals rare organelles. Because the erythrocytes of salamanders and newts complete their maturation in the peripheral circulation, the cytoplasm is not homogenous, and ultrastructural examination demonstrates clusters of granular and vacuolar bodies. Some amphibians, such as the slender salamander (*Batrachoceps attenuatus*), lack nuclei in most of their erythrocytes.

Laboratory Evaluation

The microhematocrit method is used for obtaining a PCV, which is the most common method for evaluating the red cell mass of amphibians. The cyanmethemoglobin method commonly is used to determine the hemoglobin concentration in amphibian blood. As with blood hemoglobin determinations in birds, reptiles, and fish, this procedure requires centrifugation of the blood–cyanmethemoglobin mixture to remove the free erythrocyte nuclei before the optical density is measured.

The total erythrocyte count in amphibians can be determined either by manual counting with a hemocytometer or by an electronic cell counter. Manual counting methods to obtain red-cell concentrations in amphibian blood include the erythrocyte Unopette system (Becton-Dickinson, Rutherford, NJ) and Natt and Herrick's method. These methods are the same as those described for use in avian blood (see Chapter 17).

Responses in Disease

Because newts and salamanders generally are more fish-like than toads and frogs, interpretation of their hemograms may be more like those of fish, whereas hematologic changes in toads and frogs may be more like those of reptiles. In general, amphibian PCVs are lower than those of mammals and birds, and these values vary with species, age, gender, environmental temperature, photoperiod, season, and life style of the amphibian *(Table 20.1)*. Normal erythrocytes exhibit a slight anisocytosis; however, increased anisocytosis suggests erythroid regeneration or dyscrasia caused by an increased concentration of large red cells. Because of the stability of their environments, captive amphibians may have erythron parameters that

TABLE 20.1   NORMAL HEMATOLOGIC PARAMETERS FOR THE JAPANESE NEWT (*CYNOPS PYRRHOGASTER*) AND BULLFROG (*RANA CATESBEIANA*)

	Japanese Newt[a]	Bullfrog[b]
Erythrocytes		
PCV (%)	40.0 ± 1.90	22.0 ± 5.00
Red blood cells (×10⁶ cells/µL)	22.8 ± 2.95	—
Hemoglobin (g/dL)	—	4.70 ± 0.90
Leukocytes		
White blood cells (× 10³cells/µL)	1.80 ± 0.29	5.20 ± 2.90
Neutrophils		
(%)	28.0 ± 2.60	22.0 ± 15.2
(× 10³ cells/µL)	—	1.25 ± 1.31
Lymphocytes		
(%)	3.00 ± 0.40	62.9 ± 15.0
(× 10³ cells/µL)	—	3.16 ± 1.84
Monocytes		
(%)	6.00 ± 1.00	0.64 ± 1.00
(× 10³ cells/µL)	—	27.0 ± 39.0
Eosinophils		
(%)	4.00 ± 0.70	8.90 ± 6.10
(× 10³ cells/µL)	—	0.38 ± 0.32
Basophils		
(%)	57.0 ± 3.20	2.50 ± 2.90
(× 10³ cells/µL)	—	0.13 ± 0.14
Band cells		
(%)	—	0.20 ± 0.60
(× 10³ cells/µL)	—	19.9 ± 53.0

Data from Pfeiffer CJ, Haywood P, Asashima M. Blood cell morphology and counts in the Japanese newt (*Cynops pyrrhogaster*). J Zool Wildl Med 1990;21:56–64; and Cathers T, Lewbart GA, Correa M, et al. Serum chemistry and hematology values for anesthetized American bullfrogs (*Rana catesbeiana*). J Zool Wildl Med 1997;28:171–174.
[a] Values reported as mean ± standard error.
[b] Values reported as mean ± standard deviation.

fluctuate less than those of wild amphibians. Because amphibians are ectothermic, the rapidity of their hematologic responses can be manipulated by changes in the environment, such as temperature fluctuation.

LEUKOCYTES OF AMPHIBIANS

Morphology

The leukocytes of amphibians, like those of most mammals, are classified as being neutrophils, eosinophils, basophils, lymphocytes, and monocytes. Amphibian leukocytes generally are larger than those of mammals.

Amphibian neutrophils resemble those of mammals, and they range from 10 to 25 µm in diameter for most species *(Fig. 20.3)*. They have multilobed nuclei with small cytoplasmic granules that vary in size, shape, and ultrastructure between species. Cells with small eosinophilic cytoplasmic granules often are referred to as heterophils. Amphibian neutrophils typically are peroxidase positive, but phosphatase activity varies with the species. The large, irregular cytoplasmic granules of neutrophils from the giant salamander (*Megalobatrachus* sp.) resemble those in humans with Chédiak-Higashi syndrome.

Eosinophils of amphibians are similar in size to neutrophils, and they have a slightly basophilic cytoplasm, with small to moderate-sized, round to oval, eosinophilic cytoplasmic granules *(Fig. 20.4)*. The nuclei of eosinophils are less lobed than those of neutrophils. Eosinophils are peroxidase negative, and the phosphatase activity

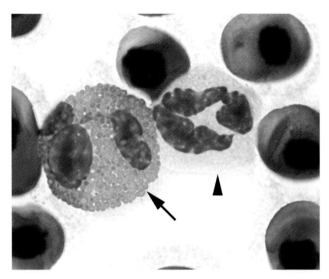

Figure 20.3 A neutrophil (arrowhead) and an eosinophil (arrow) in the blood of a salamander (*Ambystoma tigrinum*). Wright's stain, 500×.

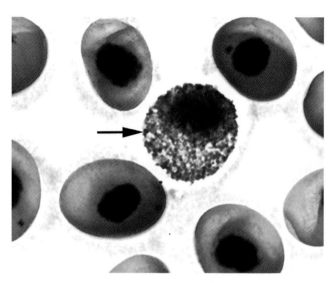

Figure 20.5 A basophil (arrow) in the blood of a salamander (*Ambystoma tigrinum*). Wright's stain, 500×.

varies with species. The eosinophils of some species, such as the Colorado River toad (*Bufo alvarus*), are negative for aryl sulfatase and β-glucuronidase activity. Some amphibian eosinophil granules have a crystalloid ultrastructure, but others, such as the Japanese newt (*Cynops pyrrhogaster*) and the slender salamander, lack the crystalloid structures that are typical of the ultrastructural morphology of eosinophils from higher vertebrates.

The size of amphibian basophils varies between species. Typically, these basophils have nonsegmented nuclei and large, metachromatic granules *(Fig. 20.5)*. The granules contain acid mucopolysaccharides (i.e., glycosaminogly-

cans) that are less sulfated than those of mammals, and the histamine content is lower than that of mammals. Ultrastructural analysis demonstrates large numbers of membrane-bound cytoplasmic granules with small numbers of organelles.

The lymphocytes of amphibians resemble those of other vertebrates. Small lymphocytes are more abundant than larger forms in the blood films of normal amphibians. The lymphocytes are round, with round nuclei, and they have dense chromatin clumping as well as a scant amount of pale blue cytoplasm *(Fig. 20.6)*. Many of the lymphocytes have distinct azurophilic granules from

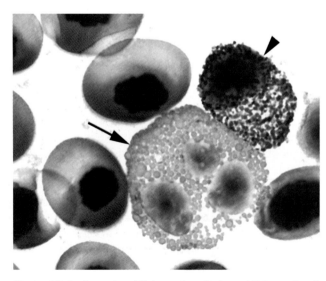

Figure 20.4 An eosinophil (arrow) and a basophil (arrowhead) in the blood of a salamander (*Ambystoma tigrinum*). Wright's stain, 500×.

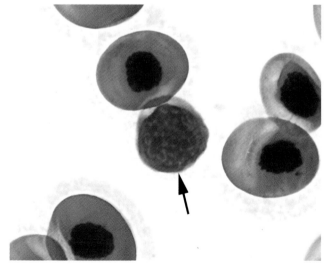

Figure 20.6 A lymphocyte (arrow) in the blood of a salamander (*Ambystoma tigrinum*). Wright's stain, 500×.

frogs of the family Ranidae. Amphibian lymphocytes, like mammalian lymphocytes, are nonspecific esterase positive and peroxidase negative but, unlike mammalian lymphocytes, are negative for β-glucuronidase and aryl sulfatase.

Monocytes in amphibian blood films are similar to those of other vertebrates, and they are characterized by their large size; abundant, blue-gray cytoplasm that may be foamy or vacuolated; and a variably shaped nucleus with less chromatin clumping than seen in lymphocyte nuclei *(Fig. 20.7)*. Amphibian monocytes may contain fine, azurophilic granulation and pseudopodia. They also contain some of the hydrolytic enzymes that are found in mammalian monocytes.

Granulopoiesis occurs in the liver, kidney, and bone marrow of amphibians; however, some species lack bone marrow. Myeloblasts and progranulocytes have not been positively described in amphibians. Immature neutrophils have small granules of various shapes that increase in both size and density with maturation, until the larger, definitive peroxidase-positive granules are formed. Some species do not develop primary granules; rather, they produce a different population of granules. Evidence suggests that in some species, eosinophils begin as round cells, with a round nucleus and scant cytoplasm that contains large, dense, and round primary granules. Further development of eosinophils results in a mixture of the larger primary granules and the smaller secondary granules.

The monocyte is the first leukocyte to appear in the peripheral blood of bullfrog (*Rana catesbeiana*) larvae, in which immature monocytes with linear nuclear chromatin appear 15 days after hatching and mature monocytes with round nuclei, which develop into kidney-shaped or lobed

nuclei, appear 22 days after hatching. Definitive neutrophils, eosinophils, and basophils in larval bullfrogs appear in the peripheral blood late during development of the frog, but all three appear at the same time.

Lymphopoiesis in amphibians resembles that in other vertebrates. Small lymphocytes are the most common, but larger lymphocytes also may be seen.

Laboratory Evaluation

As in other nonmammalian vertebrates, amphibians have nucleated erythrocytes and thrombocytes that interfere with automated methods for counting leukocytes; therefore, manual counting methods are used. The Natt and Herrick's or phloxine B method, as described for birds in Chapter 17, can be used to obtain a total leukocyte concentration in amphibian blood.

The leukocyte differential is performed using Romanowsky-stained blood films (Table 20.1). Because most blood samples from amphibians are collected into heparin, making blood films either with blood containing no anticoagulant or immediately after mixing of the blood with the heparin (to decrease cell clumping and improve staining) is best.

Responses in Disease

Little is known regarding the function of the various amphibian leukocytes. The process of interpreting the amphibian leukogram is extrapolated from that used with other vertebrates. Amphibian neutrophils have both migratory and phagocytic activity, and they participate in inflammation. Likewise, amphibian monocytes are phagocytic and, most likely, function in a manner similar to those of other vertebrates. Therefore, increases in the neutrophil and monocyte counts likely suggest an inflammatory response.

Eosinophils have an inferior ability to phagocytize particles or microorganisms compared with that of neutrophils, but they do respond to metazoan parasitic infections. Therefore, peripheral eosinophilia may suggest a parasitic infection.

Amphibian basophils may function in a manner similar to those of mammals. They rarely are found in the peripheral blood of some species, such as the Colorado River toad, but they are abundant in others. For example, the Japanese newt normally has a differential leukocyte count that includes as much as 60% basophils. In this species, basophils are considered to play a significant role in immunosurveillance.

Lymphocytes of frogs and toads demonstrate an immunologic sophistication similar to those of higher vertebrates. The lymphocytes can be classified as B cells

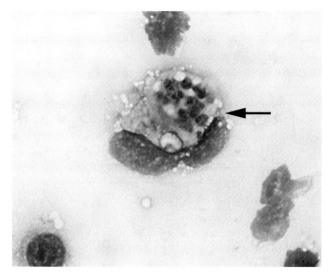

Figure 20.7 A monocyte (arrow) exhibiting leukophagocytosis in the blood of a tree frog (*Litoria caerulea*). Wright's stain, 500×.

that produce immunoglobulins or as T cells with populations of functional diversity, such as helpers and different effectors. In contrast, the lymphocytes of newts and salamanders appear to lack such refinement. Japanese newts demonstrate a transitory lymphocytosis after tail amputation for blood collection.

THROMBOCYTES OF AMPHIBIANS

Morphology

Amphibian thrombocytes are nucleated cells resembling those described for birds, reptiles, and fish. They tend to resemble small, mature lymphocytes but often are spindle-shaped, with a dense, round to oval nucleus and abundant, colorless cytoplasm *(Fig. 20.8)*. The thrombocytes of some amphibians, such as *Xenops* and *Rana* sp., are alkaline phosphatase positive, whereas the lymphocytes are negative. Anucleated thrombocytes that resemble mammalian platelets have been described in certain species.

Laboratory Evaluation

The total thrombocyte count can be obtained from the same charged hemocytometer used to obtain the total erythrocyte and leukocyte count. The thrombocytes resemble the erythrocytes in the hemocytometer, but they are smaller and appear to be round to oval, with a greater nucleus:cytoplasm ratio compared to the erythrocytes. All squares in the central large square of a Neubauer-

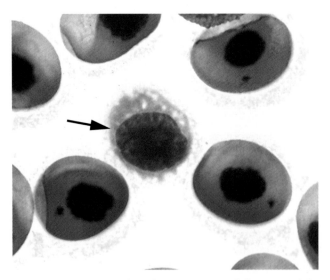

Figure 20.8 A reactive thrombocyte (arrow) with fine eosinophilic cytoplasmic granulation in the blood of a salamander (*Ambystoma tigrinum*). Wright's stain, 500×.

ruled hemocytometer are counted on both sides, and the average number of thrombocytes in one large square is calculated and multiplied by 2000 to obtain the total thrombocyte count per microliter. Accurate counts may be difficult to achieve, however, because thrombocytes tend to clump.

Responses in Disease

Functionally, thrombocytes are equivalent to mammalian platelets, and they participate in coagulation. Immature forms of thrombocytes (round cells with round nuclei) are not normally found in the peripheral blood of amphibians; therefore, their presence suggests either a regenerative response or dyscrasia. Thromboblasts have fine, nuclear chromatin, with a large, irregular, and eccentric nucleolus and weakly basophilic cytoplasm. Prothrombocytes have elongate nuclei and vacuolated cytoplasm with pale blue granules. Low and high thrombocyte counts are interpreted in the same manner as those described for other nonmammalian vertebrates.

BLOOD PARASITES

Microfilaria and trypanosomes commonly are seen in amphibian blood. Common differentials for amphibian intraerythrocytic inclusions include hemogregarines such as those described in reptiles (see Chapter 18), *Aegyptianella* sp., and a *Pirohemocyton*-like virus. Often, these organisms are considered to be an incidental finding; however, they may be pathogenic when they occur with anemia.

ERYTHROID HEMATOPOIESIS

Development of the amphibian erythrocyte is similar to that described for other vertebrates with nucleated erythrocytes. Maturation of the rubriblast to the mature erythrocyte involves a progressive change of cytoplasmic basophilia to eosinophilia, a change from a round to an elongated shape, a decrease in the nuclear and nucleolar size, and an increased chromatin density.

The liver is the predominant erythropoietic tissue of both larval and adult frogs. Larval amphibians may have two populations of morphologically different erythrocytes, which have different origins. One population, originating in the liver, has a centrally positioned nucleus; the other, originating in the kidney, has a peripherally located nucleus. The different erythrocyte populations also have different larval hemoglobins. During metamorphosis, a third population of erythrocytes appears, and this population persists in adults. Dark-field illumination can be used to differentiate larval erythrocytes, which have a white to gray, granular luminescence, from adult erythrocytes, which lack luminescence.

The metamorphosis from larval to adult amphibians is accompanied by the synthesis of hemoglobins with different oxygen affinities and various intracellular modulators of hemoglobin–oxygen affinity. Gilled larval amphibians have blood with a higher affinity for oxygen than that of air-breathing adults. The tetrameric hemoglobin of amphibians consists of two α-like and two β-like globin chains, thereby creating four larval-type and four adult-type hemoglobins. No globin chains are shared between larval and adult amphibians. Adult hemoglobin begins to appear in frogs during tail regression, and it is the only hemoglobin found 3 weeks after metamorphosis. Adult amphibians have higher hemoglobin concentrations and PCVs compared with the larval forms. Metamorphosis results in decreases in adenosine triphosphate (ATP) and guanosine triphosphate concentrations in the erythrocytes, thus suggesting a change in the phosphate regulation of hemoglobin in adults compared with larval forms.

Metamorphosis in newts and salamanders is not always associated with a transition in hemoglobin such as that occurring in frogs and toads. When newts and salamanders change from aquatic to aerobic respiration at metamorphosis, the larval and adult hemoglobins have the same affinity for oxygen. The reduced oxygen affinity of the blood in adults, however, frequently is achieved by an increased erythrocyte concentration of ATP. Even so, some species, such as the tiger salamander (*Ambystoma tigrinum*), experience no decrease in the oxygen affinity of blood at metamorphosis, and the hemoglobin and total erythrocytic organic phosphate concentrations remain unchanged.

Toads, which primarily rely on aerobic respiration, tend to have higher hemoglobin and erythrocyte phosphate concentrations and a lower blood oxygen affinity compared with frogs, which primarily rely on anaerobic respiration. Aquatic amphibians do not have the same association between high erythrocyte phosphate concentrations and dependence on aerobic production of energy for activity as terrestrial amphibians do. The exchange of gases from the blood to the surrounding water occurs through the skin of aquatic amphibians.

SUGGESTED READINGS

Barta JR, Desser SS. Blood parasites of amphibians from Algonquin Park, Ontario. J Wildl Dis 1984;20:180–189.

Cannon MS, Cannon AM. The blood leukocytes of *Bufo alvarius*: light, phase-contrast, and histochemical study. Can J Zool 1979; 57:314–322.

Cathers T, Lewbart GA, Correa M, et al. Serum chemistry and hematology values for anesthetized American bullfrogs (*Rana catesbeiana*). J Zool Wildl Med 1997;28:171–174.

Coates ML. Hemoglobin function in the vertebrates: an evolutionary model. J Mol Evol 1975;6:285–307.

Crawshaw GJ: Amphibian medicine. In: Kirk RW, Bonagura JD, eds. Kirk's current Veterinary therapy XI. Small animal practice. Philadelphia: WB Saunders 1992:1230–1231.

Curtis SK, Cowden RR, Nagel JW. Ultrastructure of the bone marrow of the salamander *Plethodon glutinosus* (Caudata: Plethodontidae). J Morphol 1979;159:151–184.

Desser SS. *Aegyptianella ranarum* sp. n. (Rickettsiales, Anaplasmataceae): ultrastructure and prevalence in frogs from Ontario. J Wildl Dis 1987;23:52–59.

Desser SS, Barta JR. The morphological features of *Aegyptianella bacterifera*: an intraerythrocytic rickettsia of frogs from Corsica. J Wildl Dis 1989;25:313–318.

Duellman WE, Trueb L. Biology of amphibians. Baltimore: Johns Hopkins University Press, 1994.

Essani K, Granoff A. Properties of amphibian and piscine iridoviruses: a comparison. In: Ahne W, Kurstak E, eds. Viruses of lower vertebrates. Berlin: Springer-Verlag, 1989:79–85.

Gruia-Gray J, Petric M, Desser SS. Ultrastructural, biochemical, and biophysical properties of an erythrocytic virus of frogs from Ontario, Canada. J Wildl Dis 1989;25:497–506.

Harris JA. Seasonal variation in some hematological characteristics of *Rana pipiens*. Comp Biochem Physiol 1972;43A:975–989.

Jerret DP, Mays CE. Comparative hematology of the hellbender (*Cryptobranchus alleganiensis*) in Missouri. Copeia 1973;2:331.

Jones RM, Woo PTK. Use of kidney impressions for the detection of trypanosomes of anura. J Wildl Dis 1989;25:413–415.

Mitruka BM, Rawnsley HM. Clinical biochemical and hematological reference values in normal experimental animals. 2nd ed. New York: Masson Publishing USA, 1981:89–145.

Pfeiffer CJ, Haywood P, Asashima M. Blood cell morphology and counts in the Japanese newt (*Cynops pyrrogaster*). J Zool Wildl Med 1990; 21:56–64.

Speare R, Freeland J, Bolton SJ. A possible Iridovirus in erythrocytes of *Bufo marinus* in Costa Rica. J Wildl Dis 1991;27:457–462.

Surbis AY. Ultrastructural study of granulocytes of *Bufo marinus*. Fla Sci 1978;41:42–45.

Turner RJ. Amphibians. In: Rowley AF, Ratcliffe NA, eds. Vertebrate blood cells. Cambridge: Cambridge University Press, 1988:129–209.

Woo PTK. Sensitivity of diagnostic techniques in determining the prevalence of anuran trypanosomes. J Wildl Dis 1983;19:24–26.

Wright KM. Amphibian husbandry and medicine. In: Mader DR, ed. Reptile medicine and surgery. Philadelphia: WB Saunders, 1996: 436–458.

FOUR

CLINICAL CHEMISTRY OF

COMMON DOMESTIC SPECIES

LABORATORY EVALUATION

OF RENAL FUNCTION

BLOOD UREA NITROGEN

Metabolism

Blood urea nitrogen (BUN) is one of the traditional blood indices of glomerular filtration. Simply stated, most of the urea produced in the body is excreted in the urine by filtration across the glomerulus. Therefore, reductions in the glomerular filtration rate (GFR) result in increases in the BUN concentration; however, the BUN is affected by both the rates of urea production by the liver and the rates of urea excretion by the renal and extrarenal routes. Factors that increase the rate of hepatic ureagenesis add urea to the blood and may increase the BUN. For instance, if dietary protein intake is increased, more amino acids are absorbed from the gastrointestinal (GI) tract after protein digestion, and if the quantity of amino acids absorbed exceeds the nutritional requirement of the animal, these excess amino acids are deaminated in the liver. Their carbon skeletons are used for gluconeogenesis or lipogenesis, and the amine groups are incorporated into the urea to eliminate this nitrogenous waste from the body.

This concept may be extended to include the effects of consuming any protein-containing meal *(Fig. 21.1)*, of upper GI tract bleeding, or of disorders that increase endogenous protein catabolism. In each of these examples,

the liver is presented with a "bolus" of amino acids that may exceed the protein anabolic functions of the body. This "excess" may undergo oxidative deamination and contribute to increased hepatic urea production. Thus, increases in the BUN caused by increased hepatic ureagenesis may lead to underestimation of the GFR. Conversely, significant liver disease resulting in impairment of the hepatic functional capacity may result in abnormally low rates of amino acid deamination and ureagenesis. In this case, a decreased BUN may be used as an index of severe liver disease. Concurrent renal disease may be obscured, however, because not enough urea is produced to be abnormally accumulated when the GFR is reduced.

Renal and Extrarenal Factors Affecting the BUN

Urinary excretion of urea is affected not only by the GFR, because urea is reabsorbed across the renal tubules to contribute to maintenance of the renal medullary concentration gradient of the kidneys. When the tubular flow rate is decreased, urea reabsorption is increased, thus increasing the concentration gradient for subsequent water reabsorption and urinary concentration by the collecting tubules. Dehydration may disproportionately reduce the tubular flow rate compared with the GFR (i.e., glomerulotubular imbalance) and, thus, result in disproportionately

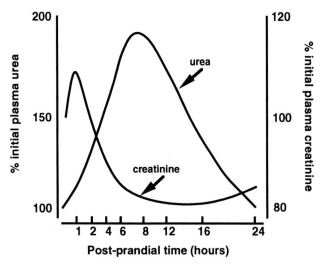

Figure 21.1 Sequential changes in plasma urea and creatinine concentrations in dogs after eating a protein-containing meal. (Adapted from Watson ADJ, Church DB, Fairburn AJ. Postprandial changes in plasma urea nitrogen and creatinine concentrations in dogs. Am J Vet Res 1981;42:1878–1880.)

greater increases of the BUN than would a reduction in the GFR alone. Therefore, increases in the BUN during dehydration may lead to underestimation of the GFR.

Laboratory Methods

Quantitative laboratory measurement of BUN typically is accomplished with reagents that are designed to react with urea in serum or plasma to produce a proportionate increase in colored products (i.e., chromogens), the concentration of which may be interpreted relative to a standardized calibration curve. One method uses a series of chemical reactions with diacetyl monoxime and thiosemicarbazide to produce a chromogen. Another employs urease to enzymatically hydrolyze the urea and to release ammonia, which then reacts with any of several possible secondary reagents to produce a chromogen (e.g., pH indicator dye, Nessler reagent, glutamate dehydrogenase and NADH). These methods have high specificity (i.e., few false positives) and high sensitivity (i.e., few false negatives). Azostix-reagent-test strips (Ames, Miles, Inc., Diagnostic Division, Elkhart, IN, USA) can be used to estimate semiquantitatively the BUN in whole blood both quickly and conveniently. The reagent zone of the strip consists of paper that is impregnated with urease and bromothymol blue (i.e., a pH indicator) and is coated with a membrane that is permeable to urea but not to blood pigments. A color chart is provided for comparative evaluation of four different shades of green to the color produced by the reaction, corresponding to discontinuous concentration ranges of 5 to 15, 15 to 26, 30 to 40, and

50 to 80 mg/dL. This test is inexpensive, easy to use, and highly specific (i.e., capable of correctly identifying low or normal values), but its sensitivity and positive predictive value (i.e., capability of correctly identifying an abnormally high value) are relatively poor. Thus, marginal increases in the BUN that may be of diagnostic significance may not be detected by this screening method.

SERUM CREATININE

Metabolism

Creatinine is formed by the spontaneous condensation and dehydration of muscle creatine into a ring structure. The amount of creatinine that is produced daily is relatively constant and is not as affected by extrarenal factors, as is urea. It has been stated that creatinine production is proportional to the muscle mass of the individual, but the results of studies in humans have shown that age and gender, but not lean body mass, influence its serum concentration. Once creatinine is formed, it is removed from the body almost entirely by renal excretion through glomerular filtration. Species and gender effects also may cause a small amount to be secreted by the renal tubules, as has been observed in human male patients, but these effects generally are not significant. Factors such as cytokines, which increase endogenous muscle catabolism during sepsis or cancer cachexia, can increase the release of creatine and, hence, the quantity of creatinine that is produced.

Renal and Extrarenal Factors Affecting Serum Creatinine

Dietary sources of creatine (e.g., cooked red meat) increase the serum creatinine concentration after absorption from the GI tract. Most meals, however, actually may result in a decreased serum creatinine concentration, because the absorbed nutrients induce a postprandial increase in the GFR (Fig. 21.1). Reductions in the GFR resulting from prerenal, renal, or postrenal causes all may increase the serum creatinine concentration, and they cannot be definitively differentiated. Postrenal azotemia, however, such as that which occurs after lower urinary tract obstruction or urinary bladder rupture, usually is associated with the largest and the most acute increases in the serum creatinine concentration.

Laboratory Methods

Quantitative laboratory measurement of creatinine typically is accomplished with the use of reagents that are designed to react with creatinine in serum or plasma to produce a proportionate increase in colored products (i.e., chromogens), the concentration of which may be interpreted relative to a standardized calibration curve. One method uses a chemical reaction with picrate ions in alkaline solution to produce a chromogen that may be measured kinetically or at the time the reaction is complete. A newer method uses a creatininase to enzymatically hydrolyze the creatinine and to release creatine (i.e., creatinine amidohydrolase) or ammonia (i.e., creatinine iminohydrolase), which then react with any of several possible secondary reagents (e.g., pyruvate kinase or glutamate dehydrogenase and NADH) to produce a chromogen. The enzymatic methods have high specificity (i.e., few false positives) and high sensitivity (i.e., few false negatives). The alkaline picrate or Jaffé reaction historically has been employed most commonly in veterinary medicine, but it has lower specificity and reacts with many noncreatinine chromogens in biologic specimens.

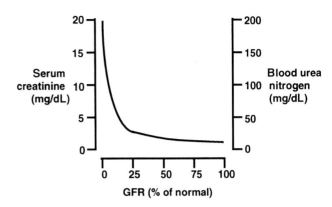

Figure 21.2 Idealized relationship between serum creatinine or blood urea nitrogen and glomerular filtration rate.

QUANTITATIVE RELATIONSHIPS BETWEEN BLOOD INDICES AND THE GFR

Reference Intervals for BUN and Creatinine

One of the drawbacks of using increases in the BUN or serum creatinine concentration to detect decreases in the GFR is the width of the reference intervals that are used in clinical laboratory medicine. Even when large numbers of healthy animals are studied to establish reference intervals, "normal values" are observed over a fairly wide range. At the Colorado State University Veterinary Teaching Hospital, reference ranges for BUN (dogs, 7–28 mg/dL; cats, 17–32 mg/dL) and serum creatinine (dogs, 0.9–1.7 mg/dL; cats, 0.9–2.1 mg/dL) are sufficiently wide that an animal may experience significant reductions in the GFR before azotemia, relative to the individual patient's values in health, is detected. For instance, if a dog has a normal BUN of 7 mg/dL, a fourfold reduction in the GFR theoretically is needed before an increase outside the reference interval is detected. Some healthy animals have values for these indices below the lower limit of the reference range; for example, a dog with a normal creatinine concentration of 0.5 mg/dL theoretically must experience a threefold reduction in the GFR before an increase outside the reference interval is detected. If one also considers the confounding effects of diet, meal consumption, endogenous metabolism, and extrarenal routes of excretion, it becomes apparent that BUN and serum creatinine are very inexact screening tests for the detection of renal dysfunction. The mathematical relationship between BUN or serum creatinine and the GFR appears to be logarithmic or hyperbolic in nature *(Fig. 21.2)*. Reductions in the GFR of 75% or more generally are considered to be nec-

essary before significant increases in the BUN or creatinine concentration above the reference interval may be detected. When renal disease causes a loss of functional nephrons, the remaining, less-affected nephrons typically undergo compensatory hypertrophy. Thus, the single-nephron GFR increases, thereby maintaining the overall GFR and keeping both BUN and creatinine within their reference ranges. Thus, renal disease may have been long-standing, and more than 75% of the individual nephrons may have been lost, before clinical detection of azotemia on the basis of standard screening methods becomes possible. Furthermore, because chronic renal disease usually is progressive, the loss of nephrons and accompanying reductions in the GFR predispose the remaining nephrons to additional damage as they undergo compensatory hypertrophy to maintain renal function.

Reciprocal of Serum Creatinine Concentration

The hyperbolic association between the serum creatinine concentration and GFR may be converted into a linear function that is described by the relationship between time and the reciprocal of the serum creatinine concentration in individuals with progressive loss of renal function *(Fig. 21.3)*. This method was first used successfully to monitor progression of renal disease in humans, and it has been applied more recently to other species. In addition to better quantitating changes in serum creatinine with progressive renal disease, the linear regression equation describing the relationship between the reciprocal of creatinine ($1/cr$ or cr^{-1}) and time can be used to predict the future progression of renal dysfunction and an approximate future time of death. In addition, the graphic representation of this regression equation can be used to illustrate to clients the rate of deterioration in renal function for an individual pet. Changes in renal function in response to specific therapeutic modalities (e.g., dietary

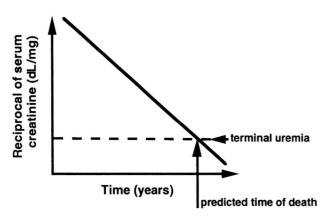

Figure 21.3 Idealized relationship between reciprocal of serum creatinine concentration and time in a canine patient with chronic progressive renal disease. (Adapted from Allen TA, Jaenke RS, Fettman MJ. A technique for estimating progression of chronic renal failure in the dog. J Am Vet Med Assoc 1987;190:866–868)

changes, control of hypertension, administration of antiuremic drugs) also may be seen as "breaks" in this line because of changes in the slope of the relationship. Thus, the reciprocal of creatinine is useful as a prognostic index as well.

BUN:Creatinine Ratio

In humans, BUN:creatinine ratios of approximately 10:1 occur in healthy individuals as well as in azotemic patients in whom extrarenal factors are absent. Ratios of greater than 10:1 are seen under conditions that cause a disproportionate increase of BUN relative to reductions in the GFR. These include factors that increase urea synthesis (e.g., increased dietary protein intake, upper GI bleeding, tissue catabolism) or that cause glomerulotubular imbalance (e.g., dehydration, hypovolemia, cardiac insufficiency). Unfortunately, a quantitative association between an increased BUN:creatinine ratio and extrarenal effects on the degree of azotemia has only been partially demonstrated in dogs or cats. Data from the Colorado State University Veterinary Teaching Hospital indicate that disproportionate increases in BUN, leading to BUN:creatinine ratios of greater than approximately 30:1, are more likely to be seen after upper GI hemorrhage. Furthermore, in a patient undergoing serial laboratory evaluation during treatment of renal disease, changes in the BUN:creatinine ratio may be used to judge hydration status and to evaluate responsiveness to treatment of uremic signs. In a patient for which finite variability in the BUN:creatinine ratio is expected, disproportionate increases in BUN may be indicative of dehydration or accumulation of uremic toxins and result from dietary treatment failure or noncompliance by the owner.

SERUM INORGANIC PHOSPHORUS

Hormonal Control

Metabolism of inorganic phosphorus (Pi) is regulated, to a very large extent, through its interactions with calcium and by the actions of parathormone (PTH), calcitonin, and calcitriol (1,25-[OH]$_2$ vitamin D). The plasma concentrations of ionic calcium and Pi tend to be reciprocally related; in fact, their solubility is defined by a pH-dependent solubility product constant. Alkaline pH or large increases in one or both of these ions promotes the precipitation of calcium phosphate salts. An increase in the plasma Pi concentration can result in a reciprocal decrease in the plasma Ca concentration and suppression of 1α-hydroxylation of 25-hydroxyvitamin D *(Fig. 21.4)*. Hypocalcemia as well as decreased hydroxylation of 25-OH vitamin D result in the release of PTH from the parathyroid glands. Parathyroid hormone stimulates bone demineralization to increase circulating Ca levels. Parathyroid hormone also increases adenylate cyclase activity in the thick ascending limb of the loop of Henle, and subsequent increases in cyclic adenosine monophosphate promote active Ca reabsorption, which is facilitated by the electrogenic Cl gradient in this segment. Parathyroid hormone stimulates renal 1α-hydroxylation of vitamin D to produce the most active form of vitamin D, calcitriol, as well. Vitamin D then promotes both intestinal absorption

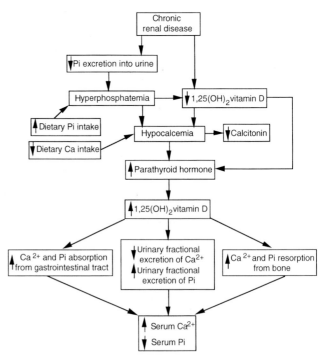

Figure 21.4 Interactions between calcium, phosphorus, and calcitriol metabolism in chronic renal disease.

and distal renal tubular reabsorption of Ca by stimulating the synthesis of a calcium-binding protein that is central to epithelial cell uptake of Ca in these organs. Calcitriol also inhibits further release of PTH by the parathyroid gland. Because Pi is only reabsorbed and not secreted by the kidneys, PTH promotes increased urinary excretion of Pi as well by inhibiting its reabsorption in the renal proximal tubules. Urinary fractional excretion of Pi usually is less than 20%, but it may increase substantially under the influence of PTH.

Other Metabolic Factors

Hyperphosphatemia also may result from redistribution between the intra- and extracellular fluid compartments. Cellular damage resulting in the release of intracellular phosphates from high-energy phosphorylated intermediates of metabolism can cause hyperphosphatemia. Acid-base imbalances also can affect the Pi distribution. Alkalosis buffers the acid that is produced during metabolism, thereby removing product feedback inhibition by protons on intermediary metabolism. In turn, this enables more rapid generation of phosphorylated intermediates, and it draws more Pi into the cells. Acidosis has the opposite effect, blocking the metabolic pathways through an accumulation of acid end products and blocking the cellular uptake of Pi. Phosphorus released from bone mineral serves an important role in buffering excess acid in the body. Given the pH-dependent solubility product relationship between Ca and Pi, it is no surprise that acidification induces bone demineralization, which in turn provides more phosphate buffer to neutralize the acid. Furthermore, the phosphates serve as the major source of "titratable acidity" in the renal tubules, wherein they act as proton acceptors where tubular cells actively secrete acid into the urine. On the other hand, phosphoric acid is used by some commercial pet food manufacturers to provide dietary phosphorus and dietary acidification in cat foods that are designed to prevent feline lower urinary tract disorders.

Because urinary Pi excretion depends on glomerular filtration and tubular reabsorption, reductions in the renal blood flow and GFR often result in hyperphosphatemia. Likewise, when the urinary bladder is ruptured, Pi excreted in the urine is reabsorbed along its concentration gradient from the abdomen and into the blood to cause hyperphosphatemia. Hyperphosphatemia also can result from excessive dietary intake of phosphorus. In any case, hyperphosphatemia can induce a secondary hypocalcemia and hypocalcitriolemia, which in turn stimulate PTH release. Thus, two forms of secondary hyperparathyroidism are induced by excessive retention of Pi: renal secondary hyperparathyroidism caused by the hyperphosphatemia of reduced excretion, and nutritional secondary hyper-parathyroidism caused by the hyperphosphatemia of increased intake. In both situations, PTH induces bone demineralization to restore blood Ca levels, thereby resulting in osteopenia and metabolic bone disease (Fig. 21.4).

Renal Disease

The endocrine responses involved in renal secondary hyperparathyroidism can maintain the serum Pi concentration within relatively normal limits for some time, and it is thought that approximately 85% of the GFR must be lost before persistent hyperphosphatemia develops. Thus, the onset of prerenal or renal hyperphosphatemia is not a very sensitive index for the detection of reductions in the GFR. The urinary fractional excretion of Pi (FE_P) has been evaluated for its ability to detect alterations in renal function, but it likewise is not as sensitive as other measures (e.g., serum creatinine concentration). It may be useful, however, to monitor changes in the serum Pi concentration over time to determine response to treatments of chronic renal failure (e.g., dietary Pi restriction, exogenous calcitriol supplementation). (Determination and interpretation of FE_P are discussed later with the urinary fractional excretion of other electrolytes.)

ESTIMATING GFR WITH URINE COLLECTION

For azotemic patients or those who are nonazotemic but have other signs of renal disease (e.g., persistent proteinuria, impaired urinary concentration capacity), a "clearance study" to estimate the GFR or effective renal plasma flow (ERPF) may be useful. These methods typically are performed only after other results of screening methods have indicated the likelihood of renal dysfunction. Clearance tests involve greater time commitment and analytic costs, and they also may require administration of an exogenous chemical. Their results, however, are more quantitative than those of any screening tests, and the results of serial evaluations can provide a more accurate appraisal of the progression of disease in an individual patient.

Regardless of the method employed, the principal is the same. A substance that is eliminated from the systemic circulation by glomerular filtration alone is used to estimate the GFR. A substance that is eliminated from the systemic circulation by both glomerular filtration and tubular secretion, so that virtually all of that substance is extracted during each pass through the kidneys, is used to estimate the ERPF. Methods that entail complete, quantitative urine collection over a defined period of time derive the clearance calculations from the following formula. If "X" is cleared by glomerular filtration only, then

C_X = GFR, and if "X" is cleared by glomerular filtration and tubular secretion, then C_X = ERPF. Thus,

$$C_X = U_X \times V/P_X$$

where C_X is the clearance (mL/kg per min) of solute "X," U_X is the urinary concentration (mg/mL) of solute "X," V is the volume of urine (mL/kg per min) collected over a defined time period, and P_X is the plasma concentration (mg/mL) of solute "X."

The two most commonly employed methods for estimating the GFR have been the traditional "endogenous" and "exogenous" creatinine clearance tests.

Endogenous Creatinine Clearance Test

For endogenous creatinine clearance, the urinary bladder first is catheterized to evacuate all preexisting urine. The animal then is placed in a metabolic cage that allows for complete collection of all voided urine during the time of the clearance study. Generally, urine is collected for 24 hours, and a single blood sample is collected in the middle or at the end of the collection period. Urine and serum are analyzed for creatinine, and the clearance is calculated to estimate the GFR.

Noncreatinine chromogens may interfere with the determination of creatinine by the alkaline picrate method. Because most noncreatinine chromogens that are identified in serum (e.g., pyruvate, acetic acid, acetoacetic acid, ascorbic acid, glucose, protein, uric acid) typically do not appear in the urine in large amounts, the denominator in the clearance formula described earlier to calculate the GFR may be spuriously high, and values for the Jaffé endogenous creatinine clearance may underestimate the GFR.

Exogenous Creatinine Clearance Test

For exogenous creatinine clearance, a creatinine solution (50 mg/mL) is injected subcutaneously at a dose of 75 to 100 mg/kg, a volume of water approximately equal to 3% of body weight is given by stomach tube, the urinary bladder is catheterized and emptied, and after an equilibration period of 40 to 60 minutes, quantitative urine collections with bladder rinsings are performed for 20-minute periods. Blood samples are drawn at the start of each collection period, urine and serum are analyzed for creatinine, and clearance is calculated to estimate the GFR. Because hydration has a marked effect on the ERPF and GFR, and because the state of hydration cannot be determined precisely on the basis of physical inspection, clearance protocols should be standardized by oral administration of a consistent amount of fluid to correct potential deficits and to promote reasonable urine production during the clearance procedure. Recent work indicates that 30 mL/kg orally gives stable GFR values for

three 20-minute collection periods after the administration of exogenous creatinine.

Exogenous creatinine is administered to artificially increase the serum concentration of creatinine relative to that of noncreatinine chromogens and to increase the concentration of excreted creatinine in the voided urine to minimize errors in urine volume quantitation. A comparison of inulin clearance (i.e., a synthetic marker for determination of the GFR) with creatinine clearances as determined from the alkaline picrate or creatininase methods has demonstrated greater accuracy with the enzymatic method. Because one published report indicates that reduction of renal mass in male dogs leads to increased tubular secretion of creatinine, the results of simultaneous clearance of exogenous creatinine and inulin have been experimentally compared to validate the use of creatinine clearance as a measure of the GFR. The clearance ratio of creatinine to inulin is not affected by the degree of renal dysfunction.

ESTIMATING GFR AND ERPF WITHOUT URINE COLLECTION

To eliminate the tedious and error-prone procedure of quantitative urine collection from methods for determination of the GFR or ERPF, newer protocols using a single-injection method of an exogenous tracer solute have employed serial blood sampling to pharmacokinetically quantitate the disappearance of the clearance solute without the need for concurrent urine collection (Fig. 21.5). These methods were first developed with radiolabeled solutes that could be administered intravenously in miniscule amounts and detected very accurately at minute concentrations in very small, serial blood samples.

Single-Injection, Double-Isotope Methods

Effective renal plasma flow has been estimated from the plasma disappearance of the organic acid ^{131}I-sodium iodohippurate or the organic base ^{3}H-tetraethylammonium bromide. Both these substances are filtered by the glomerulus and secreted via active transport by the proximal renal tubules; they are completely cleared from the blood during each pass through the kidneys. The GFR has been estimated from the plasma disappearance of ^{125}I-sodium iothalamate or ^{14}C-inulin, both of which are excreted by glomerular filtration alone. Gamma-particle emitters (e.g., iodinated compounds) or beta-particle emitters (e.g., ^{3}H, ^{14}C) may be administered together so that the GFR and ERPF can be determined simultaneously by pharmacokinetic analysis of their disappearance curves after scintillation counting of plasma samples. Concurrent analysis of the GFR and ERPF by these methods is highly accurate, and it also allows the additional determination of

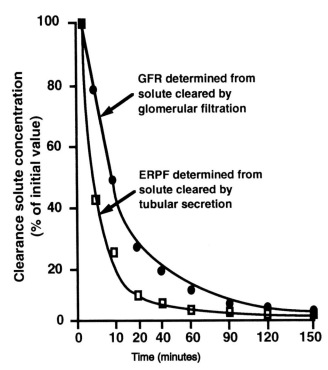

Figure 21.5 A typical renal clearance solute disappearance curve. (Adapted from Fettman MJ, Allen TA, Wilke WL, Radin MJ, Eubank MC. Single-injection method for evaluation of renal function with ^{14}C-inulin and ^{3}H-tetraethylammonium bromide in dogs and cats. Am J Vet Res 1985;46:482–485)

the "filtration fraction" as another index of renal function. The filtration fraction represents the proportion of blood flow to the kidneys that actually is filtered through the glomerulus. Alterations in the filtration fraction may reveal glomerulotubular imbalance, wherein the rate of loss of glomerular and tubular functions are unequal and may reflect the particular pathogenesis of renal disease in an individual patient. This is a time-consuming, but highly accurate, method that has been useful in the setting of a referral teaching institution.

The plasma disappearance of the gamma-emitting ^{99m}Tc-diethylenetriaminepentaacetic acid (^{99m}Tc-diethylenetriamine pentaacetic acid [DTPA]) has been validated more recently for determination of the GFR in both dogs and cats. Furthermore, the GFR can be determined noninvasively by quantitative renal scintigraphy using a gamma camera for nuclear imaging of the kidneys at serial time points after intravenous administration of ^{99m}Tc-DTPA. This is a rapid, accurate, and noninvasive method that shows much promise; however, it requires specialized equipment and training and currently is available only at referral institutions.

Nonisotopic Methods

Although these radioisotope clearance methods are impractical for routine clinical practice, they have taught us much about the pathophysiology of renal disease and the pharmacokinetics of renal clearance solutes. Most importantly, however, they have led to the development of more practical single-injection, nonradioisotopic clearance methods without urine collection that can be used to quantitatively evaluate the GFR in routine clinical patients.

One recent method uses an intravenous injection of iohexol, which is a contrast medium used for renal imaging, as the clearance solute for determination of the GFR. A single bolus (600 mg/kg) is administered, and serial blood samples are drawn at intervals of 30 to 60 minutes for 6 hours. A specialized analytic instrument is used to analyze the plasma samples for iohexol by x-ray fluorescence. These concentrations then are entered into a standard pharmacokinetic analysis program, and the clearance results are calculated. Because iohexol is nonradioactive, the clearance study can be conducted in a clinical practice and the plasma samples sent to a referral laboratory for chemical and mathematical analysis.

Alternatively, a single bolus of 20 mL of a 5% (w/v) solution of inulin dissolved in normal saline may be administered as the tracer solute. Blood samples then are drawn at 15-minute intervals for 1 to 2 hours and are analyzed for inulin either by a cumbersome anthrone colorimetric technique or by a newly available enzymatic inulinase assay. Once again, because inulin is nonradioactive, the clearance study can be conducted in a clinical practice and the plasma samples sent to a referral laboratory for chemical and mathematical analysis.

Finally, a method that shows much promise is a modification of the traditional exogenous creatinine clearance test, in which creatinine is administered as a bolus of 88 mg/kg and the serum creatinine concentration is determined (preferably by the creatininase method) at 30, 60, 120, 180, and 240 minutes after injection. Because creatinine is nonradioactive and its analysis is readily available at any referral laboratory, the clearance study can be conducted in a clinical practice and the plasma samples sent to a referral laboratory for chemical and mathematical analysis. Using the pharmacokinetic parameters as generated by the newer single-injection methods, a much older method using a single intravenous injection of sodium sulfanilate to determine half-life as an index of the GFR may be modified for use with other, more readily analyzed solutes (e.g., creatinine). In the original sodium sulfanilate method, 0.20 mL/kg of a 10% w/v solution were administered intravenously, and blood samples were drawn at 30-minute intervals for as long as 2 hours. After determination of blood sulfanilate values, the time needed for 50% of the dye to be cleared from the blood was calculated. The elimination phase for inulin or creatinine appears to begin approximately 90 to 120 minutes after administration. Thus, the half-life for creatinine or inulin

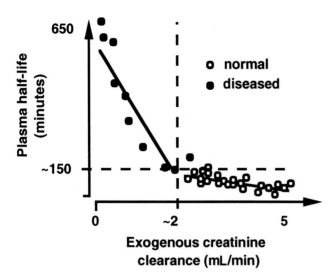

Figure 21.6   Relationship between exogenous creatinine clearance and half-life for healthy dogs (open circles) and dogs with renal disease (closed circles). (Adapted from Labato MA, Ross LA. Plasma disappearance of creatinine as a renal function test in the dog. Res Vet Sci 1991;50:253–258.)

could be determined from a small number of blood samples taken at 15- to 30-minute intervals after this time point, and the half-life could be comparatively evaluated against published reference intervals or serially evaluated in an individual patient to determine progression or response to therapy. In fact, one study has demonstrated the utility of a single plasma concentration of inulin 75 minutes after intravenous administration of 1000 mg of inulin in predicting the pharmacokinetically determined clearance of exogenous creatinine *(Fig. 21.6)*. Thus, a single plasma concentration of any exogenously administered clearance solute may be serially evaluated to determine the progression of renal dysfunction in an individual patient over time. Note, however, that this offers only a marginal advantage compared with serial evaluation of 1/cr values with time.

URINARY CONCENTRATION CAPACITY

Having discussed several methods for detecting changes in renal clearance functions, we now consider methods for detecting changes in renal "free-water" clearance, which is better known as "concentration capacity." The ability of the kidneys to concentrate urine generally is regarded as being a sensitive indicator of renal function, and it is thought to be one of the earlier signs of renal disease, often occurring before the onset of azotemia. Loss of urinary concentration capacity in dogs appears after two-thirds nephrectomy, whereas clinically detectable azotemia ap-

pears only after loss of approximately 75% of the GFR, which may represent a loss of approximately 90% of the total number of nephrons, with functional hypertrophy of remaining nephrons.

Potential causes for the loss of urinary concentration capacity include many other clinically significant extrarenal disorders that do not cause renal disease but that impair maintenance of the medullary concentration gradient or renal responsiveness to vasopressin *(Table 21.1)*. Thus, although the concurrent findings of azotemia and inappropriately low urinary specific gravity are widely stated to be indicative of renal disease, one must also consider differential diagnoses of secondary disorders arising from imbalances in electrolyte metabolism, endocrine function, or drug effects.

Specific Gravity Versus Osmolality

Urinary specific gravity is the most commonly used screening method to detect changes in the concentration capacity. Specific gravity represents the density of a fluid (i.e., the ratio of the weight of that fluid to an equal volume of water), and it may be determined either gravimetrically or refractometrically. The former represents a true measure of the fluid's weight, whereas the latter employs the physical relationship between light refraction by a fluid and the content of solutes in solution. Variations in sample temperature and the chemical nature of the solutes, however, can affect the accuracy of the refractometric estimate of density. Furthermore, the specific gravity only estimates the true urinary concentration capacity, because it merely estimates the solute content by weight rather than the absolute number of osmotically active particles in solution, which would represent the actual osmotic concentration as determined by renal function. For instance, 1 mOsm of urea weighs 28 mg, whereas 1 mOsm of glucose weighs 180 mg. Therefore, equivalent weights of urea and glucose would have a sixfold difference in osmotic activity. On the other hand, because light refraction also is affected by molecular size and the refractive index of individual solutes, each solute has a different effect on the specific gravity as determined by refractometry. The addition of any of the following to 1 mL of water is reported to increase specific gravity by 0.001: 1.47 mg NaCl, 3.6 mg urea, 2.7 mg glucose, or 4.0 mg albumin.

Sensitivity for Detection of Renal Dysfunction

Accumulation of a renal medullary concentration gradient of solutes determines the osmotic gradient for water reclamation across the collecting tubules during urine formation. Thus, a direct measure of the urine osmolality by vapor-point elevation or freezing-point depression is a more accurate representation of the osmotic concentra-

> TABLE 21.1 POTENTIAL CAUSES FOR LOSS OF URINARY CONCENTRATION CAPACITY

Disease	Mechanism
Pituitary diabetes insipidus	Lack of vasopressin production
Primary nephrogenic diabetes insipidus	Congenital lack of renal response to vasopressin
Acquired nephrogenic diabetes insipidus	Acquired lack of renal response to vasopressin
Antagonism of vasopressin action	Direct effects, which may also be accompanied by:
Hypercalcemia	Altered renal medullary blood flow Impaired sodium reabsorption Hypercalcemic nephropathy
Hypokalemia	Altered renal medullary blood flow Kaliopenic nephropathy
Hypomagnesemia	Altered renal medullary blood flow Impaired potassium reabsorption
Glucocorticoids	Impaired vasopressin release Altered renal medullary blood flow Impaired potassium reabsorption
Loss of renal medullary concentration gradient	Impaired water reabsorption regardless of vasopressin actions
Hyponatremia Hypochloremia Fluid overload Psychogenic polydipsia	
Endocrine disorders	
Acromegaly	Insulin antagonism by growth hormone leading to hyperglycemia, glucosuria, and osmotic diuresis
Diabetes mellitus	Hyperglycemia, glucosuria, and osmotic diuresis
Hypoadrenocorticism	Impaired sodium reabsorption
Hyperadrenocorticism	Effects of excessive glucocorticoids
Hyperparathyroidism	Effects of hypercalcemia
Hyperthyroidism	Effects of excessive thyroid hormones
Primary renal disease	Effects of primary morphologic or functional impairment of the kidneys, which may also be accompanied by:
Chronic renal failure	Osmotic diuresis in remnant nephrons
Nonoliguric acute renal failure	Impaired sodium reabsorption Altered medullary blood flow Impaired vasopressin sensitivity
Pyelonephritis	Altered medullary blood flow Vasopressin antagonism by Bacterial toxins
Fanconi syndrome (primary renal glucosuria)	Osmotic diuresis Impaired sodium reabsorption
Postobstructive diuresis	Osmotic diuresis Altered medullary blood flow Impaired sodium reabsorption

(continued)

TABLE 21.1 *(Continued)*	

Disease	Mechanism
Drug induced	
Anticonvulsants	Vasopressin antagonism
Calcitriol toxicity	Hypercalcemic nephropathy
Diuretics	Impaired sodium reabsorption
Glucocorticoids	Impaired vasopressin release
	Altered renal medullary blood flow
	Impaired potassium reabsorption
Lithium	Vasopressin antagonism
Methoxyflurane	Fluoride toxicity
	Vasopressin antagonism
Sodium salt supplementation	Osmotic diuresis
Thyroid-hormone toxicity	Altered medullary blood flow
	Effects of hypokalemia
Miscellaneous causes	
Hepatic insufficiency	Decreased urea synthesis and loss of renal medullary concentration gradient
	Decreased metabolism of hormones such as glucocorticoids
	Hypokalemia
Pyometra	Vasopressin antagonism by bacterial toxins
	Immune complex glomerulonephritis

tion capacity of the kidneys than is determination of the specific gravity. Mathematical comparison of urinary specific gravity and osmolality reveals a very close association, but the confidence limit for a single osmolality value as predicted from a single specific gravity is quite wide. In one study, a specific gravity of 1.005 predicted an osmolality of 185 mOsm/kg; however, the 95% confidence interval was 0 to 380 mOsm/kg. This range is too wide to be accurate in the determination of renal function.

We assume that a urinary specific gravity of approximately 1.010 (range, 1.008–1.012) represents isosthenuric urine (i.e., a concentration unaltered from that of glomerular filtrate), and that values less than this represent urinary dilution and values greater represent urinary concentration. In humans, normal kidneys should be able to concentrate urine to a specific gravity or 1.025 or greater. The maximal urinary concentration capacity in humans is approximately 1.040, whereas that in dogs is 1.060 or greater and that in cats is 1.080 or greater. Thus, a urine specific gravity of 1.025 in a human probably implies better renal tubular function than it does in dogs or cats. Therefore, we generally consider urine that

is concentrated to a specific gravity of greater than 1.030 in dogs and greater than 1.035 in cats to be evidence of acceptable renal concentrating function. In one study, healthy dogs deprived of water for 72 hours could concentrate their urine to a specific gravity of approximately 1.060. The corresponding urinary osmolality was approximately 2300 mOsm/kg, and the maximal $U:P_{osm}$ (i.e., the ratio of urine to plasma osmolality) was approximately 7.5:1. In cats, significant reductions in the GFR and ERPF, resulting in clinically detectable azotemia, may occur before loss of urinary concentration capacity. Healthy cats studied both before and after partial (58%–83%) nephrectomy could concentrate urine to an osmolality of approximately 2300 mOsm/kg before and approximately 1950 mOsm/kg after nephrectomy.

To evaluate renal function, a water deprivation test may be performed to maximally stimulate urinary concentration. This test should be performed only in animals that are neither dehydrated nor azotemic to avoid the induction of iatrogenic acute renal failure. Body weight should be monitored, and the test should be terminated when the urinary specific gravity ranges between 1.025 and 1.035, the $U:P_{osm}$ reaches 3.0:1 or greater, the plasma osmolality exceeds 320 mOsm/kg, azotemia develops, or body weight declines by 5% or more because of dehydration.

URINARY FRACTIONAL EXCRETION OF ELECTROLYTES

Definition and Calculation

Calculation of the urinary fractional excretion of electrolytes can be diagnostically useful in differentiating renal from extrarenal causes of azotemia or abnormalities in urine composition. For instance, differentiating prerenal from renal azotemia is critical for cases in which the urinary concentration capacity is impaired because of extrarenal abnormalities in the regulation of electrolyte balance and inability to maintain the renal medullary concentration gradient. Acute renal failure usually is defined as an abrupt deterioration in renal function, with resultant retention of nitrogenous waste products and loss of the ability to adequately regulate solute and water balance. Although oliguria traditionally has been emphasized as a cardinal feature of acute renal failure, nonoliguric acute renal failure is being recognized with increasing frequency in both human and veterinary patients.

The mechanism of the urine concentrating defect in nonoliguric acute renal failure is not clear. This syndrome is one manifestation of glomerulotubular imbalance, wherein glomerular function is reduced, the GFR decreases, and azotemia develops. Production of urine, however, is maintained, with varying degrees of loss of individual tubular functions, paramount of which may be the urinary concentration capacity or electrolyte reabsorptive ability. If urine is produced by an acutely azotemic patient, it can be analyzed by traditional physicochemical and microscopic methods, as described earlier for routine urinalysis. In some cases, sediment changes may be ambiguous or nondetectable, and proteinuria may be absent. In others, extrarenal causes of sodium chloride depletion, resulting in loss of the renal medullary concentration gradient, or of potassium depletion, resulting in collecting tubule refractoriness to antidiuretic hormone, may be the cause of an inappropriately low urine specific gravity. In these cases, determination of the urinary fractional excretion of electrolytes like sodium (FE_{Na}) is a reliable test for detecting renal tubular dysfunction. The urinary fractional excretion of a solute is calculated with the following formula after the analysis of random but simultaneously collected blood and urine specimens:

$$FE_X = (U_X/P_X) \times (P_{cr}/U_{cr}) \times 100\%$$

where FE_X is the fractional excretion of solute "X," U_X is the urinary concentration (mg/mL) of solute "X," P_X is the

plasma concentration (mg/mL) of solute "X," P_{cr} is the plasma concentration (mg/mL) of creatinine, and U_{cr} is the urinary concentration (mg/mL) of creatinine. This formula merely represents an arithmetic transformation of the ratio of the urinary clearance formula for "X" divided by that for creatinine. Thus, fractional excretion quantitatively describes the excretion of "X" relative to the GFR.

Fractional Excretion of Sodium

In most species that are fed a typical diet with an average sodium content, the kidneys normally reabsorb 99% or more of the sodium that is filtered by the glomerulus; hence, the normal FE_{Na} is less than 1.0%. Disorders affecting renal tubular function result in a pathologic increase in the proportion of filtered sodium that is not reabsorbed and an FE_{Na} of greater than 1.0%. Exceptions to this are seen under only a few relatively uncommon conditions, including:

1. Sodium-avid states, wherein dietary sodium restriction has been used to control systemic hypertension, resulting in decreased ERPF and enhanced sodium reabsorption disproportionate to the remaining functional tubular mass;
2. Intratubular obstruction, wherein pigmenturia or radiographic contrast media induce reductions in the tubular flow rate that promote sodium reabsorption; and
3. Glomerulotubular imbalance, wherein glomerular damage exceeds tubular dysfunction so that fractional sodium reclamation may appear to be normal.

In a study of diagnostic indices of azotemia in horses, urinary osmolality, $U:P_{osm}$, $U:P_{urea}$, and $U:P_{cr}$ ratios as well as FE_{Na} were more abnormal in renal azotemia than in prerenal azotemia (*Fig. 21.7*).

Fractional Excretion of Potassium

Reference ranges for the urinary fractional excretion of other electrolytes are more variable because of the greater effects of dietary mineral consumption on resting urinary excretory rates. For instance, the FE_K in cats that are fed a typical commercial diet (~0.65% K dry matter) ranges from approximately 5% to 20%, whereas in sheep that are fed a hay and alfalfa pellet diet (~2.25% K dry matter), the FE_K may be 100% to 180%. In llamas that are fed mixed hay (~0.22% K dry matter) or grass hay (~0.12% K dry matter) diets, the FE_K may be 45% to 125%.

In healthy cats, the FE_K decreases rapidly, to less than 5%, when such cats are fed a potassium-restricted diet. In cats with feline kaliopenic polymyopathy-nephropathy syndrome, the FE_K is pathologically increased given the degree of hypokalemia ($\leq$65%) and only returns to normal

Diagnostic Index	Prerenal Azotemia	Renal Azotemia	Normal Horses
Urine osmolality (mOsm/kg)	458–961	226–495	727–1456
U/Posm	1.7–3.4	0.8–1.7	2.5–3.4
U/Purea	15.2–43.7	2.1–14.3	34.2–100.8
U/Pcreatinine	51.2–241.5	2.6–37.0	2.0–344.4
FENa	0.02–0.50	0.80–10.10	0.01–0.70

Figure 21.7   Ranges for diagnostic indices of azotemia in three groups of horses. (Reprinted from Grossman BS, Brobst DF, Kramer JW, Bayly WM, Reed SM. Urinary indices for differentiation of prerenal azotemia and renal azotemia in horses. J Am Vet Med Assoc 1982;180:284–288.)

after treatment of the conditional dietary potassium deficiency and metabolic acidosis that are characteristic of this disorder.

Fractional Excretion of Phosphorus

The FE$_P$ has been evaluated in both acute and chronic renal failure. In experimentally induced gentamicin nephrotoxicosis in sheep, the FE$_P$ increased in parallel with increases in the FE$_{Na}$ and FE$_K$, but it offered no additional diagnostic advantage in the detection of renal tubular dysfunction. In dogs with chronic renal failure, the FE$_P$ increases in response to renal secondary hyperparathyroidism. Detection of chronic renal insufficiency by increased FE$_P$ values (>20%), however, is inferior to measurement of increased serum creatinine because of a poor quanti-

tative relationship with GFR and, thus, is neither very sensitive nor specific. Nevertheless, it may be useful to monitor changes in the FE$_P$ with time to determine the response to treatments of chronic renal failure (e.g., dietary Pi restriction, exogenous calcitriol supplementation).

Temporal Changes Compared with Azotemia

In dogs with experimentally induced gentamicin nephrotoxicosis, the FE$_{Na}$ increases within 6 to 8 days, and the FE$_K$ increases within 4 to 6 days. These changes occur after significant decreases in endogenous creatinine clearance and increases in the serum creatinine concentration, but they serve to localize the cause of azotemia to the kidneys and to identify renal tubular dysfunction. In dogs that are intoxicated experimentally with ethylene glycol, an increase in the FE$_{Na}$ occurs within 3 hours of antifreeze consumption, which is well before the onset of azotemia *(Fig. 21.8)*. Unfortunately, increased urinary fractional excretion of some electrolytes may not always be indicative of renal disease. Fractional excretions may be iatrogenically increased in patients because of exogenous fluid and electrolyte administration. Increases in the fractional excretion of sodium, potassium, and phosphorus also have been observed in dogs with Fanconi syndrome, but without discernible azotemia, because of the selective tubular transport defects that are characteristic of this syndrome. Likewise, the FE$_{Na}$ would be expected to increase during the developmental phase of hyponatremia in dogs with hypoadrenocorticism, perhaps even before the onset of azotemia or secondary renal complications. Furthermore, the association between fractional excretion and 24-hour urinary excretion of electrolytes has not always been correlated well enough to justify the use of fractional excretion as a substitute for complete mineral balance studies. Compensatory hypertrophy of remnant nephrons in animals with chronic renal failure may lead to increased fractional electrolyte excretion pursuant to decreases in creatinine clearance and increases in the individual nephron electrolyte load. Although increases in the FE$_K$ are not unusual, significant increases in the FE$_{Na}$ are uncommon, even in fairly advanced cases of chronic renal failure. Thus, an increased FE$_{Na}$ in an animal with documented chronic renal disease may be indicative of "acute-on-chronic" renal failure (i.e., an acute exacerbation superimposed on the preexisting renal disease).

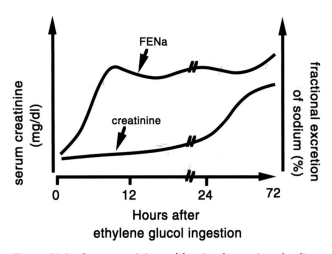

Figure 21.8   Serum creatinine and fractional excretion of sodium in experimental canine ethylene glycol nephrotoxicosis. (Adapted from Dial SM, Thrall MA, Hamar DW. Efficacy of 4-methylpyrazole for treatment of ethylene glycol intoxication in dogs. Am J Vet Res 1994;55:1762–1770.)

ENZYMURIA

Origin and Sensitivity

We routinely screen for organ damage by evaluating the serum activities of tissue-specific enzymes that are released into the circulation from damaged cells. In this manner, hepatocellular disease may be diagnosed on the basis of increases in serum aspartate aminotransferase (AST) or alanine aminotransferase activity (ALT), muscle damage may be discerned on the basis of increases in serum creatine kinase (CK) or lactate dehydrogenase (LDH) activity, and pancreatitis may be indicated on the basis of increases in amylase or lipase activity. Likewise, the urinary activity of enzymes that are released by damaged renal tubular epithelial cells may be used to screen for tubular injury in animals with nephrotoxicoses. These urinary enzymes are neither released into the systemic circulation nor filtered from the blood into the urine in meaningful amounts. Thus, increases in the measured urinary activity of these enzymes are highly specific for renal tubular disease and highly sensitive for tubular epithelial injury, even before the onset of functional disturbances affecting urinary fractional excretion of electrolytes or the glomerular filtration of nitrogenous wastes.

Two of the most commonly employed enzymes for detecting clinical enzymuria are γ-glutamyltransferase (GGT) and N-acetyl-β-D-glucosaminidase (NAG). Urinary GGT, which is a membrane-bound enzyme similar to the GGT produced by the hepatic biliary epithelium, is specific for renal tubular damage. Urinary NAG, which is a lysosomal enzyme produced by many tissues, is not filtered into the urine even during increased extrarenal release of NAG into the blood. Thus, increases in the urinary NAG activity are specific for renal tubular damage. Urinary GGT and NAG excretion may be evaluated from random urine samples by indexing the enzyme activity to the urinary creatinine concentration (U/mg creatinine) or from quantitative urine collections by determining 24-hour enzyme excretion. Urinary GGT activity is preserved during refrigeration, but it may be lost, to some extent, during freezing. Urinary NAG activity appears to be stable when frozen at −20°C for prolonged periods of time. Commercial methods for the measurement of human urinary enzyme activities perform well without modification for the detection of enzymuria in animals.

Temporal Changes Compared with Azotemia

Urinary GGT and NAG excretion increase rapidly after exposure to nephrotoxic agents. In sheep and rats, urinary GGT activity increases abruptly within 1 day of experimental exposure to mercuric chloride. In rats, dogs, and sheep, increases in urinary GGT and NAG activity have been observed experimentally after only 2 to 4 days of treatment with nephrotoxic doses of gentamicin.

Increases in urinary enzyme activity occur before changes in creatinine clearance, serum creatinine concentrations, or urinary fractional excretion of electrolytes, which develop after 4 to 8 days of exposure to nephrotoxin. Furthermore, increases in urinary enzyme excretion beyond the upper limit of the clinical reference interval

occur within 2 to 4 days of the induction of experimental gentamicin nephrotoxicosis, as opposed to increases in the serum creatinine concentration beyond the upper limit of the clinical reference interval, which occurred after only 8 to 10 days of nephrotoxic gentamicin treatment *(Fig. 21.9).*

There are some caveats in the clinical utilization of urinary enzyme excretion. Renal disease causing glomerulotubular imbalance may result in disparate changes in urinary enzyme excretion indexed to urinary creatinine,

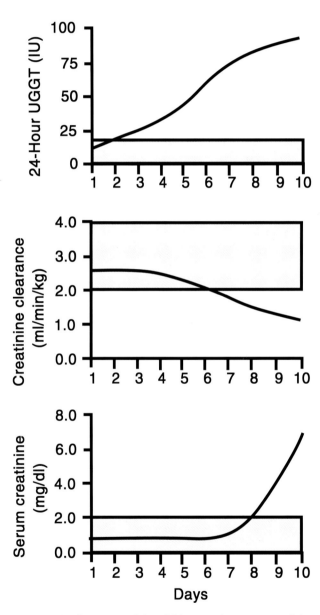

Figure 21.9 Serum creatinine, 24-hour endogenous creatinine clearance, and 24-hour urinary GGT activity in experimental canine gentamicin nephrotoxicosis. (Adapted from Greco DS, Turnwald GH, Adams R, Gossett KA, Kearney M, Casey H. Urinary γ-glutamyl transpeptidase activity in dogs with gentamicin-induced nephrotoxicity. Am J Vet Res 1985;46:2332–2335.)

as opposed to excretion quantitated during a 24-hour void. Thus, polyuric acute renal failure may be associated with lesser enzyme activities relative to creatinine than would be predicted from the increases in 24-hour enzyme excretion values. Likewise, oliguric acute renal failure may result in lesser 24-hour excretion values than would be expected from enzyme activities indexed to urinary creatinine.

The correlation of 24-hour urinary enzyme excretion of NAG and GGT with random urine sample enzyme:creatinine ratios has been examined in dogs with experimentally induced gentamicin nephrotoxicosis. Depending on the dietary protein consumption before treatment, significant correlations were observed during 0 to 8 days of gentamicin administration. This relationship became weaker with progression of the nephrotoxicosis, so that by 8 days both 24-hour excretion values and enzyme:creatinine ratios in random urine samples were significantly greater than normal. In healthy 18-month-old male Beagles, mean ± standard deviation (SD) baseline values for the urinary NAG:creatinine ratio and 24-hour urinary NAG excretion were 0.06 ± 0.04 IU/mg and 0.19 ± 0.14 IU/kg per 24 hours, respectively. Mean ± SD baseline values for the urinary GGT:creatinine ratio and 24-hour urinary GGT excretion were 0.39 ± 0.18 IU/mg and 1.42 ± 0.82 IU/kg per 24 hours, respectively.

URINALYSIS

Urinalysis is a vital component of the laboratory database for any patient ill enough to warrant a serum chemistry profile. Historically, routine urinalysis has consisted of a macroscopic or physicochemical analysis and microscopic examination of the urine sediment. The former includes an evaluation of color, turbidity, specific gravity, and qualitative chemical content by reagent strip or tablet reactions. The latter is used to identify cellular elements, microorganisms, renal tubular casts, and crystals. The value of including microscopic examination in routine urinalysis has been attributed to the identification of components that are essential to establishing the diagnosis of urogenital system disease that might not otherwise be detected by physicochemical examination. These components include leukocytes, renal tubular casts, neoplastic epithelial cells, parasitic ova, bacteria, and yeast or fungal elements.

Physical Examination of Urine

Color

Physical examination of urine includes the assessment of color, turbidity, and urine specific gravity. Normal urine varies from nearly colorless to deep amber; color inten-

sity primarily reflects the degree of urinary concentration and, therefore, the concentration of normal urinary pigments (i.e., urochromes). In general, the first urine of the day is more concentrated and, therefore, darker than later urine samples.

A number of abnormalities result in a changed urine color. Hemoglobinuria, myoglobinuria, and hemorrhage into the urinary tract all can result in red or red-tinged urine, and all are accompanied by proteinuria in the chemical examination. Further separation of these three conditions requires the evaluation of a fresh urine sediment for microscopic evidence of hemorrhage. If such evidence is lacking, then hemoglobinuria or myoglobinuria most likely are incriminated; these conditions can be differentiated by chemical means.

A greenish-brown discoloration of urine most frequently results from bilirubinuria associated either with liver disease or marked hemolysis. Urine with a high bilirubin content tends to foam when the sample is swirled. The presence of bilirubin in the urine is confirmed either by chemical means or by demonstration of bilirubin crystals in the urine sediment (discussed later). Chemical and cytologic evidence of bilirubinuria can occur together or independently. Bilirubin pigments in the urine are unstable; when bilirubinuria is suspected, urine samples should be kept in the dark and analyzed as quickly as possible.

Drug therapy also may influence the color of urine. For example, phenothiazine anthelmintics, which once commonly were used in small ruminants, turn urine pink to red. Whenever urine color is atypical and unexplained, a complete therapeutic and nutritional history of the patient should be obtained.

Turbidity

Urine turbidity reflects the amount of particulate material in the urine. Normal urine turbidity varies from species to species. Canine urine normally is clear, whereas feline urine normally may be slightly turbid because of the presence of fat. Normal horse urine generally is quite turbid because of mucus secreted by glands in the renal pelvis. Urine from normal rabbits is white and opaque because of a high content of calcium carbonate and calcium phosphate crystals. Casts, inflammatory cells, and crystals all can cause increases in turbidity. Microscopic examination of the sediment, however, is required to differentiate causes.

Specific Gravity

Evaluation of the urine specific gravity, which provides an estimate of the solute concentration, is the most important part of the physical examination. Urine specific gravity is an estimate of the ability of the kidney tubules to either concentrate or dilute urine. As such, it is a tubular function test (and is considered in more detail along with urine osmolality in a separate section).

The urine specific gravity has no normal value. The absolute isosthenuric range (i.e., where the urine specific gravity is the same as that of plasma and, therefore, the kidney has done no concentrating or diluting work) is 1.008 to 1.012. In practice, the isosthenuric range generally is considered to extend to 1.017. Specific gravities of less than 1.008 are indicative that the renal tubules are working to dilute urine; specific gravities of greater than 1.030 for dogs and greater than 1.035 for cats are indicative of the ability of the tubules to concentrate. Specific gravities of between 1.017 and these values are regarded as being ambiguous regarding tubular functional capacity.

Most commonly, the urine specific gravity is determined by refractometry. As discussed earlier, measurement by this method depends on the particle size and weight as well as the particle number. Consequently, large amounts of albumin or glucose in the urine can falsely increase the urine specific gravity, thereby creating the illusion of an ability to concentrate. From an interpretive perspective, this possibility should be considered whenever reagent strip concentrations exceed 3+.

Chemical Examination of Urine

Chemical examination of urine primarily is done on a semiquantitative basis using reagent strips *(Fig. 21.10)*. Numerous reagent strips, measuring a variety of analytes, are available, but unfortunately, all these strips have been designed for use in humans. In addition, not all the tests are relevant or accurate in animals. For example, the

reagent strip test for white blood cells is based on a specific leukocyte esterase that is found in human leukocytes but not in those of dogs and cats. Therefore, the test is of limited use in veterinary medicine.

Other tests of limited value in animals include strip tests for specific gravity and for urobilinogen. In our experience, the strip test for urine specific gravity simply does not correlate well with refractometry and should be disregarded. In humans, urinary urobilinogen is used as an indicator of biliary obstruction. If the bile duct is patent, then urobilinogen is present in the urine; if the bile duct is obstructed, then no urobilinogen is detected. In animals, however, the urobilinogen test has little relevance for several reasons. First, the test has low sensitivity, so false-negative results are common and negative tests difficult to interpret. Second, most biliary obstructions in animals are intrahepatic and incomplete, so positive urinary urobilinogen results actually are expected.

Tests that have value in animals include protein, glucose, ketones, bilirubin, occult blood, and pH. With the exception of pH, all these tests are scored as 1+ to 4+, with progressively higher scores correlating with increasing concentrations. Because the concentrations of these substances relate to the degree of overall urinary concentration, results can be interpreted only in light of the urine specific gravity. For example, a 2+ proteinuria with a 1.060 urine specific gravity is far less significant than a 2+ proteinuria with a 1.010 urine specific gravity.

Protein

Interpretation of significant proteinuria depends on findings in the sediment. Proteinuria can be expected as an accompaniment to hemorrhage, inflammation, or renal tubular degeneration. In the absence of indicators of these sediment abnormalities, the proteinuria probably results from glomerular damage and leakage. Urine reagent strip tests for protein react primarily with albumin; globulin and paraproteins (i.e., Bence-Jones proteins) do not react well. False-positive results for protein can be obtained in extremely alkaline urine samples. (Further consideration is given later to the sensitivity and specificity of detecting proteinuria in predicting urogenital tract disease.)

Glucose

Evaluation of glucose in the urine must be coupled with simultaneous evaluation of glucose in the blood. The most common cause of glucosuria is a circulating glucose concentration that exceeds the maximum renal tubular transport for glucose reabsorption. In dogs and cats, the renal threshold is approximately 180 mg/dL; in ruminants, the renal threshold is as low as 80 mg/dL. Circulating hyperglycemia that exceeds renal thresholds may

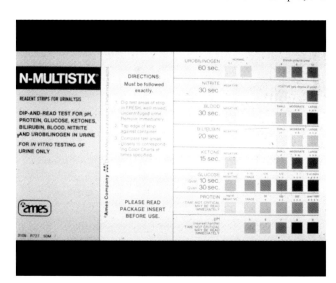

Figure 21.10 Label from a bottle of Ames Multistix. Reagent strip tests are semiquantitative and must be interpreted in light of the urinary concentration (i.e., specific gravity). Also, note that many of these tests must be read at specified time intervals.

be postprandial, the result of stress, or a reflection of true diabetes mellitus. Stress hyperglycemia most commonly is seen in cattle and cats.

There are several causes of glucosuria other than hyperglycemia, however. Both hereditary and acquired defects in proximal renal tubular glucose transport have been identified in most species and sometimes are given the appellation Fanconi syndrome (in reference to the disorder first described in humans). This syndrome may be accompanied by abnormalities in the tubular handling of several solutes, thereby resulting in the pathologic loss of amino acids, proteins, electrolytes, and glucose. A proximal renal tubular acidosis also may occur, wherein bicarbonate absorption is impaired, urinary acidification is inadequate, and systemic metabolic acidosis may ensue. Renal tubular degeneration may interfere with glucose reabsorption; for example, toxic nephropathies caused by heavy metals or aminoglycoside antibiotics may be characterized by mild to moderate glucosuria even when the blood glucose levels are normal.

Urinary glucose often is detected in the absence of hyperglycemia at the time of urine collection. Inherited or acquired disorders of renal tubular glucose transport should be considered in these cases, but one cannot exclude an earlier occurrence of hyperglycemia, thereby resulting in the appearance of glucose in urine that is stored in the bladder at some time before collection of the specimen. Examples include intermittent stress, administration of glucose-containing fluids, and postprandial hyperglycemia.

False-negative results also can occur with glucose reagent strip tests. Ascorbic acid interferes with the glucose strip test and, therefore, can cause false-negative results in the face of true glycosuria. Dogs with diabetes mellitus intermittently produce large amounts of ascorbic acid; consequently, even animals with uncontrolled hyperglycemias may yield negative results on spot checks. Clearly, urine glucose cannot be entirely relied on, either as a diagnostic test or as a monitoring device in canine diabetes.

Because protein and glucose are dissolved solutes, they can contribute to the urine specific gravity. At lower concentrations, this contribution is not significant. When concentrations exceed the 3+ indicator for either glucose or protein, however, the specific gravity can be spuriously increased beyond the isosthenuric range. Addition of 2.7 mg of glucose or 4.0 mg of albumin to 1 mL of urine increases the specific gravity by 0.001.

Ketones

Ketones appear in the urine when the magnitude of ketoacidemia exceeds the renal threshold for absorption from the glomerular filtrate. Ketoacidemia and ketonuria reflect the overproduction of ketones, which occurs when the rate of fat mobilization from peripheral adipose storage sites exceeds the metabolic capacity of the liver to oxidize this fat completely or to repackage it into lipoproteins for delivery to peripheral tissues for oxidation. This imbalance in fat metabolism principally relates to inadequate carbohydrate availability to facilitate complete oxidation, and it has been observed with a variety of conditions in which the availability of glucose is limited, including pregnancy toxemia, cachexia and starvation, and diabetes mellitus. The reagent strip tests for ketones can detect acetone and acetoacetic acid, but they cannot detect the third common ketone body, β-hydroxybutyric acid. Consequently, some cases of ketonuria may not be detected, simply because β-hydroxybutyric acid is the predominant ketone that is present. Contrary to anecdotal reports, addition of hydrogen peroxide to urine specimens containing β-hydroxybutyric acid does not convert this ketone to acetoacetic acid for subsequent detection by semiquantitative test strip or tablet methods.

Bilirubin

Urine bilirubin is an indicator of potential hepatic disease rather than of disease in the urinary system. Reagent strip tests for bilirubin use the same diazo methods that are used to identify serum bilirubin. These tests only detect conjugated bilirubin. Most of the conjugated bilirubin in urine comes from the blood and passes through the glomerulus, whereas small amounts of free bilirubin may be conjugated by the renal tubules and excreted in the urine. Increased urine bilirubin concentrations generally are indicative of cholestatic liver disease; however, other entities that cause increased formation of bilirubin conjugates by the liver (e.g., hemolytic anemias), also may increase urinary bilirubin excretion.

Occult Blood

A positive occult blood test on the urinary reagent strip results from hemorrhage in the urinary tract, hemoglobinuria, or myoglobinuria. Hemorrhage in the urinary tract may be confirmed by the finding of red blood cells in the urine sediment. Hyposthenuric urine, however, may result in hypotonic lysis of erythrocytes, thereby interfering with their detection at microscopy. In the absence of hemorrhage, hemoglobinuria and myoglobinuria must be differentiated. From a practical perspective, this can be done through evaluation of the hemogram and clinical history. Hemoglobinuria results from overwhelming intravascular hemolysis, generally is accompanied by evidence of severe anemia, and may be accompanied clinically by icterus and signs of sudden collapse. Myoglobinuria generally is seen only in cases in which there has been extreme muscle damage, and it should be accompanied by increases in the serum activity of muscle-derived enzymes (e.g., CK, LDH, AST).

pH

The pH of urine normally is acidic in carnivores and alkaline in herbivores. Increased pH in carnivores most typically results from the bacterial conversion of urea to ammonia and usually occurs in cases of cystitis caused by urease-positive organisms. Cystitis can be confirmed on the basis of evaluating the sediment (discussed later). Leukocytes and bacteria typically are present in the sediment. Decreased urine pH in ruminants may be seen in cases of abomasal displacement, where hydrochloric acid is sequestered in the abomasum, and when the animal is alkalotic, hypochloremic, and hypokalemic. Under these circumstances, bicarbonate is reabsorbed by the renal tubules because of the unavailability of chloride, and hydrogen is excreted in the urine because of the unavailability of potassium for exchange. (This condition of "paradoxic aciduria" is discussed in detail in a separate section.)

Microscopic Examination of Urine Sediment

Urine sediment examination is the most sensitive indicator of urinary tract disease and is useful in localizing injury to the kidney. Proper sediment examination depends on appropriate sample preparation and use of the microscope.

Sediment Preparation and Approach to Evaluation

Urine sediments are prepared by centrifuging a standard volume of urine (5–15 mL) at low speeds (400–700 g for 5 minutes). After decanting the supernatant, a drop of the sediment is placed on a microscope slide and then coverslipped for examination as a wet preparation. Although stains are available for sediments, their use carries several potential disadvantages. Stain penetration of cellular constituents (e.g., granulocytes, epithelial cells) may not be uniform throughout the preparation, and sediment stains often contain large amounts of stain precipitate, which may be confused with bacteria. Moreover, sediment stains are a good growth media for bacteria; therefore, they actually may contain bacteria and, thus, introduce organisms into the preparation.

To examine unstained sediment slides, the microscope is adjusted so that the margins of all cells are refractile. This is accomplished by reducing the light that reaches the stage by lowering the substage condenser and closing the iris diaphragm. If sediment slides are observed with full light, structures such as hyaline or waxy casts are easily missed. Sediments are examined at two magnifications:

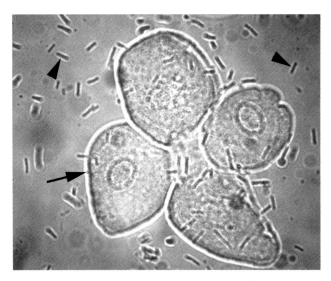

Figure 21.11   Urine sediment, unstained. Note the four transitional epithelial cells (arrow), with scattered rod-shaped bacteria (arrowheads). ×350.

×100 (i.e., low power), and ×400 (i.e., high power or high dry). Because a standard volume of urine is used to prepare sediments, they may be evaluated semiquantitatively. Numbers of casts are recorded per low-power field, and numbers of red cells and leukocytes are recorded per high-power field.

Cells in the Urine

Cells in the urine are of three major types: epithelial cells, red blood cells, and white blood cells. The numbers of cells that are present are influenced by the method of collecting

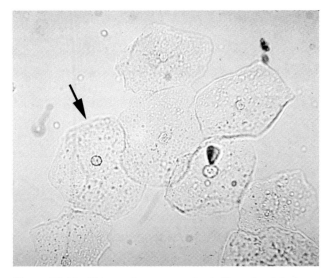

Figure 21.12   Urine sediment, unstained. Note the eight keratinized squamous epithelial cells (arrow). ×450.

the urine. In general, cystocentesis is the preferred method, and samples obtained in this manner contain the lowest number of cells in healthy animals. Catheterized samples usually contain increased numbers of transitional cells and, depending on how traumatic the collection, also may contain increased numbers of erythrocytes. Midstream free-flow samples often contain increased numbers of contaminating squamous epithelial cells.

Epithelial

Epithelial cells that are found in urine include renal tubular cells, transitional cells, and squamous cells. Renal tubular cells are the most difficult to recognize, because they are only slightly larger than leukocytes. Therefore, these two cell types may be easily confused. Renal epithelium may occur as individual cells or as epithelial cell casts. In either case, these cells, when present in significant numbers, are indicative of tubular degeneration. Epithelial cell casts are precursors of granular cell casts.

Most renal epithelial cells are round to polygonal cells with central, round nuclei. They measure approximately 20 μm in diameter. One particular type of renal epithelium, the caudate epithelial cell, differs in that they are not round but, rather, have a cytoplasmic tail. Caudate renal epithelial cells arise from the renal pelvis.

Transitional epithelial cells line the bladder and proximal urethra. They are much larger than renal epithelial cells because of more cytoplasmic volume. They are round to polyhedral, and they may be found either singly or in sheets *(Fig. 21.11)*. Nuclei are centrally located and contain one to three nucleoli, which often are visible even in unstained urine sediments. Transitional epithelium is stratified epithelium; consequently, cells may be of varying size and have some degree of variability in the nucleus:cytoplasm ratio. This is particularly true when rafts of epithelium are seen. Superficial cells are much larger than basal cells, with lower nucleus:cytoplasm ratios.

Cystocentesis samples from normal animals contain no more than one to three transitional cells per high-power field, whereas catheterized samples often have more cells, which may occur in groups or rafts. Increased numbers of transitional cells are seen in the urine from patients with cystitis (in association with increased numbers of leukocytes and, possibly, erythrocytes), and they also may be seen in cases of transitional cell carcinoma, in which the cytomorphology often is markedly aberrant even in unstained urine sediments. Neoplastic transitional cells often show marked variation in cell size. In addition, large cytoplasmic vacuoles may be recognized. Because normal transitional epithelial cells vary in size, however, and frequently contain nucleoli, one must be careful not to make an erroneous cytologic diagnosis of malignancy. Whenever transitional cell carcinoma is sus-

pected on the basis of unstained sediment morphology, a push smear may be made from the sediment, air-dried, stained with routine Romanovsky stains, and evaluated for criteria of malignancy.

Squamous cells in the urine usually are contaminants, although squamous metaplasia or neoplasia of the bladder or urethral epithelium can occur. In males, squamous cells in urine generally come from the penile sheath; in females, they desquamate from the vaginal vault or vulva. Cystocentesis samples generally contain fewer squamous cells than samples collected by other methods. Squamous cells are larger than transitional cells, and they are distinguished by their angular cytoplasmic margins and low nucleus:cytoplasm ratios *(Fig. 21.12)*. Superficial squamous cells may not contain visible nuclei.

Erythrocytes

Increased numbers of red blood cells in the urine are indicative of hemorrhage somewhere in the urogenital system, but they do not implicate a specific site of bleeding. Erythrocytes in the urine may result in a positive occult blood test and be accompanied by a mild proteinuria. Normal animals have fewer than three red blood cells per high-power field. Erythrocytes generally are recognized easily in unstained urine sediments. They are pale red-brown to yellow and, in appropriate species, contain a visible, central depression that is reflective of their normal, biconcave shape. They often have ruffled cytoplasmic margins because of crenation *(Fig. 21.13)*. Fat droplets may appear similar to erythrocytes, but they are irregular in size (whereas red blood cells are uniform).

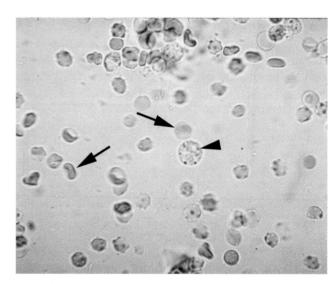

Figure 21.13   Urine sediment, unstained. Note the predominance of erythrocytes (arrows; biconcave disk shape often is discernible) with occasional leukocytes (arrowhead; larger cell size and granulated cytoplasm). ×400.

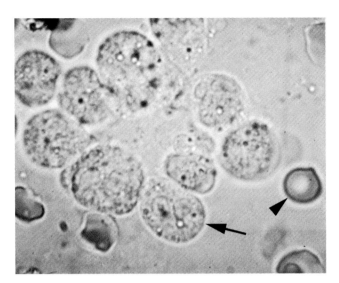

Figure 21.14   Urine sediment, unstained. Approximately 11 leukocytes (arrow) can be noted in the center and left of center. Some erythrocytes can be noted around the periphery (arrowhead). ×800.

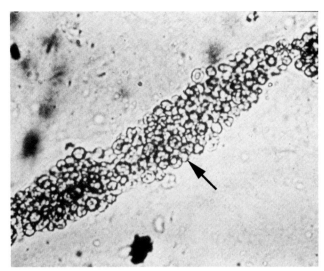

Figure 21.15   Urine sediment, unstained. Note the erythrocyte cast (arrow). ×400.

Leukocytes

Increased numbers of white blood cells in the urine are indicative of hemorrhage or inflammation in the urogenital tract, but as with red blood cells, they do not specify the site. Inflammation is differentiated from hemorrhage on the basis of the ratio of leukocytes to erythrocytes. If the two cell types are present in the proportions that are found in peripheral blood, then the process probably is hemorrhage; if leukocytes are more numerous than in the peripheral blood, then inflammation more likely is present. Normal urine contains no more than one to three leukocytes per high-power field. In unstained sediments, leukocytes are uniform, round cells that are only slightly larger than erythrocytes *(Fig. 21.14)*. In some instances, a segmented nucleus clearly is visible, but in others, the nucleus appears merely as a granular zone in the cell center.

Casts

Casts in the urine originate only from the renal tubules. They always are abnormal, regardless of how few are present. Casts are of several kinds: erythrocyte, leukocyte, epithelial, granular, waxy, and hyaline.

Erythrocyte and leukocyte casts.   Erythrocyte casts are indicative of renal hemorrhage, whereas leukocyte casts are indicative of renal inflammation. Often, they occur together, and they also may be seen in association with granular casts in cases of pyelonephritis. Red-blood-cell casts are recognized easily *(Fig. 21.15)*, but white-blood-cell casts *(Fig. 21.16)* may be difficult to differentiate from epithelial cell casts *(Fig. 21.17)*. The main difference is that epithelial cells are larger than white blood cells.

Tubular casts.   Epithelial cell, granular, and waxy casts all are indicative of renal tubular degeneration, and they result from the sloughing of dying tubular lining cells into tubular lumens. The kind of cast that is seen simply reflects how long the sloughed material stays in the kidney before passing out with the urine. Epithelial cell casts represent material that was present in the lumen for a minimal period after cast formation. As they age, epithelial cell casts transform into coarse granular *(Fig. 21.18)* and, eventually, fine granular casts *(Fig. 21.19)*. Waxy casts represent the end stage of tubular cell degeneration *(Fig. 21.20)*. All three kinds of casts can occur in the same urine sample. This is uncommon, however, because one

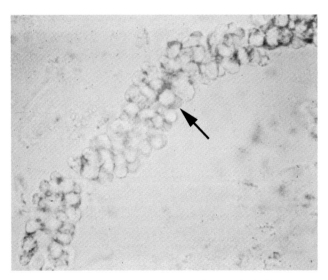

Figure 21.16   Urine sediment, unstained. Note the leukocyte cast (arrow). ×400.

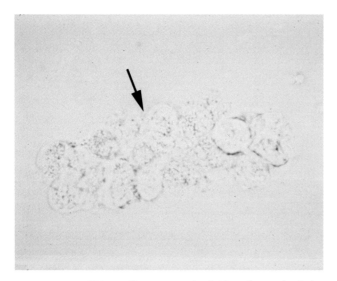

Figure 21.17 Urine sediment, unstained. Note the renal tubular epithelial cell cast (arrow). ×400.

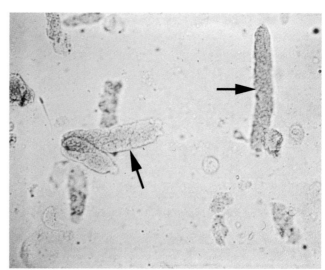

Figure 21.19 Urine sediment, unstained. Note the fine granular casts (arrows). ×100.

form usually predominates. Granular casts most commonly are seen. Epithelial cell casts are comprised of large (20–30 μm), round cells with granular nuclei. They can be confused with leukocyte casts, particularly if white blood cells are present in the sample. Granular casts are composed of amorphous granular material and usually are quite distinctive. Differentiating coarse granular from fine granular casts is an academic exercise and serves no practical purpose. Waxy casts are recognized only when the light in the microscope has been reduced to the point at which cell and cast margins are refractile. Waxy casts are devoid of internal structure and must be differentiated from hyaline casts. Differentiation is performed on the

basis of the fact that waxy casts are brittle and break and, consequently, have sharp ends, whereas hyaline casts are soft and have rounded ends.

Hyaline casts. Hyaline casts are protein casts that result from increased protein leakage across glomerular membranes into the tubules or from increased tubular protein concentration because of dehydration *(Fig. 21.21)*. When present in low numbers, they are not necessarily indicative of serious renal pathology; exercise, fever, and a variety of other nonspecific causes can increase glomerular protein leakage and result in the passage of low numbers of hyaline casts. When present in large numbers, hyaline

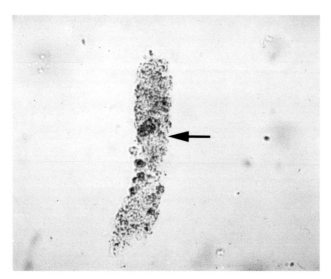

Figure 21.18 Urine sediment, unstained. Note the coarse granular cast (arrow). ×400.

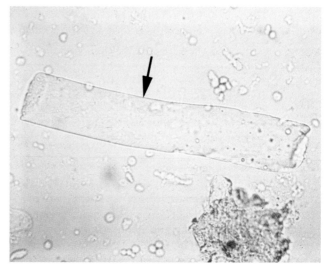

Figure 21.20 Urine sediment, unstained. Note the waxy cast (arrow). ×400.

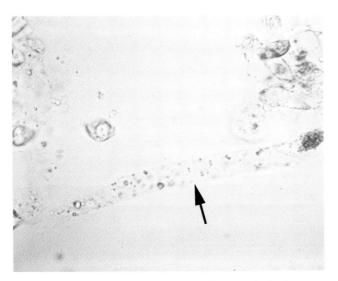

Figure 21.21   Urine sediment, unstained. Note the hyaline cast (arrow). ×400.

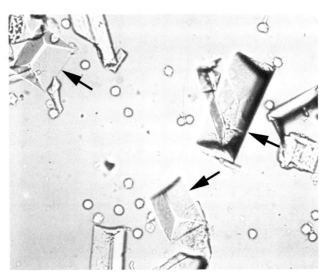

Figure 21.22   Urine sediment, unstained. Note the magnesium ammonium phosphate crystals (arrows) and the prism-like appearance. ×400.

casts generally are indicative of significant glomerular damage and are correlated with proteinuria. Like waxy casts, hyaline casts are observable only with low light, and because they are softer than waxy casts, they tend to resist fragmentation and are longer in length. Hyaline casts may contain embedded fat droplets as well.

Crystals

Crystals commonly are found in both normal and abnormal urine. Certain types of crystals are seen in a given species but also depend on diet and urinary pH. Urine crystals usually are identified on the basis of their characteristic shape and color.

Normal crystals. The predominant normal crystal in the urine of dogs and cats is the magnesium ammonium phosphate crystal *(Fig. 21.22)*. In its most common form, the phosphate crystal resembles a prism. If urine is allowed to stand, phosphate crystals may coalesce, thereby resulting in giant forms, or they may partially dissolve, thereby resulting in characteristic though less frequently observed variants.

The predominant normal crystals in the urine of horses and cows (and in most other herbivores) are calcium carbonates and calcium oxalate dihydrates. Calcium carbonate crystals occur in a variety of forms, including dumbbells, striated spheres, and so on *(Fig. 21.23)*. Calcium oxalate dihydrate crystals are recognized easily because of their "Maltese cross" or "envelope" configuration *(Fig. 21.24)*. Oxalates in the urine of herbivores derive from the high oxalate content of their diet; dogs and cats that eat plants also occasionally may pass oxalate crystals in the

urine. In most cases, however, oxalates are regarded as being pathologic crystals in dogs and cats (discussed later).

Abnormal crystals

Pigmented crystals. Two abnormal pigmented crystals that may be found in urine are bilirubin and ammonium biurate. Bilirubin crystals in the urine are a reflection of the increased urinary concentration of conjugated bilirubin. In most cases, they are found in association with cholestatic liver disease, but they also may occur in other conditions with systemic bilirubin alterations (e.g., severe hemolytic

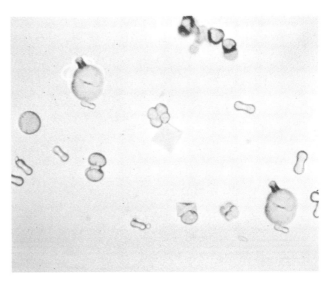

Figure 21.23   Urine sediment, unstained. Note the calcium carbonate crystals, which can be dumbbell shaped or spherical with striations. Size is somewhat variable. ×400.

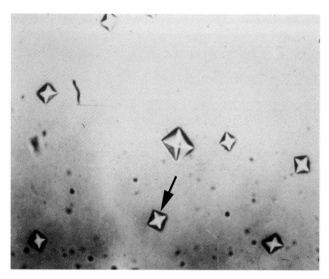

Figure 21.24   Urine sediment, unstained. Note the calcium oxalate dihydrate crystals (arrow). Oxalate dihydrate crystals are envelope-shaped and sometimes are termed the *Maltese cross crystal.* ×400.

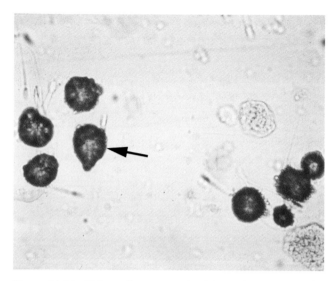

Figure 21.26   Urine sediment, unstained. Note the ammonium biurate crystals (arrow). ×400.

anemia). Although found in urine, bilirubin crystals are not associated with disorders of the urinary system. Bilirubin crystalluria may, or may not, correlate with evidence of increased urine bilirubin by reagent strip methodologies. Morphologically, bilirubin crystals are feather-like crystals with a distinct, golden-brown color *(Fig. 21.25).*

Ammonium biurate crystalluria also is associated with liver disease. Whenever the liver fails to convert ammonia to urea via the urea cycle, the increased blood and urinary ammonia levels lead to the formation of biurate crystals in the urine. Ammonium biurate crystalluria, therefore,

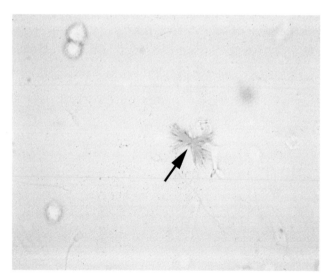

Figure 21.25   Urine sediment, unstained. Note the bilirubin crystal (arrow). ×400.

commonly is seen in portosystemic shunt disease, in which the hepatic parenchymal urea cycle is bypassed, and can occur in any hepatic disorder during which urea cycle activity is inadequate. In fresh urine, ammonium biurate crystals have a distinctive, mace-head appearance (i.e., sphere covered by irregular, projecting spikes); if urine is allowed to stand, the spikes become blunted and indistinct. Biurate crystals are brown *(Fig. 21.26).*

Amino acid crystals. Two amino acid crystals, tyrosine and cystine, occasionally can be found in the urine. Like bilirubin and biurate, tyrosine crystals generally are reflective of ongoing liver disease. Tyrosine crystals are needle-like and are arranged in aggregates, so that they may resemble bilirubin crystals. They are not, however, pigmented *(Fig. 21.27).*

Cystine crystals are extremely rare, and they are associated with an inherited disease of renal tubular cell carrier–mediated amino acid transport, thereby resulting in cystinuria. The defective carrier protein also is responsible for the transport of the dibasic amino acids, including lysine, arginine, and ornithine. Because of its poor solubility, especially in acidic urine, cystine crystals precipitate out and have the appearance of clear, hexagonal plates *(Fig. 21.28).*

Oxalate crystals. Oxalate crystalluria in dogs and cats often is associated with ethylene glycol toxicosis. Ingested ethylene glycol is metabolized by the liver to oxalic acid, which then combines with calcium to form calcium oxalate, which in turn precipitates in the renal tubules and may pass out as crystals in the urine. The morphology

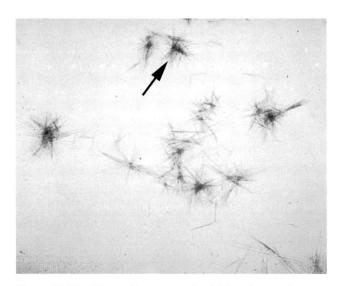

Figure 21.27   Urine sediment, unstained. Note the tyrosine crystals (arrow). ×400.

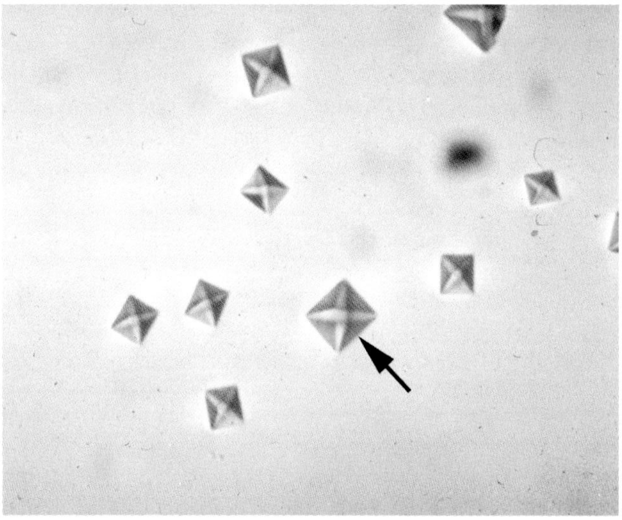

of calcium oxalate dihydrate crystals is described as a "Maltese cross" or "envelope" configuration *(Fig. 21.29)*. Calcium oxalate monohydrate crystals are "hempseed-shaped" or six-sided, "hippurate-like" prisms that were formally mischaracterized in several publications as being hippuric acid crystals *(Fig. 21.30)*.

Drug crystals. When sufficient blood and urinary concentrations of drugs such as sulfonamides are achieved, precipitation and drug crystalluria may result. Drug crystals vary in morphology, but they often resemble large, fan-like structures *(Fig. 21.31)*. Whenever unusual crys-

tals are found in a urine sample, a complete drug history should be obtained. Drug crystalluria often is associated with drug toxicity, including neomycin, gentamicin, and sulfa toxicity.

Miscellaneous Findings in the Sediment

Infectious agents. Both bacteria and parasitic structures can be found in urine sediments. As a general rule, bacteria must be present at concentrations of greater than approximately 1×10^4 organisms/mL to be seen microscopically. Rods occur either singly or in chains. Bacteria

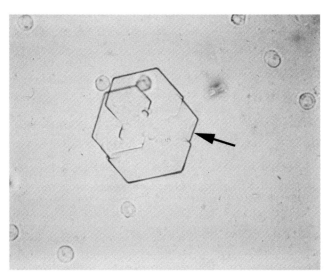

Figure 21.28   Urine sediment, unstained. Note the cystine crystal (arrow). ×400.

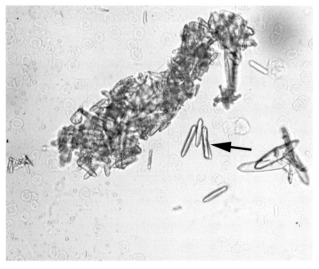

Figure 21.30   Urine sediment, unstained. Note the calcium oxalate monohydrate crystals (arrow). ×400.

Figure 21.29   Urine sediment, unstained. Note the calcium oxalate dihydrate crystals (arrow). ×400.

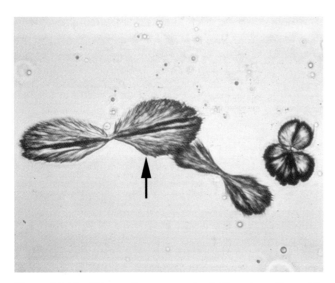

Figure 21.31   Urine sediment, unstained. Note the sulfonamide crystals (arrow). Nephrotoxic drugs may lead to the appearance of bizarre crystals in urine. ×400.

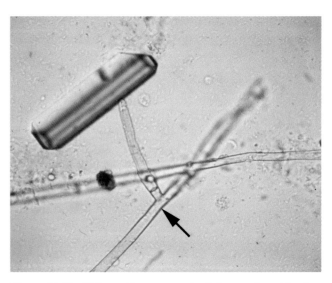

Figure 21.32   Urine sediment, unstained. Septate fungal hyphae (arrow) are relatively common urine contaminants. ×400.

in catheterized or voided samples may be contaminants and are of equivocal significance. Cystocentesis is the preferred collection technique for the evaluation of bacteriuria, because urine in the bladder normally is sterile. The observation of bacteria in urine specimens that are not fresh, or that have not been preserved properly, should be interpreted with caution. Finding increased numbers of white blood cells in association with bacteria is helpful in suggesting that the bacteriuria is clinically important. Once bacteriuria has been identified microscopically, however, culture is required to truly assess the clinical significance.

A variety of parasitic structures may be found in urine. Microfilaria of *Dirofilaria immitis* occasionally are seen. Eggs from *Capillaria plica*, *Dioctophyma renale*, and *Stephanurus dentatus* all are passed in the urine.

Contaminants and artifacts. Fungal hyphae *(Fig. 21.32)* and macroconidia *(Fig. 21.33)*, budding yeasts, and pollen grains *(Fig. 21.34)* all are common contaminants found in urine sediments, particularly if the samples are collected in a dusty environment (e.g., a barn). These findings have no clinical significance. Sperm are a frequent contaminant in male urine and may be found in urine from recently bred females. Fat droplets are common in the urine of cats. In dogs, fat droplets may be observed after a fatty meal and can be present in the urine of diabetics. Strands of mucus are a normal finding in the urine of horses. Finally, fragments of broken glass from pipettes or sample containers *(Fig. 21.35)*, talc crystals from powdered surgical gloves, and wax marking pencil fragments also may appear as urine sediment contaminants.

New Diagnostic Algorithms for Urinalysis

Macroscopic Versus Microscopic Examination

Several studies have questioned both the predictive value and the cost-effectiveness of routinely performing a microscopic examination as a component of the urinalysis in humans. The question regarding effectiveness arises on the basis of the low yield of additional information from abnormal urine specimens in which physicochemical findings are negative but in which microscopic findings are positive, as well as on the basis of the potentially inefficient use of laboratory technician time and added cost to

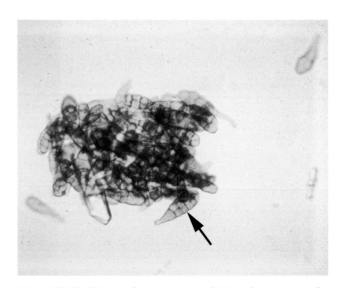

Figure 21.33   Urine sediment, unstained. Note the macroconidia of the fungus *Alternaria* sp. (arrow), which are ubiquitous in the environment and, therefore, common urine contaminants. ×400.

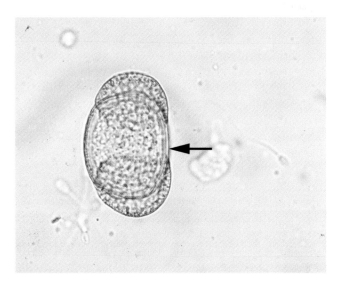

Figure 21.34 Urine sediment, unstained. Note the pine pollen (arrow). ×400.

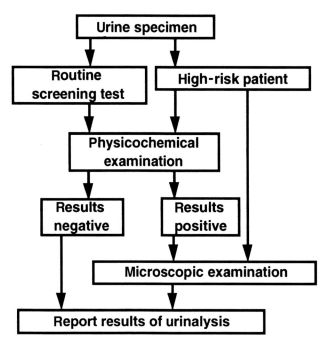

Figure 21.36 Discriminative diagnostic algorithm for the laboratory evaluation of urine specimens on the basis of physicochemical test results.

human patients. The effects of a discriminative diagnostic algorithm *(Fig. 21.36)* on macroscopic examination sensitivity have been determined.

In a retrospective study that compared macroscopic and physicochemical examinations of urine, results of 1000 consecutive canine urinalyses were reviewed and summarized. Physicochemical examination alone would have resulted in an 11.4% false negative rate for the detection of abnormal urine specimens without consideration of patient risk for genitourinary disease. Small numbers of macronegative, micropositive, or macro- and

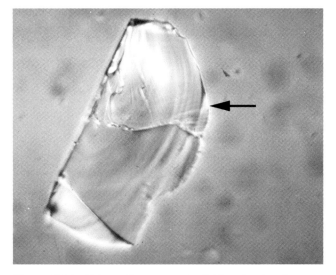

Figure 21.35 Urine sediment, unstained. Note the glass fragment (arrow). Shards of glass from urine specimen containers or environmental contamination may be mistaken for crystals of pathologic significance. ×400.

micronegative samples were obtained from higher-risk patients with history, physical signs, clinical problems, or serum biochemical analysis results that were indicative of a predisposition to genitourinary disease, which would have warranted complete urinalysis regardless of the physicochemical findings. Signs associated with a predisposition to genitourinary disease included neurologic deficits, lower vertebral disk abnormalities and hind-limb lamenesses, genitourinary abnormalities, perineal abnormalities, diarrhea, and serum biochemical abnormalities caused by renal failure. Exclusion of these patients from the evaluation of physicochemical examination sensitivity to consider the impact of such methodology as a screening procedure only on those patients in which genitourinary disease was not already suspect resulted in a significantly lower false negative rate of 3.0%.

Urinary Protein

The previously mentioned study demonstrated that use of a discriminative diagnostic algorithm to identify high-risk animals may obviate the need for routine microscopic sediment examinations. Historically, repeated detection of proteinuria with qualitative urine screening tests derived on the basis of the protein error of indicator dyes, or turbidimetric reactions with organic acids, would be verified using more precise, quantitative methods. The predominant urinary chemical abnormality detected by routine screening procedures in animals with genitourinary disease appears to be proteinuria. Quantitative analysis of urinary protein alone, as compared with a microscopic examination in screening for genitourinary disease, is quite sensitive. Although crystals, yeast, bacteria, and parasites may be present without detectable proteinuria, glomerular disease often is associated with proteinuria in the absence of urine sediment findings. Sediment analysis still provides an important tool for the localization of urinary tract lesions, however, when proteinuria is present.

Depending largely on the particular chemical method used, protein concentrations in urine from dogs without urogenital disease have been reported to range from 0.95 to 2.78 mg/mL. Because the urinary protein concentration is influenced by the quantity filtered through the glomerulus, the protein secreted by tubular cells into the filtrate, and the modification of filtrate concentration by the renal tubules, evaluation of proteinuria relies on standardization to some index of the GFR. Formerly, urinary protein loss was quantitated as 24-hour excretory rates, which preferably are standardized to body weight or surface area. Again, depending on the chemical method, 24-hour urinary protein loss in dogs without urogenital disease ranges from 53.6 to 386 mg. Values for 24-hour urinary protein loss as standardized to body weight have been reported to range from 5.1 to 22.4 mg/kg. Through many studies of human and canine proteinuria, it has become evident that protein in randomly collected urine specimens may be accurately evaluated through semi-quantitative indexing to the urinary creatinine concentration. The urinary protein:creatinine ratio (U[P:C]) correlates well with the 24-hour urinary protein excretion, and increases in this value beyond the range reported for healthy dogs have been associated with protein-losing glomerulonephropathies. Ranges for U(P:C) in healthy dogs have been reported to range from 0.01 to 0.54 mg or protein per 1 mg of creatinine. It appears from most studies that a U(P:C) of less than 1.0 is normal, whereas a U(P:C) of greater than 2.0 is abnormal. Animals with values between 1.0 and 2.0 should be evaluated further by a determination of 24-hour urinary protein excretion. Unfortunately, it has been demonstrated that large increases in U(P:C) may be observed in dogs with experimentally induced cystitis when inflammatory exudation is marked. Thus, it is recommended that U(P:C) be evaluated with caution when there is also significant pyuria, so that renal proteinuria is not mistakenly diagnosed. Blood contamination due to traumatic hemorrhage induced during the course of urine collection by cystocentesis does not significantly affect urinary protein concentration or U(P:C) even when large amounts of blood are detected by dipstick.

In another study, 500 consecutive urinalyses of canine patients at the Colorado State University Veterinary Teaching Hospital were reviewed and summarized to compare the sensitivities for detection of abnormalities indicative of urinary system disease among qualitative (i.e., sulfosalicylic acid [SSA]), quantitative (i.e., Coomassie brilliant blue [CBB]), and indexed (U[P:C]) determinations of urinary protein loss versus microscopic examination of urine sediment. The effects of a modified, discriminative diagnostic algorithm on macroscopic examination sensitivity were determined (Fig. 21.37). False-negative rates for the detection of microscopically abnormal urine specimens were 5.4% for an SSA of greater than 1+, 8.5% for a CBB of greater than 1.0 mg/ml, and 9.7% for a U(P:C) of greater than 1.0. A discriminatory U(P:C) of 2.0 would have excluded dogs with clinically relevant proteinuria in the lower ranges. Degrees of azotemia were higher (high serum creatinine or BUN concentration) and the prevalence of chronically diseased dogs was greater in patient categories with higher U(P:C) values. It was concluded that more quantitative determinations of urinary protein loss as a screening test offer potentially labor-saving and diagnostic advantages, but not greater sensitivity in the identification of urinary disease compared with more qualitative routine screening methods.

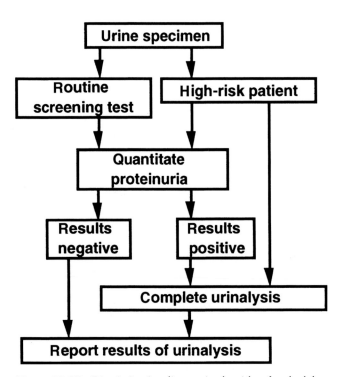

Figure 21.37 Discriminative diagnostic algorithm for the laboratory evaluation of urine specimens on the basis of the magnitude of proteinuria.

SUGGESTED READINGS

Urea Nitrogen and Creatinine
Allen TA, Jaenke RS, Fettman MJ. A technique for estimating progression of chronic renal failure in the dog. J Am Vet Med Assoc 1987;190:866–868.

Bertone JJ, Traub-Dargatz JL, Fettman MJ, et al. Monitoring the progression of renal failure in a horse with polycystic kidney disease: use of the reciprocal of serum creatinine concentration and sodium sulfanilate clearance half-time. J Am Vet Med Assoc 1987;191:565–568.

Finco DR, Duncan JR. Evaluation of blood urea nitrogen and serum creatinine concentrations as indicators of renal dysfunction: a study of 111 cases and a review of related literature. J Am Vet Med Assoc 1976;168:593–601.

Hill D, Correa MT, Stevens JB. Sensitivity, specificity, and predictive values of reagent test strip estimations of blood urea nitrogen. Vet Clin Pathol 1995;23:73–75.

Jacobs RM, Lumsden JH, Taylor JA, Grift E. Effects of interferents on the kinetic Jaffe reaction and an enzymatic colorimetric test for serum creatinine concentration in determination in cats, cows, dogs, and horses. Can J Vet Res 1991;55:150–154.

Urashima M, Toyoda S, Nakano T, et al. BUN/Cr ratio as an index of gastrointestinal bleeding mass in children. J Pediatr Gastroenterol Nutr 1992;15:89–92.

Watson ADJ, Church DB, Fairburn AJ. Postprandial changes in plasma urea nitrogen and creatinine concentrations in dogs. Am J Vet Res 1981;42:1878–1880.

Serum Inorganic Phosphorus
Chew DJ, DiBartola SP, Nagode LA, Starkey RJ. Phosphorus restriction in the treatment of chronic renal failure. Curr Vet Ther 1992;XI:853–857.

Slatopolsky E, Lopez-Hilker S, Delmez J, Dusso A, Brown A, Martin KJ. The parathyroid-calcitriol axis in health and chronic renal failure. Kidney Int 1990;38(Suppl):S41–S47.

Traditional Renal Clearance Methods
Bovee KC, Joyce T. Clinical evaluation of glomerular function: 24-hour creatinine clearance in dogs. J Am Vet Med Assoc 1979;174:488–491.

Finco DR, Brown SA, Crowell WA, Barsanti JA. Exogenous creatinine clearance as a measure of glomerular filtration rate in dogs with reduced renal mass. Am J Vet Res 1991;52:1029–1032.

Finco DR, Coulter DB, Barsanti JA. Procedure for a simple method of measuring glomerular filtration rate in the dog. J Am Anim Hosp Assoc 1982;18:804–806.

Finco DR, Tabaru H, Brown SA, Barsanti JA. Endogenous creatinine clearance measurement of glomerular filtration rate in dogs. Am J Vet Res 1993;54:1575–1578.

Tabaru H, Finco DR, Brown SA, Cooper T. Influence of hydration state on renal functions of dogs. Am J Vet Res 1993;54:1758–1764.

New Renal Clearance Methods
Allen TA, Fettman MJ, Jaenke RS, Wilke WL. Renal functional relationships in dogs with glomerulopathies. Am J Vet Res 1987;48:610–612.

Brown SA. Evaluation of a single-injection method for estimating glomerular filtration rate in dogs with reduced renal function. Am J Vet Res 1994;55:1470–1473.

Fettman MJ, Allen TA, Wilke WL, Radin MJ, Eubank MC. Single-injection method for evaluation of renal function with ^{14}C-inulin and ^3H-tetraethylammonium bromide in dogs and cats. Am J Vet Res 1985;46:482–485.

Labato MA, Ross LA. Plasma disappearance of creatinine as a renal function test in the dog. Res Vet Sci 1991;50:253–258.

Maddison JE, Pascoe PJ, Jansen BS. Clinical evaluation of sodium sulfanilate clearance for the diagnosis of renal disease in dogs. J Am Vet Med Assoc 1984;185:961–965.

Moe L, Heiene R. Estimation of glomerular filtration rate in dogs with ^{99m}Tc-DTPA and iohexol. Res Vet Sci 1995;58:138–143.

Rogers KS, Komkov A, Brown SA, Lees GE, Hightower D, Russo EA. Comparison of four methods of estimating glomerular filtration rate in cats. Am J Vet Res 1991;52:961–964.

Uribe D, Krawiec DR, Twardock AR, Gelberg HB. Quantitative renal scintigraphic determination of the glomerular filtration rate in cats with normal and abnormal kidney function, using ^{99m}Tc-diethylenetriaminepentaacetic acid. Am J Vet Res 1992;53:1101–1107.

Urinary Concentration Capacity
Bovee KC. Urine osmolarity as a definitive indicator of renal concentrating capacity. J Am Vet Med Assoc 1969;155:30–35.

Breitschwerdt EB, Verlander JW, Hribernik TN. Nephrogenic diabetes insipidus in three dogs. J Am Vet Med Assoc 1981;179:235–238.

Hardy RM, Osborne CA. Water deprivation test in the dog: maximal normal values. J Am Vet Med Assoc 1979;174:479–483.

Ross LA, Finco DR. Relationship of selected clinical renal function tests to glomerular filtration rate and renal blood flow in cats. Am J Vet Res 1981;42:1704–1710.

Urinary Fractional Excretion of Electrolytes
Adams LG, Polzin DJ, Osborne CA, O'Brien TD. Comparison of fractional excretion and 24-hour urinary excretion of sodium and potassium in clinically normal cats and cats with induced chronic renal failure. Am J Vet Res 1991;52:718–722.

Dial SM, Thrall MA, Hamar DW. Efficacy of 4-methylpyrazole for treatment of ethylene glycol intoxication in dogs. Am J Vet Res 1994;55:1762–1770.

Dow SW, Fettman MJ, Smith KR, et al. Effects of dietary acidification and potassium depletion on acid-base balance, mineral metabolism, and renal function in adult cats. J Nutr 1990;120:569–578.

Fettman MJ. Feline kaliopenic polymyopathy/nephropathy syndrome. Vet Clin North Am Sm Anim Pract 1989;19:415–432.

Garry FB, Chew DJ, Hoffsis GF. Urinary indices of renal function in sheep with induced aminoglycoside nephrotoxicosis. Am J Vet Res 1990;51:420–427.

Gleadhill A. Evaluation of screening tests for renal insufficiency in the dog. J Small Anim Pract 1994;35:391–396.

Grauer GF, Greco DS, Behrend EN, Fettman MJ, Jaenke RS, Allen TA. Effects of dietary protein conditioning on gentamicin-induced nephrotoxicosis in healthy male dogs. Am J Vet Res 1994;55:90–97.

Grossman BS, Brobst DF, Kramer JW, Bayly WM, Reed SM. Urinary indices for differentiation of prerenal azotemia and renal azotemia in horses. J Am Vet Med Assoc 1982;180:284–288.

Lackey MN, Belknap EB, Salman MD, Tinguely L, Johnson LW. Urinary indices in llamas fed different diets. Am J Vet Res 1995;56:859–865.

Enzymuria
Garry FB, Chew DJ, Hoffsis GF. Enzymuria as an index of renal damage in sheep with induced aminoglycoside nephrotoxicosis. Am J Vet Res 1990;51:428–432.

Gould DH, Fettman MJ, Daxenbichler ME, Bartuska BM. Functional and structural alterations of the rat kidney induced by the naturally occurring organonitrile 2S-1-cyano-2-hydroxy-3,4-epithiobutane. Toxicol Appl Pharmacol 1985;78:190–201.

Grauer GF, Greco DS, Behrend EN, Fettman MJ, Jaenke RS, Allen TA. Effects of dietary protein conditioning on gentamicin-induced nephrotoxicosis in healthy male dogs. Am J Vet Res 1994;55:90–97.

Grauer GF, Greco DS, Behrend EN, Mani I, Fettman MJ, Allen TA. Estimation of quantitative enzymuria in dogs with gentamicin-induced nephrotoxicosis using urine enzyme/creatinine ratios from spot urine samples. J Vet Intern Med 1995;9:324–327.

Greco DS, Turnwald GH, Adams R, Gossett KA, Kearney M, Casey H. Urinary γ-glutamyl transpeptidase activity in dogs with gentamicin-induced nephrotoxicity. Am J Vet Res 1985;46:2332–2335.

Urinalysis

Allen TA, Jones RL, Purvance J. Microbiologic evaluation of canine urine: direct microscopic examination and preservation of specimen quality for culture. J Am Vet Med Assoc 1987;190:1289–1291.

Bagley RS, Center SA, Lewis RM, et al. The effect of experimental cystitis and iatrogenic blood contamination on the urine protein/creatinine ratio in the dog. J Vet Intern Med 1991;5:66–70.

Bovee KC, Joyce T, Blazer-Yost B, Goldschmidt MS, Segal S. Characterization of renal defects in dogs with a syndrome similar to the Fanconi syndrome in man. J Am Vet Med Assoc 1979;174:1094–1099.

Comer KM, Ling GV. Results of urinalysis and bacterial culture of canine urine obtained by antepubic cystocentesis, catheterization, and the midstream voided methods. J Am Vet Med Assoc 1981;179:891–895.

Fettman MJ. Comparison of urinary protein concentration and protein/creatinine ratio vs. routine microscopy in urinalysis of dogs: 500 cases (1987–1988). J Am Vet Med Assoc 1989;195:972–976.

Fettman MJ. Evaluation of the usefulness of routine microscopy in canine urinalysis. J Am Vet Med Assoc 1987;190:892–896.

Thrall MA, Dial SM, Winder DR. Identification of calcium oxalate monohydrate crystals by x-ray diffraction in urine of ethylene glycol-intoxicated dogs. Vet Pathol 1985;22:622–628.

Vail DM, Allen TA, Weiser G. Applicability of leukocyte esterase test strip in detection of canine pyuria. J Am Vet Med Assoc 1986;189:1451–1453.

van Vonderen IK, Kooistra HS, Rijnberk. Intra- and interindividual variation in urine osmolality and urine specific gravity in healthy pet dogs of various ages. J Vet Intern Med 1997;11:30–35.

C H A P T E R

22

FLUID AND ELECTROLYTE
METABOLISM

FLUID BALANCE

Hydration

The concentration of certain blood elements may be used to evaluate the hydration status *(Table 22.1)*. Plasma protein concentration and packed cell volume (PCV) both increase as water is lost because of dehydration. These laboratory parameters provide a fairly accurate means of assessing large water losses in patients, but the wide reference ranges for these values in normal animals makes the interpretation of small changes, resulting from dehydration in previously unevaluated patients, very difficult. In addition, concurrent anemia, blood loss, or protein-losing conditions (e.g., enteropathies, nephropathies) may obscure the interpretation of water loss and hemoconcentration resulting from dehydration.

Although dehydration is associated with increased concentration of certain blood elements (e.g., erythrocytes, plasma proteins), electrolyte concentrations are not always increased. Dehydration may, or may not, be associated with changes in electrolyte concentrations, depending on the cause of the water loss. Three models of dehydration (i.e., isotonic, hypertonic, hypotonic) are differentiated predominantly on the basis of changes in the plasma concentration of sodium (Na) and chloride (Cl), which

are the principal ions of the extracellular fluid (ECF) compartment.

Water Requirements

Water is the single greatest component of the body and the most fundamental of all nutrients. It also constantly is being lost through obvious excretory routes, including feces and urine, wherein it serves as a carrier for the elimination of other waste products *(Table 22.2)*. It also is lost through inapparent routes, which are referred to as "insensible losses," including perspiration and respiratory evaporation (Table 22.2).

Metabolic Rate

An individual's daily water requirement is determined predominantly by that individual's metabolic body size, in direct proportion to the caloric requirement. In other words, the higher the energy expenditure, the higher the water requirement. Large animals have a higher total energy and water requirement than smaller animals, but when examined more closely, the caloric and water requirements are greater per unit of body weight in smaller animals. This is, in part, because smaller animals have larger surface area per unit of body weight and, thereby,

TABLE 22.1 COMPARATIVE EFFECTS OF WATER, BLOOD, OR PROTEIN LOSS ON PCV AND PLASMA PROTEIN CONCENTRATIONS

PCV	Plasma Protein Concentration	Condition
Increased	Increased	Dehydration
Decreased	No change	Anemia not caused by blood loss
Decreased	Increased	Anemia caused by chronic inflammation
Decreased	Decreased	Overhydration or anemia caused by blood loss
Increased	Decreased	Protein-losing enteropathy or nephropathy

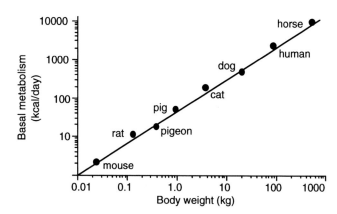

Figure 22.1 Log-linear relationship between body weight and basal metabolic rate. (Adapted from Blaxter K. Energy metabolism in animals and man. New York: Cambridge University Press, 1989.)

have a greater surface for energy loss as heat and for water loss via evaporation. The relationship between metabolic body size and caloric or water requirements is log-linear *(Fig. 22.1)*.

This relationship describes the basal energy or water requirement for an inactive animal. The logarithmic formula describing this relationship is

$$\text{Basal metabolic rate} = 70(\text{Body weight}_{kg}^{0.75})$$

TABLE 22.2 WATER BALANCE IN DOGS AT REST

Source	Body Weight (mL/kg)	% Total
Intake		
Food	10–12	35–45
Drink	15–20	50–60
Metabolic	4–5	10–20
Loss		
Urine	10–25	50–70
Feces	1–3	2–5
Insensible	10–25	40–60

Adapted from Kohn CW, DiBartola SP. Composition and distribution of body fluids in dogs and cats. In: DiBartola SP, ed. Fluid therapy in small animal practice 2nd ed. Philadelphia: WB Saunders, 2000:3–25.

The linear equivalent of this formula, which for animals weighing more than 2 kg but less than 60 kg, is 30(body weight$_{kg}$)+ 70. To convert these values to the resting energy expenditure or water requirement, one multiplies the basal value by some corrective factor, such as 1.2 for cats and 1.6 for dogs. For animals consuming a high-fiber diet (e.g., weight-loss diets in small animals or normal diets in herbivores), the dietary water requirement is higher to accommodate gastrointestinal (GI) passage and digestion.

Age-Related Changes

Stage of life, environment, and disease all may change the resting energy expenditure and water requirement. Immature animals are smaller than adults of the same species and, thus, have larger relative metabolic body sizes and requirements. In addition, they are in their rapid growth phase, which also increases their requirements. Likewise, many physiologic systems may not function as well in neonates, thereby increasing water loss through inefficient renal concentration of urine, colonic resorption of GI water, or thermoregulation and surface evaporation.

Dehydration

Small deficits in body water do not result in clinically detectable dehydration. As the loss of water increases, however, so does the magnitude of the clinical signs. Clinical signs are used to estimate what percentage of body weight may have been lost as water. Signs that are attributed to dehydration (e.g., enophthalmos, decreased skin elasticity) result predominantly from changes in the interstitial tissue consistency. Decreased peripheral vascular blood flow results in sludging and injection of capillaries and increased capillary refill time. Clinical parameters and the approx-

TABLE 22.3	CLINICAL SIGNS USED TO CLASSIFY DEHYDRATION	
Water Loss (% body wt)	**Dehydration Status**	**Signs**
1–4	Very mild	Non detectable
5–6	Mild	Skin doughy, inelastic, slight loss of skin turgor; dry mucous membranes; conjunctiva injected
7–9	Moderate	Definite loss of skin turgor, with slow return; enophthalmos; capillary refill time, 2–3 seconds
10–12	Severe	Pronounced loss of skin turgor, with incomplete return; peripheral vasoconstriction, cold extremities; capillary refill time, >3 seconds
13–15	Very severe	Vascular collapse, renal shutdown, death

imate degrees of dehydration to which they correspond are summarized in *Table 22.3*.

Total body water normally comprises approximately 60% of body weight *(Fig. 22.2)*. Anatomically, this water is divided almost equally between the intracellular fluid (ICF) and the ECF compartments.

Functionally, however, this water may be divided with two-thirds in the ICF and one-third in the ECF *(Fig. 22.3)*. Differences between the anatomic and functional distributions may result from the low rate of solute exchange between connective tissue, transcellular fluid, and bone fluid compartments. In other words, subcompartments of the ECF may function more like the ICF in their exchange of solutes.

Isotonic Dehydration

Isotonic dehydration occurs when proportionately equivalent amounts of water and solute (Na and Cl) have been lost from the body *(Fig. 22.4)*. The plasma concentrations of Na and Cl remain constant, whereas a hemoconcentration with increased PCV and plasma protein concentration may be observed. Clinical signs that are referable to dehydration are present as well. Certain types of diarrhea and renal diseases may result in proportional loss of water and solutes, thereby resulting in isotonic dehydration.

Hypertonic Dehydration

Hypertonic dehydration occurs when proportionately greater amounts of water have been lost from the body compared with solute *(Fig. 22.5)*. The plasma concentrations of Na and Cl increase as solute-free water is lost from the body. Clinical signs of dehydration and degrees of hemoconcentration may be indistinguishable from those observed with equivalent water losses because of isotonic dehydration. Diabetes insipidus is the classic example of a disease that causes hypertonic dehydration and

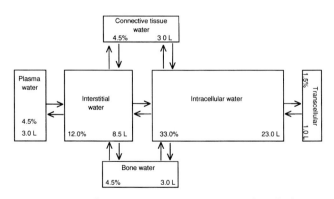

Figure 22.2 Body water compartments in a normal, 70-kg human shown as a percentage of body weight and in liters. (Adapted from Hays RM. Dynamics of body water and electrolytes: In: Maxwell MH, Kleeman CR, eds. Clinical disorders of fluid and electrolyte metabolism. 3rd ed. New York: McGraw Hill, 19080:1–36.)

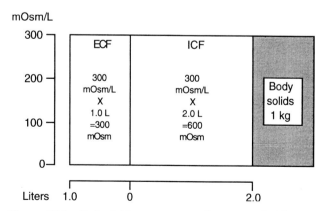

Figure 22.3 Body fluid compartments in a normal, 4-kg cat. (Adapted from Holliday M, Egan TJ. Dehydration, salt depletion, and potassium loss: theoretical considerations. Pediatr Clin North Am 1959;6:81–98.)

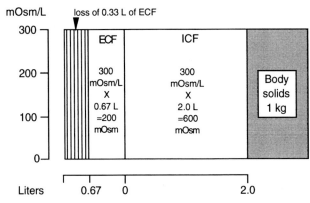

Figure 22.4   Body fluid compartments for isotonic dehydration in a normal, 4-kg cat. (Adapted from Holliday M, Egan TJ. Dehydration, salt depletion, and potassium loss: theoretical considerations. Pediatr Clin North Am 1959;6:81–98.)

increased urinary water loss because of decreased renal concentration of urine. Osmotic diarrhea resulting from oral administration of certain nonabsorbable drugs, or osmotic diuresis resulting from intravenous mannitol administration, are examples of iatrogenic causes of hypertonic dehydration.

Hypotonic Dehydration

Hypotonic dehydration occurs when proportionately greater amounts of solute (Na and Cl) have been lost from the body compared with water *(Fig. 22.6)*. The plasma concentrations of Na and Cl decrease as solute-rich water is lost. Clinical signs of dehydration may be indistinguishable from those observed with other forms of dehydration, but signs also may be referable to electrolyte deficiencies.

In hypotonic dehydration, the predominant loss of electrolytes may result in simultaneous contraction of the ECF volume and expansion of the ICF volume to restore

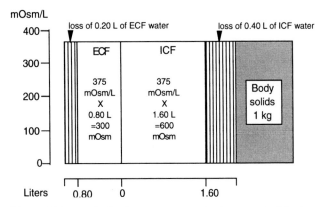

Figure 22.5   Body fluid compartments for hypertonic dehydration in a normal, 4-kg cat. (Adapted from Holliday M, Egan TJ. Dehydration, salt depletion, and potassium loss: theoretical considerations. Pediatr Clin North Am 1959;6:81–98.)

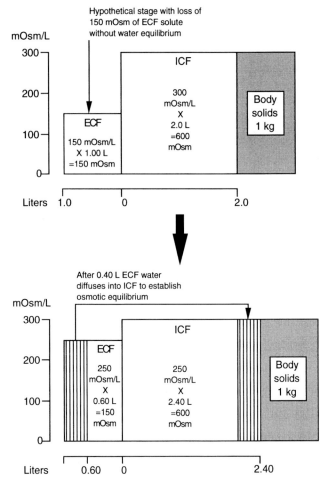

Figure 22.6   Body fluid compartments for hypotonic dehydration in a normal, 4-kg cat. (Adapted from Holliday M, Egan TJ. Dehydration, salt depletion, and potassium loss: theoretical considerations. Pediatr Clin North Am 1959;6:81–98.)

osmotic equilibrium. This is, by far, the most common type of dehydration encountered in clinical practice. Most diseases result predominantly in electrolyte loss, which induces secondary water loss. Examples include secretory diarrhea (e.g., calf scours), vomiting, and "third space" losses (e.g., displaced abomasum). The appellation "third space" is used to describe syndromes in which fluid and solutes accumulate within an anatomically unusual compartment within the body. The fluid and solutes are neither in the ECF nor the ICF; they are functionally "lost" from the body, though still within its physical confines.

Species that produce hypertonic sweat (e.g., horses) develop hypotonic dehydration with heat stress. Species that produce hypotonic sweat (e.g., cows) or little sweat but much evaporative loss with heat (e.g., dogs, cats), on the other hand, develop hypertonic dehydration under similar conditions. Whenever electrolyte secretion drives water loss in a disease condition, hypotonic dehydration may result.

Urinary Concentration

The capacity of the kidneys to concentrate urine in response to dehydration is important. When animals are dehydrated, the renal blood flow, glomerular filtration rate (GFR), and urine production should decrease. This results in the so-called "prerenal azotemia," wherein the intrinsic renal function is normal but the kidneys are inadequately perfused. This condition is identified on the basis of accumulation in the blood of nitrogenous waste products (i.e., urea, creatinine) and minerals (i.e., phosphorus [P], potassium [K]) whose excretion depends on sufficient glomerular filtration. Likewise, antidiuretic hormone (ADH) should be released, thereby promoting urinary concentration as evidenced by an increase in the urine specific gravity. Progressive dehydration may sufficiently impair the renal blood flow to cause ischemic acute renal failure, and the quantity of urine produced by dehydrated patients should be monitored. Unfortunately, in hypotonic dehydration, conflicting signals may reach the hypothalamus and posterior pituitary, where ADH secretion is controlled. Hypovolemia resulting from dehydration may stimulate ADH release, but hypotonicity may inhibit its release. Species differ in their relative sensitivity to volume versus tonicity signals. More importantly, however, if an animal is sufficiently hypotonically dehydrated, the renal medullary concentration gradient may be inadequate. That is, ADH may be released and induce collecting tubule water channels to open, but the osmotic gradient is insufficient to drive water reclamation from those tubules. This is a serious complication of hypotonic dehydration that may lead to inability of the animal to compensate. Thus, the type of dehydration should be determined to accurately interpret the urine volume in dehydrated animals, because increases in the urine volume may result from rehydration or from loss of ability of the kidneys to concentrate urine.

SODIUM METABOLISM

Physiologic Roles

Sodium is the principal cation in the ECF and a required cofactor for some metabolic reactions, but it serves predominantly as the driver behind most movements of fluid across epithelial surfaces in the body. Primary Na transport may provide the electromotive force for coupled anion movements or the osmotic gradient for water movement between compartments. Many facilitated diffusion processes for simple organic molecules also depend on Na cotransport. The gated inrush of Na across a cell membrane is the basis for the propagation of all action potential changes throughout the body, thereby resulting in neural impulses, muscle contractions, and many

secretory cell events. The Na content in the body is determined by the balance of dietary intake and excretion in the urine, feces, and sweat. Regulation of the Na balance is predominantly a function of renin-angiotensin-aldosterone effects on Na transport across epithelial surfaces in the kidneys, GI tract, and sweat glands.

Hyponatremia

Hyponatremia may be observed under three general conditions of practical importance. The first, which is termed *pseudohyponatremia*, is associated with hyperlipidemia or hyperproteinemia, and it occurs when the serum or plasma sample is diluted with an aqueous solution before analysis of the Na content by any method *(Fig. 22.7)*. The hyponatremia is artifactual; it does not result from physiologic changes in Na metabolism.

True hyponatremia may occur either from dilution by excess water retention or from loss of Na from the body *(Table 22.4)*. Excess water retention and subsequent dilution of the plasma Na concentration may occur in syndromes of inappropriate secretion of ADH, thereby resulting in excess water retention by the kidneys that, in turn, causes a syndrome of hypervolemic hypoosmolal hyponatremia. Dilution of the plasma Na concentration may occur after intravenous administration of osmotic diuretics (e.g., mannitol) that promote intravascular movement of water as a prelude to its excretion by the kidneys (i.e., hypervolemic hyperosmolal hyponatremia). Finally, Na may be lost from the body because of disorders such as secretory diarrhea, hypertonic sweating with heat stroke, or renal tubular disease causing natriuresis.

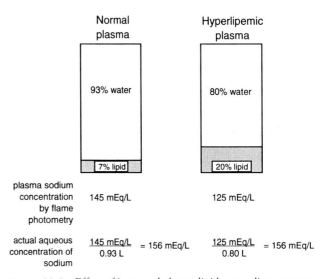

Figure 22.7   Effect of increased plasma lipids on sodium concentration. (Adapted from DiBartola SP. Hyponatremia. Vet Clin North Am Small Anim Pract 1998;28;515–532)

TABLE 22.4 POTENTIAL CAUSES OF DISTURBANCES IN SODIUM AND CHLORIDE METABOLISM

Causes of Hyponatremia/Hypochloremia	Causes of Hypernatremia/Hyperchloremia

Hyperosmolal conditions
  Hyperglycemia
  Mannitol infusion
	Pure water deficit
	  Dietary deficiency
	  Diabetes insipidus
	    Central
	    Nephrogenic
	  Primary hypodipsia
	  Heat stress or fever

Hypoosmolal hypervolemic conditions
  Nephrotic syndrome
  Severe chronic hepatic failure
  Severe chronic renal failure
  Congestive heart failure
	Hypotonic fluid loss
	  GI losses
	    Vomiting
	    Diarrhea
	  Third space syndromes
	    Peritonitis
	    Ascites

Hypoosmolal euvolemic conditions
  Hypotonic fluid infusion
  Antidiuretic drug administration
  Psychogenic polydipsia
  Inappropriate secretion of ADH
	Urinary losses
	    Osmotic diuresis
	      Diabetes mellitus
	      Mannitol
	    Chronic renal failure
	    Nonoliguric acute renal failure
	    Postobstructive nephropathy
	  Cutaneous losses
	    Burns

Hypoosmolal hypovolemic conditions
  Dietary deficiency
  Gastrointestinal losses
    Vomiting
    Diarrhea
  Third space syndromes
    GI obstruction
    Peritonitis
    Uroabdomen
    Ascites
  Urinary losses
    Hypoadrenocorticism
    Nonoliguric acute renal failure
    Diuretic administration
    Fanconi syndrome
  Cutaneous losses
    Burns
	Solute gain
	  Salt poisoning
	  Hypertonic fluid administration
	    Hypertonic NaCl or $NaHCO_3$
	    Sodium phosphate enema
	    Hyperalimentation fluids
	  Hyperadrenocorticism
	  Hyperaldosteronism

All these disorders would cause water loss as well, thereby resulting in hypovolemic hypoosmolal hyponatremia. A classic example of this syndrome occurs with hypoadrenocorticism or Addison disease, which involves deficient mineralocorticoid secretion by the adrenal cortices, excessive Na loss, and excessive K retention by the kidneys. A plasma Na:K ratio of less than 23:1 is considered to be highly suggestive for this disorder, but changes in the Na and K balance also are certainly possible with other diseases (e.g., distal renal tubular acidosis, acute renal failure) that impair the mineralocorticoid-controlled Na and K metabolism. Hyponatremia often occurs with third space syndromes, such as that resulting from a displaced abomasum in ruminants, in part because of electrolyte trapping in the distended, obstructed viscus and complex alterations in the electrolyte and acid-base balance.

Urinary Fractional Excretion of Sodium

It often is not clinically obvious by which route Na has been (or is being) lost from an ill animal. Even when diarrhea or vomiting may be obvious, evaluating the renal handling of Na is still potentially useful to determine whether the kidneys are functioning appropriately. During hyponatremia, the normal kidney response is to completely reduce Na excretion (to conserve as much as possible). Should the handling of Na by the kidneys be abnormal, a larger-than-expected fraction of the filtered Na may be lost in the urine. The urinary concentration of Na can be determined, but alterations in total urine concentration, as affected by ADH, may confound interpretation of the actual urinary Na excretion. For example, renal disease resulting in both increased Na and water loss can result in very low urinary Na concentrations, even though the total amount lost is abnormally high. A 24-hour urine collection to quantitate the total amount of Na lost per day could be performed; however, 24-hour urine collections are cumbersome and may delay both establishing the diagnosis and initiating appropriate treatment. To standardize the quantity of Na in a random sample of urine to the kidneys' ability to concentrate the urine, Na clearance can be expressed relative to something that is excreted in direct proportion to the GFR, such as creatinine clearance. The formula for calculating urinary clearance of a solute is

$$C_x = U_x/P_x \times Volume/Time$$

where Cx is the clearance of "x" (mL/min), U_x is the urinary concentration of "x," and P_x is the plasma concentration of "x." Dividing the clearance of "x" by the clearance of creatinine results in dividing out the volume and time functions, which in turn results in a ratio of urinary and plasma concentrations. This can be rearranged mathematically and multiplied by 100 to derive the urinary fractional excretion of a solute (expressed as a percentage):

$$FE_x = U_x/P_x \times P_{cr}/U_{cr} \times 100$$

For Na, the normal FE_{Na} is less than 1.0%, which corresponds to the observation that more than 99% of filtered Na normally is reabsorbed by the tubules. Renal tubular disease, hypoadrenocorticism, and certain other electrolyte imbalances can impair renal tubular Na reabsorption, thereby resulting in an increased FE_{Na}. This is an extremely useful calculation, both for evaluating disorders of Na metabolism and as a urinary marker for renal tubular disease.

Hypernatremia

Hypernatremia may be caused either by excessive Na retention or by water loss from the body in excess of Na loss (i.e., hypertonic dehydration). Excessive Na retention usually results in secondary water retention, thereby leading to volume expansion, eunatremia, and problems such as hypertension. The principal cause for hypernatremia is hypertonic dehydration; however, salt toxicity resulting from excessive dietary salt intake or iatrogenic administration also may cause hypernatremia. If the urine volume is increased, the serum Na concentration is increased, and signs of dehydration are observed, the hypernatremia may result from Na loading. The urinary FE_{Na} may be useful in determining the role of the kidneys in the disorder. If the urine volume is reduced, the FE_{Na} is decreased or normal, and clinical signs of dehydration are observed, the hypernatremia may result from hypertonic

dehydration caused by extrarenal water loss. If the urine volume is increased, the FE_{Na} is normal, and clinical signs of dehydration are observed, the hypernatremia may result from hypertonic dehydration caused by osmotic diuresis.

CHLORIDE METABOLISM

Physiologic Roles

Chloride, which is the principal anion in the ECF, functions predominantly in transport processes integral to cation and water balance and as a conjugate anion in acid-base metabolism. Because its movement is coupled with the transport of other ions, Cl is central to cerebrospinal fluid production, loop of Henle electrolyte absorption, and GI fluid and electrolyte absorption and secretion. Its metabolism usually is regulated secondary to that of Na, but Cl is a required nutrient, the importance of which often is overlooked.

Hypochloremia and Hyperchloremia

Both decreases and increases in the serum Cl concentration may occur by the same mechanisms as those described for Na, because Cl usually accompanies the cation Na to maintain electrical neutrality (*Table 22.4*). Just as the FE_{Na} is used to evaluate renal handling of Na, so the FE_{Cl} is used to evaluate Cl metabolism. Normal FE_{Cl} values usually are less than 1.0%. Values greater than 1.0%, however, sometimes are seen in large animals that are fed a diet higher in Cl. Results of some studies in human beings have indicated that increases of the FE_{Cl} may be more sensitive in detecting renal tubular disease than increases of Na, but this has not been substantiated in veterinary patients.

Because the facilitated transport of Cl contributes to the movement of water and other electrolytes such as Na in the rumen, distal ileum, proximal colon, and loop of Henle, drugs that block Cl transport can affect the overall fluid and electrolyte balance. Likewise, most enterotoxins induce diarrhea by stimulating enterocyte prostaglandin E_2 synthesis and adenylate cyclase activity, increasing cellular cyclic adenosine monophosphate (cAMP) levels, and switching on active Cl secretion. Loss of other electrolytes and water follows secondarily. Thus, drugs that block facilitated Cl absorption or active Cl secretion play a central role in fluid and electrolyte management during disease.

Because of the central role of Cl in electrolyte metabolism, disorders that primarily affect the Cl balance can induce many secondary imbalances. For example, following dietary Cl deficiency in lactating dairy cows, primary depletion of body Cl leads to secondary losses of Na and K as well as to induction of a metabolic alkalosis. The same train of events probably is central to the third space metabolic disturbances of abomasal displacement, distal ileal obstruction, and urinary bladder rupture.

POTASSIUM METABOLISM

Physiologic Roles

Potassium (K) is the principal cation of the ICF—and of the whole body. Its distribution across cell membranes, between the ICF and ECF compartments, is the primary determinant of resting cell membrane potential. Rapid Na entry into cells characterizes the changes in electrical potential that are necessary to many cell signals, but K distribution determines the ease with which this occurs. In addition, K redistribution repolarizes the membrane after an action potential event. Potassium is specifically central to normal cardiac rhythm and rate, renal Na handling, acid-base metabolism, and many processes in intermediary metabolism.

Hypokalemia

Redistributional Hypokalemia

Certain hormones, including insulin and catecholamines, can induce cellular K uptake, thereby producing a redistributional hypokalemia (*Table 22.5*). Thus, bolus administration of glucose may lead to hyperinsulinemia and hypokalemia. Likewise, excitement and adrenal medullary activation also may result in hypokalemia. The distribution of K between the ICF and ECF compartments is influenced greatly by the acid-base balance. With metabolic alkalosis and deficiency of extracellular protons (H$^+$), intracellular proteins may donate protons from the protonated amine groups for transfer to the ECF (*Fig. 22.8*). To maintain electrical neutrality as protons exit the cells, another cation (K$^+$) must enter those cells; this explains the redistribution hypokalemia that often, but not always, is observed with alkalosis.

Absolute Potassium Depletion

Potassium is actively absorbed throughout much of the small intestine, but if the load of Na reaching the large bowel is increased by some pathologic process, compensatory Na absorption coupled to K secretion in the colon can result in significant fecal loss of K. Thus, depletion of K may occur in association with almost any diarrheic process (*Table 22.5*). Concurrent metabolic acidosis may obscure this depletion of K because of redistributional hyperkalemia (discussed later); however, depletion of K associated with GI losses may be quite severe.

TABLE 22.5 POTENTIAL CAUSES OF DISTURBANCES IN POTASSIUM METABOLISM

Causes of Hypokalemia

Decreased intake
  Anorexia
  Administration of potassium-free fluids
  Dietary deficiency

Translocation between ECF and ICF
  Metabolic or respiratory alkalosis
  Glucose/insulin administration
  Catecholamines

Increased loss
  GI losses
    Vomiting
    Diarrhea
  Third space syndromes
    Gastrointestinal obstruction
    Peritonitis
    Ascites
  Urinary losses
    Hyperadrenocorticism
    Nonoliguric acute renal failure
    Postobstructive diuresis
    Chronic renal failure in cats
    Potassium-losing diuretics
    Fanconi syndrome
    Renal tubular acidosis
  Cutaneous losses
    Burns

Causes of Hyperkalemia

Pseudohyperkalemia
  In vitro translocation to plasma
    Thrombocytosis
    Leukemia
    Hemolysis (equids, bovids)
    Akita anomaly

Increased intake
  Excessive infusion of potassium-containing fluids

Translocation between ICF and ECF
  Metabolic or respiratory acidosis
  Hyperkalemic periodic paralysis
  Ischemia/reperfusion injury

Decreased urinary excretion
  Hypoadrenocorticism
  Anuric or oliguric renal failure
  Urinary tract obstruction
  Ruptured urinary bladder
  Potassium-sparing diuretics
  Nonsteroidal anti-inflammatory drugs
  Angiotensin-converting enzyme inhibitors

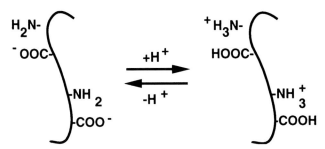

Figure 22.8 Buffering of proton imbalances by intracellular proteins results in net charge alterations that affect the distribution of potassium between fluid compartments.

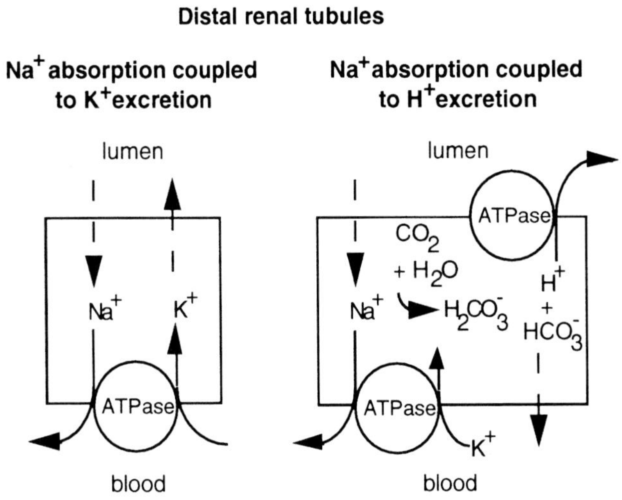

In the kidneys, 80% or more of the filtered K is reabsorbed by the time the modified glomerular filtrate reaches the distal nephron. There, continued K absorption or secretion by distal tubular epithelium depends on numerous other factors. Increased tubular fluid flow increases the gradient for K secretion, thereby increasing its urinary loss. Because distal Na reabsorption is coupled to K secretion, increased Na presentation to the distal tubule also can increase the urinary K loss. Nonreabsorbable anions in the distal tubular fluid may increase K excretion as well. That is, anions that were not reabsorbed in the proximal tubules (including sulfates, phosphates, ketoacids, or lactate) and that are impermeant in the distal tubules remain in the tubular lumina, increase both tubular flow rate and luminal negativity, and, thereby, cause decreased K absorption and increased K secretion. The urinary FE_K normally is less than 20% in small animals but may be as high as 100% in large animals, because their herbivorous diet contains much more K than is required and, subsequently, they excrete more K in their urine and feces.

Acid-base metabolism influences handling of K by the distal tubule as well *(Fig. 22.9)*. As described, intracellular proton and K concentrations have a reciprocal relationship throughout the body. With metabolic alkalosis and fewer protons in the distal tubular cells, more K can be secreted in exchange for Na. Thus, what may have originated as a redistributive change in K balance between the ICF and ECF compartments may develop, with time or severity of the disturbance, into a true hypokalemia.

Mineralocorticoid activity also plays a major role in regulating the handling of K by the kidneys. Aldosterone secretion may occur in response to hypovolemia or Na depletion, as mediated by renal renin release and systemic angiotensin activation. Alternatively, decreased blood pH (i.e., increased proton concentrations) also may directly stimulate aldosterone release by the adrenal cortex. Increased mineralocorticoid levels are necessary to promote distal renal tubular Na reabsorption to restore Na balance

Distal renal tubules

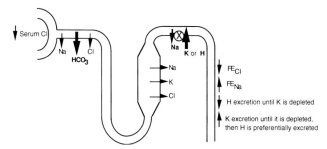

Figure 22.9 Conceptual cell models for distal renal tubular absorption of sodium coupled to cation secretion. The relative intracellular abundance of potassium and hydrogen ions determines which mechanism predominates. (Adapted from Fettman MJ. Feline kaliopenic polymyopathy/nephropathy syndrome. Vet Clin North Am Small Anim Pract 1989;19:415–432.)

or to promote distal renal tubular proton secretion to restore acid-base balance. Mineralocorticoid release initiated during eukalemic conditions, however, may result in enhanced renal excretion of K, depletion of K, and hypokalemia.

Third Space Syndromes

Electrolyte imbalance may result in paradoxic changes in renal tubular electrolyte handling *(Fig. 22.10)*. The classic model for this is the displaced abomasum, but any syndrome resulting in primary Cl depletion can set the wheels in motion. With a displaced abomasum, particularly one that has undergone torsion or volvulus, secretion

Figure 22.10 The principle sites of electrolyte flux along the nephron that are influenced by Cl depletion. In the proximal nephron, bicarbonate (HCO_3) is absorbed, thereby propagating the alkalosis. In the distal nephron, K is preferentially excreted until severe K depletion occurs; proton (H^+) excretion then increases, resulting in paradoxic aciduria.

of HCl acid continues into the lumen, but duodenal outflow and intestinal reabsorption are blocked. This leads to an effective loss of both acid (i.e., protons) and Cl from the body into what is termed a third space (i.e., neither the ICF nor the ECF, though the fluid and solutes remain within the physical confines of the body). The loss of protons leaves behind much bicarbonate that normally would be used for acid neutralization in the intestine, thereby resulting in metabolic alkalosis, which is characterized by hyperbicarbonatemia and an increase in the blood pH. The loss of Cl ions creates a hypochloremia. When blood is filtered through the glomerulus, the filtrate that is produced is high in bicarbonate and low in Cl. Proximal tubules normally reabsorb Na coupled to HCO_3, as facilitated through the action of carbonic anhydrase. A certain amount of proximal tubular Na absorption, however, normally is coupled to Cl once most of the HCO_3 has been reabsorbed. Under the conditions of a hypochloremic metabolic alkalosis, more HCO_3 and less Cl are available for coupled Na absorption, so the proximal tubule tends to propagate the alkalosis by absorbing more HCO_3, even in the face of a metabolic alkalosis. As the tubular fluid moves along the nephron, the remaining Na is reabsorbed, mostly coupled to facilitated Cl absorption in the loop of Henle. With hypochloremia, however, not enough Cl is available to complete the usual amount of Na reabsorption, and a larger quantity of Na ions is presented to the distal tubules. Concurrent hypovolemia and decreased renal tubular fluid flow elicit renin-angiotensin-aldosterone secretion, which in turn stimulates distal tubular Na absorption coupled to either K or proton secretion. Because there is an alkalosis, the distal tubular cells tend to couple K rather than proton secretion to Na absorption, thereby compensating for the diminished Na reabsorption in the earlier nephron and alkalinizing the urine. As the syndrome progresses, however, the hypokalemia may become so severe that K no longer is preferentially exchanged for Na in the distal nephron. Instead, protons may be secreted in the face of a metabolic alkalosis, thereby resulting in urinary acidification (i.e., "paradoxic aciduria"). Any cause of significant Cl depletion can result in this syndrome of hypokalemia and paradoxic aciduria. In fact, should the syndrome progress further, the distal nephron may become incapable of adequate Na reabsorption, in which case the FE_{Na} would increase and a hyponatremia would occur—all for lack of adequate Cl.

Feline Kaliopenic Nephropathy-Polymyopathy Syndrome

A disorder peculiar to cats in which chronic depletion of K is paradoxically linked to metabolic acidosis results in the feline kaliopenic nephropathy-polymyopathy syn-

TABLE 22.6 KEY FEATURES OF THE FELINE KALIOPENIC NEPHROPATHY-POLYMYOPATHY SYNDROME

Predisposing factors	Low dietary potassium Dietary acidification Chronic renal failure
Clinical signs	Cervical ventroflexion Generalized muscle weakness Signs of renal failure
Diagnosis	Hypokalemia Hyperkaliuria (increased FE_K) Azotemia Metabolic acidosis (low blood pH and HCO_3, variable pCO_2)
Treatment	Potassium repletion Alkalinizing therapy Dietary change

drome *(Table 22.6)*. Hypokalemia traditionally has been associated with alkalosis, and hyperkalemia with acidosis, because of translocation between compartments and alterations in urinary excretion as described earlier. The duration of acid-base imbalance and the degree to which cellular buffering participates in its defense are important in determining the net, long-term effect on K metabolism. Chronic depletion of K may result in secondary hypoadrenocorticism (i.e., hypoaldosteronism), which in turn leads to an acquired distal renal tubular acidosis. Conversely, chronic metabolic acidosis may result in secondary hyperadrenocorticism (i.e., hyperaldosteronism), which in turn leads to an acquired K-losing nephropathy. In addition, cats with chronic renal failure appear to be defective in their renal and GI management of K metabolism.

Clinical Signs of Hypokalemia

Potassium is required for many important physiologic processes, so true hypokalemia can have significant—and potentially life-threatening—results. Hypokalemia can result in cardiac arrhythmias that develop because of hyperpolarization of the cardiocyte membranes. Hypokalemia also causes generalized muscle weakness, including the characteristic cervical ventroflexion as observed in kaliopenic cats. Other effects of hypokalemia may include carbohydrate intolerance, because the pancreatic beta-cell K influx that must precede normal insulin release and the target-cell K influx that must accompany glucose uptake cannot occur. Depletion of K may acutely result in metabolic alkalosis, both through redistributive effects on protons and effects on distal tubular H^+ ion handling.

Hyperkalemia

Pseudohyperkalemia

Potassium normally is found at much higher concentrations inside cells than in the ECF compartment. This concentration difference is maintained by expenditure of energy for the activity of Na/K–adenosine triphosphatase (ATPase), which pumps Na outside the cells and K into the cells. Thus, factors that cause widespread cell membrane disruption can result in the release of K into the ECF and hyperkalemia. Regarding species in which erythrocytes actively accumulate K, hemolysis can result in artifactual increases, or pseudohyperkalemia, because of the release from damaged erythrocytes. Humans, horses, and pigs normally accumulate high intraerythrocytic K levels and display hemolysis-induced pseudohyperkalemia. Cows and sheep exhibit a genetically determined polymorphism, wherein some animals accumulate high erythrocytic K levels and others do not. Cats and dogs typically do not have high erythrocytic K concentrations, but some Akitas appear to have a unique Na/K-ATPase that produces high erythrocytic K concentrations. If serum or plasma from these dogs is not quickly separated from the cells, pseudohyperkalemia may result because of K leakage from the erythrocytes.

Redistributional Hyperkalemia

With metabolic acidosis resulting in a surplus of ECF protons (H^+), these protons can enter the cells, in which they may be buffered by anionic carboxyl sites on intracellular proteins (Fig. 22.8). To maintain electrical neutrality as protons enter the cells, however, another cation (K^+) must leave the cells. This explains the redistribution hyperkalemia that often, but not always, is observed with acidosis (*Table 22.5*).

Equine hyperkalemic periodic paralysis is an inherited syndrome of episodic muscular paralysis associated with hyperkalemia that has been identified in certain quarter horses, Appaloosas, and Paints. It is characterized by intermittent episodes of muscular fasciculations, weakness, myotonia, hindquarter paresis, and involuntary recumbency. In addition, it is accompanied by moderate to marked hyperkalemia ($\leq$12 mEq/L), and it appears to relate to a defect in resting membrane electrical potential, Na gating, and K distribution between the ICF and ECF.

Absolute Potassium Excess

As described earlier, acid-base metabolism influences K handling by the renal distal tubules (Fig. 22.9). Because of the reciprocal relationship between intracellular proton and K concentrations throughout the body, when metabolic acidosis is present, relatively more protons are present in the distal tubular cells, which effectively compete against K for secretion, coupled to Na absorption (Fig. 22.9). Thus, what may have originated as a redistributive change in the K balance between the ICF and ECF compartments, may develop, with time or severity of the disturbance, into a true hyperkalemia. In addition to the stimulation of mineralocorticoid secretion by angiotensin or by decreased blood pH, hyperkalemia also may elicit aldosterone release. The distal tubular cell response to mineralocorticoids is biphasic; that is, there is an immediate increase in passive K leakage back into the tubular lumina, followed by induction over several days of increased Na/K-ATPase activity and enhanced K secretion. Mineralocorticoids thus promote distal renal tubular K secretion and increased urinary FE_K to restore the K balance. Any condition that restricts urine production may cause hyperkalemia, including terminal chronic renal failure or severe acute renal failure.

In patients with a ruptured urinary bladder, the urine that is produced by normal renal processes leaks through the rupture and into the abdominal cavity, thereby creating a third space accumulation of fluid and electrolytes *(Fig. 22.11)*. Unlike the third space syndrome caused by a displaced abomasum, however, acid is not lost from the body. Urine has low concentrations of Na and Cl and high concentrations of K and nitrogenous waste products (e.g., urea, creatinine). The peritoneal surface acts like a dialysis machine, thereby allowing equilibration of solute concentrations between the urine and blood. Thus, Na and Cl diffuse from the blood into the abdomen, whereas K and nitrogenous waste products diffuse from the urine in the abdominal cavity into the blood, thereby resulting in

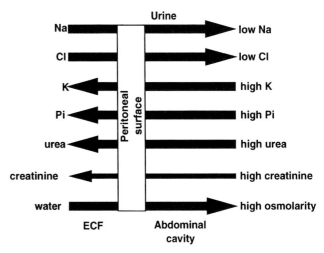

Figure 22.11   Movement of fluid and urinary components in the pathogenesis of ruptured bladder syndrome. (Adapted from Sockett DC, Knight AP, Fettman MJ, Kiehl AR, Smith JA. Metabolic alterations following induced urinary bladder rupture in steers. Cornell Vet 1986;76:198–212.)

hypochloremia, hyponatremia, and hyperkalemia. In animals that excrete alkaline urine (i.e., herbivores), equilibration of buffers tends to produce a metabolic alkalosis. In animals that excrete acid urine (i.e., carnivores), buffer equilibration tends to produce a metabolic acidosis.

Clinical Signs of Hyperkalemia

Hyperkalemia can result in disturbances of electrical conduction because of hypopolarization of the cell membrane. For example, hyperkalemia causes hypopolarization and decreases the threshold for elicitation of an action potential in cardiocytes, thereby increasing their excitability. The amplitude of the resting membrane potential, however, also determines the force of contraction once an action potential is elicited, and the ease of repolarization once it is terminated, so that whereas hypokalemia is associated with spastic contraction, hyperkalemia causes cardiac flaccidity and dilatation. Acutely, Excess K may result in metabolic acidosis, both through redistributive effects on protons and effects on distal tubular H⁺ ion handling.

PHOSPHORUS METABOLISM

Physiologic Roles

Phosphorus is found principally in the ICF compartment, as a component of hydroxyapatite in bone, in high-energy phosphoryl units of many metabolic intermediates, and as an integral part of structural phosphoproteins and phospholipids. Inorganic P occurs as one of three phosphate anions: PO_4^{3-}, HPO_4^{2-}, and $H_2PO_4^-$. Thus, like HCO_3^-, inorganic phosphates play a role in acid-base metabolism through varying degrees of protonation.

Hormonal Control and Other Metabolic Factors

Phosphorus metabolism is regulated, to a very large extent, through its interactions with calcium (Ca) and by the actions of parathormone (PTH), calcitonin, and calcitriol (1,25-[OH]₂-vitamin D) *(Fig. 22.12)*. The plasma concentrations of ionic Ca and inorganic phosphate tend to be related reciprocally. In fact, their solubility is defined by a pH-dependent solubility product constant:

$$[Ca^{2+}][P_i]/[H^+] = K$$

Alkaline pH or large increases in one or both of these ions will promote precipitation of Ca phosphate salts. An increase in the plasma P concentration can result in a reciprocal decrease in the plasma Ca concentration, which in turn leads to release of PTH from the parathyroid glands.

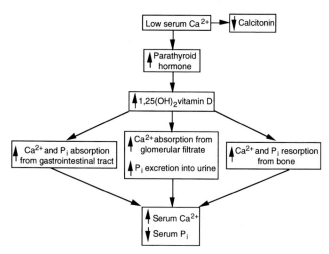

Figure 22.12 Hormonal control of calcium and phosphorus metabolism.

Parathormone stimulates bone demineralization to increase circulating Ca levels. It also increases adenylate cyclase activity in the thick ascending limb of the loop of Henle, and subsequent increases in cAMP promote active Ca reabsorption, which is facilitated by the electrogenic Cl gradient in this segment. PTH also stimulates renal 1α-hydroxylation of vitamin D to produce the most active form (i.e., calcitriol). Vitamin D then promotes both intestinal absorption and distal renal tubular reabsorption of Ca by stimulating the synthesis of a Ca-binding protein that is central to epithelial cell uptake of Ca in these organs. Because P is only reabsorbed and is not secreted by the kidneys, PTH also promotes increased urinary excretion of P by inhibiting its reabsorption in the renal proximal tubules. Urinary fractional excretion of inorganic P usually is less than 20%, but this may increase substantially under the influence of PTH. The mechanism by which PTH inhibits P reabsorption while simultaneously promoting net renal Ca absorption is circuitous. PTH inhibits proximal renal tubular coupled Na and Pi absorption. Parathormone also inhibits proton secretion and carbonic anhydrase activity in the proximal tubules, thereby blocking bicarbonate generation and Na reabsorption. Under normal circumstances, Na and HCO_3 absorption in the early proximal tubules is accompanied by water absorption and an increase in the relative concentrations of solutes remaining in the tubular lumina. In turn, this facilitates the coupled absorption of various solutes (e.g., glucose, amino acids, Ca, Cl, inorganic P) with Na. Thus, by impairing the development of this concentration gradient, the absorption of P is further decreased. Unfortunately, the proximal tubular absorption of Ca also is impaired, but this is more than compensated for by the stimulation of Ca transport in the thick ascending limb of the loop of Henle and by vitamin D–mediated increases in Ca-binding protein as well as distal nephron Ca uptake.

Hypophosphatemia

Hypophosphatemia may result from increased cellular uptake of P, such as when metabolism is accelerated and more high-energy phosphorylated intermediates are formed. Hypophosphatemia, therefore, can result in an insulin-resistant form of carbohydrate intolerance if inadequate P is available with which to make phosphorylated intermediates of glucose metabolism. Likewise, intravenous glucose may be used in the emergency treatment of hyperphosphatemia by promoting its cellular uptake. Acid-base imbalances can affect the distribution of P as well. Alkalosis buffers the acid that is produced during metabolism, thereby removing product feedback inhibition by protons on intermediary metabolism. In turn, this enables more rapid generation of phosphorylated intermediates and draws more P into the cells. Changes in blood pH caused by respiratory alkalosis appear to be associated with lower serum P concentrations than are equivalent degrees of metabolic alkalosis. Metabolic acidosis may be associated with hypophosphatemia because of enhanced urinary excretion of phosphates as the "titratable acidity" necessary for renal elimination of excess acid. Hypophosphatemia often is observed in patients with diabetic ketoacidosis because of increased urinary P loss. This may result both from the acidosis and from the osmotic diuresis induced by glucosuria.

Abnormalities in renal tubular phosphate reabsorption from the glomerular filtrate may result in P depletion and hypophosphatemia. Examples include hyperparathyroidism and renal tubular transport disorders (e.g., Fanconi syndrome, aminoglycoside nephrotoxicosis). In addition to dietary deficiency of P, abnormalities in GI function (e.g., vomiting, diarrhea, intestinal malabsorption syndromes) may inhibit the absorption of P. Excessive administration of phosphate-binding resins during treatment for chronic renal failure, or of antacids with phosphate-binding capacity, also may result in P depletion and hypophosphatemia.

Hyperphosphatemia

Hyperphosphatemia may result from redistribution between the ICF and ECF compartments. Cellular damage resulting in release of intracellular phosphates from high-energy phosphorylated intermediates of metabolism can cause hyperphosphatemia. Acute acidosis has the opposite effect of alkalosis as described earlier, inhibiting metabolic pathways through accumulation of acid end products and, thereby, blocking phosphorylation of metabolic intermediates and decreasing cellular uptake of P. Metabolic acidosis of greater intensity or duration, however, may enhance urinary phosphate loss because of increased urinary titratable acidity buffering of proton excretion

and, thereby, lead to hypophosphatemia. The principal treatment of disorders of P metabolism is to correct the underlying disorder and to allow the plasma P concentration to correct itself. If P is administered in fluids, however, the appropriate ratio of HPO_4^{2-} to $H_2PO_4^-$ of $4:1$ should be used to maintain the blood pH near 7.40 and, thus, to avoid adverse redistributional changes because of acid-base imbalance.

Because urinary P excretion depends on glomerular filtration and tubular reabsorption, reductions in renal blood flow and GFR often result in hyperphosphatemia *(Fig. 22.13)*. Likewise, in patients with a ruptured urinary bladder, P excreted in the urine is reabsorbed along its concentration gradient from the abdomen and into the blood to cause hyperphosphatemia. Acute hyperphosphatemia has been observed in cats after administration of hypertonic Na phosphate enemas, and it is further characterized by clinical signs of depression, ataxia, vomiting, and bloody diarrhea as well as by additional laboratory findings of hypocalcemia, hyperglycemia, and metabolic acidosis. Chronic hyperphosphatemia can result from excessive dietary intake of P, which induces a secondary hypocalcemia and inhibits 1α-hydroxylation of 25-hydroxyvitamin D by the kidneys, which in turn stimulates PTH release (Fig. 22.13).

Thus, two forms of secondary hyperparathyroidism are induced by excessive retention of P: renal secondary hyperparathyroidism because of the hyperphosphatemia

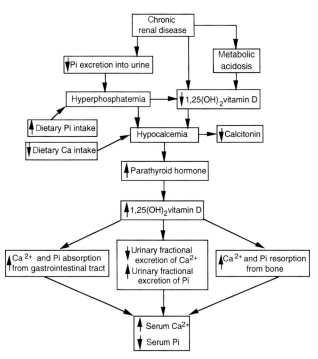

Figure 22.13. Effects of chronic renal disease on calcium and phosphorus metabolism.

of reduced excretion during chronic renal failure, and nutritional secondary hyperparathyroidism because of the hyperphosphatemia of chronic increased intake. In both cases, PTH induces bone demineralization to restore the blood Ca levels, and this may result in osteopenia and metabolic bone disease.

Phosphorus released from bone mineral serves an important role in buffering excess acid in the body. Given the pH-dependent solubility product relationship between Ca and P, it is no surprise that acidification induces bone demineralization, which in turn provides more phosphate buffer to neutralize the acid. The phosphates serve as the major source of titratable acidity in the renal tubules, wherein they act as proton acceptors where the tubular cells actively secrete acid into the urine. On the other hand, phosphoric acid is used by some commercial pet food manufacturers to provide both dietary P and dietary acidification in cat foods designed to prevent feline lower urinary tract disorders.

MAGNESIUM METABOLISM

Physiologic Roles

Magnesium (Mg) serves as a cofactor for many important enzymes of intermediary metabolism but perhaps is best known for its role in facilitating normal Na/K-ATPase activity in cell membranes throughout the body. Magnesium serves some structural role in bone formation, and it also may play a role in regulating PTH release by the parathyroid gland. In addition, it influences cell membrane properties that are vital to nerve conduction, Ca channel activity, and P transport. The handling of Mg by the body is very similar to that of K and disorders that cause hypo- or hyperkalemia generally also may cause hypo- or hypermagnesemia.

Hypomagnesemia

Clinically important hypomagnesemia most often is seen after excessive Mg losses from either the GI tract or kidneys. Malabsorption syndromes or diarrhea account for the former, whereas fluid diuresis, diuretic therapy, or renal disease lead to the latter. Because many fluids that are used to replace volume and electrolyte deficits contain little or no Mg, iatrogenic Mg deficiency is a significant concern, and this may be compounded by diuretic drug use, hyperglycemia, or inhibitory effects of hypercalcemia on renal Mg reabsorption. A number of metabolic and endocrine disorders are associated with hypomagnesemia, including diabetes mellitus (e.g., glucosuria, diuresis), primary hyperparathyroidism (e.g., hypercalcemia, inhibited Mg uptake), hyperaldosteronism (e.g., plasma volume ex-

pansion, diuresis, increased distal nephron Mg leakage), third space syndromes (e.g., reduced cation absorption secondary to Cl deficiency), and hypophosphatemia (e.g., idiopathic renal Mg wasting).

Biochemical manifestations of hypomagnesemia include renal K wasting and secondary hypokalemia, as well as impaired PTH release and calcitriol resistance leading to secondary hypocalcemia. Clinical signs are referable to these secondary electrolyte disorders as well as to the primary neuromuscular and cardiac abnormalities of hypomagnesemia. Normally, Mg stabilizes the nerve axon and competes with Ca entry into the presynaptic nerve terminal. Neuromuscular signs, therefore, include hyperexcitability, muscular tremors, fasciculations, spasms, ataxia, and vertigo. In addition, Mg regulates the release of Ca from the sarcoplasmic reticulum of muscle cells, and it promotes the reuptake of Ca after contraction. Frank tetany may result from severe depletion because of the increased excitability, rapid development of contraction, and decreased ability to recover from a contraction.

Hypomagnesemia may result in cardiac arrhythmias from direct effects on Na/K-ATPase activity or myocytic Ca release and from indirect effects of secondary hypokalemia or hypocalcemia. A deficiency of Mg sensitizes the heart to the toxic effects of many drugs, including isoproterenol and the cardiac glycosides. Results of epidemiologic studies have demonstrated a strong association between Mg depletion and myocardial disease in humans. Depletion of Mg predisposes to vascular spasms, including coronary artery spasm, and it may contribute to acute myocardial infarctions. Recently, hypomagnesemia or decreased plasma ionized Mg concentrations have been observed in a significant number of critical care patients in veterinary practice, and this is now thought to possibly play a role in cardiac dysfunction and refractoriness to inotropic agents in animal as well as human patients.

Hypomagnesemia most often is seen in ruminants under one of two conditions. The first is "milk tetany" in calves fed milk-only diets that are low in Mg. The other is "grass tetany" in adults fed on lush, green pasture, the high K content of which blocks normal Mg absorption from the rumen. In both cases, neuromuscular excitability, clonus, and contractures progressing to tetany may be observed. Hypomagnesemia most often is treated empirically with Mg salt solutions and without calculating the actual quantitative deficit. One must be careful in this regard, because excessive or rapid Mg administration may result in cardiac arrest, in which Mg blocks the Ca uptake needed by cardiocytes for normal contraction.

Hypermagnesemia

Clinically significant hypermagnesemia most often is seen when renal function or urinary elimination of excess Mg is compromised. Both dietary excess and iatrogenic overload usually are dealt with effectively by excretion in the feces and urine. Both acute and chronic renal failure may result in hypermagnesemia if the GFR is sufficiently reduced. Renal tubular reabsorption of Mg from the glomerular filtrate may be increased during conditions of ECF volume contraction, including dehydration, salt depletion, and hypoadrenocorticism. An alternative cause of hypermagnesemia in nonoliguric patients is overadministration of Mg-containing antacids or laxatives, particularly in concert with a reduced GFR.

Clinical signs of hypermagnesemia rarely develop unless the serum Mg concentration exceeds approximately 2 mmol/L. When they do occur, clinical signs are characterized by neuromuscular dysfunction (e.g., paresis, paralysis), cardiovascular depression (e.g., hypotension, arrhythmias, heart block), and GI upset (e.g., nausea, vomiting).

CALCIUM METABOLISM

Physiologic Roles

In addition to its major structural role in the skeletal system, Ca serves multiple roles in the regulation of ion gating across cell membranes, in the activation of cell secretory and contractile functions, and as a cofactor for reactions during intermediary metabolism. The most critical signs of an imbalance in Ca metabolism relate predominantly to its role in synaptic neural signal transmission, skeletal muscle contraction, and cardiovascular muscle function.

Serum Protein and pH Effects

Of the total amount of Ca circulating in the blood, approximately 50% is bound to plasma proteins (principally albumin), less than 10% is in mineral complexes with inorganic phosphates, and the remainder exists in the ionized form. Just as a pH-dependent solubility product relationship exists between Ca and P, so does a pH dependency on the relative ionization of Ca in the blood. During acidosis, larger numbers of protons compete with Ca (and with other cations) for binding to the anionic sites of plasma proteins such as albumin *(Fig. 22.14)*. This drives more protein-bound Ca into solution, thereby increasing the ionized Ca concentrations. Conversely, alkalosis decreases the ionized Ca concentrations.

Another important aspect of this Ca–protein interaction relates to the effects of changes in the albumin concentration on the total Ca concentration in the blood. Most conventional automated chemistry analyzers determine the total Ca concentration in the plasma. Typically, the ionized Ca level is ordered as a special test to be

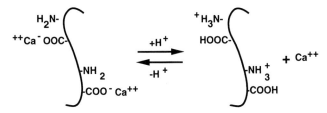

Figure 22.14 Acid-base dependent interactions between plasma albumin and blood ionized calcium distribution.

analyzed by a specific analyzer, apart from the routine chemistry panel. Thus, alterations in the albumin concentration can have significant effects on the apparent Ca concentration as reported in the standard diagnostic panel. Hypoalbuminemia is the most common cause of apparent hypocalcemia. Under such circumstances, the ionized Ca level is maintained in a normal range, because this is the value that actually determines the release of PTH and calcitonin. The fraction of Ca that is bound to albumin, however, is decreased, because the absolute amount of albumin that is available is decreased. To correct our interpretation of the total Ca concentration for the change in albumin, two formulas have been derived:

$$\text{Adjusted [Ca] (mg/dL)} = \text{Total [Ca] (mg/dL)} - \text{[Albumin] (g/dL)} + 3.5$$
$$\text{Adjusted [Ca] (mg/dL)} = \text{Total [Ca] (mg/dL)} - 0.4\text{[Total protein] (g/dL)} + 3.3$$

These formulas have been successfully validated only for use in dogs, and the derivation of similar formulas in other species has, thus far, been unsuccessful. These formulas may be accurate only under conditions of relatively normal acid-base balance; therefore, their results should be interpreted with caution. They do, however, offer a guideline for adjusting the apparent hypocalcemia that often is observed with hypoalbuminemia.

Acid-Base Metabolic Effects

Acid-base imbalances also alter the overall metabolism of Ca in predictable ways. Acidosis increases the ionization of Ca and promotes bone demineralization. Acidosis also promotes the bone effects of PTH on Ca release but inhibit its Ca reabsorptive effects in the kidneys. Likewise, renal 1α-hydroxylation of vitamin D is inhibited by acidosis. Thus, acidosis has a pronounced tendency to cause Ca loss from the body. In humans, this has been proposed as being one mechanism by which a Western-style diet, which is high in protein and other acidifying substances (e.g., carbonated beverages), may predispose to osteoporosis.

In studies regarding the effects of dietary acidification to prevent lower urinary tract disorders in cats, increased

Ca loss, net negative Ca balance, and small changes in bone mineralization have been noted after the addition of ammonium Cl to a typical feline diet. Adult cats appear to adapt fairly well to the higher dietary acid load, however, and soon return to a normal Ca balance without pathologic bone loss. Manipulation of dietary cation–anion balance or dietary acid-base balance also has been used successfully to prevent parturient paresis in lactating dairy cows. Shortly before parturition, a dry cow may be fed a more acidifying diet to promote Ca mobilization from bones, so that once lactation ensues, there is less likelihood of Ca availability being impaired. This is a safe and cost-effective means for preventing milk fever and does not require exact prediction of the due date or administration of vitamin D analogues with potentially adverse side effects.

Hypocalcemia

Hypocalcemia often is accompanied by hyperphosphatemia if there is nutritional or renal secondary hyperparathyroidism. Dietary Ca or vitamin D deficiency can induce a similar condition of secondary hyperparathyroidism without hyperphosphatemia, and primary hypoparathyroidism can cause hypocalcemia but is an unusual disorder. Ethylene glycol (i.e., antifreeze) can induce hypocalcemia secondary to binding and precipitation of ionized Ca by oxalates produced through metabolism of the antifreeze. Massive tissue degeneration, such as might occur during circulatory shock or heat stress, also may cause Ca precipitation. Hypocalcemia sometimes is seen with acute pancreatitis because of the release of lipase into the peritoneal cavity and saponification of hydrolyzed fats with Ca.

Hypercalcitoninism is a rare disorder that may cause hypocalcemia as well. Many years ago, when bulls were first gathered for artificial insemination stud farms, those bulls were mistakenly fed a standard lactating cow concentrate mixture that included Ca levels necessary for milk production. This induced secondary hypercalcitoninism and promoted osteopetrosis, ankylosing spondylosis deformans, soft-tissue mineralization, and renal disease, and it was followed in some by hypocalcemia because of the persistently high calcitonin levels.

Clinical signs of hypocalcemia referable to the musculoskeletal system include tetany in most species, but paresis in ruminants. Apparently, this results from differences in the role of Ca in controlling acetylcholine release and gating neuromuscular junction signal propagation.

It is useful to evaluate the urinary FE_{Ca} in determining the cause of hypocalcemia. If the urinary Ca loss is appropriately reduced, it is indicative of normal functioning of both the kidneys and the hormonal axis that regulates Ca reabsorption. An increased FE_{Ca} during hypocalcemia may be indicative of disturbances in either hormonal control or renal responsiveness to the disorder. As discussed earlier, chronic renal disease may result not only in P retention and reduced vitamin D hydroxylation but also in impaired tubular Ca reabsorption. Treatment of hypocalcemia usually is empiric with a Ca salt (using gluconate, borogluconate, or Cl) solution being administered to effect and without exact quantitation of the deficit. Caution is advisable during intravenous administration of Ca solutions to reverse hypocalcemia, however, because this may rapidly alter the distribution between the ICF and ECF compartments, thereby provoking cardiac arrhythmias, vascular spasm, or skeletal muscle dysfunction. Calcium cannot be administered in bicarbonate-containing solutions, because mixing of the two can result in Ca carbonate precipitation.

Hypercalcemia

The most commonly observed causes for hypercalcemia include pseudohyperparathyroidism (from a paraneoplastic condition), hypoadrenocorticism, chronic renal failure, primary hyperparathyroidism, and vitamin D toxicosis (Table 22.7) Pseudohyperparathyroidism caused by neoplasia, which commonly is referred to as humoral hypercalcemia of malignancy, has been reported with many tumor types but most often is associated with lymphoma, apocrine adenocarcinomas of the anal sac, and sporadic adenocarcinomas of other tissues. Detection of persistent hypercalcemia should lead to a "tumor hunt," because this is the most common cause for this electrolyte abnormality. The exact cause of the hypercalcemia may vary; mechanisms include secretion of PTH or PTH-like peptides by the tumor as well as release of inflammatory cytokines or prostaglandin E_2 by the tumor or inflammatory cells responding to the tumor. These cytokines include colony-stimulating factors, transforming growth factors, tumor necrosis factor, and interleukins. Rarely, a syndrome of pseudohyperparathyroidism is seen in granulomatous inflammatory conditions, that similarly elicit inflammatory cytokine release. Treatment is aimed at removal of the primary tumor or treatment of the inflammatory condition.

Hypoadrenocorticism is the next most frequent cause of hypercalcemia observed clinically and is reported in as much as one-third of dogs with this disorder. The hypercalcemia may result from hypocalciuria caused by concurrent renal failure, but there also may be changes in plasma protein binding of calcium that lead to absolute hypercalcemia even though ionized calcium concentrations may be normal.

Chronic renal failure is an important cause of hypercalcemia, which may be observed in as many as 10% of dogs and cats with renal disease. Hypercalcemia more often is associated with chronic renal failure in horses and may be accompanied by hypophosphatemia, although

TABLE 22.7 POTENTIAL CAUSES OF DISTURBANCES IN CALCIUM METABOLISM

Causes of Hypocalcemia

Distributional changes
  Hypoalbuminemia
  Acid-base imbalances

Decreased intake
  Dietary imbalance (Ca:P)
  Administration of calcium-free fluids

Endocrine disorders
  Nutritional second-degree hyperparathyroidism
  Renal second-degree hyperparathyroidism
  Hypercalcitoninism
  Hypoparathyroidism
  Hypovitaminosis D

Increased loss
  Acute renal failure
  Onset of lactation
  Stress (glucocorticoids)
  Loop diuretics

Toxicity/chelation
  Ethylene glycol
  Acute pancreatitis

Causes of Hypercalcemia

Endocrine disorders
  Primary hyperparathyroidism
  Hypervitaminosis D
    Plants
    Rodenticides
  Hypoadrenocorticism

Malignancy associated
  Pseudohyperparathyroidism (humoral hypercalcemia)
    Lymphoma
    Anal sac apocrine gland adenocarcinoma (ACA)
    Others sporadically
  Local osteolytic
    Myeloma
    Lymphoma
    Osteosarcoma

Iatrogenic
  Excess calcium carbonate
  Excess vitamin D
  Excess vitamin A
  Thiazide diuretics
  Thyrotoxicosis

Miscellaneous
  Acute renal failure
  Chronic renal failure
    Horses
    Some dogs
  Skeletal lesions
    Osteomyelitis
    Hypertrophic osteodystrophy
  Granulomatous inflammation
    Blastomycosis

hyperphosphatemia in other species is the usual result of a reduction in the GFR. The exact mechanism for development of hypercalcemia in renal failure is not known but may relate to altered control of PTH release or increased sensitivity to PTH by renal tubular and intestinal epithelial cells. Regardless, hyperparathyroidism and hypocalciuria often are observed in affected equine patients.

Primary hyperparathyroidism is an uncommon disorder that may be diagnosed by determining serum PTH concentrations and identifying abnormal parathyroid gland morphology. It is treatable by excision of the neoplastic gland, but precipitous postoperative declines in the plasma Ca concentration may occur. Vitamin D toxicosis has been observed in animals fed a diet inadvertently oversupplemented with the vitamin. Consumption of certain wild plants that accumulate vitamin D–like substances also has resulted in intoxication. These include *Cestrum diurnum* and *Solanum malacoxylon*. Dry cows treated with vitamin D analogues shortly before parturition may become intoxicated if the due date is miscalculated and the number of doses needs to be increased. Finally, vitamin D toxicosis may result from consumption of rodenticides that employ calciferol analogues.

Clinical signs of hypercalcemia include anorexia, weakness, vomiting, and polyuria/polydipsia. Polydipsia may result functionally from hypercalcemia-related antagonism of antidiuretic hormone action in the kidneys, or it may result from Ca deposition in the renal tubules (i.e., hypercalcemic nephropathy). Should emergency treatment be indicated because of significant signs that are referable to hypercalcemia (e.g., hypercalcemic nephropathy, muscle clonus, cardiac arrhythmias), the single best therapy is fluid diuresis to encourage excretion of Ca in the urine. Diuretics such as furosemide increase the Ca loss further. Oral Ca binders (to reduce GI absorption), synthetic calcitonin (to promote bone deposition), nonsteroidal anti-inflammatory drugs (to block prostaglandin and cytokine release), bisphosphonates (to block bone demineralization), and glucocorticoids (to reduce GI uptake) are ancillary treatments for chronic hypercalcemia. The greatest short-term danger of hypercalcemia is heart dysfunction, whereas the greatest long-term danger is renal disease because of precipitation of Ca salts in the kidneys.

ACID-BASE METABOLISM

Maintaining pH within certain bounds is vital to the functioning of any biologic system so that chemical reactions may proceed at desirable rates and the balance of all electrolytes can be maintained. Disorders of acid-base metabolism most commonly are manifested by the disruption of normal intermediary metabolism or by clinical signs that are referable to the electrolyte disorders that may accompany acid-base imbalance.

Definitions and Characterizations

Descriptions of acid-base metabolism are founded on the Bronsted-Lowry concept of acids and bases, wherein an acid dissociates in solution to yield a proton or hydrogen ion (H^+) and a conjugate base as follows:

$$HA \rightleftharpoons H^+ + A^-$$

From the rate constants describing this reaction, we can derive a formula that predicts the hydrogen ion concentration, or its logarithmic reciprocal, pH. A decrease in pH is characterized as an acidosis, whereas an increase in pH is characterized as an alkalosis:

$$pH = pK_a + \log [A^-]/[HA]$$

Any acid-conjugate base system may be described by this so-called Henderson-Hasselbach equation. It should be apparent that the conjugate base of an acid is a proton acceptor and, in doing so, neutralizes the proton by recreating the nondissociated acid. Therefore, salts of conjugate bases are used as buffers in chemistry, and they are especially important for maintaining pH in biologic systems.

The pH of blood can be described with any of the dissolved acid-conjugate base pairs in the plasma. Because of its quantitative and qualitative importance in acid-base management as well as the ease with which it can be measured in the laboratory, the carbonic acid–bicarbonate system is routinely used:

$$pH = pK_a + \log [HCO_3^-]/[H_2CO_3]$$

in which HCO_3^- (i.e., bicarbonate) is the conjugate base and H_2CO_3 (i.e., carbonic acid) is the nondissociated acid. By substituting the actual value for pK_a of the carbonic acid system and the concentration of dissolved carbon dioxide (pCO_2) that becomes hydrated to form carbonic acid, the form of this equation that is used routinely to describe acid-base balance is derived:

$$pH = 6.1 + \log [HCO_3^-]/0.03(pCO_2)$$

Metabolic Versus Respiratory Disorders

Changes in pH depend on the ratio of dissolved HCO_3 and CO_2. Because the HCO_3 concentration is determined principally by alterations in metabolic function (i.e., renal, GI, and bone systems), acid-base disorders caused by changes in HCO_3 are termed *metabolic* disorders. Because CO_2 concentration is determined principally by alterations in respiratory function, acid-base disorders caused by changes in CO_2 are termed *respiratory* disorders. Proteins constitute the principal buffer source throughout the body, and their importance in the ICF compartment for assimilating excess protons during an acidosis was described previously. In the blood, hemoglobin accounts for 80% and albumin for 20% of the nonbicarbonate buffering capacity. The bicarbonate–carbonic acid system is particularly important: quantitatively, it is the principal buffer in the ECF compartment; and qualitatively, it provides a means for regulation of acid-base balance by complementary actions of the metabolic (i.e., kidneys) and respiratory (i.e., lungs) systems. The bicarbonate-carbonic acid system is important clinically, because measurement with a blood gas analyzer of blood pH, HCO_3, and pCO_2 is the principal means employed in routine laboratory evaluation of acid-base balance.

Simple, Compensated, and Combined Disorders

The goal of the body's buffer systems is to "neutralize" excess acid or base until those excess ions can be eliminated by the renal or the respiratory system. Under most circumstances, the specific adjustments that follow are alterations in the excretion of acid through changes in ventilation (to alter pCO_2) or changes in urinary acidification (to alter HCO_3). All characterizations of acid-base disturbances reflect these elemental processes *(Fig. 22.15)*. Thus, a primary disturbance in respiratory control of the acid-base balance usually results in buffering, followed by metabolic compensation for primary changes in the excretion of CO_2. A primary disturbance in metabolic control of the acid-base balance usually results in buffering, followed by respiratory compensation for primary changes

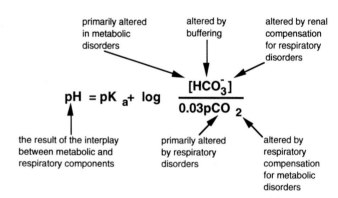

Figure 22.15   Modified Henderson-Hasselbach equation, portraying the effects of the primary acid-base disturbances and the defense mechanisms on pH. (Adapted from Kaehny WD. Pathogenesis and management of metabolic acidosis and alkalosis. In: Schrier RW, ed. Renal and electrolyte disorders. Boston: Little Brown, 1976:79–120)

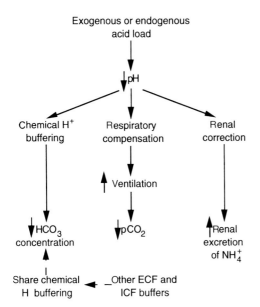

Figure 22.16 Defense mechanisms in compensated metabolic acidosis. (Adapted from Kaehny WD. Pathogenesis and management of metabolic acidosis and alkalosis. In: Schrier RW, ed. Renal and electrolyte disorders. Boston: Little Brown, 1976: 79–120).

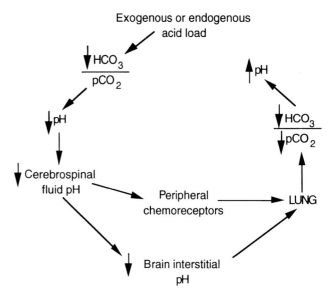

Figure 22.17 Respiratory compensation in metabolic acidosis. (Adapted from Kaehny WD. Pathogenesis and management of metabolic acidosis and alkalosis. In: Schrier RW, ed. Renal and electrolyte disorders. Boston: Little Brown, 1976:79–120).

in the excretion of HCO_3. Respiratory adaptations usually are relatively rapid, whereas metabolic changes require additional time so that transport processes in the kidneys (and GI tract) as well as bone buffer mobilization may be induced.

"Simple" acid-base disorders occur when there are changes in the primary system with little or no compensatory responses by the complementary system. "Compensated" acid-base disorders are characterized by changes in the primary system along with counteracting changes in the opposing system *(Fig. 22.16)*. "Combined" acid-base disorders are distinguished by concurrent pathologic changes in the same direction by both systems. "Complex" acid-base imbalances are more difficult to interpret but may include primary, opposing disorders in the respiratory and metabolic systems or within the metabolic system alone. They may appear to be neutralizing each other's effects on pH, but this effect on pH is purely coincidental to concurrent disorders that are not deliberately compensatory.

To characterize an acid base disorder fully, one must consider three variables: blood pH, HCO_3, and pCO_2. A decrease in pH is defined as an acidosis, whereas an increase is defined as an alkalosis. The next step is to look at the other two variables to determine which may account for the change in pH. If HCO_3 (an alkaline buffer) is decreased and the pCO_2 is normal, the disturbance is labeled as a metabolic acidosis, because HCO_3 is controlled principally by metabolic events and kidney function. If HCO_3 is unchanged and the pCO_2 (a "respiratory

acid" when hydrated to H_2CO_3 or carbonic acid) is increased, the disturbance is labeled as a respiratory acidosis, because pCO_2 is controlled principally through gas exchange by the lungs. Combined acidoses also may occur wherein both HCO_3 is decreased and pCO_2 is increased because of concurrent disorders of the metabolic and respiratory systems.

If HCO_3 is increased and the pCO_2 is normal, the disturbance is labeled as a metabolic alkalosis. If HCO_3 is unchanged and the pCO_2 is decreased, the disturbance is labeled as a respiratory alkalosis, because H_2CO_3 concentrations would be lower. Combined alkaloses also may occur wherein both HCO_3 is increased and pCO_2 is decreased because of concurrent disorders of the metabolic and respiratory systems. Most commonly, a primary event is accompanied by a compensatory event. For instance, if there is a metabolic acidosis, as defined by a decrease in blood pH and HCO_3 concentration, one also might expect to observe a decrease in the pCO_2 because of respiratory compensation *(Fig. 22.17)*. One could call this a metabolic acidosis with respiratory compensation or a compensated metabolic acidosis.

The blood pH need not return to normal. The term *compensation* indicates the response by the body in attempting to correct the pH, but the pH rarely returns to normal because of compensation. Thus, one usually may identify the primary cause and the secondary effect *(Table 22.8)*. If there is a respiratory acidosis as defined by a decrease in blood pH and an increase in the pCO_2, one also might observe an increase in the HCO_3 concentration

TABLE 22.8 ALTERATIONS IN HENDERSON-HASSELBACH PARAMETERS WITH VARIOUS ACID-BASE CONDITIONS

Condition	HCO₃ (mmol/L)	pCO₂ (mmHg)	H₂CO₃ (mmol/L)	Ratio	pH (units)
Normal	24	40	1.2	20:1	7.40
Metabolic acidosis	10	40	1.2	8.3:1	7.02
Respiratory acidosis	24	60	1.8	13.3:1	7.22
Metabolic alkalosis	36	40	1.2	30:1	7.57
Respiratory alkalosis Compensated	24	20	0.6	40:1	7.70
Metabolic acidosis	10	20	0.6	16.7:1	7.32
Combined acidosis	14	47	1.4	10:1	7.10

because of metabolic compensation. This is a respiratory acidosis with metabolic compensation or a compensated respiratory acidosis. If there is a metabolic alkalosis as defined by an increase in blood pH and HCO₃ concentration, one also might observe an increase in the pCO₂ because of respiratory compensation. This is a metabolic alkalosis with respiratory compensation or a compensated metabolic alkalosis. If there is a respiratory alkalosis as defined by an increase in blood pH and a decrease in the pCO₂, one also might observe a decrease in HCO₃ concentration because of metabolic compensation. This is a respiratory alkalosis with metabolic compensation or a compensated respiratory alkalosis. To assist in the differentiation of compensated from combined acid-base disorders, the magnitude of the expected compensatory responses for typical primary acid-base disorders has been estimated (Table 22.9).

Specimen Requirements

The ideal sample for blood gas analysis is whole arterial blood that is collected anaerobically into a gas-

TABLE 22.9 EXPECTED METABOLIC AND RESPIRATORY COMPENSATIONS TO PRIMARY ACID-BASE DISORDERS IN DOGS

Disorder	Primary Change	Compensatory Response
Metabolic acidosis	Decreased HCO₃	0.7 mm Hg decrement in pCO₂ for each 1.0 mEq/L decrement in [HCO₃]
Metabolic alkalosis	Increased HCO₃	0.7 mm Hg increment in pCO₂ for each 1.0 mEq/L increment in [HCO₃]
Acute respiratory acidosis	Increased pCO₂	1.5 mEq/L increment in [HCO₃] for each 10 mm Hg increment in pCO₂
Chronic respiratory acidosis	Increased pCO₂	3.5 mEq/L increment in [HCO₃] for each 10 mm Hg increment in pCO₂
Acute respiratory alkalosis	Decreased pCO₂	2.5 mEq/L decrement in [HCO₃] for each 10 mm Hg decrement in pCO₂
Chronic respiratory alkalosis	Decreased pCO₂	5.5 mEq/L decrement in [HCO₃] for each 10 mm Hg decrement in pCO₂

Adapted from deMorais HAS, DiBartola SP. Ventilatory and metabolic compensation in dogs with acid-base disturbances. J Vet Emerg Crit Care 1991;1:39–49.

impermeable container, treated with heparin as an anti-coagulant, chilled in ice water during transport for longer than 5 minutes, and analyzed as quickly as possible after collection. This is not always possible. Values for blood gas concentrations and acid-base parameters differ significantly between arterial and venous blood. Arterial blood values reflect systemic changes in acid-base balance and pulmonary gas exchange capability. Venous blood samples reflect modifications of systemic values by the tissues from which the sample has been collected. Blood pH and oxygen tension typically are higher in arterial samples, whereas pCO_2 and HCO_3 concentration typically are greater in venous samples. Variation in regional blood flow and tissue metabolism between individuals affected by different health disorders produces greater variability in venous blood gas and acid-base parameters. Thus, reference ranges for arterial blood gas parameters should be applied to venous blood samples only with the greatest caution. Likewise, representative reference ranges for venous blood gas parameters are difficult to generate.

Capillary blood samples may be used instead of arterial blood samples for blood gas analysis when circulation is not impaired. Furthermore, "arterialized" capillary blood specimens, which are obtained by warming the site before sampling, offer a closer approximation of arterial blood gas values. Comparisons of blood collected simultaneously from the carotid artery and the posterior medial margin of the ear of dogs revealed no significant differences in pH, pO_2, pCO_2, or HCO_3. In cats, blood samples collected simultaneously from the femoral artery and cut claw and warmed to 42–45°C, were not significantly different in pO_2 or pCO_2, but the pH was higher in the claw sample.

A complete blood gas panel may be inaccessible, but most automated chemistry analyzer diagnostic panels include total CO_2. The total CO_2 is derived from the total of HCO_3 and dissolved CO_2 in the blood, and it usually is approximately 1 to 2 mmol/L greater than the HCO_3 value as derived from a blood gas analyzer. From this, changes in the metabolic side of the acid-base balance can be identified. Because total CO_2 usually is determined in serum that derives from blood that is not been collected anaerobically and is allowed to clot at room temperature for a variable period of time, this value may not match the actual total CO_2 as would be determined with whole blood that had been appropriately collected and handled before analysis. Exposure to ambient air after incomplete filling of evacuated blood collection tubes or in uncapped specimen containers facilitates diffusion of gaseous CO_2 from the serum, whereas exposure to room temperatures facilitates continued metabolism and acid production by the blood cells. Thus, serum total CO_2 concentrations should be interpreted with caution.

Base Excess and Base Deficit

"Base excess" and "base deficit" are calculated parameters from a blood gas analysis that may be used, in addition to the HCO_3 concentration, to assess the metabolic component of the acid-base balance. These parameters derive from an equation that accounts for the contribution of hemoglobin and HCO_3 to the buffering capacity of whole blood. In healthy humans, the value for these parameters is approximately 0 ± 2.5 mEq/L. Positive values greater than this reflect a base excess, which corresponds to a metabolic alkalosis. Negative values less than this reflect a base deficit, which corresponds to a metabolic acidosis. This calculation would appear to improve assessment of the acid-base balance, but its derivation depends on the specific character of the usual acid-base "nomogram" in each species. This nomogram describes the relationship between pH, pCO_2, and HCO_3 in whole blood, which depends not only on the hemoglobin concentration but also on the species-specific pKa for hemoglobin. Other plasma proteins also might affect this relationship and, likewise, would depend on species-specific differences in their pKa. The acid-base nomogram for dogs is approximately the same as that for humans. For other species, however, either comparisons have not been made or significant differences from humans have been identified. Because the human nomogram is incorporated into the software for most commercial blood gas analyzers, base excess or base deficit values in other species should be interpreted with caution.

Anion Gap

Definition and Calculation

Calculating and interpreting the "anion gap" is useful when analyzing acid-base disorders. The anion gap is calculated on the basis of the assumption that the body is in electrical neutrality. That is, the total number of anions equals the total number of cations, so that the charges balance. Sodium and K are commonly measured cations, and Cl and HCO_3 (commonly reported in serum chemistry panels as total CO_2) are commonly measured anions. These cations and anions are used in an equation to calculate the anion gap. The remaining cations and anions are referred to as "unmeasured," and the objective of this calculation is to estimate changes in the concentrations of these unmeasured ions without actually analyzing them:

$$(Na + K) - (Cl + HCO_3) = \text{Anion gap}$$

Unmeasured anions include inorganic ions such as sulfate (SO_4^{2-}) and phosphates (HPO_4^{2-} and PO_4^{3-}) and organic ions such as lactate, pyruvate, ketoacids, metabolites of some toxicants, and plasma proteins such as albumin with deprotonated carboxyl groups (COO⁻). Unmeasured cations include inorganic ions such as Ca^{2+} and Mg^{2+} and organic ions like plasma proteins such as immunoglobulin A with protonated amine groups (NH_3^+). There are normally, a few more unmeasured anions than unmeasured cations in the blood. If some typical values for a healthy dog are inserted into the equation, the basis for a reference range for anion gap becomes apparent. For instance, for Na of 152 mEq/L, K of 5.0 mEq/L, Cl of 117 mEq/L, and HCO_3 of 21 mEq/L, the anion gap is 20 mEq/L. Another way of looking at this value is that the number of unmeasured anions in the blood exceeds the number of unmeasured cations by 20 mEq/L. At the Colorado State University Veterinary Teaching Hospital, reference intervals are 8 to 25 mEq/L for dogs and 10 to 27 mEq/L for cats.

Acid-Base Disorders

If an animal has a metabolic acidosis resulting in a decreased HCO_3 concentration, the anion gap may either increase or remain unchanged, depending on the accompanying changes that occur in the concentrations of other ions. For instance, if the HCO_3 concentration is decreased along with an increased concentration of organic anions, the anion gap will be higher than normal, resulting in an "increased anion gap acidosis". Unmeasured anions that may accumulate under such circumstances include phosphates or sulfates in uremia, lactate in hypovolemia, or ketoacid anions in diabetes mellitus. Phosphate or sulfate anions arise from phosphoric or sulfuric acid derived from the catabolism of phospholipids or sulfur-containing amino acids. Lactate anions arise from lactic acid derived from anaerobic glycolysis subsequent to reduced tissue oxygenation. Ketoacid anions (e.g., acetoacetate, β-hydroxybutyrate) arise subsequent to disorders of carbohydrate and lipid metabolism in diabetes mellitus. The protons of these acids are neutralized by HCO_3, and their conjugate, or unmeasured, anions replace HCO_3 ions to maintain electrical neutrality. As another example, the anion gap is increased significantly with ethylene glycol (i.e., antifreeze) toxicosis because of the accumulation of glycolic and oxalic acid byproducts of ethylene glycol metabolism. In experimental ethylene glycol intoxication in dogs, the anion gap increased significantly within 1 hour of antifreeze consumption, which was well before the onset of recognizable acute renal failure as indicated by increases in blood urea nitrogen (BUN) or serum creatinine (Fig. 22.18).

If, on the other hand, the HCO_3 concentration is decreased because of simple loss by the kidneys, as might occur with a disorder of proximal or distal renal tubular

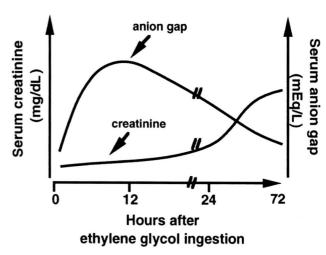

Figure 22.18 Alterations in serum creatinine and anion gap in dogs after experimental intoxication with ethylene glycol. (Adapted from Dial SM, Thrall MA, Hamar DW. Efficacy of 4-methylpyrazole for treatment of ethylene glycol intoxication in dogs. Am J Vet Res 1994;55:1762–1770.)

proton secretion, the number of unmeasured anions remains the same, but the kidney might reabsorb more Cl to maintain electrical neutrality when Na is reabsorbed. In other words, the kidneys can substitute Cl for HCO_3 absorption to maintain normal Na reclamation. The calculated anion gap remains the same, but now there is a hyperchloremia, resulting in a "normal anion gap acidosis". This change is typical of the renal tubular acidosis syndromes observed in humans and other animals.

Calculating the anion gap allows one to make an important distinction regarding the nature of the acidosis. In these cases, the pH, HCO_3, and pCO_2 may be the same, but the cause of the disorder may be characterized as a metabolic abnormality, a reduction in GFR, or a disorder of renal tubular function. Furthermore, serial evaluation of the anion gap in a patient undergoing treatment of renal failure can be indicative of relative control of uremic toxin accumulation. The anion gap also may be useful in discerning coexistent acid-base disorders that obscure alterations in blood pH or HCO_3. One example in early lactation dairy cattle is metabolic alkalosis because of a third space syndrome (associated with a right displacement of the abomasum) and simultaneous metabolic acidosis because of ketosis (associated with energy imbalance). Although blood pH and HCO_3 may be within the reference ranges for healthy individuals, identification of an increased anion gap may be indicative of concurrent metabolic disorders. Unfortunately, because albumin is a major source of "unmeasured anions" in the plasma, changes in hydration, plasma protein content, or degree of protein buffering through deprotonation can alter the calculated anion gap as well. For example, hyperprotein-emia concurrent to a simple metabolic alkalosis can result in an increased anion gap.

Strong Ion Difference

Definition and Calculation

Strong ion difference (SID) is a calculated parameter employed in a unique, quantitative approach to the interpretation of acid-base metabolism. Conceptually, it is based on the physicochemical properties of charged solutes in aqueous solution; practically, it is applied by quantitating the relative contribution of strong and weak ions in determining the proton concentration in the blood. In traditional or "Henderson-Hasselbach" acid-base calculations, pCO_2 and HCO_3 are independent variables that determine the pH. In SID or "Stewart" acid-base calculations (named for its first proponent, Peter A. Stewart), the independent variables include pCO_2, net SID, and total weak acid (A_{tot}) concentrations, and the dependent variables include pH and the concentrations of H^+, OH^-, HCO_3^-, weak acids (HA), conjugate anions of weak acids (A^-), and carbonate (CO_3^{2-}). Strong ions are blood solutes that are completely dissociated in the physiologic pH range, and they include Na, K, Ca, Mg, Cl, lactate, ketoacid anions, and sulfate (SO_4^{2-}). Similar to the anion gap, the SID is derived by the difference in concentration between the strong cations and the strong anions. Unlike the anion gap, Stewart calculations include the determination of A_{tot} (e.g., albumin, inorganic phosphates). To maintain electrical neutrality, changes in the SID and A_{tot} must be counterbalanced by changes in the dissociation of water and the relative concentrations of H^+ and OH^- Thus, alterations in the SID and A_{tot} can be used to interpret the cause of changes in the blood pH. To interpret changes in the SID and A_{tot}, one must calculate the individual differences from normal in their component solute concentrations. To compile the net effects of changes in the SID and A_{tot}, one must further adjust ion differences for the plasma free-water content and for the relative degree of ionization of each species in aqueous solution. The reader is referred to two other sources in the veterinary literature for different versions of these formulas (DiBartola, 2000; Whitehair et al., 1995)

Acid-Base Disorders

The SID quantitative approach to acid-base metabolism has several advantages. Changes in nonrespiratory factors that contribute to acid-base equilibrium are better differentiated than they are by use of the anion gap alone.

Effects of alterations in plasma albumin concentration can be distinguished from changes in other organic acids from which "unmeasured anions" typically are derived, and confounding effects of simultaneous changes in hydration and electrolyte concentrations can be resolved. Mathematically derived indices improve the quantitation of relative degrees of organ dysfunction, which heretofore could be evaluated only qualitatively. Unfortunately, the necessary calculations are complex, require the analysis of additional laboratory parameters, and depend on several assumptions regarding species-specific differences in analyte reference ranges, plasma free-water content, and relative degree of ionization of each ion species in aqueous solution. These assumptions and the arithmetic corrections factors recommended for the SID calculations in different species have not been validated experimentally.

OSMOLALITY

Osmolality is defined as being the concentration or the number of osmotically active particles in an aqueous solution. The osmolality of a solution is numerically equal to the molality of an ideal solution of nondissociable solutes or ions. It is estimated either by the quotient of the freezing-point depression of an aqueous solution below that of water or by the quotient of the vapor-point elevation of an aqueous solution above that of water. Isotonic saline solution (0.9% or 9 g/L NaCl) contains approximately 155 mmol/L each of Na and Cl and, therefore, has an osmolality of approximately 310 mOsm/L, which is roughly equivalent to the osmolality of normal ECF. Disorders of hydration, as described earlier by changes in serum Na and Cl concentration, also can be characterized by concomitant changes in serum osmolality. Hence, isotonic, hypertonic, and hypotonic dehydration alternatively can be called isosmolal, hyperosmolal, and hypoosmolal dehydration, respectively. Disorders of Na and Cl metabolism as described earlier may be characterized more completely by the concomitant determination of serum osmolality. Hence, hyponatremia may accompany hypoosmolal hypovolemia (i.e., hypotonic dehydration), hypoosmolal hypervolemia (i.e., overhydration), or hyperosmolal hypervolemia (after osmotic diuretic administration). Hypernatremia may accompany hyperosmolal hypovolemia after hypotonic fluid loss from the body, as occurs with polyuria.

Osmolal Gap

The osmolal gap is defined as being the difference between the actual measured serum osmolality and a calculated estimate of serum osmolality. The calculated osmolality is determined by accounting for the principal osmotically active solutes that typically are measured in serum, and it may be derived from an equation such as

$$\text{Calculated osmolality (mOsm/L)} = 1.86[\text{Na (mmol/L)}] \\ + [\text{Glucose (mg/dL)}/18] + [\text{BUN (mg/dL)}/2.8] + 9$$

The denominators in the glucose and BUN terms of this equation represent correction factors derived from these solutes' molecular weights (180 and 28 mg/mmol, respectively), which are used to convert their concentrations from mg/dL to mmol/L. Because the calculated osmolality cannot account for all osmotically active solutes in serum, this value usually is less than that of the measured osmolality. The difference between the actual osmolality and that estimated by a formula increases when unmeasured osmotically active solutes increase in concentration. Thus, the osmolal gap may be expected to increase whenever the anion gap is pathologically increased. Relative changes in the osmolal gap can be used to monitor the degree of uremia in patients with chronic renal failure, wherein the excretion of small, unmeasured solutes, including sulfates, phosphates, or other waste products of intermediary metabolism that normally are eliminated in the urine, may be altered. Changes in the osmolal gap also may be used to represent the elimination of ethylene glycol by metabolism and excretion in patients who have consumed antifreeze. Because ethylene glycol is a relatively small-molecular-weight, osmotically active substance, the osmolal gap correlates well with the quantity of ethylene glycol in the serum.

SUGGESTED READINGS

Fluid Balance
Blaxter K. Energy metabolism in animals and man. New York: Cambridge University Press, 1989.
Fettman MJ, Allen TA. Developmental aspects of fluid and electrolyte metabolism and renal function in neonates. Comp Cont Educ Prac Vet 1991;13:392–403.
Hays RM. Dynamics of body water and electrolytes. In: Maxwell MH, Kleeman CR, eds. Clinical disorders of fluid and electrolyte metabolism. 3rd ed. New York: McGraw Hill, 1980:1–36.
Holliday M, Egan TJ. Dehydration, salt depletion, and potassium loss: theoretical considerations. Pediatr Clin North Am 1959;6:81–98.
Kohn CW, DiBartola SP. Composition and distribution of body fluids in dogs and cats. In: DiBartola SP, ed. Fluid therapy in small animal practice. Philadelphia: WB Saunders, 2000:3–25.

Sodium
Crawford MA, Kittleson MD, Fink GD. Hypernatremia and adipsia in a dog. J Am Vet Med Assoc 1984;184:818–821.
DiBartola SP, Johnson SE, Johnson GC, Robertson GL. Hypodipsic hypernatremia in a dog with defective osmoregulation of antidiuretic hormone. J Am Vet Med Assoc 1994;204:922–925.
Dow SW, Fettman MJ, LeCouteur RA, Allen TA. Hypodipsic hypernatremia and associated myopathy in a hydrocephalic cat with transient hypopituitarism. J Am Vet Med Assoc 1987;191:217–221.

Heath SE, Peter AT, Janovitz EB, Selvakumar R, Sandusky GE. Ependymoma of the neurohypophysis and hypernatremia in a horse. J Am Vet Med Assoc 1995;207:738–741.
Lakritz J, Madigan J, Carlson GP. Hypovolemic hyponatremia and signs of neurologic disease associated with diarrhea in a foal. J Am Vet Med Assoc 1992;200:1114–1116.
Tyler RD, Qualls CW, Heald D, Cowell RL, Clinkenbeard KD. Renal concentrating ability in dehydrated hyponatremic dogs. J Am Vet Med Assoc 1987;191:1095–1100.

Chloride
Fettman MJ, Chase LE, Bentinck-Smith J, Coppock CE, Zinn SA. Effects of dietary chloride restriction in lactating dairy cows. J Am Vet Med Assoc 1984;185:167–172.
Fettman MJ, Chase LE, Bentinck-Smith J, Coppock CE, Zinn SA. Nutritional chloride deficiency in early lactation Holstein cows. J Dairy Sci 1984;67:2321–2335.
Hall JA, Fettman MJ, Ingram JT. Sodium chloride depletion in a cat with fistulated meningomyelocele. J Am Vet Med Assoc 1988;192:1445–1448.

Potassium
Degen M. Pseudohyperkalemia in Akitas. J Am Vet Med Assoc 1987;190:541–543.
Dow SW, Fettman MJ, LeCouteur RA, Hamar DW. Potassium depletion in cats. Renal and dietary influences. J Am Vet Med Assoc 1987;191:1569–1575.
Dow SW, LeCouteur RA, Fettman MJ, Spurgeon TL. Potassium depletion in cats. Hypokalemic polymyopathy. J Am Vet Med Assoc 1987;191:1563–1568.
Fettman MJ. Feline kaliopenic polymyopathy/nephropathy syndrome. Vet Clin North Am Small Anim Pract 1989;19:415–432.
Naylor JM, Robinson JA, Bertone J. Familial incidence of hyperkalemic periodic paralysis in quarter horses. J Am Vet Med Assoc 1992;200:340–343.
Spier SJ, Carlson GP, Holliday TA, Cardinet GH, Pickar JG. Hyperkalemic periodic paralysis in horses. J Am Vet Med Assoc 1990;197:1009–1017.

Third Space Syndromes
Garry FB, Hull BL, Rings DM, Hoffsis G. Comparison on naturally occurring proximal duodenal obstruction and abomasal volvulus in dairy cattle. Vet Surg 1988;17:226–233.
Gingerich DA, Murdick PW. Experimentally induced intestinal obstruction in sheep: paradoxical aciduria in metabolic alkalosis. Am J Vet Res 1975;36:663–668.
Gingerich DA, Murdick PW. Paradoxic aciduria in bovine metabolic alkalosis. J Am Vet Med Assoc 1975;166:227–230.
Smith DF. Right-side torsion of the abomasum in dairy cows: classification of severity and evaluation of outcome. J Am Vet Med Assoc 1978;173:108–111.
Sockett DC, Knight AP, Fettman MJ, Kiehl AR, Smith JA. Metabolic alterations following induced urinary bladder rupture in steers. Cornell Vet 1986;76:198–212.

Phosphorus
Fettman MJ, Coble JM, Hamar DW, et al. Effect of dietary phosphoric acid supplementation on acid-base balance and mineral and bone metabolism in adult cats. Am J Vet Res 1992;53:2125–2135.
Finco DR, Barsanti JA, Brown SA. Influence of dietary source of phosphorus on fecal and urinary excretion of phosphorus and other minerals by male cats. Am J Vet Res 1989;50:263–266.
Ogawa E, Kobayashi K, Yoshiura N, Mukai J. Bovine postparturient hemoglobinemia: hypophosphatemia and metabolic disorder in red blood cells. Am J Vet Res 1987;48:1300–1303.

Calcium
Ching SV, Fettman MJ, Hamar DW, Nogade LA, Smith KR. The effect of chronic dietary acidification using ammonium chloride on acid-

base and mineral metabolism in the adult cat. J Nutr 1989;119: 902–915.

Ching SV, Norrdin RW, Fettman MJ, LeCouteur RA. Trabecular bone remodeling and bone mineral density in the adult cat during chronic dietary acidification with ammonium chloride. J Bone Miner Res 1990;5:547–556.

Flanders JA, Scarlett JM, Blue JT, Neth S. Adjustment of total serum calcium concentration for binding to albumin and protein in cats: 291 cases (1986–1987). J Am Vet Med Assoc 1989;194:1609–1611.

Kohn CW, Brooks CL. Failure of pH to predict ionized calcium percentage in healthy horses. Am J Vet Res 1990;51:1206–1210.

Meuten DJ, Chew DJ, Capen CC, Kociba GJ. Relationship of serum total calcium to albumin and total protein in dogs. J Am Vet Med Assoc 1982;180:63–67.

Oetzel GR, Fettman MJ, Hamar DW, Olson JD. Screening of anionic salts for palatability, effects on acid-base status, and urinary calcium excretion in dairy cows. J Dairy Sci 1991;74:965–971.

Oetzel GR, Olson JD, Curtis CR, Fettman MJ. Ammonium chloride and ammonium sulfate for prevention of parturient paresis in dairy cows. J Dairy Sci 1988;71:3302–3309.

Schenck PA, Chew DJ, Brooks CL. Effects of storage on serum ionized calcium and pH values in clinically normal dogs. Am J Vet Res 1995; 56:304–307.

Szenci O, Brydl E, Bajcsy CA. Effect of storage on measurement of ionized calcium and acid-base variables in equine, bovine, ovine, and canine venous blood. J Am Vet Med Assoc 1991;199:1167–1169.

Acid-Base Metabolism

James KM, Polzin DJ, Osborne CA, Olson JK. Effects of sample handling on total carbon dioxide concentrations in canine and feline serum and blood. Am J Vet Res 1997;58:343–347.

Levraut J, Labib Y, Chave S, Payan P, Raucoules-Aime M, Grimaud D. Effect of sodium bicarbonate on intracellular pH under different buffering conditions. Kidney Int 1996;49:1262–1267.

Narins RG, Cohen JJ. Bicarbonate therapy for organic acidosis: the case for its continued use. Ann Intern Med 1987;106:615–618.

Ritter JM, Doktor HS, Benjamin N. Paradoxical effect of bicarbonate on cytoplasmic pH. Lancet 1990;335:1243–1246.

Stacpoole PW. Lactic acidosis: the case against bicarbonate therapy. Ann Intern Med 1986;105:276–279.

Anion Gap

Bristol DG. The anion gap as a prognostic indicator in horses with abdominal pain. J Am Vet Med Assoc 1982;181:63–65.

Dial SM, Thrall MA, Hamar DW. Efficacy of 4-methylpyrazole for treatment of ethylene glycol intoxication in dogs. Am J Vet Res 1994;55:1762–1770.

Garry FB, Hull BL, Rings DM, Kersting K, Hoffsis GF. Prognostic value of anion gap calculation in cattle with abomasal volvulus: 58 cases (1980–1985). J Am Vet Med Assoc 1988;192:1107–1112.

Gossett KA, French DD. Effect of age on anion gap in clinically normal quarter horses. Am J Vet Res 1983;44:1744–1745.

Hauptman JG, Tvedten H. Osmolal and anion gaps in dogs with acute endotoxic shock. Am J Vet Res 1986;47:1617–1619.

Lotekha PH, Lolekha S. Value of the anion gap in clinical diagnosis and laboratory evaluation. Clin Chem 1983;29:279–283.

Strong Ion Difference

DiBartola SP. Introduction to acid-base disorders. In: DiBartola SP, ed. Fluid therapy in small animal practice. 2nd ed. Philadelphia: WB Saunders, 2000:189–210.

Stewart PA. How to understand acid-base. A quantitative acid-base primer for biology and medicine. New York: Elsevier, 1981.

Whitehair KJ, Haskins SC, Whitehair JG, Pacoe PJ. Clinical applications of quantitative acid-base chemistry. J Vet Intern Med 1995;9:1–11.

Osmolal Gap

Feldman BF. Clinical use of anion and osmolal gaps in veterinary medicine. J Am Vet Med Assoc 1981;178:396–398.

Sklar AH, Linas SL. The osmolal gap in renal failure. Ann Intern Med 1983;98:481–482.

LABORATORY EVALUATION

OF THE LIVER

The liver functions in many body processes, including carbohydrate, fat and protein metabolism, detoxification and excretion of waste products and other toxic substances, digestion (especially fats), and production of several clotting factors. Because of the central role the liver plays in these and other processes, pathologic changes in the liver can produce many alterations in clinical biochemistry test results. This chapter discusses these alterations and their interpretations.

LIVER DISEASE VERSUS
LIVER FAILURE

Liver disease includes any of several processes resulting in hepatocyte injury, cholestasis, or both. These include hypoxia, metabolic diseases, toxicoses, inflammation, neoplasia, mechanical trauma, and intrahepatic or extrahepatic bile duct blockage. Liver failure usually results from some type of liver disease, and it is recognized both by failure to clear the blood of those substances normally eliminated by the liver and by failure to synthesize those substances normally produced by the liver. Liver disease, however, does not always result in liver failure. The liver has a marked reserve capacity, and 70% to 80% of the functional he-

patic mass must be lost before liver failure occurs. Tests for liver disease or failure fall into three categories:

- Serum enzyme assays that detect hepatocyte injury.
- Serum enzyme assays that detect cholestasis.
- Tests that evaluate or are indicative of liver functions.

INTRODUCTION TO ENZYMOLOGY

To interpret the results of serum enzyme assays used to detect liver disease, a basic understanding of diagnostic enzymology is necessary. Basic principles of diagnostic enzymology include:

- Different organs, tissues, or cells contain different enzymes. In some cases, only a few organs or tissues contain a given enzyme, and these "tissue-specific" enzymes tend to be the most useful diagnostically.
- Increased serum activities of diagnostic enzymes result when increased quantities of these enzymes pass into the blood, either because of leakage from injured cells or because of increased production.
- Detection of increased activities of these enzymes in the serum, therefore, is suggestive of an injury to the

- organ, tissue, or cell type of origin or stimulation of the organ, tissue, or cell type of origin to produce increased quantities of the enzyme.
- Diagnostic enzymology is a means of locating where tissue injury or stimulation of increased enzyme production has occurred.
- Results of diagnostic enzymology, in combination with other clinical and laboratory data, are helpful in understanding the disease process and in making a diagnosis.

Enzymes are assayed by measuring their activities, because enzymes catalyze biochemical reactions by converting a substrate into a product. For example,

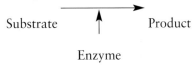

Substrate ⟶ Product

Enzyme

In measuring enzyme activity, a standard quantity of serum containing the enzyme to be measured is mixed with a solution containing the substrate for that enzyme. The reaction is then allowed to occur, and the enzyme's activity is measured by the rate of either substrate disappearance or product formation. The more rapidly that either one occurs, the greater the patient's serum enzyme activity. Frequently, the product is not measured directly; rather, it is incorporated into a second reaction, which often involves the conversion of NAD⁺ (or NADP⁺) to NADH (or NADPH), or vice versa. Because this second reaction is common to many enzyme assays, the rate of these reactions can be measured spectrophotometrically at a standard ultraviolet wavelength.

Currently, enzyme activities are reported in terms of international units per liter (IU/L). Concentrations of these enzymes are not measured directly, but the serum activity of an enzyme is considered to be directly proportional to its concentration. If serum samples are not properly handled, however, the relationship between the enzyme activity and the enzyme concentration can change, thus leading to erroneous results. Basic concepts and information that must be considered to properly interpret the results of serum enzyme assays include:

- The difference between "leakage" enzymes and "induced" enzymes.
- The duration of enzyme activity after passage into the blood (i.e., the enzyme's biologic half-life in the blood).
- The tissue specificity of enzymes.
- The proper handling and storage of serum for enzyme assays.

Increased serum enzyme activities can result from either leakage or induction. Leakage of enzymes from cells re-

sults from cell injury, and diagnostic enzymes that pass into the extracellular space and then into the serum by this mechanism are termed *leakage enzymes (Fig. 23.1)*. Induction, however, involves the increased production of an enzyme by cells that normally produce the enzyme in smaller quantities. This increased production is induced by some type of stimulus, and it results in increased release of the enzyme from the cells and increased activity of the enzyme in serum. Diagnostic enzymes that pass into the serum by this mechanism are termed *induced enzymes (Fig. 23.2)*.

Leakage enzymes are present in the cytosol, organelles, or both. These enzymes escape from cells as a result of injury to the cell membrane and, in some cases, injury to organelles. This injury can be as severe as cell death (i.e., necrosis), or it can be mild, sublethal damage that simply causes the cell membranes to leak. Because this process does not require increased enzyme production, it can happen very quickly, and increased serum enzyme activities can be detected within hours of the injury.

Induced enzymes are attached to cell membranes; therefore, their serum activities usually do not increase as a result of cell injury or death. Because increased serum activities of induced enzymes depend on increased production, these increases develop more slowly than those of leakage enzymes (i.e., days rather than hours).

The concept of "leakage" versus "induced" enzymes is important, but the difference is not entirely clear-cut. Some evidence is suggestive that loss of leakage enzymes from sublethally injured cells induces these cells to produce more of these enzymes. In addition, the serum ac-

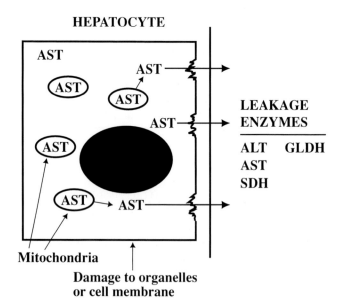

Figure 23.1 Leakage enzymes escape from the cell because of alteration of the plasma membrane. Some leakage enzymes, such as AST, are also present in the organelles. More severe damage is required to cause leakage from these organelles.

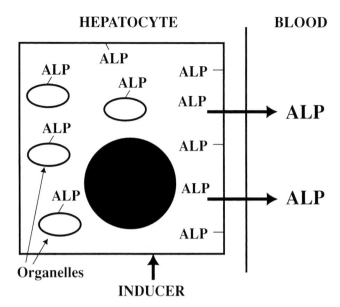

HEPATOCYTE   **BLOOD**

Figure 23.2   Increased serum activities of induced enzymes result, in part, from increased production of these enzymes, with a subsequent increase in secretion. This increased production is caused by some type of inducer.

tivities of some induced enzymes can increase rapidly after acute cell injury. In such cases, small fragments of membrane, to which the induced enzyme is attached, are theorized to be released, to pass into the serum, and to result in the detection of increased serum activity for this enzyme. It also is theorized that the release of induced enzymes can occur secondary to less acute membrane alterations. The increased serum activities of alkaline phosphatase (ALP) and γ-glutamyltransferase (GGT), as a result of cholestasis, are one example. A portion of the increase in the serum activities of these enzymes probably results from increased enzyme production, but the bile acids sequestered in bile canaliculi and ducts may cause the cell membranes of hepatocytes and bile duct epithelial cells to become more soluble, thereby resulting in increased release of both these enzymes.

After leakage or secretion from cells, the enzymes eventually are degraded or excreted from the body (or both). Some enzyme molecules also might lose their activity and, therefore, not be detected before either of these events. The rate at which the loss of activity, degradation, or excretion occurs determines the length of time during which the enzyme activity is detectable in the serum after leakage or secretion. The disappearance rate of enzyme activity typically is measured as the biologic half-life of the enzyme, which is the time required, after leakage or secretion of the enzyme, for one-half of that enzyme's activity to disappear from the serum. Enzymes with short biologic half-lives, therefore, are quickly inactivated, degraded, or excreted from the serum; the opposite is true

of enzymes with long biologic half-lives. Knowledge of the average biologic half-life of an enzyme is helpful when assessing how recently leakage or increased production has occurred and whether either process is continuing. (The biologic half-lives of various diagnostic enzymes and examples regarding the use of enzyme half-lives in assessing tissue injury are reviewed in the later discussions of specific enzymes.)

Regardless of which type of enzyme is being assayed, it is important to know from which tissues the enzyme most likely originated. This knowledge of tissue specificity allows the diagnostician to narrow the list of possible tissues that are involved in a disease process. Tissue specificity is a function of:

- **The presence or absence of the enzyme in the tissue.** An enzyme can be absent from some tissues and present in other tissues. When increased serum activity of an enzyme is detected, only the tissues in which that enzyme is present are considered to be potential sites of injury.
- **The concentration of the enzyme in tissues.** An enzyme can be present in many tissues but have high concentrations in only one or a few. When increased serum activity of an enzyme is detected, the tissues in which that enzyme is found at the highest concentrations are the most likely sites of injury.
- **Where the enzyme goes after leakage or secretion.** Enzymes that are detected in serum have either leaked or been secreted into the extracellular spaces and then passed into the serum. Injury to some tissues containing high concentrations of certain enzymes can result in leakage or secretion of these enzymes into areas of the body that result in these enzymes being immediately eliminated rather than passing into the serum. In such cases, increased serum activities are not detected. For example, injury to renal epithelial cells results in leakage of the enzyme GGT. This enzyme leaks from the brush border of the cell into the lumens of the renal tubules, rather than into the extracellular space. Thus, increased GGT activity can be detected in the urine, but the serum activity does not increase.
- **The half-life of the enzyme.** Enzymes with the same catalytic activity might be produced in several different tissues, but these enzymes can vary regarding other properties. These different forms of enzymes are termed *isoenzymes*. Some isoenzymes can have different half-lives compared with those of others. If an isoenzyme has a very short half-life (e.g., minutes to a few hours), it is less likely to accumulate in the serum after leakage or secretion and, therefore, is less likely to be detected. If an enzyme originates from two different tissues but the half-life of the isoenzyme from one tissue is minutes and that of the isoenzyme from the second

tissue is days, then the increased serum activity of that enzyme is more likely to have originated from the second tissue. For example, in dogs, the placenta contains large quantities of the enzyme ALP, but the half-life of the placental isoenzyme is minutes. Therefore, the placenta is not considered to be a likely source when an increased serum ALP activity is detected in a dog.

The ideal diagnostic enzyme would be specific for only one tissue. Increased serum activities of such an enzyme would direct the diagnostician to that tissue as the site of a disease process. Almost no diagnostic enzymes are found in only one tissue; however, some of these enzymes are found in only a few tissues.

Diagnosticians commonly attempt to relate the magnitude of increased serum enzyme activities with the type or degree of injury in a tissue. Assuming that higher enzyme activities are indicative of more severe tissue injury (especially in the case of leakage enzymes) is tempting, but this assumption also is not always true *(Fig. 23.3)*. Dead cells leak all of their enzymes, and they produce no additional enzymes. Sublethally injured cells, however, leak only a portion of their enzyme content and continue to produce enzymes (possibly at an increased rate). Such cells, therefore, ultimately can leak more enzyme than dead cells do. In other words, necrosis in a tissue can produce high serum enzyme activity, but diffuse, sublethal injury to the same tissue can result in even higher activity. As a result, the magnitude of the serum enzyme activity is not a reliable indicator regarding the type or degree of tissue injury.

Unlike substances in which absolute quantities are measured in the serum (e.g. urea, creatinine, electrolytes), the assay of enzymes involves measuring serum activities and assuming that these activities are proportional to the serum concentrations of the enzymes. After obtaining

a blood sample, enzyme molecules remain in harvested serum for a long period of time under various storage conditions; however, the activity of these molecules can be lost. Enzymes are proteins that can be denatured by heat, changes in pH, and exposure to various chemicals. This denaturation results in loss of activity. In addition, substances that normally are present in the serum (e.g., sulfhydryl inhibitors) can gradually inactivate enzyme activity over time. Different enzymes vary in their susceptibility to these inactivating factors.

Regardless of whether serum enzyme activities are assayed in a practice laboratory or a reference laboratory, some variable delay usually occurs in performing these assays. Therefore, handling these samples properly during this time is important to reduce the effects of enzyme inactivators. Serum to be used in these assays should be harvested as soon as possible. Hemolysis, icterus, and lipemia should be avoided, because these can affect some enzyme assays or, in the case of hemolysis, result in erythrocyte enzymes leaking into the serum and erroneously increasing some enzyme activities (see Chapter 3).

TESTS DETECTING HEPATOCYTE INJURY

Hepatocyte injury is detected by measuring the serum activities of enzymes that have leaked from hepatocytes. Four such leakage enzymes are liver specific, though to varying degrees. In veterinary medicine, use of these enzymes to detect hepatocyte injury varies from common to rare depending on the enzyme.

Alanine Aminotransferase

Alanine aminotransferase (ALT), which previously was called serum glutamic pyruvic transaminase (SGPT), is a leakage enzyme that is free in the cytoplasm. The highest concentrations of ALT occur in the hepatocytes of dogs and cats, and the ALT assay commonly is included in the serum biochemical profiles of these species. This enzyme has been considered to be very liver specific in these species, but reports of dogs and cats with severe muscle damage are indicative that serum ALT activities may be increased in these animals without apparent liver damage. Muscle ALT activity is less than that of the liver (~5% and 25% of liver activity in skeletal and cardiac muscle, respectively). Because the total mass of muscle is much greater than that of the liver, however, muscle is a significant potential source of ALT leakage. Increased serum ALT activity in dogs and cats usually is suggestive of either hepatocyte death or sublethal hepatocyte injury, but necrosis or sublethal damage to muscle cells must be considered as well. Measurement of a serum enzyme ac-

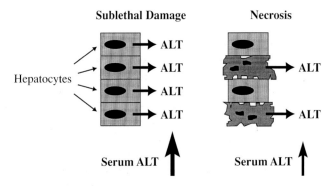

Figure 23.3 The magnitude of serum enzyme activity is not necessarily related to the severity of tissue injury. Serum ALT leaks from hepatocytes when their plasma membranes are injured. The resultant serum ALT activity can be greater after sublethal injury to many hepatocytes than after necrosis of a few hepatocytes.

tivity that is more muscle specific (e.g., creatine kinase [CK]) in dogs and cats with increased ALT activity is helpful in determining if muscle damage is a possible source of the increased ALT.

A wide variety of liver diseases can produce increased serum ALT activity. Any disease that causes hepatocyte injury, ranging from membrane injury to hepatocyte death, can result in increased serum ALT activity. Hypoxia, metabolic alterations resulting in hepatocyte lipid accumulation, bacterial toxins, inflammation, hepatic neoplasia, and a multitude of toxic chemicals and drugs can cause hepatocyte injury, thereby resulting in ALT leakage. Increased blood glucocorticoid concentrations commonly result in increased serum ALT activity in dogs; such increases in glucocorticoid concentrations may result from treatment with glucocorticoids or from increased endogenous glucocorticoid synthesis secondary to hyperadrenocorticism. Serum ALT activity typically increases by two- to fivefold as a result of increased blood glucocorticoid concentration, and this increase may result from a glucocorticoid-induced increase in enzyme production as well as from hepatocyte injury. Such increases are not necessarily indicative that glucocorticoids have caused hepatocyte injury of the degree occurring in glucocorticoid hepatopathy. Serum ALT activity may increase by as much as 40-fold in dogs with glucocorticoid hepatopathy. Anticonvulsant drugs also cause increased serum ALT activity in dogs, possibly as a result of hepatocyte injury as well as of increased enzyme production.

Acutely, the serum activity of ALT probably is proportional to the number of cells that are injured, but as illustrated in Figure 23.3, the magnitude of ALT activity is not indicative of the cause of the injury or of the type of damage to the hepatocytes (e.g., sublethal damage or necrosis). Serum ALT activity increases approximately 12 hours after a liver injury, and it peaks approximately 1 to 2 days after a single acute injury. Serum ALT activity also can be increased during recovery from liver injury, when active hepatocyte regeneration is occurring. Dogs and cats may have significant liver disease but either normal or only slightly increased serum ALT activity. In at least some cases of severe liver disease, the hepatic mass is markedly decreased, and the number of hepatocytes remaining might be too few to result in a markedly increased serum activity, even if the remaining cells are injured and leaking ALT. In addition, if the liver disease is chronic, the degree of active hepatocyte injury possibly may be mild; if so, the remaining hepatocytes do not leak a large amount of ALT. The half-life of ALT in dogs is uncertain with estimates ranging from a few to 60 hours. The half-life of ALT in cats also is uncertain but may be shorter than that in dogs.

The ALT concentration in the hepatocytes of horses and ruminants is low; consequently, the serum ALT activity is not useful for detecting liver disease in these

species. Moderate amounts of ALT are present in the muscle of horses and ruminants, and moderate increases in the serum ALT activity occur with muscle injury in these species. Because the serum ALT activity rarely is measured in horses and ruminants, these increased activities secondary to muscle injury seldom are noted. Other muscle-specific enzymes (e.g., CK) more commonly are used for detecting muscle injury in these species.

Aspartate Aminotransferase

Aspartate aminotransferase (AST), which previously was called serum glutamic oxaloacetic transaminase (SGOT), is present at highest concentrations in the hepatocytes and muscle cells (both skeletal and cardiac) of all species. Therefore, AST is not a liver-specific enzyme. Aspartate aminotransferase is a leakage enzyme, some of which is free in hepatocyte cytoplasm but more of which is associated with mitochrondrial membranes. Increased serum AST activities can result from hepatocyte death, sublethal hepatocyte injury, muscle cell death, and sublethal muscle cell injury.

In dogs and cats, the serum ALT activity sometimes is used as the only test to detect hepatocyte injury, because ALT is more liver specific than AST. Serum AST activity increases because of the same variety of liver diseases previously listed for ALT in dogs and cats, but the magnitude of its activity usually is less than that of ALT. Although AST is less liver specific than ALT, it is more sensitive than ALT for detecting certain types of hepatocyte injury in dogs and cats.

As previously noted, high concentrations of AST are present in the skeletal and cardiac muscle of dogs and cats, and muscle injury in these species results in increased serum AST activities. Diagnostic enzymes that are more specific for muscle injury (e.g., CK [see Chapter 27]), however, are available for dogs and cats and, therefore, are more reliable for detecting such injury.

Because the ALT activity in the livers of horses and ruminants is low, ALT is not a useful enzyme for detecting hepatocyte injury in these species. Aspartate aminotransferase, sorbitol dehydrogenase (SDH), and glutamate dehydrogenase (GLDH), however, have been used to detect such injury in these species. Whereas SDH and GLDH are more liver specific than AST, the assays for these enzymes are not as widely available as that for AST. Therefore, AST often is the enzyme of choice for the routine detection of hepatocyte injury in horses and ruminants. In these species, an increased serum AST activity can result from the same spectrum of liver diseases (both sublethal and necrotic) as that listed for ALT. The major problem with AST in detecting hepatocyte injury is its lack of liver specificity. As in dogs and cats, increased serum AST activity in horses and ruminants can result not only from hepatocyte injury but also from muscle injury. This problem can be mitigated (to a certain extent) by assaying a muscle-specific enzyme such as CK along with AST. Increased AST activity with normal CK activity could be suggestive both that the source of the AST is the liver and that hepatocyte injury has occurred. Uncertainty remains in such a case, however, because the half-life of CK is shorter than that of AST *(Fig. 23.4)*. Serum activities of both enzymes could have increased as a result of muscle injury, but the CK activity might have returned to normal earlier than the AST activity. These problems with use of AST in detecting hepatocyte injury in horses and ruminants have led to attempts to use more liver-specific enzymes in these species.

As noted with ALT, the serum activity of AST might be normal or only slightly increased with significant liver diseases that are chronic and low-grade, that have resulted in markedly decreased hepatic mass, or both. The half-life of AST is estimated to be approximately 5 hours in dogs, 1 to 2 hours in cats, and 50 hours in horses.

Sorbitol Dehydrogenase

Sorbitol dehydrogenase (SDH) is a leakage enzyme that is free in the cytoplasm. It is present at high concentrations in the hepatocytes of dogs, cats, horses, and ruminants, but its concentration in other tissues in these species is low. Therefore, SDH is a liver-specific enzyme. Increased serum SDH activity is suggestive of either hepatocyte death or sublethal hepatocyte injury. Even so, SDH is not superior to ALT for detecting hepatocyte injury in dogs and cats, and it is not commonly used in

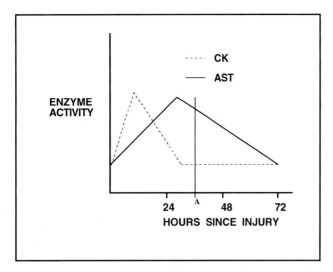

Figure 23.4 Serum activities of both AST and CK increase because of muscle injury. As illustrated here, however, these activities increase and decrease at different rates. Depending on when a blood sample is analyzed after muscle injury, it is possible to detect increased serum AST activity and normal serum CK activity (note time A) and to erroneously interpret this as being an indication of hepatic injury.

these species. In horses and cattle, however, SDH is much more specific than AST for detecting hepatocyte injury. The half-life of SDH is very short (<2 days); after acute hepatocyte injury, serum activities may return to normal within 4 to 5 days. The in vitro stability of SDH is less than that of many other diagnostic enzymes. In both horses and cattle, however, SDH is stable in serum for as long as 5 hours at room temperature and for as long as 48 hours (72 hours in cattle) when frozen. In most cases, these time periods should be sufficient to allow the delivery of serum to a laboratory for an SDH assay. Because SDH is preferable to AST for detecting hepatocyte injury in horses and ruminants, one should identify a laboratory that can perform this assay within the appropriate time frames.

Glutamate Dehydrogenase

Glutamate dehydrogenase (GLDH) is a leakage enzyme that is free in the cytoplasm. It is present at high concentrations in the livers of dogs, cats, horses, and ruminants and at low concentrations in other tissues in these species. Therefore, GLDH is a liver-specific enzyme. An increased serum GLDH activity is suggestive of either hepatocyte death or sublethal hepatocyte injury. In vitro, GLDH is more stable than SDH, but this period of stability is short compared with those of most other diagnostic enzymes. In addition, the assay for GLDH activity is difficult and not widely available. Because of these problems, ALT is considered to be superior to GLDH for detecting hepatocyte injury in dogs and cats. In horses and ruminants, however, GLDH is potentially useful, because it is more liver specific than AST and has better storage stability than SDH. Whereas the serum GLDH activity might be a sensitive indicator of acute hepatocyte damage in ruminants, it is not very sensitive for more chronic liver diseases.

TESTS DETECTING CHOLESTASIS

Cholestasis can be detected by measuring the serum activities of enzymes whose increased production is induced by cholestasis or by measuring the serum concentrations of substances (either endogenous or exogenous) that normally are excreted through the biliary system. The latter tests are actually tests of liver function and are discussed later. The two serum enzymes used to detect cholestasis are ALP and GGT.

Alkaline Phosphatase

Alkaline phosphatase (ALP) is an induced enzyme that is synthesized by the liver, osteoblasts, intestinal epithelium, renal epithelium, and placenta. Most of the normal serum activity of ALP, however, originates from hepatocytes. The half-life of intestinal, renal, and placental ALP in dogs is approximately 6 minutes, and the half-life of intestinal ALP in cats is approximately 2 minutes. These ALP isoenzymes are not, therefore, considered to be likely sources of increased serum ALP activity in these species. Increased ALP production and increased serum ALP activity can occur with increased osteoblastic activity, cholestasis, induction by certain drugs (in dogs, but this is questionable in other species), and a variety of chronic diseases, including neoplasia.

Alkaline Phosphatase of Bone Origin

Increased serum ALP activity associated with increased osteoblastic activity occurs in all species. These increases usually are mild, however, and most often are detected in young, growing animals when the results of ALP assays are compared with adult reference intervals for ALP. For instance, the serum activity of alkaline phosphatase of bone origin (BALP) in kittens younger than 5 months old ranges from 63 to 150 IU/L, whereas serum BALP activity in adult cats ranges from 2 to 20 IU/L. These age-related differences in serum BALP activities result in a serum ALP activity of 33 to 303 IU/L in kittens and of 6 to 106 IU/L in adult cats. Therefore, it is best to use age-specific reference intervals, if available, when interpreting serum ALP activities. If such intervals are not available, then remember that young animals commonly have serum ALP activities moderately greater than adult reference intervals. Osteosarcoma and other bone neoplasms (both primary and secondary) inconsistently result in increased serum ALP activity because of osteoblast proliferation in these processes. Bone healing usually results in very localized increases in osteoblastic activity and very mild (if any) increases in serum ALP. Hyperparathyroidism (primary or secondary) can result in increased bone turnover and increased osteoblastic activity. Mild increases in serum ALP may be detected in patients with these diseases.

Alkaline Phosphatase of Liver Origin

Increases in serum ALP can be marked with cholestasis in dogs but more variable in other species. Increased intrabiliary pressure induces an increased ALP production by hepatocytes and, possibly, bile duct epithelial cells. In addition, sequestration of bile in the biliary system causes solubilization of ALP molecules attached to cell membranes, then increased release of these molecules into the blood. The half-life of the cholestasis-induced ALP isoenzyme, which is termed *liver ALP (LALP)*, is approximately 72 hours in dogs and approximately 6 hours in cats. Serum bilirubin and bile acid concentrations

also might be increased simultaneously with cholestasis-induced ALP increases, unlike other causes of increased serum ALP. With cholestasis, serum ALP often increases before the serum bilirubin concentration does. Even if the serum bilirubin concentration is normal, an increased urinary bilirubin concentration may accompany cholestasis-induced increases in ALP (discussed later). Whereas lesions primarily involving the intra- or extra-hepatic biliary system are common causes of cholestasis, hepatocytic diseases resulting in significant hepatocyte swelling (e.g., lipidosis or inflammation of the hepatic parenchyma) can obstruct small bile canaliculi and also induce increased ALP production and release.

Alkaline Phosphatase Induced by Drugs

Serum ALP activities also can be markedly increased when greater production is induced by drugs, particularly in dogs. Drug-induced ALP production is not well documented in other species, but glucocorticoids (exogenous or endogenous) induce increased ALP production by hepatocytes in dogs. In the case of glucocorticoid-induced production, the isoenzyme produced is distinct from that produced by hepatocytes in response to cholestasis. The half-life of the glucocorticoid-induced isoenzyme, which is termed *glucocorticoid-induced* or *corticosteroid-induced ALP (CiALP)*, is approximately 72 hours in dogs. In animals with increased blood glucocorticoid concentrations, the magnitude of serum CiALP activity is not consistently related to the presence or absence of steroid hepatopathy. Anticonvulsants (e.g., phenobarbitol, phenytoin, primidone) also induce increased ALP production in dogs. Because most clinically significant increases in serum ALP in dogs not being treated with anticonvulsants result from either cholestasis or steroid induction, distinguishing the LALP isoenzyme from the CiALP isoenzyme in dogs with increased serum ALP is desirable. Several tests are available for distinguishing LALP from CiALP.

Even if the LALP isoenzyme can be distinguished from CiALP, the significance of this distinction can be uncertain. During the first week or more after an increase in the blood glucocorticoid concentrations in dogs, increased serum ALP activity primarily results from LALP. No evidence is suggestive that cholestasis has occurred during this time, and it appears that glucocorticoids induce an increased production of LALP. Isoenzyme identification during this period would erroneously suggest a cholestatic problem. After a week or more, however, the serum CiALP activity increases, and at this time, isoenzyme determination would potentially be helpful in identifying the cause of the increased serum ALP activity. Moreover, because chronic diseases, including chronic hepatobiliary disease, cause long-term stress, these diseases may cause increased glucocorticoid production and increased blood glucocorticoid concentration, which in turn may cause increased activities of CiALP. In this situation, detecting increased activities of this isoenzyme might be misleading. Increased CiALP activity can occur with a variety of chronic diseases in dogs; therefore, the specificity of increased CiALP activity in dogs is limited. If the chronic disease involves the hepatobiliary system, the LALP also should be increased.

To distinguish cholestasis-induced from corticosteroid-induced increases in serum ALP in dogs, other tests can be performed. These tests include serum and urinary bilirubin concentrations, serum bile acid concentration, and those to detect hyperadrenocorticism. A suggested approach to distinguishing cholestasis-induced from glucocorticoid-induced increases in serum ALP activity in dogs is presented in *Figure 23.5*. The concurrent presence of hyperbilirubinemia is strongly suggestive of a cholestatic cause for the increased ALP, but as noted earlier, the serum bilirubin concentration may be normal in some cases of cholestasis. This can happen early during cholestatic diseases or when only a portion of the biliary tree is obstructed. In the latter situation, the unobstructed portion of the biliary system excretes enough bilirubin that serum concentrations remain within the reference interval.

Increased serum ALP activity can occur secondary to a variety of neoplasms, and the underlying mechanisms of these increases vary with different neoplasms. Bone neoplasms result in increased ALP production by osteoblasts. Primary or metastatic neoplasms of the liver or the biliary system can cause cholestasis with resultant increases in serum ALP. Neoplasms of the pituitary or adrenal glands can result in increased glucocorticoid production and, as a result, increased hepatocyte production of ALP. The mechanism leading to increased ALP activity associated with other neoplasms is uncertain, but it may be increased production of CiALP. Mammary adenocarcinoma, squamous cell carcinoma, and hemangiosarcoma are neoplasms that have been associated with such increases in serum ALP activity. Neoplasia always should be considered in older animals with unexplained increases in the serum ALP. Subclinical liver disease also is common in older animals (e.g., dogs), however, and this also can result in increased serum ALP.

Interpretation of serum ALP values in cats requires some special considerations. Whereas the half-life of serum ALP in dogs is approximately 3 days, that in cats is estimated to be 6 hours. In addition to this short half-life, the potential of the feline liver to produce ALP is significantly less than that in other species. As a result, the increases of serum ALP in cats with cholestatic liver disease are lower than those in other species (e.g., dogs). In other words, mild increases in serum ALP are more significant in cats than in other species. γ-Glutamyltransferase has been recommended as an alternative to ALP for the detection of cholestasis in cats. Glucocorticoid-induced increases in serum ALP activity, if any, are very mild in cats, and exogenous administration of glucocorticoids to cats produces inconsistent, mild increases in serum ALP activity. Hyperthyroidism in cats can produce moderate increases in ALP activity as well. The cause of this is not clear, but both liver and bone isoenzymes are increased. These increases possibly may result from the effects of thyroxine on liver and bone.

In horses, glucocorticoid-induced increases in ALP are not well documented. Most increases in ALP detected in horses have been associated with cholestasis or osteoblast production of the bone isoenzyme. Wide reference intervals for equine ALP contribute to the reduced sensitivity of the serum ALP assay for the detection of liver disease in horses.

Increases in the serum ALP in ruminants most commonly result from cholestasis or increased osteoblastic activity (e.g., young, growing animals or nutritional secondary hyperparathyroidism). Wide reference intervals for ALP in ruminants contribute to the reduced sensitivity of the serum ALP assay for the detection of liver disease in these species.

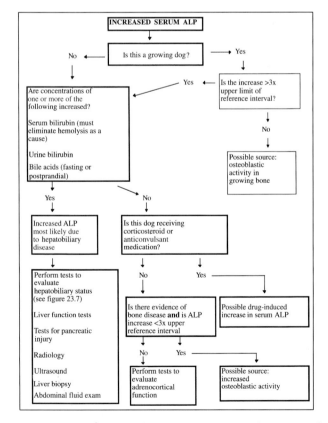

Figure 23.5 Flow chart for evaluating the possible causes of increased serum ALP activities in dogs.

γ-Glutamyltransferase

γ-Glutamyltransferase (GGT) is considered to be an induced enzyme. Acute hepatic injury, however, can produce rapid increases in serum GGT activity, possibly because of the release of membrane fragments to which GGT is attached. γ-Glutamyltransferase is synthesized by most body tissues, with the highest concentrations occurring in the pancreas and kidney. It also is present at lower concentrations in the hepatocytes, bile duct epithelium, and intestinal mucosa and at high concentrations in the mammary glands of cattle, sheep, and dogs. Most of the serum GGT originates in the liver. Release from renal epithelial cells results in increased urinary GGT activity, but not increased serum GGT activity (see Chapter 21). When GGT is released by pancreatic cells, it apparently passes out with pancreatic secretions rather than into the blood.

Increased GGT production, release, and the resultant increased serum GGT activity occur with cholestasis. In dogs, these also occur with induction by glucocorticoids.

The increased serum GGT activity in cholestasis may result from both increased production and solubilization of GGT attached to cell membranes. In the latter case, solubilization from cell membranes is induced by the detergent action of bile acids that have not passed at a normal rate through the bile ducts to the intestine.

With cholestasis, serum GGT activity increases at approximately the same rate as serum ALP activity. For the detection of liver disease in dogs, GGT is more specific, but less sensitive, than ALP. For the detection of liver disease in cats, GGT is more sensitive, but less specific, than ALP. In both dogs and cats, results of serum ALP and GGT assays performed in combination to detect hepatobiliary disease are more diagnostically valid than those of either enzyme assay used alone.

In dogs, glucocorticoid-induced increases in serum GGT activity appear to be associated with increased enzyme production by the liver. When the increase in GGT activity is induced by glucocorticoids, the increase in serum GGT parallels that in the serum ALP activity. Increased serum GGT activity also has been reported in dogs that are receiving anticonvulsant medication, but these increases usually are mild (i.e., two- to threefold the upper end of the reference interval). If such increases are of greater magnitude, they are more likely the result of cholestasis. Marked increases in the serum GGT activity of an animal being treated with anticonvulsant medication may be indicative of an idiosyncratic reaction resulting in a cholestatic liver disease with life-threatening implications.

The narrower reference intervals for serum GGT in horses and ruminants make this enzyme superior (i.e., more sensitive and specific) to ALP for the detection of

cholestasis. Thus, GGT, rather than ALP, often is used in these species.

High serum GGT activity in the colostrum of cattle and sheep can result in extremely high activities in the serum of young calves and lambs that have consumed colostrum. In calves, the GGT activity can be more than 200-fold the upper limit of the adult reference interval during the first 3 days after birth. Typically, a three- to fourfold decrease occurs in this activity by the end of the first week, and the activity gradually continues decreasing, to within the adult reference interval by 6 to 13 weeks of age. Lambs also have markedly increased serum GGT activity after colostrum consumption, with this activity falling to within the adult reference intervals by approximately 30 days of age. Although pups have high serum GGT activity after colostrum ingestion as well, this activity rapidly falls to within the adult reference intervals by approximately 10 days of age. High serum GGT activity also occurs in foals, but this enzyme activity apparently is not of colostral origin, because mares do not have significant GGT activity in their colostrum.

LEAKAGE VERSUS INDUCED ENZYMES IN DETERMINING TYPES OF LIVER DISEASES

The serum activities of both the leakage and induced enzymes discussed earlier tend to increase during most types of liver disease, but the relative magnitudes of these increases can provide a hint regarding the primary liver lesions. In diseases that are characterized primarily by hepatocyte injury, the activities of leakage enzymes tend to be increased relatively more than those of induced enzymes. In diseases that are characterized primarily by cholestasis, the activities of induced enzymes tend to be increased relatively more than those of leakage enzymes. Because many liver diseases, especially as they become more chronic, result in both hepatocyte injury and cholestasis, this differentiation does not always yield useful information.

TESTS OF LIVER FUNCTION

Tests of liver function include measurement of the serum concentrations of substances that normally are removed from the blood by the liver and then metabolized or excreted (or both) via the biliary system (e.g., bilirubin, bile acids, cholesterol, exogenous substances, ammonia). In addition, these tests include measurement of the serum concentrations of blood constituents that normally are synthesized by the liver (e.g., albumin, globulins, urea, cholesterol, coagulation factors). Abnormal blood concentrations of these substances can result from nonhepatic factors, but the detection of abnormal concentrations in addition to evidence of liver injury (as detected via changes in leakage or induced enzyme activities) can supply further evidence of significant liver disease, liver failure, or both.

Bilirubin

Normal Bilirubin Metabolism

Bilirubin is a byproduct of hemoglobin breakdown *(Fig. 23.6)* and, to a lesser extent, of the breakdown of other porphyrin-containing compounds (e.g., myoglobin, cytochrome P_{450}, peroxidase, catalase). Erythrocytes normally are destroyed at a constant rate because of aging, but they also can be destroyed at an increased rate because of hemolytic processes (discussed later). Senescent erythrocytes, which have reached the end of their normal life span, are phagocytized by cells in the mononuclear phagocyte system. This occurs primarily in the spleen but also in the liver and the bone marrow. These phagocytized erythrocytes are broken down, and their hemoglobin is dismantled. The globin portion then is converted to amino acids, and the heme portion is split into iron and protoporphyrin. The iron is recycled, but the protoporphyrin is converted first to biliverdin and then to bilirubin. This

bilirubin is released from macrophages and then transported, attached to a protein (e.g., albumin, globulin, or other proteins) to the liver, where it is extracted from the carrier protein and then enters hepatocytes. Passage through the hepatocyte membrane is facilitated by a carrier, the capacity of which can be saturated if too much bilirubin is presented to the liver. This saturation does not occur under normal conditions, but it can occur under those of increased erythrocyte destruction.

Bilirubin that has been carried into hepatocytes attaches to a binding protein, ligandin, which prevents the efflux of bilirubin from the hepatocyte back into the blood and, therefore, influences the net uptake of bilirubin. Free fatty acids compete with bilirubin for ligandin-binding sites. In the hepatocyte, bilirubin is conjugated to sugar groups. In many mammals, the major sugar group to which bilirubin is conjugated is glucuronic acid, and this results in the formation of bilirubin glucuronide. This reaction is catalyzed by the membrane-associated enzyme uridine diphosphoglucuronoside glucuronosyltransferase. Both monoglucuronides and diglucuronides are formed in mammals, with the latter being the predominant form of conjugated bilirubin in bile. In addition to glucuronides, alternate conjugates (e.g., glucosides, glucoside-glucuronide mixed conjugates, xylosides) are produced in some species. Most conjugated bilirubin is secreted into bile canaliculi and excreted in the bile. This form of bilirubin is not protein bound, however, and is more water soluble than the protein-bound, unconjugated bilirubin. A small portion of the bilirubin conjugated in hepatocytes normally passes through the sinusoidal side of the hepatocyte membrane and back into the blood. If this conjugated bilirubin remains unbound to protein, it is quickly excreted by the kidney via glomerular filtration. A portion of the conjugated bilirubin in the blood is bound to protein and is termed *biliprotein* or *delta bilirubin*. This form of conjugated bilirubin does not pass through the glomerular membrane and remains in the blood for a longer period of time. (The implications of delta bilirubin in the assessment of cholestatic disease are discussed later.)

As a result of the processes just described, two types of bilirubin, unconjugated and conjugated, can be found in the blood. Numerous terms are used to describe these two types of bilirubin, and these are summarized in *Table 23.1*.

Conjugated bilirubin that is secreted into bile canaliculi passes with the bile into the small intestine, where conjugated bilirubin is converted to urobilinogen by bacterial reduction. Approximately 90% of the urobilinogen is excreted with the feces as stercobilinogen. The remaining 10% of urobilinogen is reabsorbed and enters the blood. A portion of this urobilinogen then is removed from the blood by the hepatocytes and is reexcreted. Another portion of the urobilinogen circulates to the kidneys, where

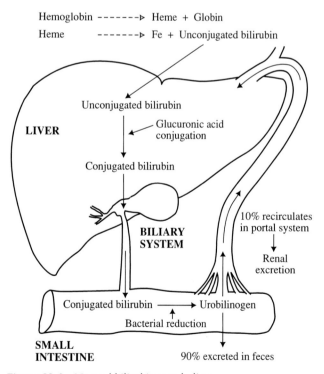

Figure 23.6   Normal bilirubin metabolism.

TABLE 23.1 FORMS OF BILIRUBIN

Bilirubin before Conjugation	Bilirubin after Conjugation
Unconjugated bilirubin	Conjugated bilirubin
Protein-bound bilirubin	Bilirubin glucuronide
Indirect (or indirect-reacting) bilirubin[a]	Direct (or direct-reacting) bilirubin[a]
Prehepatic bilirubin	Posthepatic bilirubin

[a] The terms *indirect-reacting* and *direct-reacting bilirubin* refer to characteristics of the assay for each of these fractions.

it passes through the glomerular membrane and is excreted in the urine.

Abnormalities of Bilirubin Metabolism

Increased serum bilirubin concentrations (i.e., hyperbilirubinemia) can result from any of three alterations in the previously described processes. These abnormalities are increased production of hemoglobin because of increased erythrocyte destruction, decreased uptake or conjugation of bilirubin by hepatocytes, and disruption of bile flow.

Increased production of hemoglobin because of increased erythrocyte destruction usually results from extra- or intravascular hemolysis (see Chapter 8), but it can also result from massive internal hemorrhage and subsequent breakdown of erythrocytes in the area of that hemorrhage. During the process of extravascular hemolysis, macrophages remove and destroy erythrocytes, just as they do senescent erythrocytes but at an accelerated rate. Hemoglobin breakdown and bilirubin delivery to the liver then occurs in a manner identical to that described earlier for normal bilirubin metabolism. During the process of intravascular hemolysis, erythrocytes lyse within the blood, and the free hemoglobin that is released into the blood forms complexes with haptoglobin (i.e., hemoglobin–haptoglobin complexes). These complexes then are removed from the circulation by hepatocytes, and the breakdown of hemoglobin and resulting unconjugated bilirubin production as described earlier occurs in the hepatocytes.

An increased rate of erythrocyte destruction can result in the production of increased amounts of unconjugated bilirubin, which can overwhelm the capacity of carriers in the hepatocyte membrane or the hepatocyte itself. The result is an accumulation of bilirubin in the blood and an increased serum bilirubin concentration. This is termed *prehepatic*, *hemolytic*, or *retention hyperbilirubinemia*.

Decreased uptake or conjugation of bilirubin by hepatocytes can result from decreased delivery of bilirubin

to hepatocytes secondary to decreased hepatic blood flow, a marked decrease in the numbers of hepatocytes because of acute or chronic hepatocyte destruction, or defects in either bilirubin uptake or conjugation by hepatocytes. This is another form of retention hyperbilirubinemia, and it also is termed *hepatic bilirubinemia*.

Retention hyperbilirubinemia of variable magnitudes occurs with decreased food intake because of anorexia or starvation in several species, and it also is referred to as fasting hyperbilirubinemia. This type of hyperbilirubinemia is most marked in horses and can result in serum bilirubin concentrations that plateau at greater than 5 mg/dL by 64 to 136 hours after initial food deprivation. In fasted cattle, as much as threefold increases in the serum total bilirubin concentration can occur after cessation of food intake. Small increases in the serum bilirubin concentration occur in other species when deprived of food. These increases result from an increased serum concentration of unconjugated bilirubin, but they do not appear to relate to increased bilirubin production. Experimental data in horses are suggestive that fasting hyperbilirubinemia relates to increased free fatty acid release from depot fat during food deprivation. Free fatty acid molecules in the blood then are transported to the liver, where they enter hepatocytes and attach to the binding protein, ligandin. The free fatty acids may compete with bilirubin for ligandin-binding sites, thereby resulting in decreased ligandin binding of bilirubin after its uptake by hepatocytes. The net effect is decreased retention of unconjugated bilirubin by hepatocytes, regurgitation of this bilirubin into the blood, and an increased serum unconjugated bilirubin concentration. Other possible mechanisms of fasting hyperbilirubinemia include decreased hepatic blood flow, decreased affinity of hepatocyte membrane carriers for bilirubin molecules, and competition for hepatocyte bilirubin uptake by substances other than free fatty acids that accumulate during fasting.

Disruption of bile flow can be either intra- or extrahepatic. Such disruption usually results from a blockage (partial or complete) in the biliary system. Such blockage causes cholestasis and accumulation of bile in the biliary system (i.e., bile inspissation). Cholestasis most often is associated with inflammation or neoplasia either in or near the biliary system, but it also can occur, though less commonly, secondary to calculi in the biliary system. Blockage of bile flow results in regurgitation of conjugated bilirubin into the blood. Liver diseases that primarily affect the parenchyma rather than the biliary system also can result in cholestasis. In such diseases (e.g., lipidosis, parenchymal inflammation), hepatocyte swelling blocks the small bile canaliculi in the liver and prevents the normal flow of bile. Blockage resulting in increased serum bilirubin concentration can also occur secondary to blockage of the upper small intestine. Leakage of bile into the abdominal cavity resulting from rupture of the gall bladder or bile duct also can result in hyperbilirubinemia. Hyperbilirubinemia resulting from disrupted bile flow is termed *regurgitation hyperbilirubinemia*, though it also is termed *posthepatic* or *cholestatic hyperbilirubinemia*. In theory, most of the increased serum bilirubin in this type of hyperbilirubinemia is conjugated.

If obstruction is the cause of hyperbilirubinemia, the serum ALP and GGT activities are more sensitive indicators of the resultant cholestasis than the serum bilirubin concentration, because these enzyme activities tend to increase more quickly than the serum bilirubin concentration. Because conjugated bilirubin is not bound to protein, it is water soluble and readily passes the glomerulus. An increased urinary bilirubin concentration (i.e., hyperbilirubinuria) is a sensitive indicator of cholestasis or bile leakage, especially in species with a low renal threshold for bilirubin. In dogs, hyperbilirubinuria can precede increases in serum bilirubin concentrations, because conjugated bilirubin that regurgitates into the blood is efficiently excreted by the kidneys and does not immediately accumulate in the blood.

In diseases producing an increased serum conjugated bilirubin concentration, a portion of the conjugated bilirubin is tightly bound to serum protein. This bilirubin has been termed *delta bilirubin* or *biliprotein*. Delta bilirubin is not removed from the serum as quickly as nonprotein-bound, conjugated bilirubin; rather, it is eliminated at a rate approximately equal to the half-life of albumin (~2 weeks). Delta bilirubin is a portion of the serum total bilirubin as measured by routine chemistry methods. The prolonged half-life of delta bilirubin can cause misleading interpretations, however, when these interpretations are made only on the basis of the serum total bilirubin concentration. During cholestatic disease, delta bilirubin tends to accumulate, and the percentage of the serum total bilirubin that is in the delta bilirubin form increases as the disease persists. If cholestasis is eliminated, delta bilirubin still persists in the serum, despite the fact that conjugated bilirubin no longer is escaping into the serum from the biliary system. This results in a persistently increased serum total bilirubin concentration and may lead the clinician to erroneously believe that the cholestasis persists. Such animals may have increased serum total bilirubin concentrations but normal urinary bilirubin concentrations. Practical laboratory methods for the measurement of delta bilirubin concentration exist, and some authors have suggested that serum total bilirubin measurements in dogs should be routinely supplemented with measurement of the serum delta bilirubin concentrations.

Historically, the measurement of serum bilirubin involved not only the measurement of total bilirubin but also the determination of the concentrations of both conjugated and unconjugated bilirubin. In theory, hyperbili-

rubinemia associated with hemolysis or reduced hepatic uptake of bilirubin should produce marked increases in unconjugated bilirubin and smaller, if any, increases in conjugated bilirubin. In addition, and also in theory, cholestasis or leakage of bile should produce marked increases in conjugated bilirubin and smaller, if any, increases in unconjugated bilirubin. Such determinations, however, have been unreliable indicators regarding the cause of hyperbilirubinemia. As a result, most veterinary laboratories now measure only the total bilirubin concentration. If hyperbilirubinemia is detected, then the patient history, physical findings, and results of other laboratory tests can be helpful in differentiating the potential causes. A flow chart for the evaluation of hyperbilirubinemic animals is presented in *Figure 23.7*.

Species differences also should be considered when evaluating serum bilirubin concentrations. Such differences include:

1. Dogs have a low renal threshold for bilirubin. In all species, renal tubules reabsorb conjugated bilirubin that passes the glomerulus. In most species, the tubular epithelial cells efficiently reabsorb this bilirubin; therefore, bilirubin seldom is detected in the urine before

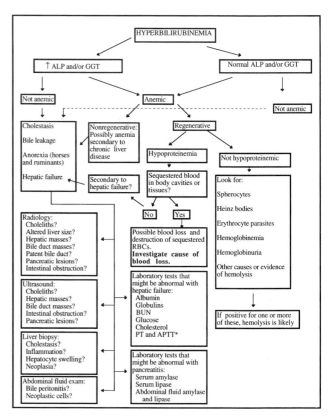

Figure 23.7 Flow chart for the evaluation of hyperbilirubinemic animals. *PT, prothrombiotime; APTT, activated partial thromboplastin time.

hyperbilirubinemia. In dogs, the tubular reabsorptive capacity (i.e., the renal threshold) for bilirubin is low This reabsorptive capacity is lower in male dogs than in female dogs, so a trace of bilirubin is normal in the urine of dogs, especially male dogs, with urine specific gravities of greater than 1.040. In addition, hyperbilirubinuria in dogs frequently occurs before hyperbilirubinemia.

2. Hyperbilirubinemia that is associated with hemolysis, decreased hepatocyte numbers, decreased hepatic blood flow, and cholestasis also can occur in horses. With hemolysis, extreme hyperbilirubinemias can occur (e.g., serum bilirubin concentrations >50 mg/dL). As noted earlier, anorexia or starvation can result in serum bilirubin concentrations of greater than 5 mg/dL in horses. Regardless of the cause of hyperbilirubinemia in horses, most of the bilirubin in the blood is unconjugated.

3. In ruminants, bilirubin concentrations are not consistently increased in animals with liver disease. Significant hyperbilirubinemias most often result from hemolysis. Cholestasis in ruminants can result in moderate increases of serum bilirubin, but this is not a consistent finding. Hyperbilirubinemia, possibly related to anorexia and rumen stasis, has been noted in several ruminant diseases (discussed earlier), and two forms of inherited hyperbilirubinemias have been identified in sheep. Mutant Southdown sheep can have hyperbilirubinemia associated with defective hepatocyte uptake of bilirubin from the serum. This is similar to Gilbert syndrome in humans, and it produces an increased serum unconjugated bilirubin concentration. Mutant Corredale sheep can have hyperbilirubinemia associated with defective hepatic excretion of conjugated bilirubin, and this produces an increased serum conjugated bilirubin concentration and is similar to Dubin-Johnson syndrome in humans. The renal threshold for bilirubin is low in cattle, and as many as 25% of normal cattle can have traces of bilirubin in their urine.

Bile Acids

Measurement of serum bile acid concentrations has been a useful liver function test in several species. Normally, small amounts of bile acids are present in the blood. Increased serum bile acid concentrations, however, can occur with several different hepatic and biliary abnormalities. Such increases are very sensitive and specific indicators of these abnormalities.

Bile acids are synthesized in hepatocytes from cholesterol *(Fig. 23.8)*. Cholic acid and chenodeoxycholic acid are the primary bile acids in most animals. After their synthesis, bile acids are conjugated to amino acids (primar-

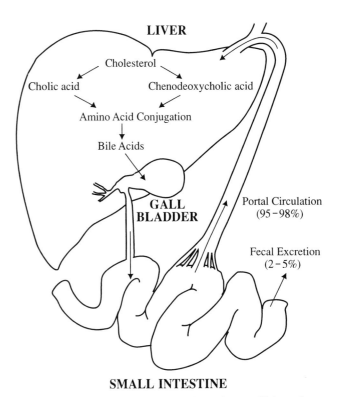

Figure 23.8 Normal production and circulation of bile acid.

ily taurine in most animals). This conjugation makes bile acids more soluble in water, and these bile acids then are secreted into the biliary system. In animals with gallbladders, the bile acids are stored and concentrated there. At the time of a meal, hormonal and neurohormonal factors stimulate gallbladder contraction and passage of bile acids into the small intestine, where dehydroxylation by anaerobic microorganisms results in the conversion of the primary bile acids to secondary bile acids. Thus, cholic acid is converted to deoxycholic acid, and chenodeoxycholic acid is converted to lithocholic acid. Bile acids emulsify fat and, therefore, promote both the digestion and absorption of fat as well as of fat-soluble vitamins. Most of the bile acids are reabsorbed into the blood from the ileum (<5% of the bile acid pool is lost in the feces each day). Normally, the liver very efficiently clears bile acids from the portal circulation on their first pass through the liver; as a result, only a slight postprandial increase in serum bile acid concentrations is seen in healthy animals. Bile acids that are cleared by hepatocytes are secreted into the biliary system and recirculate; a bile acid molecule recirculates several times after a meal.

Possible causes of increased bile acid concentrations include:

1. Deviation of the portal circulation, which causes it to merge abnormally with the systemic circulation (e.g.,

portosystemic shunts, severe cirrhosis). In this situation, blood is shunted away from hepatocytes, which, therefore, cannot perform first-pass clearing of bile acids.

2. Decrease in the intrinsic hepatocyte uptake of bile acids. This is a major factor in many liver diseases (e.g., hepatitis, necrosis, glucocorticoid hepatopathy) and, in some, relates to decreased functional hepatic mass.
3. Decreased bile acid excretion via the biliary system and subsequent regurgitation into the systemic circulation. This most often results from cholestasis (e.g., cholangitis, bile duct blockage, intestinal obstruction, neoplasia) but also could occur with leakage from the bile duct or gallbladder.

Bile acid assays are most useful for animals in which liver disease is suspected but not unequivocally proven on the basis of routine biochemical profile tests. Such tests may shows results, for instance, of increased serum ALP or GGT activities but normal serum bilirubin, or increased serum bilirubin but normal or equivocally increased liver enzyme activities. Although assaying bile acid concentrations in animals with icterus or hyperbilirubinemia usually does not add useful information, serum bile acid assay may be helpful in differentiating hemolytic hyperbilirubinemia from hepatic or cholestatic hyperbilirubinemia in those rare cases in which a hemolytic cause is not obvious and liver enzyme activities are equivocal. Bile acids do not compete with bilirubin for uptake or metabolism by hepatocytes; therefore, a hemolytic hyperbilirubinemia possibly may occur without a concurrent increase in serum bile acid concentrations.

Bile acid assays are readily available. Bile acids are stable at room temperature for several days, and serum for bile acid assays can be frozen. Hemolysis can result in falsely decreased bile acid concentrations, however, and lipemia can result in falsely increased bile acid concentrations.

In dogs and cats, fasting (i.e., preprandial) and postprandial samples usually are collected for bile acid assays. A standard procedure is the following:

1. The patient is fasted for 12 hours before collection of the serum sample (i.e., fasting sample).
2. A fat-containing diet is fed. This diet must be of adequate volume and contain adequate fat to stimulate cholecystokinin secretion by the small intestine and subsequent gallbladder contraction. Growth diets with higher fat content are recommended. In animals with potential hepatoencephalopathy, a restricted-protein diet can be used but should be supplemented with corn oil to increase the fat content to approximately 5%.
3. A serum sample is collected at 2 hours after feeding (i.e., postprandial sample).

4. Both fasting and postprandial bile acid concentrations are measured.

Fasting bile acid concentration of greater than 20 μmol/L and postprandial bile acid concentration of greater than 25 μmol/L are very specific for liver disease in dogs and cats. A fasting bile acid concentration of less than 5 μmol/L is normal in dogs and cats, and concentrations from 5 to 20 μmol/L are suggestive of hepatic disease. Fasting bile acid concentrations of as great as 20 μmol/L, however, occasionally occur in normal dogs and cats. Fasting bile acid concentrations from 5 to 20 μmol/L in dogs and cats should be interpreted in light of the patient history, clinical signs, and results of diagnostic imaging as well as other laboratory tests for hepatic disease or function.

In dogs, an increased fasting or postprandial serum bile acid concentration (or both) can occur with a variety of liver diseases, including portosystemic shunts, cholestasis, cirrhosis, necrosis, hepatitis, hepatic lipidosis, glucocorticoid hepatopathy, and neoplasia. In most of these diseases, postprandial bile acid concentrations are markedly increased compared with fasting bile acid concentrations, but this is not consistently true in all liver diseases. Exaggerated increases in postprandial bile acid concentrations are most consistent and marked in animals with portosystemic shunts. Extremely high fasting or postprandial bile acid concentrations are more likely to be associated with some types of liver diseases compared with others, but defining the type of liver disease on the basis of the bile acid concentrations alone is not possible. Abnormal bile acid concentrations are an indication for further testing (e.g., liver biopsy, radiologic studies, ultrasound) aimed at identifying the specific type of liver disease that is present. In general, either fasting or postprandial bile acid concentrations are more sensitive for the detection of liver disease in dogs than most other tests for liver injury or function.

In cats, increased serum bile acid concentrations in either fasting or postprandial samples are suggestive of hepatic disease, including portosystemic shunts, cholestasis, cirrhosis, necrosis, hepatitis, hepatic lipidosis, and neoplasia. Results of bile acid assays are useful in identifying the presence of liver disease in cats, but they do not reliably differentiate the different types of liver diseases. Bile acid measurement in cats should be performed only if other serum biochemical results are suggestive of possible liver disease. Increased postprandial bile acid concentrations are more sensitive for the detection of hepatic lipidosis, portosystemic shunts, and various causes of cholestasis than either liver enzyme tests (e.g., ALT, AST, ALP, GGT) or other liver function tests (e.g., albumin, blood urea nitrogen [BUN], cholesterol, bilirubin). Fasting bile acid concentrations in cats with these diseases are less consistently increased, and measuring both fasting and postprandial bile acid concentrations in cats suspected of having liver disease is desirable.

Postprandial bile acid concentrations occasionally are lower than fasting bile acid concentrations in dogs and cats. This may result from spontaneous emptying of the gallbladder during the fasting period, before the fasting blood sample was obtained, thereby causing a high fasting serum bile acid concentration.

In horses, ruminants, and llamas, a single sample usually is collected for a bile acid assay. Reference intervals in these species tend to be wider than those in dogs and cats. In nonfasted dairy cattle, bile acid reference intervals range from 27 to 323 μmol/L and from 18 to 79 μmol/L at the point of peak milk production and at the end of the lactation period, respectively. The reference interval is narrower in some, but not all, fasted dairy cattle, ranging from 3 to 31 μmol/L reported after a 14-hour fast. The importance of fasting cattle before measurement of the serum bile acid concentration, however, is not clearly documented. The reference interval for serum bile acid concentration in beef cattle ranges from 9 to 126 μmol/L. Hour-to-hour fluctuations of serum bile acid concentrations as high as 250 μmol/L occur in lactating dairy cattle. In llamas older than 1 year, the reference interval for serum bile acid concentration ranges from 1 to 23 μmol/L. Wider reference intervals occur in llamas younger than 1 year (2–50 μmol/L). Fluctuations over time and after feeding are minimal in llamas.

In horses, the serum bile acid reference interval has varied in different studies, but the upper limit of this interval is less than 20 μmol/L. Horses continuously secrete bile into the intestinal tract because of their lack of a gallbladder and the weakness of the sphincter of the common bile duct. Fasting may increase serum bile acid concentrations in horses, with values as great as 25 μmol/L being reported after 3 to 4 days of fasting.

Because only one sample is collected in horses, ruminants, and llamas, an increased bile acid concentration is suggestive of hepatic disease. Results, however, must be correlated with other laboratory findings and clinical signs. Basic abnormalities that may cause increased bile acid concentrations are similar to those listed for dogs and cats.

Decreased serum bile acid concentrations can result from:

1. Delayed gastric emptying after a meal, which leads to delayed emptying of the gallbladder and results in a lower postprandial increase in dogs and cats.
2. Delayed intestinal transit time, which delays the delivery of bile acids to the ileum, where most bile acid reabsorption occurs and results in a lower postprandial increase in dogs and cats.

3. Diseases of the ileum, which can result in decreased reabsorption of bile acids.

Failure of hepatic synthesis does not result in decreased serum bile acid concentrations.

Plasma Ammonia Concentration and Ammonia Tolerance Test

Ammonia is produced in the digestive tract and absorbed from the intestine into the blood. It then is carried by the portal circulation to the liver, where it is removed. Alterations in blood flow to the liver or markedly decreased numbers of functional hepatocytes can result in increased blood ammonia concentrations. Blood ammonia measurement or performance of the ammonia tolerance test may be used to assess liver function. These tests are useful, but measurement of fasting and postprandial bile acid concentrations is both more sensitive for the detection of abnormalities in hepatic blood flow or hepatocyte numbers and easier to perform.

Ammonia concentrations typically are measured using plasma. Ammonia concentrations in blood are very unstable after collection, however, which may preclude routine use of this test in clinical practice. A procedure for the collection and storage of plasma for an ammonia assay is as follows:

1. Simple-stomached animals are fasted for at least 8 hours before sampling.
2. Blood is collected (check with the laboratory being used for specific sample requirements) and immediately placed in an ice bath, and the plasma is separated within 30 minutes of collection. Erythrocytes contain two- to threefold as much ammonia as plasma, and prolonged contact can produce falsely increased plasma ammonia concentrations.
3. Plasma is refrigerated (0–5°C) and assayed within 60 minutes. Plasma should not be frozen, because blood ammonia is unstable in frozen plasma.

Increased plasma ammonia concentrations most commonly are found in animals with portosystemic shunting of blood (either congenital shunts or shunting secondary to severe cirrhosis), but these results are not considered to be very sensitive for establishing the diagnosis of these disorders. Increased blood ammonia concentrations also can occur with the loss of 60% or more of the hepatic functional mass.

The ammonia tolerance test generally is performed on animals in which portosystemic shunts are suspected but high baseline blood ammonia concentrations are not present. If the ammonia tolerance test is performed on animals with high blood ammonia concentrations, a markedly increased blood ammonia concentration could result and, in turn, produce adverse clinical effects. A suggested procedure is as follows:

1. A fasting heparinized (preadministration) blood sample is collected. Ammonia-free heparin must be used.
2. Ammonium chloride solution (20 mg/ml) at a dosage of 100 mg/kg body weight is administered via a stomach tube.
3. A total dose of 3 g should not be exceeded.
4. A 30-minute postadministration heparinized blood sample is collected.

The preadministration-to-postadministration increase of blood ammonia in normal dogs is from 2.0- to 2.5-fold. Most dogs with portosystemic shunts have postadministration increases of three- to 10-fold the preadministration concentrations.

Because of technical difficulties with the blood ammonia and ammonia tolerance tests, an assay of the serum bile acid concentration usually is preferable to these tests.

Bromosulfophthalein Excretion

Bromosulfophthalein (BSP) is a dye that is administered intravenously and that circulates bound to protein (primarily albumin) until removed from the blood by hepatocytes. In hepatocytes, BSP is conjugated and then excreted in the bile. Measurement of BSP excretion, therefore, is a test of the hepatic blood flow. In addition, this test measures the ability of hepatocytes to remove BSP from the blood for conjugation and excretion as well as the patency and integrity of the biliary system.

Historically, the BSP excretion test has been useful for assessing liver function in animals, but this dye has caused occasional anaphylactic reactions in humans and, therefore, no longer is commercially available. Measurement of the serum bile acid concentration is more specific for hepatic disease than the BSP excretion test, because BSP excretion by the liver is affected by several nonhepatic factors that do not affect the bile acid concentration. Serum bile acid concentrations also are more sensitive indicators of hepatobiliary disease in dogs and cats. In addition, bile acid measurement is easier to perform than the BSP excretion test, because it does not require the injection of a dye.

Indocyanine Green Excretion

Indocyanine green (ICG) is a dye that is administered intravenously and that circulates bound to protein (primarily albumin and β-lipoprotein) until removed from the blood by hepatocytes. Indocyanine green dye is excreted in the bile in an unconjugated form. The ICG excretion test assesses the hepatic blood flow and the ability of hepatocytes to remove ICG from the blood as well as the patency and integrity of the biliary system. Indocyanine green dye is commercially available, but the test requires several timed blood collections to be performed after the injection of the dye. The ICG excretion test, therefore, is more complicated to perform than a bile acid measurement, and it offers no significant advantages compared with measurement of bile acid concentrations, being affected by more interfering factors than bile acids are. Therefore, this test seldom is performed in clinical settings.

Albumin

Hypoalbuminemia usually is not noted until 60% to 80% of hepatic function is lost. There appear to be some species differences, however, in the incidence of hypoalbuminemia accompanying liver disease. Hypoalbuminemia is quite common in dogs with chronic liver diseases (>60% have hypoalbuminemia), but it does not appear to be as common in horses with chronic liver diseases (~20% have hypoalbuminemia).

Globulins

Although most globulins functioning in the immune system are synthesized in lymphoid tissue, several other types are synthesized in the liver. Hepatic failure can result in decreased synthesis and, therefore, decreased serum concentrations of these globulins. The globulin concentration usually does not decrease as much as the albumin concentration, and the albumin:globulin ratio commonly decreases because of hepatic failure. In some cases, globulin concentrations may increase with chronic liver disease. Frequently, both beta and gamma globulin concentrations increase, resulting in a bridging (beta–gamma bridging) between the peaks of these two fractions on an electrophoretogram (Fig. 23.9). This has been especially well documented for horses, in which more than 50% of those with chronic hepatic disease also have increased globulin concentrations. In animals with severe liver disease, the clearance of foreign proteins by the Kupffer cells of the liver is theorized to be decreased. Such foreign proteins are thought to be absorbed from the intestine and carried to the liver by the portal circulation. Thus, when Kupffer cells fail to efficiently clear these proteins on their first passage through the liver, they come in contact with the immune system in other parts of the body, and an immune response to these proteins then occurs, thereby resulting in hyperglobulinemia.

Glucose

The liver plays a key role in glucose metabolism. Glucose that has been absorbed by the small intestine is transported to the liver via the portal circulation and then en-

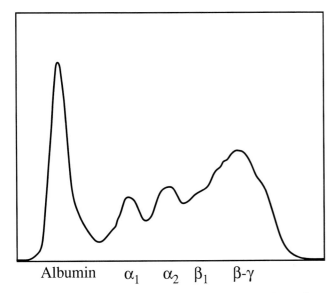

Figure 23.9 Electrophoretogram from a horse with chronic liver disease. Both the beta globulin and gamma globulin concentrations are increased, which has resulted in bridging between the beta and gamma globulin peaks (beta–gamma bridging).

Albumin   α₁   α₂   β₁   β-γ

ters hepatocytes. The hepatocytes convert glucose to glycogen, which helps to regulate the blood glucose concentration. Hepatocytes also synthesize glucose via gluconeogenesis and release stored glucose via glycogenolysis. In animals with hepatic failure, glucose concentrations can vary from decreased to increased. These concentrations may be increased because of decreased hepatic glucose uptake, thereby resulting in prolonged postprandial hyperglycemia. Conversely, these concentrations may be decreased because of reduced hepatocytic gluconeogenesis or glycogenolysis.

Urea

Urea is synthesized in hepatocytes from ammonia. In animals with liver failure, the decrease in hepatocyte numbers results in decreased conversion of ammonia to urea. Consequently, the blood ammonia concentration increases, and the BUN concentration decreases. However, BUN concentrations also may decrease because of numerous other disorders (see Chapter 21).

Cholesterol

Bile is a major route of cholesterol excretion from the body. Therefore, interference with bile flow (i.e., cholestasis) can result in increased serum cholesterol concentrations (i.e., hypercholesterolemia). Many other nonhepatic disorders, however, also can result in hypercholesterolemia (see Chapter 28).

The liver also is a major site of cholesterol synthesis. In some forms of hepatic failure, decreased cholesterol syn-

thesis can lead to decreased blood cholesterol concentrations (i.e., hypocholesterolemia). The balance between decreased cholesterol synthesis and decreased cholesterol excretion appears to vary with different types of liver disease. If decreased synthesis of cholesterol is the major alteration in hepatic failure, hypocholesterolemia can result. If, however, cholestasis is the major alteration, hypercholesterolemia may occur. In many animals with liver failure, the serum cholesterol concentrations are normal.

Coagulation Factors

The liver synthesizes most of the coagulation factors (i.e., factors I, II, V, IX, and X). In addition, the blockage of bile flow can result in decreased absorption of vitamin K and decreased production of vitamin K–dependent coagulation factors (i.e., factors II, VII, IX, and X). In patients with liver failure, reduced synthesis of these factors can prolong the one-stage prothrombin time and the activated partial thromboplastin time. These test results are prolonged if the concentration of any factor involved in that test decreases to less than 30% of normal. Coagulation disorders are common in dogs with liver failure, but they are rare in large animals with liver failure. If an animal has a coagulation disorder and evidence of hepatic disease, the coagulation disorder should be fully evaluated using the tests discussed in Chapter 14, because causes other than hepatic failure (e.g., disseminated intravascular coagulation) should be considered.

TYPICAL LABORATORY CHANGES IN VARIOUS TYPES OF HEPATIC DISEASE

The spectrum and potential magnitude of changes in laboratory test results for common liver diseases are summarized in *Table 23.2*. The most typical changes in different types of liver diseases are listed, but one should be aware that these changes are inconsistent, that a good deal of overlap is seen in different liver diseases, and that characterization of the specific type of liver disease often is not possible on the basis of laboratory results alone. In many cases, laboratory results simply reveal the presence of liver disease, and other tests (e.g., liver biopsy, radiographic studies, ultrasound) are necessary to more specifically characterize the disease.

Portosystemic Shunt

Portal systemic shunting of blood can be acquired because of severe cirrhosis, and if this is the case, test results similar to those described for end-stage liver disease are expected. Early congenital portosystemic shunts usually

TABLE 23.2 LABORATORY TESTS FOR LIVER DAMAGE AND FUNCTION

Disease Process	Leakage Enzymes	Induced Enzymes	Bilirubin	Bile Acids	Other Function Tests	Other Abnormalities
Congenital portosystemic shunt	ALT = N to ↑ AST = N to ↑	ALP = N to ↑ (possible bone origin in young dogs) GGT = N	N	Fasting = N to ↑↑ Postprandial = ↑↑ to ↑↑↑	Ammonia = N to ↑ Ammonia tolerance = abnormal Albumin = N to ↓ BUN = N to ↓ Glucose = N to ↓ Cholesterol = N to ↓	Microcytosis in 33%–72% of dogs
Focal to multifocal necrosis	N to ↑↑	N	N	N	N	
Diffuse necrosis	↑↑ to ↑↑↑	N to ↑↑	N to ↑↑	Fasting = N to ↑↑ Postprandial = N to ↑↑	Variable	
Hypoxia or mild toxemia	↑ to ↑↑	N to ↑	N	Fasting = N to ↑ Postprandial = N to ↑	N	
Focal lesions Abscesses Infarcts Neoplasms	N to ↑	N to ↑↑	N to ↑	Fasting = N to ↑ Postprandial = N to ↑	N	
Diffuse lipidosis	ALT = N to ↑↑↑ AST = N to ↑↑↑	ALP = N to ↑↑↑ GGT = N to ↑	N to ↑↑↑	Fasting = N to ↑↑↑ Postprandial = ↑ to ↑↑↑	Pro time = ↑ in ≈ 45% ACT = ↑ in ≈ 35%	Glucose = ↑↑ if diabetes mellitus Poikilocytosis in RBCs common in red blood cells
Steroid hepatopathy (dogs)	ALT = N to ↑↑ AST = N to ↑↑	ALP = ↑ to ↑↑↑ GGT = ↑ to ↑↑↑	N to ↑	Fasting = N to ↑ Postprandial = N to ↑↑	N	
Cholangitis, cholangiohepatitis, bile duct obstruction	ALT = ↑ to ↑↑ AST = ↑ to ↑↑	ALP = ↑ to ↑↑↑ GGT = N to ↑↑↑	N to ↑↑↑	Fasting = N to ↑↑↑ Postprandial = ↑ to ↑↑↑	N, unless at end stage	
Chronic liver disease (including diffuse neoplasia)	ALT = N to ↑↑ AST = N to ↑↑	ALP = N to ↑↑↑ GGT = N to ↑↑	N to ↑↑	Fasting = N to ↑↑↑ Postprandial = N to ↑↑↑	Variable	
End-stage liver disease (liver failure)	ALT = N to ↑↑ AST = N to ↑↑	ALP = N to ↑↑↑ GGT = N ↑↑↑	↑↑ to ↑↑↑	Fasting = N to ↑↑↑ Postprandial = N to ↑↑↑	Ammonia = N to ↑ Albumin = N to ↓ Globulins = ↓, N or ↑ BUN = N to ↓ Glucose = N to ↓ Cholesterol = N to ↓ Coagulation tests = prolonged	

ACT, activated clotting time. *Pro time*, prothrombin time.
a May be normal in rare cases of end-stage liver disease.

do not produce a high degree of active hepatocyte damage. Consequently, leakage enzyme activities often are normal or only slightly increased. Cholestasis is not a feature of congenital portosystemic shunts, and increased production of ALP and GGT is not induced by this disease. Because congenital shunts most commonly occur in young animals with growing bones, however, mildly increased serum ALP activity, which probably is osteoblastic in origin, is common. Because blood delivery to the liver is impaired, increased fasting or postprandial bile acid concentrations are common, and these changes may be marked. Liver atrophy is a common sequela to portosystemic shunts; therefore, tests of hepatic function can be abnormal in more chronic cases. Microcytic anemia is a common occurrence in dogs with portosystemic shunts and appears to relate to the sequestration of iron in tissues such as the liver and to low serum iron concentrations in many of these dogs. Abnormal lipid metabolism producing alterations in erythrocyte membrane cholesterol and triglyceride content also may play a role in the development of microcytosis in dogs with portosystemic shunts.

Hepatic Necrosis

Hepatic necrosis can vary from focal to multifocal to diffuse. Focal to multifocal hepatic necrosis can result in increased activities of leakage enzymes, but these increases are less frequent and of lesser magnitude than those resulting from diffuse necrosis. Focal necrosis usually does not cause significant cholestasis, and induced enzyme activities usually remain normal. Diffuse necrosis is more likely to compromise the flow of bile and, therefore, to cause cholestasis. Thus, activities of induced enzymes may increase with diffuse necrosis. Bile acid concentrations usually are not affected by focal necrosis, but diffuse necrosis can produce increases in bile acid concentrations because of decreased hepatocyte removal of bile acids from the portal circulation as well as cholestasis. Tests of hepatic function are not affected by focal necrosis, but if more than 60% to 80% of the hepatic mass is lost because of diffuse necrosis, results of liver function tests (i.e., albumin, BUN, glucose, cholesterol, coagulation) may be abnormal.

Hypoxia or Mild Toxic Damage

Hypoxia or mild toxic damage (possibly secondary to endotoxins, mycotoxins, or other toxicants) can result in mild injury to many hepatocytes. As a result, activities of leakage enzymes can be mildly to moderately increased. These changes usually do not cause cholestasis, and the activities of induced enzymes usually are normal. If the cell swelling resulting from these conditions is severe enough, however, swollen hepatocytes may impinge on bile canaliculi and cause cholestasis as well as increased activities of induced enzymes. This cholestasis usually is not severe enough to result in increased serum bilirubin concentrations, but in conjunction with decreased bile acid clearance by hepatocytes, it can result in mild increases of fasting or postprandial bile acid concentrations.

Focal Lesions

Focal lesions such as abscesses, infarcts, or localized neoplasms may only cause local hepatocyte damage, in which case the activities of leakage enzymes are normal or mildly increased. The activities of these enzymes depend on the time and the extent of hepatocyte damage. Expansion of abscesses or neoplasms into the surrounding tissue may be slow and result in only a few hepatocytes being damaged during any given period of time. Activities of induced enzymes usually are normal but may be increased if the focal lesion causes significant cholestasis. Serum bilirubin concentrations or fasting and postprandial bile acid concentrations occasionally are increased. The pathogenesis of this is not clear, however, because these lesions seldom occlude bile ducts that are large enough to interfere significantly with bile flow. Other tests of hepatic function usually are normal, because 60% to 80% of the hepatic mass is not lost with focal lesions.

Hepatic Lipidosis

Hepatic lipidosis occurs in many species, but the syndrome has been documented best in cats. Serum activities of leakage enzymes are mildly to markedly increased in more than 75% of cats with hepatic lipidosis, and this increase probably results from marked lipid accumulation in hepatocytes. More than 80% of cats with hepatic lipidosis have increased serum ALP activities, varying from mild to marked, whereas approximately 15% have increased serum GGT activities. Serum activities of these induced enzymes probably are increased because of swollen hepatocytes that impinge on bile canaliculi, with resultant cholestasis. The serum bilirubin concentrations are increased in a high percentage of cats (~75%) with this disease, probably because of cholestasis. Fasting or postprandial serum bile acid concentrations often are increased, probably resulting from impaired hepatocyte removal of bile acids from the portal blood as well as cholestasis. Other tests of hepatic function are inconsistently abnormal. If diabetes mellitus is the underlying problem in cats with hepatic lipidosis, blood glucose concentrations may be very high. A relatively high percentage of affected cats with hepatic lipidosis also have prolonged prothrombin times (40%) and activated coagulation times (35%), but only approximately 10% have prolonged activated partial thromboplastin times.

Steroid (Glucocorticoid) Hepatopathy

Steroid hepatopathies are most common in dogs, and they produce moderate damage to hepatocytes. The serum activities of leakage enzymes usually are mildly increased in dogs with steroid hepatopathies. The serum activities of induced enzymes are markedly increased in this disease because of corticosteroid-mediated induction of the synthesis of these enzymes. Occasionally, serum bilirubin concentrations are mildly increased. Fasting or postprandial serum bile acid concentrations are inconsistently increased in dogs with steroid hepatopathies, and other tests of hepatic function usually are normal.

Biliary Abnormalities

Cholangitis, cholangiohepatitis, and extrahepatic bile duct obstruction can occur in many different species. Because lesions usually are centered in the portal areas of the liver or outside of the liver, increased serum activities of leakage enzymes usually are mild and result from secondary damage to hepatocytes caused by increased intrabiliary pressure. The serum activities of induced enzymes are markedly increased and become progressively higher as the disease becomes more severe. Increased intrabiliary pressure induces hepatocytes and biliary epithelial cells to produce increased amounts of these enzymes. Serum bilirubin concentrations are moderately to markedly increased because of the blockage of bile flow. Both fasting and postprandial serum bile acid concentrations usually are increased, and sometimes markedly so, resulting from the blockage of bile flow. Other tests of hepatic function usually are normal, unless these diseases progress to end-stage liver disease.

Chronic Progressive Liver Diseases

Chronic progressive liver diseases can occur in many species but are most common in dogs. Moderate to severe inflammation is a common feature, and variable degrees of hepatocyte necrosis, fibrosis, and cirrhosis also can occur. Several dog breeds are predisposed to such diseases. In some, such as Bedlington and West Highland White Terriers, chronic hepatitis may result from inherited disorders, thereby resulting in abnormal copper accumulation in the liver. In others, such as Doberman pinschers, Skye terriers, and cocker spaniels, familial predispositions toward chronic hepatitis exist, but the causes and relationships of these diseases to hepatic copper accumulation are not clear. Certain drugs (e.g., anticonvulsants) and infectious agents also may cause chronic hepatitis in dogs. Serum activities of leakage enzymes often are mildly or moderately increased because of progressive hepatocyte damage. If progression of the disease is slow, the release of these enzymes within a given period of time may be minimal, with normal serum activity of the leakage enzymes. Many of these diseases ultimately result in varying degrees of hepatic fibrosis, however, which may compromise bile flow. Serum activities of induced enzymes, therefore, often are mildly or moderately increased. Serum bilirubin concentrations are normal in animals with the early, less severe forms but can be increased in those with later, more advanced disease. Fasting and postprandial serum bile acid concentrations are inconsistently increased, depending on how far the disease has advanced. These increases probably relate to impaired blood flow to the liver, impaired clearance of bile acid by hepatocytes, and cholestasis. Other tests of hepatic function are normal, unless the disease has resulted in the loss of 60% to 80% of functional capacity.

End-Stage Liver Disease

End-stage liver disease occurs when more than 60% to 80% of the hepatic functional mass has been lost. The serum activities of leakage enzymes are normal or moderately increased. Normal serum activities of these enzymes may result from markedly decreased numbers of hepatocytes or minimal active hepatocyte damage. Serum activities of induced enzymes are moderately to markedly increased because of cholestasis. Serum bilirubin concentrations are moderately to markedly increased. Fasting or postprandial serum bile acid concentrations are increased, and sometimes markedly so, and result from decreased hepatic blood flow, impaired hepatocyte uptake of bile acids from portal blood, and cholestasis. Many other hepatic function tests are abnormal, including increased blood ammonia concentrations, decreased blood glucose concentrations, decreased BUN concentrations, and decreased serum albumin concentrations. Serum globulin concentrations vary from mildly decreased to increased. Coagulation tests also often are abnormal in animals with end-stage liver disease.

SUGGESTED READINGS

Anderson JG, Washabau RJ. Icterus. Comp Cont Educ 1992;14: 1045–1059.

Bostwick DR, Twedt DC. Intrahepatic and extrahepatic portal venous anomalies in dogs: 52 cases (1982–1992). J Am Vet Med Assoc 1995;206:1181–1185.

Cebra CK, Garry FB, Getzy DM, Fettman MJ. Hepatic lipidosis in anorectic, lactating Holstein cattle: a retrospective study of serum biochemical abnormalities. J Vet Intern Med 1997;11:231–237.

Center SA, Baldwin BH, Dillingham S, et al. Diagnostic value of serum gamma glutamyl transferase and alkaline phosphatase activities in hepatobiliary disease in the cat. J Am Vet Med Assoc 1986;188: 507–510.

Center SA, Crawford MA, Guida L, et al. A retrospective study of 77 cats with severe hepatic lipidosis: 1975–1990. J Vet Intern Med 1993;7: 349–359.

Center SA, Erb HN, Joseph SA. Measurement of serum bile acids concentrations for diagnosis of hepatobiliary disease in cats. J Am Vet Med Assoc 1995;207:1048–1054.

Center SA, Manwarren T, Slater MR, et al. Evaluation of twelve-hour preprandial and two-hour postprandial serum bile acids concentrations for diagnosis of hepatobiliary disease in dogs. J Am Vet Med Assoc 1991;199:217–226.

Center SA, Slater MR, Manwarren T, et al. Diagnostic efficiency of serum alkaline phosphatase and gamma glutamyl transferase in dogs with histologically confirmed hepatobiliary disease: 270 cases (1980–1990). J Am Vet Med Assoc 1992;201:1258–1264.

Garry FB, Fettman MJ, Curtis CR, Smith JA. Serum bile acid concentrations in dairy cattle with hepatic lipidosis. J Vet Intern Med 1994; 8:432–438.

Engelking LR. Evaluation of equine bilirubin and bile metabolism. Comp Cont Educ 1989;11:328–336.

Hoffman WE, Rengar WE, Forner JL. Alkaline phosphatase and alkaline phosphatase isoenzymes in the cat. Vet Clin Pathol 1977;6:21–24.

Hoffman WE, Sanecki RK, Dorner JL. A technique for automated quantification of canine glucocorticoid-induced isoenzyme of alkaline phosphatase. Vet Clin Pathol 1988;17:66–70.

Meyer DJ, Williams DA. Diagnosis of hepatic and exocrine pancreatic disorders. Semin Vet Med Surg Small Anim 1992;7:275–284.

Neer TM. A review of disorders of the gallbladder and extrahepatic biliary tract in the dog and cat. J Vet Intern Med 1992;6:186–192.

Parraga ME, Carlson GP, Thurmond M. Serum protein concentrations in horses with severe liver disease: a retrospective study and review of the literature. J Vet Intern Med 1995;9:154–161.

Rothuizen J, van den Ingh T. Covalently protein-bound bilirubin conjugates in cholestatic disease of dogs. Am J Vet Res 1988;49:702–704.

Simpson KW, Meyer DJ, Boswood A, et al. Iron status and erythrocyte volume in dogs with congenital portosystemic vascular anomalies. J Vet Intern Med 1997;11:14–19.

Solter PE, Hoffman WE, Hungerford LL, et al. Assessment of corticosteroid-induced alkaline phosphatase isoenzyme as a screening test for hyperadrenocorticism in dogs. J Am Vet Med Assoc 1993; 203:534–538.

Swenson CL, Graves TK. Absence of liver specificity for canine alanine aminotransferase (ALT). Vet Clin Pathol 1997;26:26–28.

24

LABORATORY EVALUATION

OF THE EXOCRINE PANCREAS

The primary function of the exocrine pancreas is the synthesis and secretion of digestive enzymes. These enzymes include trypsinogen, chymotrypsinogen, proelastase, and procarboxypeptidases, all of which hydrolyze protein when activated; lipase, which hydrolyzes lipids; and amylase, which hydrolyzes starches.

Two major disorders of the exocrine pancreas can be detected by laboratory evaluation:

- **Injury to the pancreatic parenchyma,** resulting in the leakage of pancreatic enzymes into the pancreatic interstitium and peritoneal cavity. These enzymes ultimately pass into the blood, as evidenced by their increased activities in serum. Pancreatic injury most commonly results from inflammation of the pancreas (i.e., pancreatitis). Intraperitoneal release of pancreatic enzymes causes tissue damage in the area of the pancreas, thereby increasing both the severity and the extent of the inflammation.
- **Insufficient production and secretion of pancreatic enzymes,** resulting from loss of pancreatic acinar cells. This disorder is termed *exocrine pancreatic insufficiency*, and it results in inadequate digestive function (i.e., maldigestion).

DETECTION OF PANCREATIC INJURY

The diagnosis of pancreatitis can be extremely difficult to establish. Clinical signs and patient history often are suggestive, but laboratory testing as well as radiologic or ultrasound studies (or both) are necessary to confirm the diagnosis. Unfortunately, laboratory tests often are neither sensitive nor specific indicators of pancreatitis. The most commonly used tests for detecting pancreatic injury are serum assays for the activities of pancreatic digestive enzymes that have leaked from injured pancreatic acinar cells. Serum amylase and lipase activities are the most common of these assays, but more recently, serum trypsin-like immunoreactivity also has been used.

Serum Amylase

Serum Amylase in Dogs

Amylase is present in several tissues in dogs. The highest concentrations occur in the pancreas and the small intestinal mucosa. The source of serum amylase activity in normal dogs is controversial. Some authors report it to be of pancreatic origin, whereas others indicate that a source other than the pancreas is more likely. Dogs with azotemia commonly have increased serum amylase activities, and the kidneys appear to play a key role in determining these activities. The exact mechanism by which this occurs, however, is controversial (discussed later). Causes of increased serum amylase activity in dogs include:

▪ **Pancreatic injury.** Injury or death of pancreatic acinar cells results in the leakage of amylase from these cells. Pancreatitis is the most common cause of such injury. In some cases, blockage of the pancreatic duct also may cause increased serum amylase activity because of the resorption of pancreatic secretions from the pancreatic duct system.

▪ **Renal dysfunction.** Approximately 60% of dogs with renal failure have increased serum amylase activity. Dogs with prerenal or postrenal azotemia also may have increased serum amylase activity. In normal animals, steady amounts of amylase leak from the pancreatic acinar cells or other tissues (or both) and enter the blood. If this amylase is not excreted or inactivated at a steady rate, the serum amylase activity increases. Glomerular filtration has been considered to be an important route of amylase excretion, and if this is the case, a decreased glomerular filtration rate (GFR) could produce an increased serum amylase activity in otherwise normal animals (e.g., animals without pancreatic injury). Studies of renal amylase excretion in dogs, however, have yielded conflicting results. Results of at least one study strongly suggest that amylase does not pass through the normal canine glomerulus and, therefore, that reduced glomerular excretion cannot explain the increased serum amylase activity occurring with renal dysfunction. This failure of small amylase molecules (molecular weight, 54,000 daltons) to pass the normal glomerular filter likely results from formation of macroamylases. Macroamylases usually are complexes of amylase molecules with other plasma proteins, but they also may be complexes of polymerized amylase molecules. The resulting complexes are too large to pass the normal canine glomerular filter. Lack of correlation between serum urea or creatinine concentrations, both of which depend on the glomerular filtration rate, and serum amylase activities also argues against decreased glomerular filtration as the only mechanism leading to increased serum amylase activity in dogs with azotemia. Increased serum amylase activity with renal dysfunction may result from pancreatic injury secondary to uremia. This occurs in humans, but it has not been well documented in dogs. In addition, the kidneys possibly may inactivate amylase by a process not dependent on the passage of amylase through the glomerular filter. At present, evidence for this type of renal inactivation of amylase is lacking.

Hepatic inactivation of amylase is an important mechanism of amylase elimination in dogs. A decrease in this hepatic inactivation also may contribute to the hyperamylasemia in uremic dogs, but at present, no evidence supports this view. Regardless of the mechanism leading to increased serum amylase activity in dogs with renal dysfunction, such dysfunction (prerenal, renal, or postrenal) can result in increased serum amylase activity, and this increase does not necessarily result from pancreatic injury.

▪ **Gastrointestinal disease.** Increased serum amylase activity has been reported in dogs with enteritis, small intestinal obstruction, and intestinal perforation. These increases may result from the leakage of amylase from mucosal epithelial cells, in which amylase normally is present, into lymphatics and blood vessels of the intestinal mucosa. In patients with intestinal rupture, amylase in the intestinal tract probably leaks directly into the peritoneal cavity and then diffuses into the blood.

▪ **Hepatic disease.** The cause of increased serum amylase activity in patients with hepatic disease is not clear. The mononuclear phagocyte system of the liver is a major pathway of amylase degradation, and compromise of this system, thereby resulting in decreased clearance of amylase from the blood, could result in increased serum amylase activity. Amylase normally is present in hepatocytes, and increased serum amylase activities may be caused by leakage from injured hepatocytes. The concentration of amylase in hepatocytes is lower than the concentration of amylase in the blood of normal dogs, however, and this leakage alone cannot account for hyperamylasemia. Increased production of amylase by hepatocytes has not been documented.

▪ **Neoplasia.** Increased serum amylase activity has been reported in dogs with lymphoma or hemangiosarcoma, but the cause of this increased activity and the frequency with which it occurs in dogs with these neoplasms is not known.

As evident from the previous discussion, increased serum amylase activity is not a specific indicator of pancreatic injury in dogs, and several disease processes can result in such an increase. Although not definitive, the magnitude of increased serum amylase activity may be helpful in distinguishing increases caused by pancreatic injury from those caused by other processes. A commonly used "rule of thumb" is that a serum amylase activity threefold greater than the upper limit of the reference range is very suggestive of pancreatic injury and is less typical of other potential causes. Serum amylase activity less than threefold the upper limit of the reference range, however, commonly occurs with pancreatic injury, and amylase activity greater than threefold the upper limit of the reference range has been reported in dogs with azotemia. The severity of clinical signs in dogs with pancreatitis does not necessarily correlate with the amylase activity.

Serum Amylase in Species Other than Dogs

Both the usefulness and interpretation of serum amylase activity varies with the species. Serum amylase activity in cats with pancreatic injury usually is not increased and occasionally is decreased *(Table 24.1)*, and, therefore, is not a reliable indicator of pancreatic injury. The increase in serum amylase activity, if any, usually is slight in horses with pancreatic injury (Table 24.1). Serum amylase activity is reported to increase in more than 50% of horses with proximal enteritis and in more than 25% of horses with other causes of intestinal colic. The intestinal mucosa may be the source of serum amylase in these cases. Many of these horses also have prerenal azotemia, and increased serum amylase activity resulting from renal dysfunction is possible in these cases as well.

Serum Lipase Activity

Serum Lipase in Dogs

Lipase is present in several tissues, including pancreas, adipose tissue, gastric mucosa, and duodenal mucosa in dogs. The source of serum lipase activity in normal dogs is controversial, with the results of some studies suggesting this activity is of pancreatic origin but others suggesting extrapancreatic sources are more likely. The kidneys may play an important role in the excretion or inactivation (or both) of serum lipase, because serum lipase activity commonly is increased in dogs with azotemia. Causes of increased serum lipase activity in dogs include:

- **Pancreatic injury.** Injury or death of pancreatic acinar cells results in the leakage of lipase from these cells. Pancreatitis is the most common cause of such injury. Blockage of the pancreatic duct also may cause increased serum lipase activity because of the resorption of pancreatic secretions from the pancreatic duct system.

- **Renal dysfunction.** Approximately 50% of dogs with renal failure have increased serum lipase activities. Dogs with prerenal or postrenal azotemia also may have increased serum lipase activity. A possible mechanism for these increases is failure of the kidneys to excrete lipase, which normally enters the blood from the pancreatic acinar cells or other tissues (or both). Glomerular filtration may be an important route of lipase excretion; however, the role of the kidneys in lipase excretion has not been clearly demonstrated. The lack of correlation between the magnitude of decrease in the GFR and the increase in serum lipase activity has led to speculation that other factors are involved in the hyperlipasemia occurring with renal failure. Decreased renal tubular degradation of lipase and pancreatic injury secondary to uremia may result in increased serum lipase activity in dogs with a decreased GFR. These possible causes have not been documented, however. Regardless of the mechanism, serum lipase activity may increase in dogs with a decreased GFR and in which significant pancreatic damage has not occurred.

- **Hepatic disease.** The mechanism producing increased serum lipase activity and the frequency with which increased activity occurs in dogs with hepatic disease is not known.

- **Corticosteroid therapy.** Dexamethasone therapy can produce as much as a fivefold increase in canine serum lipase activity, and prednisone therapy can cause a smaller increase. The mechanism of this increase is not known, and no concurrent increase in serum amylase activity occurs because of treatment with these drugs. Neither dexamethasone nor prednisone causes detectable pancreatic lesions in dogs. Because of potential corticosteroid-related increase in serum lipase activity, serum amylase activity is a more specific indicator of pancreatic injury than serum lipase activity in dogs receiving corticosteroid treatment.

- **Gastrointestinal disease.** Gastrointestinal disease should always be considered as a differential diagnosis in dogs with increased serum lipase activity. Serum lipase activity was reported to increase to levels between two-

TABLE 24.1   CHANGES EXPECTED IN SERUM AMYLASE AND LIPASE ACTIVITIES AND IN SERUM TRYPSIN-LIKE IMMUNOREACTIVITY IN PANCREATIC INJURY

Species	Amylase	Lipase	Trypsin-Like Immunoreactivity
Dog	Increased	Increased	Increased
Cat	Normal to decreased	Normal	Increased
Horse	Inconsistently increased	?	?

to fivefold greater than the upper limit of the reference range in young dogs with gastroenteritis of probable viral origin, although pancreatitis was not completely ruled out in these dogs. Increased serum lipase activity also has been reported in dogs with duodenal obstruction. As noted, lipase is present in both the gastric and duodenal mucosa, either of which may have been the source of the increased serum lipase in these dogs.

- **Neoplasia.** Increased serum lipase activity has been reported in dogs with lymphoma and hemangiosarcoma, but the cause of this increased activity or the frequency with which it occurs in dogs with these neoplasms is not known.

As evident from the previous discussion, increased serum lipase activity is not a specific indicator of pancreatic injury, because several other disease processes can produce such increases in dogs. As with serum amylase activity, the magnitude of the increased serum lipase activity may be helpful in distinguishing increased activity caused by pancreatic injury from increased activity caused by other processes. A commonly used "rule of thumb" is that a serum lipase activity greater than twofold the upper limit of the reference range is very suggestive of pancreatic injury and less typical of the other potential causes of increased activity. This rule does not apply, however, in dogs receiving corticosteroid therapy, especially if the corticosteroid is dexamethasone, because dexamethasone treatment can produce increases in lipase activity as large as fivefold. Serum lipase activity less than twofold greater than the upper limit of the reference range commonly occurs with pancreatic injury in dogs, and the severity of clinical signs does not necessarily correlate with the lipase activity.

Serum Lipase in Species Other Than Dogs

The usefulness and interpretation of serum lipase activity varies with the species. Like amylase, lipase is not a reliable indicator of pancreatitis in cats. Cats with pancreatitis commonly have a serum lipase activity within the reference range (Table 24.1). The usefulness of serum lipase activity for the detection of pancreatic injury in horses has not been reported.

Serum Amylase Versus Serum Lipase in Dogs

Pancreatitis and, therefore, pancreatic injury occur most commonly in dogs, and the validity of serum enzyme assays for the diagnosis of pancreatic injury has been most thoroughly evaluated in this species. Several studies have compared the usefulness of serum amylase and lipase activities in dogs. The sensitivity and specificity of these serum enzymes, as well the rates at which they increase and then decrease after pancreatic injury, also have been studied.

Neither serum amylase nor serum lipase activity is sensitive for detecting pancreatic injury in dogs, and dogs with pancreatitis can have normal serum amylase and lipase activities. Serum amylase and lipase activities also are not specific for detecting pancreatic injury in dogs. As noted, increased serum amylase or lipase activity can occur in dogs with a variety of other disorders not related to pancreatic injury. Despite the poor level of sensitivity and specificity of these enzyme assays, serum lipase activity appears to be more sensitive and specific for pancreatic injury than serum amylase activity.

Studies regarding the relative rates at which serum amylase and lipase activities increase after pancreatic injury have produced conflicting results. The prevailing opinion is that serum amylase and lipase activities increase at approximately the same rates after pancreatic injury. Activities of both enzymes usually increase within the first 24 hours and then peak at approximately 4 to 5 days after injury. Both enzymes appear to have very short half-lives in serum (3–6 hours). The serum lipase activity may remain increased for a longer period of time than the serum amylase activity. The short half-lives of these enzymes partially explains why serum activities sometimes are normal in animals with pancreatic injury, in that the injury may have been acute and leakage may have stopped by the time serum enzyme activities were measured. From the information available concerning these enzymes, both serum amylase and lipase activities should be assayed if pancreatitis is suspected. If either serum amylase or lipase activity is markedly increased (i.e., greater than a three- or twofold increase above the upper limit of the reference range, respectively) and the dog is not azotemic and has not been treated with corticosteroids, pancreatitis is likely. In dogs treated with corticosteroids, especially dexamethasone, the serum amylase activity is more reliable.

In summary, serum amylase and lipase activities can be helpful in establishing the diagnosis of pancreatic injury in dogs if used in combination with patient history, clinical signs, and other laboratory tests. A flow chart for the interpretation of increased serum amylase and lipase activities in dogs is presented in *Figure 24.1*.

Peritoneal Fluid Amylase and Lipase Activities

If peritoneal fluid can be obtained from animals suspected of having pancreatic injury, measurement of amylase and lipase activities in this fluid may be diagnostically useful. With active pancreatic damage, these enzymes leak into the cavity, and peritoneal fluid activities may be increased *(Fig. 24.2)*. Peritoneal fluid amylase or lipase activity that is higher than serum amylase or lipase activity is suggestive of pancreatic injury. This test is most appropriate in dogs with suspected pancreatic injury but in which serum enzyme activities are not strongly suggestive of such in-

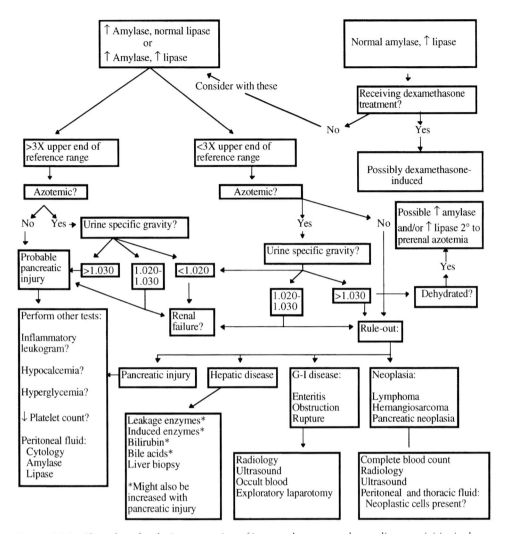

Figure 24.1 Flow chart for the interpretation of increased serum amylase or lipase activities in dogs.

jury. This test also should be considered for any cat or horse with suspected pancreatic injury, because serum activities might not be reliable indicators of such injury in these species. Duodenal perforation, however, also can result in increased peritoneal fluid amylase and lipase activities. The sensitivity and specificity of peritoneal fluid amylase and lipase activities for detecting pancreatic injury have not been determined.

Serum Trypsin-Like Immunoreactivity

Serum trypsin-like immunoreactivity (TLI) is proportional to serum trypsinogen and trypsin concentrations. Trypsinogen is synthesized only by the pancreas, and it is converted to the active proteolytic enzyme, trypsin, in the small intestine *(Fig. 24.3)*. Measurement of TLI by radioimmunoassay detects both trypsinogen and trypsin (hence, trypsin-like immunoreactivity). In normal animals, a small portion of trypsinogen, which is the principle form of TLI produced by pancreatic acinar cells, leaks into the

extracellular space and then diffuses via the lymphatics into the blood. Normal serum TLI activity is a good indicator of adequate pancreatic trypsinogen production. (For a discussion of serum TLI in detecting exocrine pancreatic insufficiency, see Chapter 25).

Injury to pancreatic parenchymal cells results in the leakage of large amounts of trypsinogen from acinar cells into the extracellular space *(Fig. 24.4)*. Trypsinogen is quickly activated to form trypsin, which then diffuses into the blood, where despite binding to serum protease inhibitors, it is detected as increased serum TLI. The serum TLI assay, therefore, is potentially useful for detecting pancreatic injury. The assay for serum TLI is species specific, however, and is only readily available for dogs and cats.

The potential superiority of serum TLI over serum amylase and lipase activities for detecting pancreatitis awaits evaluation in clinical trials. Because trypsinogen and trypsin are produced only by the pancreas, TLI is a potentially more specific test for pancreatic injury in dogs

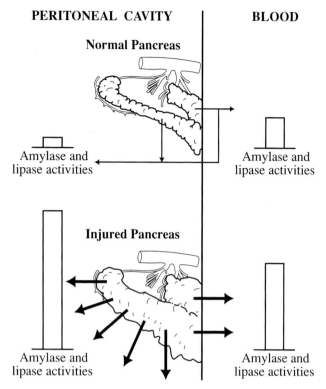

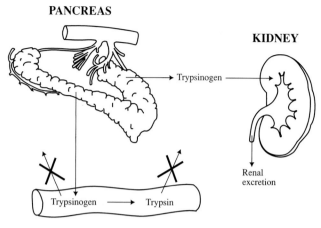

Figure 24.2 Peritoneal fluid amylase or lipase activities can be used to confirm pancreatic injury. Normally, small quantities of these enzymes pass from the blood or pancreatic interstitium into the peritoneal cavity, and enzyme activities in the peritoneal cavity do not exceed those of blood. When pancreatic acinar cells are injured, large amounts of amylase and lipase may leak from the injured pancreas directly into the peritoneal cavity. Peritoneal fluid amylase or lipase activities higher than serum amylase or lipase activities may result, and this is suggestive of pancreatic injury.

Figure 24.3 Trypsinogen normally is secreted by pancreatic acinar cells. It then passes via the pancreatic duct to the small intestine, where it is converted to the activated proteolytic enzyme, trypsin. Neither trypsinogen nor trypsin are reabsorbed from the intestine. Small amounts of trypsinogen normally leak from pancreatic acinar cells into the pancreatic interstitium and then into the blood. This trypsinogen is the serum trypsin-like immunoreactivity found in the blood of normal animals. Trypsinogen is partially removed from the blood by renal excretion.

Other Laboratory Abnormalities Associated With Pancreatic Injury

Because serum amylase and lipase activities are not highly sensitive or specific for pancreatic injury, the results of these tests should be considered in light of other physical and laboratory abnormalities that commonly occur with

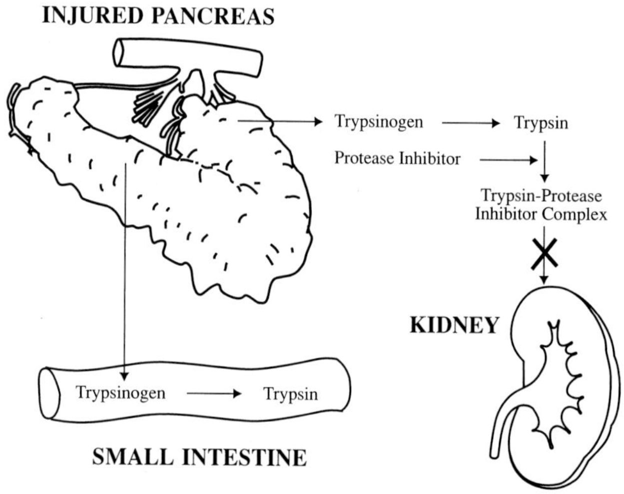

than serum amylase and lipase activities. In dogs with pancreatic injury induced by pancreatic duct ligation, the serum TLI increased and decreased more rapidly than serum amylase and lipase activities; therefore, serum TLI also is a potentially more sensitive indicator of early pancreatitis. Trypsinogen is cleared by glomerular filtration; thus, decreased renal function could cause increased serum TLI, just as it causes increased serum amylase and lipase activities. Activated trypsin, on the other hand, is quickly complexed with protease inhibitors in the blood, and these complexes do not pass through the glomerulus but are removed by the mononuclear phagocyte system.

In cats, pancreatitis is the most common disease of the pancreas, but it is not commonly diagnosed. This relates partly to the absence of the typical clinical signs seen in dogs with pancreatitis, but it also relates to the low sensitivity of serum amylase and lipase for feline pancreatitis. Serum TLI measurements have been investigated in cats with suspected pancreatic injury. Preliminary studies suggest that the serum TLI is a much more sensitive and specific indicator of pancreatitis in cats than either serum amylase or lipase activities (Table 24.1).

Figure 24.4 Pancreatic injury results in the leakage of large amounts of trypsinogen from injured pancreatic acinar cells. This trypsinogen is quickly converted to trypsin, which enters the blood and then is complexed to serum protease inhibitors. Most of the serum trypsin-like immunoreactivity found in the blood of animals with pancreatitis is trypsin. The trypsin–protease inhibitor complex does not readily pass the glomerulus, and it is not excreted by the kidneys.

such injury. The presence of several of these abnormalities increases the reliability of increased serum amylase or lipase activities as indicators of pancreatic injury. Laboratory abnormalities that can accompany pancreatic injury are discussed here.

Leukocytosis

Leukocytosis and neutrophilia often are present and usually result from the inflammation (i.e., pancreatitis) accompanying pancreatic injury. A left shift is inconsistently present and depends on the degree of tissue demand for neutrophils. Because pancreatitis is very painful, both neutrophilias induced by epinephrine (excitement) and corticosteroids (stress) also can occur. Lymphopenia may be present if stress is a major factor.

Hemoconcentration

Increased hematocrit, hemoglobin concentration, and red-blood-cell count occur if the animal is significantly dehydrated. Vomiting and lack of appropriate fluid intake can lead to dehydration and resultant hemoconcentration.

Anemia

Anemia of unknown origin occurs infrequently. Hemorrhage or hemolysis (or both) in the area of the pancreas may be responsible.

Azotemia

Azotemia, which usually is prerenal, is common in severe cases of pancreatitis and is caused by a combination of factors, including dehydration and hypovolemia, that result in a decreased GFR. Tubular concentrating ability usually is normal, and urine specific gravity usually is high.

Hyperthenuria

Urine specific gravity helps to differentiate prerenal azotemia–associated nonrenal diseases, such as pancreatitis, from renal azotemia associated with renal failure. This is an important distinction, because increases in the serum amylase and lipase activities similar in magnitude to those caused by pancreatitis can occur with renal failure. In addition, the clinical signs of pancreatitis and renal failure sometimes can be similar. In animals with azotemia and increases in serum amylase and lipase activities, the urine specific gravity may be the most important laboratory test for verifying primary renal failure (Table 24.2). Analysis of urine collected at the time of blood sampling is important for animals in which pancreatitis or renal failure (or both) are possibilities. Measurement of the urine specific gravity is a not valid indicator of concentrating ability, however, if the urine is obtained after fluids have been administered.

TABLE 24.2   HYPOTHETIC DATA FROM TWO DOGS WITH SIMILAR CLINICAL SIGNS (VOMITING, ANOREXIA, AND DEPRESSION)[a]

	Dog 1	Dog 2	Reference Range
BUN (mg/dL)	110	100	7–28
Creatinine (mg/dL)	2.8	2.5	0.9–1.7
Amylase (IU/L)	2800	2600	20–1250
Lipase (IU/L)	950	910	30–560
Urine-Specific Gravity	1.010	1.050	
Probable Diagnosis	Renal failure	Prerenal azotemia, with or without pancreatitis	

BUN, blood urea nitrogen.

[a] The BUN, creatinine, and serum amylase and lipase activities are similar in both dogs, but the urine specific gravity is low in dog 1 (in the isosthenuric range) but high in dog 2. Assuming that dog 1 has not received fluid therapy, the combination of serum biochemical results with a low urine specific gravity suggests renal failure with secondary retention of urea and creatinine and with renal-associated increases in serum amylase and lipase activities. In dog 2, the combination of serum biochemical results with high urine specific gravity suggests a prerenal azotemia. In this dog, the increased BUN and creatinine concentrations probably result from a glomerular filtration rate that has decreased secondary to dehydration and hypovolemia caused by the vomiting. The urine specific gravity has increased, however, because this dog needs to conserve fluids. Increased serum amylase and lipase activities may be the result of renal dysfunction (i.e., prerenal azotemia) or pancreatitis (or both). This dog may have pancreatitis, and a portion of the serum amylase and lipase activities may have originated from this process. This same combination of results, however, could occur with other diseases causing similar clinical signs and subsequent prerenal azotemia.

Hyperglycemia

Hyperglycemia is common in animals with acute pancreatic injury and, acutely, is the result of increased serum concentrations of corticosteroids, epinephrine, and glucagon. In patients with chronic or recurring pancreatitis, hyperglycemia may be caused by diabetes mellitus resulting from islet cell injury.

Hypocalcemia

Hypocalcemia is inconsistently present in animals with pancreatic injury. In such cases, hypocalcemia usually is mild to moderate. The exact pathogenesis of this hypocalcemia is not known, but it may relate to deposition of calcium in saponified intra-abdominal fat. Fat saponification results from the breakdown of peripancreatic fat by pancreatic lipase. In dogs with marked hypoproteinemia, hypoalbuminemia resulting in decreased protein-bound calcium also may contribute to the hypocalcemia.

Increased Serum Enzyme Activities

Increased serum activities of leakage or induced liver enzymes (i.e., alanine aminotransferase, aspartate aminotransferase, alkaline phosphatase, and γ-glutamyltransferase) can occur. Increased serum activities of leakage enzymes result from ischemic or toxic damage to hepatocytes secondary to pancreatic damage and release of pancreatic enzymes. Increased serum activities of induced enzymes result from blockage of the common bile duct secondary to inflammation of tissue near both the pancreas and the bile duct. Hepatic lipidosis can occur with pancreatitis in anorexic cats, and it results in increased serum activities of hepatic leakage and induced enzymes.

Hyperbilirubinemia

Increased serum bilirubin concentration occasionally occurs in dogs with pancreatic injury. The most likely cause is cholestasis secondary to blockage of the common bile duct. Hyperbilirubinemia occurs in more than 50% of cats with pancreatitis and may result from secondary hepatocyte injury.

Hyperlipidemia

Hypercholesterolemia and hypertriglyceridemia are common in patients with pancreatitis, and they often are accompanied by gross hyperlipemia. Mobilization of lipids by the action of pancreatic lipase on abdominal fat may lead to these increased levels. Increased serum cholesterol concentration also can result from cholestasis, thereby leading to decreased cholesterol excretion by the liver.

Hyperlipemia with hypercholesterolemia and hypertriglyceridemia may precede the onset of pancreatitis and predispose animals to development of this disease.

Hypoproteinemia or Hyperproteinemia

Serum and plasma protein concentrations are variable in patients with pancreatitis. Exudation of protein-rich fluid into the peritoneal cavity, as a component of peritonitis, can decrease the serum protein concentration, but dehydration tends to increase the serum protein concentration. In some cases, these changes counterbalance each other.

Abnormal Hemostasis

Disseminated intravascular coagulation can be a sequela to acute pancreatitis. Alterations in hemostatic function tests that occur with disseminated intravascular coagulation are discussed in Chapter 14.

DETECTION OF EXOCRINE PANCREATIC INSUFFICIENCY

Exocrine pancreatic insufficiency results in inadequate digestion of food (i.e., maldigestion). The clinical signs are similar to—and must be distinguished from—intestinal disorders that result in inadequate absorption of adequately digested nutrients (i.e., malabsorption). Because several of the tests used to diagnose and distinguish these two syndromes are the same, laboratory testing for exocrine pancreatic insufficiency is discussed in Chapter 25.

SUGGESTED READINGS

Corraza M, Tognetti R, Guidi G, Buonaccorsi A. Urinary α-amylase and serum macroamylase activities in dogs with proteinuria. J Am Vet Med Assoc 1994;205:438–440.

Fittschen C, Bellamy JEC. Prednisone treatment alters the serum amylase and lipase activities in normal dogs without causing pancreatitis. Can J Comp Med 1984;48:136–140.

Hill RC, Van Winkle TJ. Acute necrotizing pancreatitis and acute suppurative pancreatitis in the cat. J Vet Intern Med 1993;7:25–33.

Hudson EB, Strombeck DR. Effects of functional nephrectomy on the disappearance rates of canine serum amylase and lipase. Am J Vet Res 1978;39:1316–1321.

Jacobs RM. Relationship of urinary amylase activity and proteinuria in the dog. Vet Pathol 1989;26:349–350.

Jacobs RM. Renal disposition of amylase, lipase and lysozyme in the dog. Vet Pathol 1988;25:443–449.

Jacobs RM. The origins of canine serum amylases and lipase. Vet Pathol 1989;26:525–527.

Murtaugh RJ, Jacobs RM. Serum amylase and isoamylases and their origins in healthy dogs and dogs with experimentally induced acute pancreatitis. Am J Vet Res 1985;46:742–747.

Parent J. Effects of dexamethasone on pancreatic tissue and on serum amylase and lipase activities in dogs. J Am Vet Med Assoc 1982;180:743–746.

Polzin DJ, Osborne CA, Stevens JB, et al. Serum amylase and lipase activities in dogs with chronic primary renal failure. Am J Vet Res 1983;44:404–410.

Simpson KW, Batt RM, McLean L, et al. Circulating concentrations of trypsin-like immunoreactivity and activities of lipase and amylase after pancreatic duct ligation in dogs. Am J Vet Res 1989;50:629–632.

Simpson KW, Simpson JW, Lake S, Morton DB, Batt RM. Effect of pancreatectomy on plasma activities of amylase, isoamylase, lipase and trypsin-like immunoreactivity in dogs. Res Vet Sci 1991;51:78–82.

Steiner JM, Medinger TL, Williams DA. Development and validation of a radioimmunoassay for feline trypsin-like immunoreactivity. Am J Vet Res 1996;10:1417–1420.

Steiner JM, Williams DA. Feline trypsin-like immunoreactivity in feline exocrine pancreatic disease. Comp Cont Educ 1996;18:543–547.

Strombeck DR, Farver T, Kaneko JJ. Serum amylase and lipase activities in the diagnosis of pancreatitis in dogs. Am J Vet Res 1981;42:1966–1970.

Wagner AE, Macy DW. Nephelometric determination of serum amylase and lipase in naturally occurring azotemia in the dog. Am J Vet Res 1982;43:697–699.

LABORATORY EVALUATION OF DIGESTION AND INTESTINAL ABSORPTION

Diarrhea, vomiting, and weight loss are clinical signs that commonly are seen with diseases of the digestive system. These signs are not, however, indicative of a specific disease or cause. Laboratory tests that specifically evaluate the digestive system can provide important diagnostic information in these cases. Before performing these tests, the patient history and clinical signs should be assessed. In addition, physical examination, basic laboratory tests (e.g., hematology, biochemical profile, and urinalysis), and, in some cases, radiologic and ultrasound studies should be performed. The choice of laboratory tests to evaluate the digestive system depends on whether clinical signs are suggestive of acute or chronic disease.

Two important abnormalities that cause signs of chronic digestive system disease are maldigestion and malabsorption syndromes. Maldigestion is a failure to adequately digest food and usually results from inadequate secretion of digestive enzymes by the pancreas. In turn, this usually results from decreased numbers of pancreatic acinar cells and is known as exocrine pancreatic insufficiency (EPI). Malabsorption is a failure of the intestinal tract to absorb adequately digested nutrients and results from a variety of small intestinal lesions. The clinical signs caused by these two syndromes may be similar, and they include increased fecal volume and abnormally formed feces, varying from poorly formed stools to diarrhea. Because the treatment and prognosis differ, distinguishing maldigestion from malabsorption is important. This chapter describes the use of laboratory tests to diagnose maldigestion and malabsorption and to distinguish between these entities. In addition, several other laboratory tests to evaluate the digestive system are discussed. The appropriateness of each test for the evaluation of acute or chronic digestive tract disease is also noted.

SCREENING TESTS IN A VETERINARY PRACTICE

Several screening tests can be performed in a veterinary practice on animals with clinical signs and history that are suggestive of digestive system disease. The results of these tests can be suggestive—but usually not confirmatory—of a specific diagnosis or cause. Confirmatory tests usually must be performed at a reference laboratory (discussed later).

Fecal Parasites

The potential role of GI parasites should be considered in animals with chronic diarrhea, and fecal examination for evidence of parasitism should be a routine part of laboratory testing in these cases. This examination should be performed on fresh feces. If a fecal sample cannot be examined within 2 hours after collection, it should be refrigerated at 4°C. Basic methods to detect parasitic ova, larvae, oocysts, cysts, and trophozoites are discussed here; a parasitology textbook should be consulted for more detailed descriptions and interpretations of these techniques.

Direct, unstained fecal smears may be helpful in detecting parasitic ova, larvae of metazoan parasites (e.g., *Strongyloides* sp.), coccidial oocysts, and cysts or trophozoites of protozoa (e.g., *Giardia*, *Balantidium*, *Entamoeba*, and *Trichomonas* sp.) Such smears also may be stained with routine hematologic stains (e.g., Wright-Giemsa or Diff-Quik stain [Dade Diagnostics of P.R., Inc., Aquada, PR]). In many cases, however, low concentrations of these structures preclude their detection in direct fecal smears. Wet mounts produced by mixing a small amount of feces with a few drops of isotonic saline can be used to detect motile parasites (e.g., trophozoites of *Giardia*, *Balantidium*, and *Entamoeba* sp.)

Fecal examination for parasitic ova and oocysts is best performed using fecal flotation. The typical fecal flotation technique involves mixing feces with water, straining this mixture to remove large debris, centrifuging the strained feces, and then mixing the resulting sediment with flotation solutions composed of varying concentrations of sugar or salts, including sodium chloride, magnesium sulfate, zinc sulfate, or sodium nitrate. Instructions for preparing commonly used flotation solutions are provided in *Table 25.1*. The fecal sediment/flotation solution mixture then is centrifuged for 5 to 10 minutes or is allowed to stand for 30 minutes. Because most parasitic ova and oocysts have a lower density than the flotation solution, they float to the surface of the mixture, where they are collected by touching a coverslip to the surface. Microscopic observation of the material collected (×10 objective) reveals the presence of parasitic ova or oocysts. This technique can be modified to allow the counting of ova and oocysts and, therefore, to indicate their concentration in the feces. Cysts of parasites such as *Giardia* also float in many of these solutions but may be distorted.

Fluke ova float in some flotation solutions (e.g., zinc sulfate), but the fecal sedimentation technique generally is preferred for their detection. In its simplest form, this technique involves mixing feces with water, straining the feces to remove large debris, and centrifuging the strained feces. Centrifugation of this mixture sediments the fluke ova, and microscopic examination of a few drops of this sediment reveals the presence or absence of fluke ova.

> ### TABLE 25.1 PREPARATION OF COMMONLY USED FLOTATION SOLUTIONS
>
> *Sugar Solution*
> Dissolve 454 g of granulated sugar (sucrose) in 355 mL of hot (not boiling) water. Check the solution's specific gravity with a hydrometer. Specific gravity should be 1.200 to 1.250. Add more water or sugar to adjust the specific gravity. Six milliliters of formaldehyde may be added to inhibit fungal growth in the solution.
>
> *Sodium Chloride Solution*
> Dissolve 400 g of sodium chloride in 1000 mL of tap water. This should produce a saturated sodium chloride solution. Check the specific gravity with a hydrometer. Specific gravity of a saturated sodium chloride solution should be 1.180 to 1.200. If the specific gravity is less than this range, add more sodium chloride until this specific gravity is attained.
>
> *Magnesium Sulfate Solution*
> Dissolve 400 g of magnesium sulfate in 1000 mL of tap water. Use a hydrometer to adjust the specific gravity to 1.200 by adding water or magnesium sulfate.
>
> *Zinc Sulfate Solution*
> Dissolve 371 g of zinc sulfate in 1000 mL of tap water. Heating the water speeds dissolution of the zinc sulfate. Use a hydrometer to adjust the specific gravity to 1.018 by adding water or zinc sulfate.
>
> *Sodium Nitrate Solution*
> Dissolve 400 g of sodium nitrate in 1000 mL of tap water. Use a hydrometer to adjust the specific gravity to 1.200 to 1.250 by adding water or sodium nitrate.

A modification of this technique using formalin and ether in the sedimented mixture has been described as well.

Some GI parasites (e.g., *Strongyloides* sp.) produce larvae rather than ova. Such larvae are not readily detected using the flotation technique, but they may be detected using the sedimentation technique. The most sensitive technique for the detection of larvae in feces, however, is the Baermann technique, in which warm water is placed in a glass funnel that is plugged by a stopcock or rubber hose clamped at its end. A small amount of feces, which is wrapped in a double layer of gauze, is placed in the water and allowed to remain there for 8 hours. During this period, any larvae that are present leave the feces, pass into the water, and fall to the bottom of the funnel. After 8 hours, a small amount of fluid is collected from the bottom of the funnel and centrifuged. The resulting sediment then is examined microscopically for the presence of larvae.

Fecal Occult Blood

The occult blood test detects the presence of blood in the feces at concentrations 20- to 50-fold less than those resulting in grossly visible blood. Loss of 30% to 50% of blood volume into the GI tract can occur without gross evidence of blood in the feces. The occult blood test is a simple test that is available for in-practice use. This test detects the pseudoperoxidase activity of hemoglobin in feces. When present, this activity results in formation of a blue color on a paper square onto which the feces has been applied *(Fig. 25.1)*.

Two types of fecal occult blood test are available. The modified quaiac slide test is based on detection of the chemical oxidation of guaiaconic acid to a conjugated quinone, and the orthotolodine tablet test is based on the oxidation of tetramethylbenzidine. In either test, formation of a blue color is considered to be indicative of blood in the feces. These tests appear to have similar sensitivities as well. The fecal occult blood test should be performed in animals with:

▪ Unexplained acute diarrhea, chronic diarrhea, or loose stools.
▪ Microcytic anemia, in which the cause of chronic blood loss is not obvious.

The test also can be used to monitor animals with a high risk of developing hemorrhage in the GI tract because of treatment with ulcerogenic drugs (e.g., nonsteroidal anti-inflammatory agents) or a history of GI tract tumors.

The fecal occult blood test is very sensitive. Peroxidase activity from myoglobin and hemoglobin in meat diets and from certain plants in vegetable diets can potentially cause false-positive results. The guaiac slide test may be more prone to such false positive results than the orthotolodine tablet test, but this difference also may vary with different diets. Dietary restriction for several days before the occult blood test is performed decreases the number of false-positive results. Such restrictions should include feeding meat-free, low-peroxidase diets (e.g., rice and cottage cheese).

False-negative results on the fecal occult blood test can occur with high concentrations of vitamin C in the feces. Consumption of a high fiber diet is variably reported to increase or decrease the number of false-negative results. High-fluid content in the feces decreases the sensitivity of the occult blood test by diluting any blood that might be present.

Positive results on the fecal occult blood test in the absence of grossly visible blood in the feces is suggestive of upper GI tract inflammation, ulceration, or neoplasia. If blood is grossly visible in the feces, these same disorders may be present in the colon rather than the upper GI tract, because blood from the upper GI tract usually is digested and not grossly visible in the feces. Blood from the lower GI tract is not digested, however, and is grossly visible in the feces. Loss of large quantities of blood in the upper GI tract can cause rapid transit times and, occasionally, result in grossly visible blood in the feces.

Fecal Cytology

Fecal cytology is most useful for identifying potentially pathogenic organisms and for confirming the presence of active inflammation in the GI tract. Fecal cytology is indicated in animals with acute or chronic diarrhea. Such cytologic specimens usually are prepared by making a thin film of the feces and then staining this film with either Wright-Giemsa or some type of quick Romanowsky stain (e.g., Diff-Quik). These preparations also can be made using Gram stain. Whereas Gram stain is necessary to determine the Gram-negative or -positive features of various bacteria, it is inadequate for distinguishing cell types and other infectious organisms in the feces.

The initial step in fecal cytology is assessment of the bacterial flora. The flora *(Fig. 25.2)* is mixed in normal animals. If one type of bacteria clearly predominates, this organism may be pathogenic, and a bacterial culture is indicated. In animals with maldigestion or malabsorption, a mixed flora usually is observed. Two types of bacteria that can predominate and cause digestive problems are *Clostridium* and *Campylobacter* sp. *Clostridium* sp. *(Fig. 25.3)* are bacilli that can be recognized only when in their sporulated form, in which these bacteria have a "safety pin" appearance, because a spore causes a large

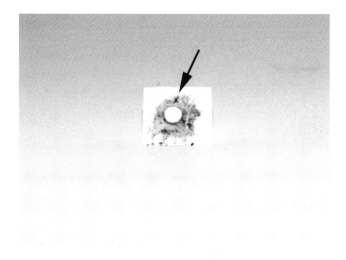

Figure 25.1   The occult blood test. This test is positive for occult blood, as indicated by the blue color on the filter pad.

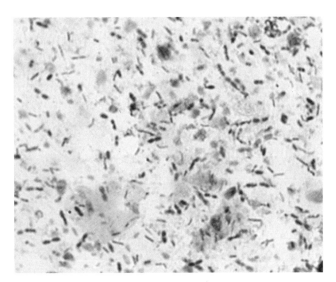

Figure 25.2 Wright-Giemsa–stained fecal smear from a dog showing a mixture of bacteria representing the mixed bacterial flora typical of normal animals. ×1000.

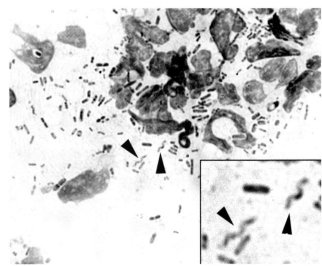

Figure 25.4 Wright-Giemsa–stained fecal smear from a dog showing an overgrowth of *Campylobacter* sp., which are recognized by a distinctive "sea gull" morphology (arrows). ×1000.

portion of the bacillus to appear swollen and clear. More than five sporulated bacteria per ×100 oil field is considered to be excessive and suggestive of clostridial overgrowth. *Campylobacter* sp. are recognized by their "sea gull" or W shape *(Fig. 25.4)*. Pathogenic protozoa (e.g., *Giardia* sp.) occasionally are visible in direct fecal preparations *(Fig. 25.5)*. Fecal films or colon scrapings also may reveal other infectious agents (e.g., fungal organisms).

Very small numbers of epithelial cells *(Fig. 25.6)* can be found in fecal films from normal animals. Neutrophils

(Fig. 25.7) are abnormal in fecal films and, when present, often appear to be degenerate. Neutrophils in fecal films are suggestive of inflammation in the colon, because neutrophils migrating into the lumen of the small intestine do not survive intact during transit to the terminal colon. Invasive bacteria (e.g., *Salmonella* and *Campylobacter* sp.) should be considered as possible causes when neutrophils are present in feces. Eosinophils also are abnormal in fecal films and, when present, are suggestive of eosinophilic colitis.

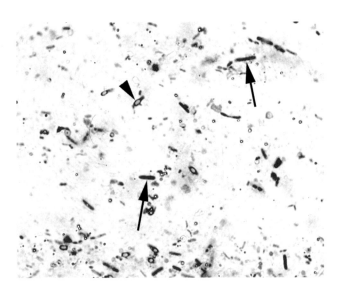

Figure 25.3 Wright-Giemsa–stained fecal smear from a dog showing an overgrowth of *Clostridium* sp. (arrows) that are recognized in the sporulated form ("safety pin" form). ×1000.

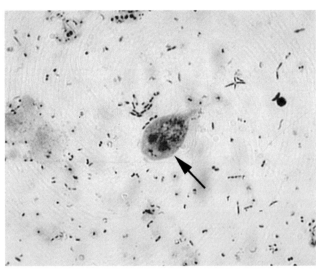

Figure 25.5 Wright-Giemsa–stained fecal smear from a dog showing a *Giardia* organism (arrows). ×1000.

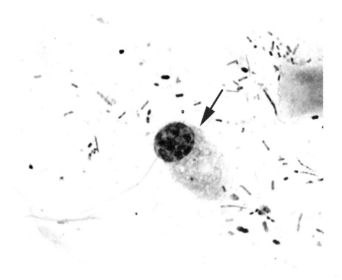

Figure 25.6 Wright-Giemsa–stained fecal smear from a dog. Epithelial cells (arrow) are interspersed with a variety of bacteria and amorphous material. Small numbers of epithelial cells are a normal finding in fecal smears. ×1000.

Digestion/Absorption Screening Tests

Digestion/absorption screening tests performed on feces are intended to detect either failure to digest nutrients because of EPI or failure to absorb digested nutrients (i.e., malabsorption syndrome) because of intestinal disease. Fresh feces (i.e., feces directly from the rectum or within 15 minutes of defecation) always should be used in these tests, which have low sensitivity and specificity. If abnormalities are detected, repeating the test increases reliabil-

ity. The serum trypsin-like immunoreactivity (TLI) test (discussed later) is a much more specific and sensitive test for EPI.

Fecal Starch

Undigested starch in the feces is detected by staining feces with Lugol solution, which is a stain that is specific for starch. A small amount of feces (~1–2 drops) is mixed with one to two drops of Lugol solution (i.e., a 2% iodine solution) on the surface of a microscopic slide. A coverslip is placed over the mixture, which then is observed microscopically. Undigested starch appears as dark, blue to black granules (Fig. 25.8). The presence of undigested starch is suggestive of a deficiency in starch-digesting enzymes or an increase in intestinal motility, thereby resulting in decreased intestinal transit time. Starch-digesting enzymes (i.e., amylases) are produced by the pancreas, and a deficiency in these enzymes is suggestive of EPI. This test is insensitive and nonspecific, however, because it depends on the quantity of starch in the diet. If a normal animal has ingested a large amount of starch, its ability to digest starch could be overwhelmed, thereby resulting in a false-positive fecal starch test. If an animal with EPI is receiving a diet that is very low in starch, a negative fecal starch test could result despite a deficiency in starch digestion.

Fecal Fat

Both undigested and digested fat in the feces can be detected by a stain that selectively stains fat (i.e., Sudan III or IV). This test is performed in two steps, direct and indirect, to detect both undigested and digested fat.

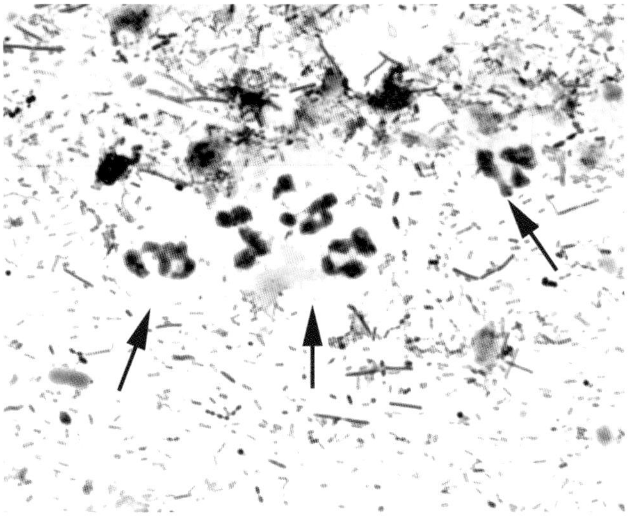

Figure 25.7 Wright-Giemsa–stained fecal smear from a dog. Large numbers of degenerate neutrophils are present (arrows). Neutrophils are abnormal in fecal smear from all species. ×1000.

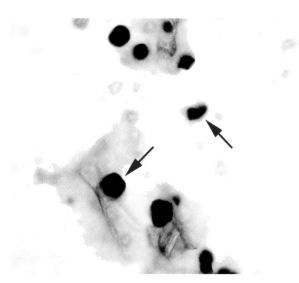

Figure 25.8 Canine fecal smear stained with Lugol solution and positive for undigested starch. Starch granules appear as dark-blue to black spheres. ×400.

The direct fecal fat test is performed by mixing a small amount of feces (~1–2 drops) with one to two drops of Sudan III or IV stain on the surface of a microscopic slide. A coverslip is placed over the mixture, and the slide then is examined microscopically. Undigested fat appears as large, refractile, orange droplets *(Fig. 25.9)*. The presence of 10 or more large, refractile, orange droplets per ×40 microscopic field is considered to be a positive result, thereby indicating a deficiency of fat-digesting enzymes (i.e., lipases). Because these enzymes are produced by the pancreas, a deficiency of these enzymes is suggestive of EPI. The quantity of fat in the diet can affect the results of this test. Normal animals on high-fat diets may have positive fecal fat tests; animals with EPI that are receiving low-fat diets may have negative fecal fat tests.

The indirect fecal fat test can detect the presence of digested fat in fecal samples that are negative on the direct fecal fat test (i.e., samples that do not appear to contain undigested fat). The test is performed by mixing a small amount of feces (~1–2 drops), one to two drops of 36% acetic acid solution, and one to two drops of Sudan III or IV stain on the surface of a microscopic slide. The mixture then is brought to a boil twice by heating the slide over a flame and is examined immediately. A positive result is the presence of 10 or more large, refractile, orange droplets per ×40 microscopic field. As the slide cools, these lipid droplets begin to form orange-yellow spicules. Both undigested and digested fat are detected by this procedure. Because the direct test should have initially confirmed the absence of undigested fat, however, a positive result on the indirect test is suggestive of the presence of digested fat. A negative result with the direct test and a positive

result with the indirect test are suggestive that fat is being digested (i.e., that adequate lipases are being produced by the pancreas), but that digested fat is not being absorbed by the intestine. An intestinal problem (i.e., malabsorption) rather than EPI, therefore, should be suspected.

Performing the indirect fecal fat test on a sample that clearly is positive on the direct fecal fat test probably does not add any significant diagnostic information. If the indirect test is performed on a fecal sample that was positive on the direct test (i.e., undigested fat is present), then the indirect test might appear to be more strongly positive than the direct test. This does not necessarily imply an intestinal problem, however, because with EPI, the indirect test occasionally is slightly more strongly positive than the direct test.

A positive direct fecal fat test is very specific for EPI; however, this is not a sensitive indicator (e.g., >50% of dogs with EPI do not have large amounts of fecal fat detectable by this test). Analysis of undigested versus digested fat via the direct and indirect fecal fat tests is not considered to be reliable for differentiating EPI from intestinal malabsorption.

Fecal Proteolytic Activity

Fecal proteolytic enzymes include trypsin, chymotrypsin, elastase, and carboxypeptidase A and B. The feces can be screened for protease activity in practice laboratories, and more sensitive tests for fecal protease activity can be performed at some reference laboratories. The serum TLI test, however, appears to be a more reliable test of pancreatic protease enzyme production, and it has nearly replaced testing for fecal protease activity in the assessment of pancreatic protease production. Two screening tests for fecal protease activity, the x-ray film digestion test and the gelatin digestion test, have been commonly used.

The x-ray film digestion test is performed by mixing one part feces with nine parts 5% sodium bicarbonate solution in a test tube. A strip of x-ray film, which must be gelatin coated, is inserted into the tube and then incubated at 37°C for 1 hour or at room temperature for 2.5 hours. At the end of the incubation period, the film is examined to detect digestion of the film coating. If the coating has been digested, the feces are considered to be positive for protease activity. Lack of digestion is suggestive of decreased fecal protease activity.

The gelatin digestion test is performed by mixing 1 mL of the described feces–bicarbonate solution with 2 mL of melted 7.5% gelatin and incubating this mixture for 1 hour at 37°C. After the incubation period, the tube is allowed to cool and then is checked for solidification. If the gelatin remains liquid, the feces are considered to be positive for protease activity (i.e., proteases in the feces digested the gelatin). Solidification of the gelatin indi-

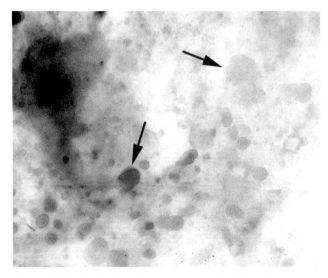

Figure 25.9 Canine fecal smear stained with Sudan IV and positive for lipids, which appear as yellow-orange globules. ×400.

cates that it was not digested and that fecal protease activity is low. The gelatin digestion test is considered to be more sensitive than the x-ray film test for detecting deficient protease activity in feces.

Deficient protease activity in the feces is suggestive of deficient protease production by the pancreas and, therefore, of possible EPI. Feces can produce a false-negative result for protease activity because of:

▪ Daily fluctuations in fecal protease activities.
▪ Protease inhibitors in the feces.
▪ Complete use of proteases in digestion.

Feces can produce a false-positive result for protease activity because of bacterial protease activity in the feces.

Fecal Muscle Fibers

Undigested, striated muscle fibers stain light brown with Lugol stain *(Fig. 25.10)*. Muscle fibers also might be seen when performing cytologic examination of the feces. Muscle fibers in the feces are suggestive of defective digestion of these fibers, most likely resulting from EPI (e.g., inadequate fecal protease activity). Muscle fibers also can be present in the feces because of increased intestinal motility and subsequent decrease in intestinal transit time.

Plasma Turbidity Test (Fat Absorption Test)

The plasma turbidity test assesses the ability to digest fat and to absorb digested fat. Oral administration of fat to normal dogs and cats results in lipemic serum, which is recognized by cream-colored turbidity. If such turbidity does not develop, then maldigestion or malabsorption of fat is possible. This test should be considered in animals with a history and clinical signs that are suggestive of maldigestion or malabsorption.

The procedure for the plasma turbidity test is as follows:

1. The animal is fasted for 12 hours.
2. A blood sample using ethylenediaminetetraacetic acid (EDTA) anticoagulant is collected and centrifuged, and the plasma then is examined to determine whether it is clear.
3. Fat is administered orally (3 mL of corn oil per 1 kg body weight).
4. Blood samples using EDTA anticoagulant are collected at 1-hour intervals for 2 to 3 hours after fat administration, centrifuged, and then examined for plasma turbidity.

Turbidity in one or more of the post–fat administration blood samples is normal *(Fig. 25.11)*. Lack of turbidity is suggestive of either maldigestion or malabsorption of fat. Possible causes include deficient production of fat digesting enzymes (i.e., lipases) by the pancreas because of EPI or impaired absorption of digested fat by the intestine (i.e., malabsorption). The test (as described) does not distinguish between maldigestion and malabsorption.

If the plasma turbidity test is negative (i.e., fat is not absorbed), then a second, modified form of this test can be performed to differentiate EPI from malabsorption. This second test is performed as described earlier, but the corn oil is incubated with pancreatic enzymes for 30 minutes

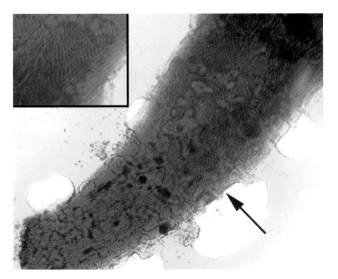

Figure 25.10   Canine fecal smear stained with Lugol solution and containing intact, striated muscle fibers (arrow). Muscle fibers in feces suggest deficient fecal protease activity. ×400.

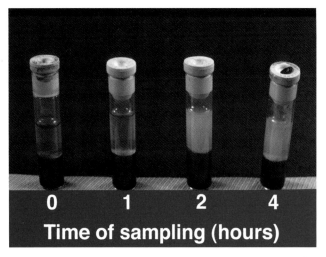

Figure 25.11   The plasma turbidity test. In this test, a dog was fed corn oil, and blood was sampled at 1, 2, and 4 hours. The plasma was slightly turbid by 1 hour and cloudy by 2 hours, indicating normal fat digestion and absorption.

before being administered. This incubation results in digestion of the fat. If the plasma remains clear for 2 to 3 hours after the predigested fat has been administered, then an intestinal absorption problem is more likely. If the plasma becomes turbid after previously remaining clear following administration of corn oil alone, then EPI is more likely (i.e., the animal can apparently absorb fat once it has been digested, and its problem is a lack of fat digestion).

The plasma turbidity test does have several potential problems. The sensitivity is poor (i.e., 80% or more of ingested fat is still absorbed in dogs with EPI). There can be marked variation in the degree of lipemia that develops and in the length of time required for lipemia to develop in normal animals. This probably relates to variations in gastric emptying times and in plasma lipid clearance rates. Dogs with EPI also may not absorb digested fat in normal quantities and, therefore, may remain negative for turbidity even if the fat is predigested with pancreatic enzymes.

TESTS IN A REFERENCE LABORATORY

As noted in the previous section, most screening tests for digestive tract diseases are both insensitive and nonspecific. As a result, practitioners may not perform these screening tests. In other cases, such screening tests may be performed and the results suggest a specific digestive system disease. In either case, laboratory tests that are more sensitive and specific are needed to confirm the diagnosis of these diseases. These tests are discussed here.

Serum TLI

Serum TLI is the most sensitive and specific laboratory test for EPI. As noted in Chapter 24, the serum TLI also is potentially useful for detecting pancreatic injury in dogs and cats. The TLI is a species-specific test and, at present, is only available for dogs and cats. Trypsinogen is synthesized only by pancreatic acinar cells and is converted to the active proteolytic enzyme, trypsin, in the small intestine.

Measurement of TLI by radioimmunoassay detects both trypsinogen and trypsin, thus the term *trypsin-like immunoreactivity*. In normal animals, small amounts of trypsinogen continually escape from pancreatic acinar cells. Absorption of detectable trypsin from the intestine does not occur; therefore, this is not a source of serum TLI. In normal animals, the TLI that is detected in the blood is trypsinogen. Pancreatitis causes leakage of increased amounts of trypsinogen from pancreatic acinar cells, and this trypsinogen quickly is converted to trypsin, which then enters the blood. The TLI detected in the blood as a result of pancreatitis, therefore, primarily is trypsin.

In the absence of active pancreatic injury, serum TLI is a good indicator of pancreatic trypsinogen production, and it is a much simpler and more specific test of pan-

creatic enzyme production than all the other alternatives. As a result, TLI has become the most widely used laboratory test for detecting EPI.

The following information should be considered when testing for TLI:

- Animals should be fasted for 12 hours before collecting a blood sample.
- At least 1 mL of nonhemolyzed serum is required.
- The TLI is stable for several days at room temperature and for several years when frozen. Serum samples for TLI analysis, therefore, can be sent to a laboratory through the mail. Because heat destroys TLI, high temperatures should be avoided.
- Oral supplementation with pancreatic extracts does not affect the TLI results.

The serum TLI concentration is dramatically decreased in dogs with EPI (<2.5 µg/L) but is normal (>5.0 µg/L) in dogs with small intestinal diseases. Therefore, serum TLI is nearly 100% specific for EPI. If the serum TLI concentration in a dog is less than 5.0 µg/L but greater than 2.5 µg/L, the test should be repeated within a few weeks; retesting usually places the dog clearly in the normal or the EPI category. Possible causes for results in this "gray" zone (2.5–5.0 µg/L) include:

- The dog is in the process of recovering pancreatic function after an episode of pancreatitis, and the results may be normal at retesting.
- The sample had a normal TLI when collected but was exposed to extreme heat during transit. Results may be normal at retesting.
- Food was not withheld for an appropriate length of time. Retesting may indicate that the dog has EPI.
- The dog has an early EPI and reduction of pancreatic secretory capacity that is not yet sufficient to cause clinical signs. The TLI test appears to be extremely sensitive for pancreatic acinar cell dysfunction and might be below normal before microscopic lesions in the pancreas are visible and before clinical signs that are suggestive of EPI appear. The TLI can decrease from the "gray" zone to a confirmatory level within a few weeks.

The serum TLI also appears to be useful for identifying EPI in cats. Serum concentrations of 8 µg/L or less are highly specific for TLI in cats.

BT-PABA (Bentiromide) Absorption Test

Although *N*-benzoyl-L-tyrosyl-*p*-aminobenzoic acid (BT-PABA ; bentiromide) absorption tests pancreatic function and, therefore, is potentially useful for detecting EPI, it rarely is performed. The BT-PABA absorption test is sensitive for detecting EPI (~95%) but is not specific for

EPI (~60%), and it has few advantages compared with the TLI test for detecting EPI. In animals with EPI caused by pancreatic duct blockage, the TLI test often is normal, but the BT-PABA absorption test might be abnormal. Pancreatic blockage, however, is a rare cause of EPI.

The basis of the BT-PABA test is that the molecule is split by the enzyme chymotrypsin in the intestinal tract *(Fig. 25.12)*. The result is production of free *p*-amino-benzoic acid (PABA). After its production, PABA is absorbed by the small intestine, enters the blood, and then is excreted in the urine. Measurement of either blood PABA concentration or urinary PABA excretion, therefore, can gauge chymotrypsin activity in the small intestine. In turn, this chymotrypsin activity provides a gauge of pancreatic production of the chymotrypsin precursor, chymotrypsinogen.

To perform the test, BT-PABA is administered orally, and either blood or urine PABA concentration then is measured. If blood is analyzed, collection and analysis of multiple samples during a 3-hour period is required. Peak blood PABA concentration in dogs typically occurs at 2 to 3 hours after oral administration of BT-PABA (16.7 mg/kg). Peak blood concentration of less than 85 mg/dL is suggestive of inadequate chymotrypsinogen production and, therefore, EPI.

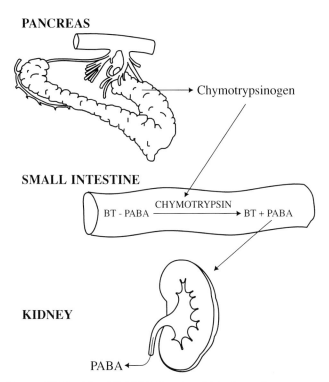

Figure 25.12 The BT-PABA (bentiromide) absorption test assesses pancreatic production of chymotrypsinogen. Blood and urine PABA concentrations are proportional to the amount of PABA produced in the small intestine, which in turn is proportional to the rate of chymotrypsinogen production by the pancreas.

Because the rate of urine production affects the urinary PABA concentration, urine must be collected in a metabolism cage over several hours. The total volume of urine produced as well as the concentration of PABA in that urine then is used to calculate the total amount of PABA excreted in the urine as follows:

Urine volume (mL) × Urinary PABA concentration (mg/mL) = Total PABA produced (mg)

Because a metabolism cage is required, this procedure is impractical in many settings, and blood PABA concentrations more commonly are used as the gauge of BT-PABA digestion.

The BT-PABA absorption test has several disadvantages compared with the TLI test. Some animals with small intestinal disease do not adequately absorb PABA; therefore, despite adequate chymotrypsinogen production by the pancreas, blood concentrations of PABA might be suggestive of this production being inadequate. This partially explains the test's lack of specificity for EPI, and it is one rationale for performing the xylose absorption and BT-PABA absorption tests simultaneously (discussed later). Some animals with EPI have normal BT-PABA absorption tests, possibly resulting from BT-PABA hydrolysis by bacterial enzymes or from compensatory production of intestinal enzymes with chymotrypsin-like activity.

D-Xylose Absorption Test

The D-xylose absorption test is a measure of the intestinal absorptive ability. It most often is used in dogs and horses when malabsorption is suspected. In normal cats, D-xylose absorption curves are widely variable, and peak values are lower and less predictable than those in dogs. In addition, D-xylose absorption may not be abnormal in cats with severe intestinal disease. D-Xylose is a pentose monosaccharide that is absorbed undigested in the jejunum by both passive and active mechanisms, is not significantly metabolized after absorption, and, eventually, is excreted (>50%) by the kidneys. These features appear to make the oral D-xylose absorption test a good choice for evaluating intestinal absorptive ability, but some reports indicate the test is insensitive for establishing the diagnosis of malabsorption in dogs.

The recommended dosages and concentrations of D-xylose used in this test vary with different authors. The normal D-xylose absorption curves described in this section are appropriate for the protocols listed. The D-xylose absorption test is performed as follows:

- The animal is fasted for 12 hours.
- D-Xylose is administered orally at a dosage of 0.5 g/kg (5%–10% solution) in dogs and 1.0 g/kg (10% solution) in horses.

■ In dogs, blood samples for D-xylose determination are collected before D-xylose administration and at 30, 60, 90, and 120 minutes after administration. For routine diagnostic purposes, the 60- and 90-minute samples are the most important.

■ In horses, blood samples for D-xylose determination are collected before D-xylose administration and at 30, 60, 90, 120, 180, 240, and 300 minutes after administration. For routine diagnostic purposes, the 60- through 180-minute samples are the most important.

In dogs, D-xylose concentrations should peak at greater than 60 mg/dL at 60 to 90 minutes *(Fig. 25.13)*. In horses, D-xylose concentrations should peak at greater than 20 mg/dL at 90 to 180 minutes *(Fig. 25.14)*. A flattened D-xylose absorption curve (i.e., a lower peak blood D-xylose concentration) is suggestive of malabsorption. The D-xylose absorption test is insensitive. Therefore, a normal D-xylose absorption test does not rule out malabsorption.

D-Xylose absorption can be falsely decreased (i.e., a falsely flattened curve or delay in reaching peak value) with delayed gastric emptying, bacterial overgrowth resulting in intraluminal bacterial breakdown of xylose, and sequestration of xylose in patients with abnormal extravascular fluid accumulations (e.g., edema, hydrothorax, or ascites). Moreover, D-xylose absorption commonly is decreased in dogs with EPI, possibly because of abnormalities in the intestinal mucosa secondary to EPI or to bacterial overgrowth associated with EPI.

Falsely elevated D-xylose absorption peaks can occur with decreased urinary D-xylose excretion because of renal failure.

Whereas D-xylose is readily available, not all reference laboratories perform D-xylose assays. Therefore, one should determine the availability of this assay before performing the D-xylose absorption test.

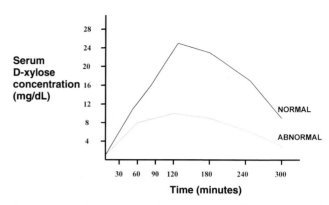

Figure 25.14   The D-xylose absorption curves from normal and abnormal horses. A normal D-xylose absorption curve in a horse peaks at greater than 20 mg/dL at 90 to 180 minutes after D-xylose administration.

Combined BT-PABA/D-Xylose Absorption Test

Performing the BT-PABA and D-xylose absorption tests simultaneously helps to determine whether decreased bentiromide absorption is caused by intestinal malabsorption or is secondary to EPI. Interpretation of the results from this combined test in animals with decreased BT-PABA absorption is illustrated in *Table 25.2*. Absorption of BT-PABA is abnormal in animals with EPI because of abnormal digestion of BT-PABA and in animals with malabsorption because of abnormal absorption of PABA. Absorption of D-xylose may be either normal or abnormal in animals with EPI depending on the degree of malabsorption accompanying this syndrome. D-Xylose absorption is abnormal with malabsorption. Therefore, both the BT-PABA and D-xylose absorption tests possibly could be abnormal in animals with EPI as well as in animals with malabsorption. As a result, EPI cannot be distinguished from malabsorption when both tests are abnormal. If only the BT-PABA test is abnormal, however, then EPI is the appropriate interpretation.

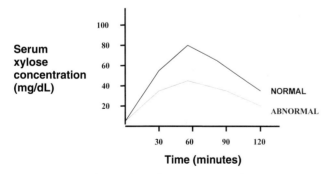

Figure 25.13   The D-xylose absorption curves from normal and abnormal dogs. A normal D-xylose absorption curve in a dog peaks at greater than 60 mg/dL at 60 to 90 minutes after oral D-xylose administration.

TABLE 25.2	INTERPRETATION OF COMBINED TEST RESULTS	
BT-PABA Absorption	**D-Xylose Absorption**	**Interpretation**
Abnormal	Normal	Exocrine pancreatic insufficiency
Abnormal	Abnormal	Malabsorption or exocrine pancreatic insufficiency

Serum Vitamin B₁₂ and Folate Assays

Serum vitamin B_{12} and folate concentrations after a 12-hour fast may be helpful in identifying which areas of the intestinal tract are affected by a disease resulting in malabsorption. Vitamin B_{12} is released from dietary proteins in the stomach by acid gastric secretions. It then is bound to proteins (called R proteins) and passes into the small intestine, in which pancreatic proteases digest the R protein, thereby releasing vitamin B_{12}. The free vitamin B_{12} then binds to intrinsic factor, which is produced by the gastric mucosa in humans but appears to be produced primarily by the pancreas in dogs and cats. The vitamin B_{12}–intrinsic factor complex is absorbed by the distal small intestine, especially the ileum. Folate is present in the diet but is conjugated with glutamate residues and is poorly absorbable. Enzymes in the brush border of the proximal small intestine remove all but one of these residues, and folate then is absorbed. Therefore, folate is absorbed by the proximal small intestine, especially the jejunum. If malabsorption primarily occurs in the proximal small intestine, then serum folate concentrations may be decreased, but serum vitamin B_{12} concentrations should be normal. If malabsorption primarily occurs in the distal small intestine, then serum vitamin B_{12} concentrations may be decreased, but serum folate concentrations should be normal. If malabsorption is generalized, then both serum vitamin B_{12} and folate concentrations may be decreased.

Misleading results can occur in cats or dogs with EPI and in patients who have bacterial overgrowth or are receiving vitamin supplements. Decreased vitamin B_{12} and folate concentrations have been reported in cats with EPI. In most of these cats, the serum vitamin B_{12} concentration was undetectable, and in more than 50%, the folate concentration was below normal. The decreased serum vitamin B_{12} is theorized to result from decreased secretion of pancreatic intrinsic factor, which is necessary for vitamin B_{12} absorption in cats. Decreased folate concentrations are thought to result from intestinal disease concurrent with EPI and the resultant decrease in folate absorption. Detection of decreased vitamin B_{12} and folate concentrations in cats warrants consideration of EPI as well as of intestinal disease. In dogs with EPI, serum vitamin B_{12} concentrations may be slightly to moderately decreased, (the stomach secretes some intrinsic factor in dogs). The serum folate concentrations, however, usually are normal to increased because of bacterial overgrowth, which is a common sequela of EPI. Bacterial overgrowth increases serum folate concentrations because of bacterial synthesis of folate, and it decreases serum vitamin B_{12} concentrations because of bacterial binding of vitamin B_{12}. Bacterial overgrowth should always be considered with this combination of results. If both vitamin B_{12} and folate concentrations are increased, then vitamin supplementation before sampling is the most likely explanation, because no disease process should cause this change.

Fecal Biochemistry Analysis

Although not commonly performed, fecal biochemistry analysis can be useful in animals with chronic diarrhea. Analysis of fecal proteolytic activity and of fecal fat excretion can be helpful in assessing the adequacy of digestive enzyme production by the pancreas. Fecal electrolyte concentrations in combination with fecal osmolarity can be useful in distinguishing the type of diarrhea (e.g., osmotic versus secretory) in animals with acute or chronic diarrhea.

Fecal Proteolytic Activity

The azocasein hydrolysis test and the radial enzyme diffusion test are more sensitive and specific than screening tests for fecal protease enzyme activity (e.g., x-ray film digestion test or gel digestion test) in animals with possible EPI. Fecal protease activity varies in different portions of the fecal specimen. In addition, day-to-day as well as diet-related fluctuations in fecal protease activities occur. These tests must be performed on multiple specimens that have been collected on different days; on a pooled, 3-day fecal collection; or after dietary supplementation with soybean meal. Protease activities in the feces are labile, and fecal samples for such analysis must be frozen immediately and shipped overnight to avoid false-negative results.

Measurement of azocasein hydrolysis is a spectrophotometric test that gauges the color change in a reaction mixture of feces and azocasein dye substrate. Proteolytic activity in the feces causes a color change in this mixture, resulting from digestion of the azocasein dye substrate. The degree of this color change is proportional to the fecal proteolytic activity. This is a more reliable test for EPI in dogs than either the x-ray film or gelatin digestion tests, but it also can erroneously indicate low fecal proteolytic activity in normal dogs because of fluctuations in fecal proteolytic activity. The sensitivity is approximately 95%, and the specificity is approximately 80%. The availability of this test is limited.

The radial enzyme diffusion test measures fecal proteolytic activity by assessing the distance over which fecal solution induces hydrolysis and clearing after diffusion into agar gel containing calcium paracaseinate substrate. This distance is proportional to the proteolytic activity of the feces. Like the azocasein dye digestion test, this test is affected by fluctuations in fecal proteolytic activity, and multiple sampling is recommended. The availability of this test also is limited.

Fecal Fat Quantitation

The total quantity of fecal fat produced during a 24- to 72-hour period is a more specific and sensitive test of fecal lipase activity than Sudan staining of feces. Fecal fat is quantitated in animals that are being fed a diet with a known fat content. In normal animals, less than 10% of ingested fat is excreted in feces. Normal 24-hour fat excretion is less than 0.3 g/kg per day in dogs and less than 0.4 g/kg per day in cats. Increased fecal fat excretion can occur in animals with either EPI or malabsorption. Fecal fat quantitation is not offered by most veterinary reference laboratories.

Fecal Electrolytes and Osmolarity

The osmolarity of the fecal supernatant is the result of electrolytes and other osmotic substances that have not been absorbed (e.g., volatile fatty acids, other fats, other fermented ingesta, amino acids, protein, carbohydrates, and bile acids). The fecal concentration of Na plus K multiplied by two provides an estimate for the contribution of these two electrolytes and their anions to the fecal osmolarity.

Animals with osmotic diarrheas, in which osmotically active substances other than Na, K, and their anions are retained in the gut contents and the feces, show a wide gap (>50 mOsmol/L) between the osmolarity estimated from the electrolyte concentrations and the measured osmolarity. This gap represents these other unmeasured, osmotically active substances. In secretory diarrheas, most of the osmolarity of the feces results from Na, K, and their anions, because most of the other osmotically active substances are digested and absorbed. The gap between the osmolarity estimated from the electrolyte concentrations and the measured osmolarity, therefore, is small (<30 mOsmol/L). If these principles are applied, then measurement of fecal osmolarity and fecal Na and K concentrations in animals with diarrhea can be indicative of whether that diarrhea is osmotic or secretory.

To determine the fecal electrolyte concentrations and fecal osmolarity on a fecal supernatant, fecal liquid must comprise at least one-third of the fecal volume. The osmolar gap of the feces then is calculated as follows:

$$\text{Osmolar gap} = \text{Measured fecal osmolarity} - 2(\text{Na} + \text{K})$$

Diarrheas with large osmolar gaps (>50 mOsmol/L) probably are osmotic diarrheas. Diarrheas with low osmolar gaps (<30 mOsmol/L) probably are secretory diarrheas. Examples of osmotic and secretory diarrheas are listed in *Table 25.3*.

TABLE 25.3 EXAMPLES OF OSMOTIC AND SECRETORY DIARRHEAS

Osmotic Diarrheas	Secretory Diarrheas
Johne's disease Granulomatous colitis Eosinophilic gastro-enteritis Intestinal lymphosarcoma Lymphangiectasis Protein-losing enteropathies Proximal enteritis (horses) Magnesium cathartics Other maldigestion/malabsorption syndromes	Salmonellosis (depends on protein loss, i.e., higher protein loss = higher gap) Enterotoxic colibacillosis Endotoxemia

OTHER LABORATORY ABNORMALITIES ASSOCIATED WITH DIGESTIVE SYSTEM DISEASES

Laboratory test abnormalities associated with GI system disease vary with the area of the system affected, the cause of the disease, and the acuteness or chronicity of the disease. Common abnormalities associated with acute or chronic diarrheas are discussed here.

Other Laboratory Abnormalities Associated With Acute Diarrheas or Vomiting

1. Increased hematocrit, hemoglobin concentration, and erythrocyte count, as well as increased plasma and serum protein concentrations, can occur with acute diarrhea or vomiting. These occur because of the loss of fluid via the GI tract and the resulting dehydration and hemoconcentration.
2. Variable abnormalities in the leukocyte concentration can occur with acute diarrhea. If the diarrhea results from an infectious agent that produces toxins, then sequestration of neutrophils as well as strong tissue demand can result in marked neutropenia and leukopenia. Less severe endotoxemia or tissue demand can result in neutrophilia with a left shift.
3. Acid-base and electrolyte abnormalities can occur in animals with diarrhea or vomiting. These abnormalities, however, are variable and unpredictable. Assessment of acid-base and serum electrolyte status is important in such animals. In patients with secretory diarrheas, loss of Na, Cl, and occasionally, K can result in decreased serum concentrations of these electrolytes.

Bicarbonate also is lost in diarrhea, which can produce a metabolic acidosis. In turn, this can result in a shift of K from intracellular to extracellular spaces as well as retention of K by the kidneys. Potassium shifts can lead to a normal or increased serum K concentration despite a loss of K in the feces. Vomiting animals may lose significant amounts of HCl in the vomitus, which often leads to hypochloremia and metabolic alkalosis. If the vomitus includes alkaline small intestinal contents, however, such animals may have normal acid-base results or metabolic acidosis. Metabolic alkalosis in vomiting animals often is associated with obstruction of the pyloric area, thereby resulting in loss of HCl without loss of alkaline intestinal contents.

4. Increases in blood urea nitrogen and creatinine can occur secondary to dehydration (i.e., prerenal azotemia).

5. Increased activities of hepatic leakage enzymes can occur with acute diarrhea, possibly because of hepatocyte damage resulting from toxins absorbed from the injured GI tract.

Other Laboratory Abnormalities Associated With EPI or Malabsorption Syndrome

Other hematologic and serum biochemical tests usually are not helpful in establishing the diagnosis of EPI. Routine hematologic tests and biochemical profiles, however, may help to differentiate EPI from other disorders. Serum amylase and lipase activities may decrease slightly with EPI, but these decreases usually are not recognized as being significant. Increased alanine aminotransferase (ALT) activities and decreased cholesterol concentrations occasionally are seen in dogs with EPI.

Other laboratory abnormalities that can occur with malabsorption syndrome include:

1. Microcytic anemia associated with iron deficiency, which commonly results from chronic blood loss via the GI tract.

2. An inflammatory leukogram, which may be suggestive of significant inflammation or deep ulceration in the intestinal wall.

3. Neutropenia. If, in addition, neutrophils are toxic, then endotoxin absorption from the GI tract secondary to Gram-negative enteritis, intestinal stasis, septicemia, severe bacterial peritonitis secondary to intestinal perforation, or viral enteritis are possible.

4. Eosinophilia, which may be associated with eosinophilic gastroenteritis or parasitism.

5. Abnormal serum protein, albumin, or globulin concentrations. Serum albumin and globulin concentrations are important in screening for protein-losing enteropathies. With these enteropathies, both albumin and globulin concentrations usually are decreased. In other types of malabsorption or maldigestion, the only decrease, if any, occurs in the albumin concentration.

An exception is immunoproliferative enteropathy of Basenjis, in which globulin concentrations increase as part of an immune response. Similar immunoproliferative enteropathies with hyperglobulinemia may occur in other breeds of dogs, especially German Shepherds.

6. Prolonged prothrombin times, prolonged activated partial thromboplastin times, and prolonged activated clotting times because of vitamin K deficiency may be seen in animals with malabsorption syndrome. A probable vitamin K–deficient bleeding syndrome has been reported in cats with malabsorption syndrome. Malabsorption of vitamin K, which is a fat-soluble vitamin, probably plays an important role in this syndrome, but the vitamin K deficiency in such animals also is potentiated by secondary hepatic diseases, thereby resulting in decreased production of vitamin K–dependent clotting factors; possible antibiotic therapy, thereby altering small intestinal bacterial flora and reducing bacterially-derived vitamin K_2 production; and in some cases, severe dietary fat restriction, thereby reducing vitamin K uptake still further, because it is dependent on fat absorption. Because the activities of vitamin K–dependent clotting factors must fall to less than 35% of normal before these changes occur, animals with such abnormalities are markedly deficient and should receive parenteral vitamin K supplementation.

SUGGESTED READINGS

Carro T, Williams D. Relationship between dietary protein concentration and serum trypsin-like immunoreactivity in dogs. Am J Vet Res 1989;50:2105–2107.

Cook AK, Gilson SD, Fischer WD, Kass PH. Effect of diet on results obtained by use of two commercial test kits for detection of occult blood in feces of dogs. Am J Vet Res 1992;53:1749–1751.

Dill-Macky E. Pancreatic diseases of cats. Comp Cont Educ 1993;15:589–598.

Edwards DF, Russel RG. Probable vitamin K–deficient bleeding in two cats with malabsorption syndrome secondary to lymphocytic-plasmacytic enteritis. J Vet Intern Med 1987;1:97–101.

Gilson SD, Parker BB, Twedt DC. Evaluation of two commercial test kits for detection of occult blood in feces of dogs. Am J Vet Res 1990;51:1385–1387.

Nix BE, Leib MS, Zajac A, et al. The effect of dose and concentration on D-xylose absorption in healthy, immature dogs. Vet Clin Pathol 1993;22:10–16.

Rice JE, Ihle SL. Effects of diet on fecal occult blood testing in healthy dogs. Can J Vet Res 1994;58:134–137.

Steiner JM, Williams DA. Feline trypsin-like immunoreactivity in feline exocrine pancreatic disease. Comp Cont Educ 1996;18:543–547.

Strombeck DR, Harrold D. Evaluation of the 60-minute blood p-aminobenzoic acid concentration in pancreatic function testing of dogs. J Am Vet Med Assoc 1982;180:419–421.

Williams D, Batt RM. Sensitivity and specificity of radioimmunoassay of serum trypsin-like immunoreactivity for the diagnosis of canine exocrine pancreatic insufficiency. J Am Vet Med Assoc 1988;192:195–201.

Williams DA, Reed SD. Comparison of methods for assay of fecal proteolytic activity. Vet Clin Pathol 1990;19:20–24.

Williams E. New tests of pancreatic and small intestinal function. Comp Cont Educ 1987;12:1167–1174.

LABORATORY EVALUATION OF PLASMA AND SERUM PROTEINS

Laboratory evaluation of plasma and serum protein concentrations typically is a part of both basic hematology and biochemistry testing in animals. Alterations in plasma or serum protein concentrations are the most important laboratory abnormalities in a small number of diseases, and protein alterations commonly are observed as secondary changes in a large number of diseases. Measurement of plasma and serum protein concentrations often yields important information that can be helpful in narrowing the list of diseases to be considered and, in some cases, in revealing the presence of a specific disease. This chapter discusses the types of proteins that normally are present in plasma and serum, the methods for analyzing these proteins, and the significance of abnormal plasma and serum protein concentrations.

CLASSIFICATION OF PLASMA AND SERUM PROTEINS

The two major types of proteins in plasma are albumin and the globulins. Albumin is the smallest of these proteins, and the concentration of albumin molecules in the blood is greater than that of globulin molecules. As a result, albumin accounts for approximately 80% of the oncotic pressure of the blood. This oncotic pressure prevents water from diffusing from the blood into the tissues. Albumin also is an important carrier protein and plays a role in the transport of free fatty acids, bile acids, bilirubin, calcium, hormones, and drugs. Albumin is synthesized by the liver, enters the blood, and is catabolized by most tissues. The half-life of a circulating albumin molecule varies in different species, ranging from approximately 8 days in dogs to approximately 20 days in horses.

Globulins are a heterogeneous group of proteins that are large but variable in size. Globulins include various types of antibody molecules, other proteins that are active in the immune system (e.g., complement), clotting factors, many different enzymes, and a variety of proteins that carry lipids, vitamins, hormones, extracellular hemoglobin, and metal ions (e.g., iron, copper). Globulins typically are classified as being alpha, beta, or gamma on the basis of their electrophoretic mobility. (The separation and measurement of these globulins are discussed later.)

The alpha globulin fraction includes thyroxine-binding globulin (transports thyroxine), transcortin (transports cortisol), lipoproteins (transport lipids), ceruloplasmin (transports copper), haptoglobin (hemoglobin binding), antithrombin III (thrombin inhibitor), and alpha$_2$-macroglobulin (binds insulin and inhibits trypsin). These proteins are produced in the liver.

The beta globulin fraction includes other lipoproteins (transport lipids), transferrin (transports iron), ferritin (transports iron), C-reactive protein, complement components (C3 and C4), plasminogen (converts to plasmin and then lyses fibrin), and in plasma, fibrinogen. Most of these proteins are produced in the liver. Fibrinogen is a large protein molecule that plays a key role in coagulation (see Chapter 14) as well as in the inflammatory response (discussed later). Immunoglobulin molecules of the IgM and IgA type also may migrate during electrophoretic analysis in the beta fraction, and these are produced in the lymphoid tissues in response to antigenic stimulation.

The gamma globulin fraction is composed of immunoglobulins. All types of immunoglobulins can be found in this fraction. These proteins are produced in the lymphoid tissues in response to antigenic stimulation.

MEASUREMENT OF PLASMA AND SERUM PROTEINS

Plasma Versus Serum

The two types of samples that commonly are used for clinical biochemistry analyses are plasma and serum. Plasma is the liquid portion of blood that has not clotted, and to collect a plasma sample, some type of anticoagulant must be used. Plasma contains all the proteins described earlier.

Serum is the liquid portion of the blood that remains after clotting, which requires the conversion of fibrinogen to fibrin. When a blood sample is collected without use of an anticoagulant, the subsequent clotting in that sample results in the conversion of all fibrinogen to fibrin. Therefore, serum is devoid of fibrinogen and contains albumin and the remaining globulins.

Total Protein Concentration

The total plasma or serum protein concentration can be estimated using a refractometer. Protein molecules in plasma or serum increase the refractive index of that fluid in proportion to their concentration. Because the protein concentration is estimated on the basis of the refractive index, however, anything that increases the refractive index of a fluid also increases the estimated protein concentration of that fluid. Increased concentrations of lipids, hemoglobin, or bilirubin in serum or plasma may result in spuriously high protein estimates via refractometry. Increased concentrations of solutes (e.g., glucose, urea, sodium, chloride) also spuriously increase the estimated protein concentration.

The total protein concentration of serum is measured routinely in reference laboratories by spectrophotometric methods. The most widely used of these methods is the biuret method, which is very accurate. The total protein concentration as derived by this method does not necessarily match the estimated protein concentration derived from a refractometer, even if the fibrinogen concentration is considered when comparing the plasma protein concentration via refractometry with the serum protein concentration via spectrophotometry.

Albumin Concentration

The albumin concentration is measured spectrophotometrically using dye-binding methods, usually with bromcresol green (BCG) dye. At very low concentrations, however, the BCG method may overestimate the albumin concentrations, because this dye binds slightly with other proteins. Other dye-binding methods for assay of the serum albumin concentration have been less reliable than the BCG method because of species variability in binding of the dye with albumin.

Globulin Concentrations

Calculated Globulin Concentration

The serum protein and albumin concentrations are measured routinely as part of serum biochemical profiles. The globulin concentration as reported on these profiles is not measured, however, but rather is calculated by subtracting the serum albumin concentration from the total protein concentration.

Serum Protein Electrophoresis

Both serum albumin and globulin concentrations can be determined by serum protein electrophoresis (see Chapter 1). Electrophoresis is performed by placing a small amount of serum on the end of a thin sheet of gel. An electrical current then is passed through the gel for a constant period of time. This current causes the proteins in the serum to migrate in the gel at variable rates, as determined by the net negative charge and size of that type of protein. The film next is submersed in a stain that attaches to protein. The stained film is scanned by a spectrophotometric device (i.e., a scanning densitometer) that produces an electrophoretogram (i.e., a hard copy depiction of the distribution of the proteins on the film) (Fig. 26.1).

Modern scanning densitometers also calculate the concentration of protein in each fraction after the operator inputs the total protein concentration of that sample. This method separates globulins into several fractions, including alpha, beta, and gamma globulins. Albumin and globulin concentrations that are derived using this method do not necessarily match those that are derived using spectrophotometric methods. The number of fractions separated by serum protein electrophoresis varies both with the species and with the type of film that is used. Albumin and

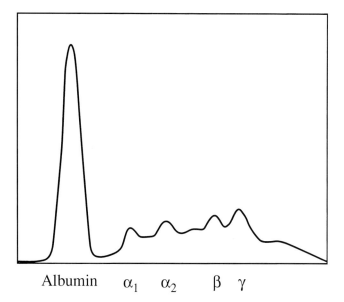

Figure 26.1 An electrophoretogram from a serum protein electrophoresis separation.

the alpha, beta, and gamma globulin fractions can be separated in specimens from all species and on all types of films. In some species and on some types of films, however, the alpha, beta, and gamma globulins are separated into alpha$_1$ and alpha$_2$, beta$_1$ and beta$_2$, or gamma$_1$ and gamma$_2$ fractions, respectively. (Causes for altered concentrations of these protein fractions are discussed later.)

Qualitative and Semiquantitative Estimation of Immunoglobulin Concentrations

Several screening tests for the estimation of immunoglobulin concentrations are available. These tests can be performed in clinical practice, and they can provide qualitative or semiquantitative estimates of immunoglobulin concentrations. They primarily are used to screen neonates (especially calves, foals, and crias) for possible failure to ingest colostrum or to absorb immunoglobulins from colostrum; this failure results in increased susceptibility to infection and is referred to as failure of passive transfer (FPT). These tests are not as sensitive or specific as more sophisticated tests (e.g., radioimmunodiffusion), but the results usually are available immediately and allow for treatment decisions to be made without delay. These test results are most valid as indicators of adequate passive transfer or FTP when performed within a few days of birth.

Total protein measurement by refractometry. Immunoglobulins absorbed from colostrum are the major determinant of the total plasma protein concentrations in neonates. Total plasma protein concentrations in calves increase by approximately 2 g/dL after the ingestion of

colostrum. Measurement of the plasma protein concentration, therefore, has been evaluated as an indicator of plasma immunoglobulin concentration and as a gauge for the adequacy of passive transfer. Refractometry is a simple procedure that requires only a microhematocrit centrifuge for separating plasma from cells and a refractometer (preferably heat compensated).

In calves, use of the plasma protein concentration as an indicator for the plasma immunoglobulin concentration has been evaluated using different plasma protein values. A plasma protein concentration greater than a certain predetermined limit is considered to be indicative of adequate immunoglobulin concentration and, therefore, of adequate passive transfer. Plasma protein concentrations from 4.2 to 5.5 g/dL have been evaluated as limits. Dehydration, which often accompanies neonatal diseases, results in relative increases in plasma protein concentrations and may result in plasma protein concentrations that are suggestive of adequate passive transfer in calves that actually have FPT.

Using the plasma protein concentration for estimating the adequacy of passive transfer in foals appears to be unreliable. This might result, in part, from wide variations in precolostral plasma protein levels in foals.

Sodium sulfite precipitation test. The sodium sulfite precipitation test is based on the fact that immunoglobulins can be selectively precipitated from serum using concentrations of anhydrous sodium sulfite ranging from 14% to 18%. A higher sodium sulfite concentration is required to cause precipitation in serum containing lower immunoglobulin concentrations. As a result, sera with high immunoglobulin concentrations undergo precipitation when mixed with a sodium sulfite solution of low concentration (e.g., 14%), whereas sera with low immunoglobulin concentrations do not undergo precipitation when mixed with this same solution of sodium sulfite. The latter sera may undergo precipitation when mixed with sodium sulfite solutions of higher concentrations (e.g., 16%–18%), depending on the immunoglobulin concentration of the serum. Sera with very low immunoglobulin concentrations do not undergo precipitation when mixed with any sodium sulfite solutions in the 14% to 18% range. Fibrinogen also is precipitated by these concentrations of sodium sulfite; thus serum, rather than plasma samples, should be used.

A procedure for performing the sodium sulfite precipitation test in ruminants is presented in Appendix 26.1. In this test, the immunoglobulin concentration is determined by judging the presence or absence of precipitation in three concentrations of sodium sulfite: 14%, 16%, and 18%. The test can distinguish three ranges of immunoglobulin concentrations: <500 mg/dL, 500–1500 mg/dL, and >1500 mg/dL. Using this procedure, classification into these categories is more than 90% accurate for predicting the three immunoglobulin ranges in calves. Immunoglobulin concentrations of less than 1000 mg/dL generally are considered to be the indicator of FPT in calves , and the cutoffs in this test do not correlate with that concentration. Thus, either less than 500 mg/dL or less than 1500 mg/dL must be used as the determinant of FPT. Using the less than 500 mg/dL limit makes the test more specific for detecting FPT (e.g., calves negative for precipitation are likely to have FPT) but less sensitive for detecting FPT (e.g., will miss many calves with FPT). Using the less than 1500 mg/dL limit makes the test more sensitive for detecting FPT but reduces the specificity (e.g., will indicate FPT in calves with adequate transfer of immunoglobulin). Using the less than 500 mg/dL limit appears to correctly predict the highest percentage of calves with FPT (~86%). The sodium sulfite precipitation test appears to be unreliable for estimating serum immunoglobulin concentrations in foals.

Zinc sulfate turbidity test. The zinc sulfate turbidity test is based on the fact that immunoglobulins are selectively precipitated by zinc sulfate in solution. This occurs over a wide range of zinc sulfate concentrations.

A procedure for this test in ruminants is presented in Appendix 26.2. Like the sodium sulfite precipitation test, a positive reaction (i.e., turbidity) in sera with low immunoglobulin concentrations occurs when a solution with a high zinc sulfate concentration is used, but not when a solution with a low zinc sulfate concentration is used. In sera with high immunoglobulin concentrations, turbidity occurs when zinc sulfate solutions of lower concentrations are used. Thus, different sensitivities and specificities for detecting FPT result when different concentrations of zinc sulfate are used (see Appendix 26.2). The highest proportion of calves being correctly classified as having FPT (i.e., true immunoglobulin concentration < 1000 mg/dL) occurs when either 350 or 400 mg/L concentrations of zinc sulfate are used (83% and 88% correctly classified, respectively). The actual concentrations most appropriate for this test depend on whether high sensitivity or high specificity is most important in the specific situation.

A procedure for the zinc sulfate turbidity test in horses is presented in Appendix 26.3. Turbidity can be gauged using a spectrophotometer and standards that are indicative of known immunoglobulin concentrations, but this precludes use of the test for quick screening. Simply observing any visible turbidity in the reaction solution after 1 hour of incubation is a good indication that the foal has a serum immunoglobulin concentration of greater than 400 mg/dL. This procedure, however, does not distinguish foals with immunoglobulin concentrations of between 400 and 800 mg/dL. This is important, because immunoglobulin concentrations of less than 800 mg/dL sometimes

are considered to be suggestive of FPT in foals. Correlations between zinc sulfate turbidity results and those of more specific tests for immunoglobulin concentrations in foals are not strong.

Glutaraldehyde coagulation test. The glutaraldehyde coagulation test is based on the fact that at low concentrations, glutaraldehyde forms insoluble complexes with immunoglobulins, thereby resulting in coagulation of the test mixture. Glutaraldehyde also forms insoluble complexes with fibrinogen; therefore, serum rather than plasma is preferred. This test has been evaluated in neonatal calves and foals.

A procedure for this test in ruminants is presented in Appendix 26.4. In neonatal calves, use of a 10% glutaraldehyde solution results in no coagulation in almost all calf sera with immunoglobulin concentrations of less than 400 mg/dL and complete or partial coagulation in almost all calf sera with immunoglobulin concentrations of greater than 600 mg/dL. Calves with immunoglobulin concentrations of between 400 and 600 mg/dL have results that vary from no coagulation to complete coagulation. A disadvantage of this procedure is that whereas it adequately identifies animals with immunoglobulin concentrations of less than 400 mg/dL and less adequately identifies animals with immunoglobulin concentrations of less than 600 mg/dL, immunoglobulin concentrations of greater than 1000 mg/dL generally are considered to be indicators of adequate passive transfer in calves. Thus, this test usually is normal at immunoglobulin concentrations of between 600 and 1000 mg/dL, and calves with such concentrations might, in fact, have FPT. This low detection limit makes this test extremely specific (e.g., calves with immunoglobulin concentrations of less than 400 mg/dL most likely have FPT) but less sensitive (e.g., many calves with immunoglobulin concentrations of 400–1000 mg/dL because of FTP will not be detected).

A procedure for performing the glutaraldehyde coagulation test in horses is presented in Appendix 26.5. Immunoglobulin concentrations that are considered to be indicative of FPT in foals range from less than 200 to less than 800 mg/dL. This procedure has a sensitivity of 100% and a specificity of 89% for detecting foal sera with immunoglobulin concentrations of less than 400 mg/dL, and of 94% and 94%, respectively, for detecting foal sera with immunoglobulin concentrations of less than 800 mg/dL (using radial immunodiffusion as standard). The glutaraldehyde coagulation test is an excellent test for detecting FPT in foals.

Other screening tests for estimating immunoglobulin concentrations. Screening tests for serum immunoglobulin concentrations also are commercially available as kits. Some of these tests are based on the methods described earlier, but others use antibody-based methods (e.g., enzyme-linked immunoadsorbent assay) to estimate immunoglobulin concentrations. These tests are semi-quantitative; however, they offer the convenience of pre-packaged reagents and may require less time to perform than the previously discussed screening tests. Sensitivity, specificity, and ability to accurately predict either adequate passive transfer or FPT vary with the different test methods.

These commercially available tests are not necessarily superior to the screening tests described earlier. In foals, the glutaraldehyde coagulation test is equal or superior to commercially available semiquantitative tests in terms of sensitivity, specificity, and both negative and positive predictive ability.

Measurement of Immunoglobulin Concentrations by Reference Laboratories

Reference laboratories offer more sophisticated antibody-based methods for quantitating specific immunoglobulins (e.g., radial immunodiffusion, immunoelectrophoresis, immunochemistry). Use of these methods is indicated when a detailed examination regarding the status of the immune system is desired. These methods are more expensive, however, and the results usually are delayed (incubation periods of 18–24 hours are required) compared with those of the screening methods discussed earlier.

Fibrinogen Concentration

Plasma fibrinogen concentrations can be determined by two methods. One assesses the conversion of fibrinogen to fibrin in the presence of thrombin and requires instrumentation that is somewhat expensive for routine use in clinical practice. Such measurement of plasma fibrinogen concentrations also requires citrated plasma that has been harvested from a mixture of nine parts fresh, whole blood and one part 3.8% sodium citrate anticoagulant. Special evacuated blood collection tubes containing sodium citrate anticoagulant are available for this purpose; these tubes draw the appropriate amount of blood to ensure a 9:1 ratio of blood to anticoagulant. This method is not routinely used to measure plasma fibrinogen concentrations.

The most common method for measuring plasma fibrinogen concentration is heat precipitation. This method is less expensive and simpler than the method described earlier, and it is summarized in Appendix 26.6. It requires simple equipment, and it can be performed at a basic in-practice laboratory.

ABNORMAL PROTEIN CONCENTRATIONS

Both decreased and increased total protein concentrations are commonly detected laboratory abnormalities

in animals. Decreases or increases result from alterations in the albumin or globulin concentration (or both). In plasma, an increased concentration of fibrinogen, which is a globulin, occasionally can produce an increased protein concentration. Interpretation of altered protein concentrations depends on determining which major protein constituents of the serum or plasma (i.e., albumin, globulin, and in plasma, fibrinogen) are abnormal. A decreased or increased albumin or globulin concentration does not always result in detectable alterations of the total protein concentration. Therefore, albumin and globulin as well as total protein concentrations should be assessed when interpreting such alterations. Causes of decreased or increased total protein, albumin, globulin, and fibrinogen concentrations are summarized here.

Causes of Decreased Protein Concentrations

Decreased total protein concentrations can result from decreased concentrations of albumin, globulin, or both. A diagnostic algorithm for evaluating variations in these decreases is presented in *Figure 26.2*.

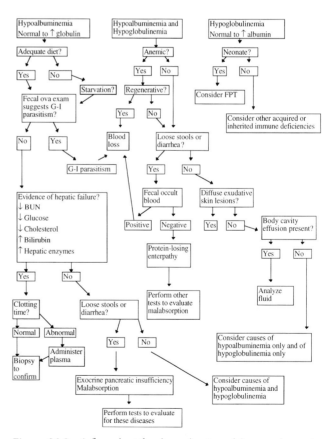

Figure 26.2 A flow chart for the evaluation of decreased protein concentrations. First, determine whether the animal has hypoalbuminemia, hypoglobulinemia, or both, and then follow the appropriate pathway.

Hypoalbuminemia with Hypoglobulinemia

Concurrent hypoalbuminemia and hypoglobulinemia can result from overhydration (e.g., excessive fluid therapy, excessive water intake) or from proportional loss of both protein fractions. The latter occurs in the following disorders:

- **Blood loss.** This results in proportional loss of all blood constituents. Albumin and globulin, therefore, are lost in concentrations equal to their concentrations in the blood. After blood loss, interstitial fluid moves into the circulatory system and dilutes the remaining blood constituents, thereby resulting in decreased plasma and serum concentrations of both albumin and globulin.
- **Protein-losing enteropathy.** This results from a variety of intestinal lesions, including inflammatory infiltrates in the lamina propria and submucosa and blockage of lymphatic drainage that leads to dilation of lymphatics (i.e., lymphangiectasia). Regardless of the underlying cause, both albumin and globulin leak from the intestinal wall into the intestinal lumen and then are digested or excreted. The result is decreased plasma and serum concentrations of both albumin and globulin. In some types of protein-losing enteropathies, a concurrent immune response results in increased, rather than decreased, serum globulin concentrations. This has been documented in Basenji dogs, but it also can occur in other breeds.
- **Severe exudative skin disease.** This results from increased vascular permeability that allows both albumin and globulin to escape from the blood.
- **Severe burns.** These cause increased vascular permeability that can result in loss of both albumin and globulin from the blood. Globulins, however, sometimes are increased in animals with severe burns.
- **Effusive disease.** This results in the accumulation of body-cavity fluids with high protein concentrations that can result in decreased serum albumin and globulin concentrations. Such decreases depend on the degree of increased vascular permeability accompanying these disorders.

Hypoalbuminemia With Normal to Increased Globulin Concentration

Decreased albumin concentrations that are not accompanied by decreased globulin concentrations can result from either decreased production or increased loss of albumin. If the globulin concentration is concurrently increased, a decreased albumin concentration may not result in a decreased total protein concentration.

   Decreased production of albumin can occur in the following disorders:

- **Hepatic failure.** The liver is the site of albumin production, and because of the liver's reserve capacity, most types of liver damage do not result in decreased albumin production. If more than 80% of the functional liver mass is lost, however, decreased albumin production can occur, eventually leading to hypoalbuminemia. Other evidence of hepatic failure (see Chapter 23) is present when this failure is the cause of hypoalbuminemia. Globulin concentrations may be increased in patients with hepatic failure (discussed later).
- **Starvation.** The liver uses amino acids in the production of albumin, and starvation can lead to a deficient supply of amino acids and, therefore, to decreased hepatic albumin production. Deficiency of amino acids, however, seldom causes a decrease in globulin production severe enough to produce detectable hypoglobulinemia.
- **Gastrointestinal parasitism.** This can cause hypoalbuminemia by at least two mechanisms. If the parasites absorb significant amounts of nutrients, including amino acids, the animal is deprived of the amino acids needed to produce albumin. If the parasites attach to the gastric or the intestinal wall and consume the host's blood, albumin and globulin are lost. Gastrointestinal parasitism seldom results in a deficiency of amino acids that is severe enough to lead to hypoglobulinemia. Fecal examination for parasite ova is helpful in establishing the diagnosis of this potential cause of hypoalbuminemia.
- **Intestinal malabsorption.** Decreased albumin production can occur if intestinal malabsorption results in deficient absorption of amino acids. Animals with malabsorption syndrome often have a history of chronic diarrhea or loose stools. If malabsorption syndrome is considered to be a possible cause of hypoalbuminemia, tests to verify this syndrome should be performed (see Chapter 25).
- **Exocrine pancreatic insufficiency (EPI).** Inadequate digestion of dietary proteins can result from EPI, in which amino acids are not liberated by protein digestion in the intestine and, therefore, are not available for absorption, thus resulting in amino acid deficiency and decreased albumin production. Animals with EPI often have a history of chronic diarrhea or loose stools. If EPI is suspected, tests to verify this disease should be performed (see Chapter 25).

Increased loss of albumin can occur in the following disorders:

- **Glomerular disease.** Because albumin molecules are smaller than globulin molecules, they leak more readily through damaged glomerular membranes. (The net negative charge of albumin molecules compared with globulin molecules also plays a part in this selective leakage.) Severe glomerular disease, therefore, can result in hypoalbuminemia with a normal serum globulin concentration. Both urinary protein concentrations and urinary protein:creatinine ratios should be increased in animals with glomerular disease. In animals with glomerular disease resulting in nephrotic syndrome, increased serum globulin concentrations may occur because of increased concentrations of alpha globulins, such as alpha$_2$-macroglobulin and alpha$_2$-lipoprotein, and beta globulins, such as transferrin and beta$_2$-lipoprotein. These increases result from a combination of increased hepatic synthesis and decreased hepatic catabolism of proteins and lipoproteins. The hypercholesterolemia that occurs in animals with nephrotic syndrome results from increased serum concentrations of cholesterol-rich lipoproteins.

- **Gastrointestinal parasitism** (discussed earlier).
- **Diseases listed as being possible causes of decreased albumin and decreased globulin** (discussed earlier). Loss of both albumin and globulin typically occurs with these diseases, but a concurrent immune response may cause increased production of globulins and, therefore, result in normal to increased globulin concentrations. These diseases also should be considered when hypoalbuminemia and normal to increased globulin concentrations are detected. When an increased globulin concentration accompanies a decreased albumin concentration, a compensatory increase in globulin concentration may have occurred.

Hypoglobulinemia with Normal to Increased Albumin Concentration

Hypoglobulinemia in the absence of hypoalbuminemia almost always results from a decreased beta or gamma globulin concentration. A decreased alpha globulin concentration alone does not result in a decreased globulin concentration. A decreased beta or gamma globulin concentration in the absence of hypoalbuminemia almost always results from a decreased immunoglobulin concentration. Such a decrease can occur in the following disorders:

- **Failure of Passive Transfer (FPT).** Ingestion of colostrum and absorption of immunoglobulins from colostrum are termed *passive transfer*. Because most animals are born with minimal immunoglobulin concentrations, this process plays an important role in transferring resistance to infection during the neonatal period. Failure to ingest colostrum or to absorb immunoglobulins from colostrum is termed *failure of passive transfer (FPT)* and is well documented in domestic animals. This failure is of concern in all

neonates, regardless of the species. Several screening tests are available to assess the adequacy of passive transfer (discussed earlier).

- **Inherited or acquired immune deficiency.** Immune deficiency involving B lymphocytes or plasma cells can result in low concentrations of immunoglobulins and, in some cases, low concentrations of globulins. Immune deficiencies resulting in low globulin concentrations have been reported in foals (e.g., transient hypogammaglobulinemia, combined immunodeficiency, selective IgM deficiency, selective IgA deficiency, agammaglobulinemia, and selective IgM, IgG(T), and IgA deficiency), calves (e.g., selective IgG2 deficiency), and puppies (e.g., combined immune deficiency and selective IgA deficiency).

Causes of Increased Protein Concentrations

Increased total protein concentrations can result from increased concentrations of albumin, globulin, or both. An increased albumin or globulin concentration, however, does not always produce detectable increases in total protein concentrations. A diagnostic algorithm for evaluating the variations in these increases is presented in *Figure 26.3*.

Hyperalbuminemia

Hyperalbuminemia occurs only with dehydration. Loss of water from the blood causes an increased concentration of albumin molecules. Globulin concentrations also may be increased in some patients with dehydration (discussed later).

Hyperalbuminemia and Hyperglobulinemia

Concurrent increases in albumin and globulin concentrations most commonly result from dehydration, which causes loss of water from the blood that, in turn, usually causes relative increases in both protein fractions. The albumin:globulin ratio is not altered, however, because both fractions are concentrated equally. The hematocrit usually is at the upper limit of the reference range or increased (unless there was a preexisting anemia). Other causes of hyperglobulinemia in dehydrated patients also should be considered (discussed later).

Hyperglobulinemia

The significance of hyperglobulinemia depends on the type of globulin that is increased.

Increased alpha globulin concentrations. Increased alpha globulin concentrations are nonspecific and of limited

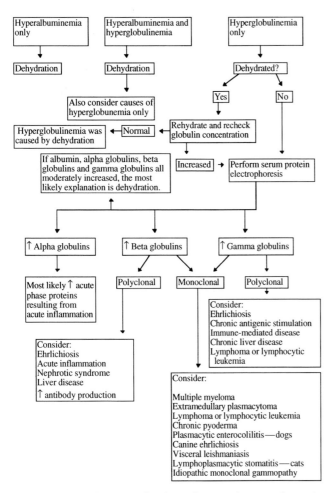

Figure 26.3 A flow chart for the evaluation of increased protein concentrations. First, determine whether the animal has hyper-albuminemia, hyperglobulinemia, or both, and then follow the appropriate pathway.

diagnostic importance. Acute inflammation is the most common cause. Concentrations of several proteins in the alpha globulin fraction (e.g., ceruloplasmin, haptoglobin, and alpha$_2$-macroglobulin) increase during acute inflammatory disease, and these proteins collectively are termed *acute-phase proteins*. Increased concentrations of lipoproteins and alpha$_2$-macroglobulin occur with nephrotic syndrome and also can result in increased alpha globulin concentrations.

Increased beta globulin concentrations. Increased beta globulin concentrations can occur with acute inflammation, nephrotic syndrome, active liver disease, and immune responses. Concentrations of several acute-phase proteins in this fraction (e.g., C-reactive protein, complement, ferritin) increase during acute inflammation. Increased beta globulin concentrations can occur with nephrotic syndrome because of increased lipoprotein con-

centrations. Transferrin, hemopexin, and complement concentrations increase during active liver disease and may result in increased beta globulin concentrations. Increased beta globulin concentrations also can result from many types of antigenic stimulation with subsequent antibody production. Monoclonal immunoglobulin peaks in the beta globulin region are possible (discussed later).

Increased gamma globulin concentrations. The gamma globulin fraction includes most of the immunoglobulins. Increases in gamma globulin concentrations are termed *gammopathies*, and they are divided into polyclonal and monoclonal gammopathies, which are distinguished on the basis of the width of the globulin peak in an electrophoretogram. Polyclonal gammopathies have broad-based peaks (i.e., wider than the base of the albumin peak, or peak height less than fourfold the peak width) on the electrophoretogram *(Fig. 26.4)*, and they represent increased quantities of immunoglobulins produced by a heterogeneous population of B lymphocytes, plasma cells, or both. Polyclonal gammopathies result from chronic antigenic stimulation associated with a variety of infectious, hepatic, and immune-mediated diseases. Monoclonal gammopathies, however, have narrow-based peaks (i.e., similar in width to the base of the albumin peak, or peak height at least fourfold the peak width) on the electrophoretogram *(Fig. 26.5)*, and they result from increased immunoglobulin production by a single clone of B lymphocytes or plasma cells. Rarely, two clones of plasma cells or B lymphocytes may proliferate, thereby resulting in production of two separate, but homogeneous,

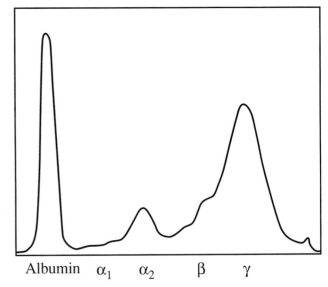

Figure 26.4 An electrophoretogram from a dog with a polyclonal gammopathy. Note the broad-based peak in the gamma region.

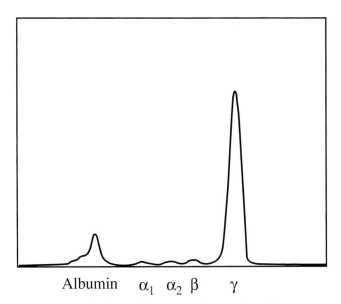

Figure 26.5 An electrophoretogram from a dog with a monoclonal gammopathy. Note the narrow-based peak in the gamma region.

types of immunoglobulins. In such cases, two narrow-based peaks are found by electrophoresis (i.e., biclonal gammopathy).

Polyclonal gammopathies. Polyclonal gammopathies can occur with the following disorders:

- **Chronic antigenic stimulation.** This can result from chronic infection or chronic presence in the body of any type of foreign substance. This stimulation leads to production of immunoglobulins by B lymphocytes, plasma cells, or both. Because more than one antigen usually is involved, the immunoglobulins that are produced are heterogeneous and, electrophoretically, migrate to produce a broad-based (i.e., polyclonal) peak. Canine ehrlichiosis and feline infectious peritonitis are diseases in which chronic antigenic stimulation by infectious agents commonly results in polyclonal gammopathies. Canine ehrlichiosis, however, also occasionally causes monoclonal gammopathies (discussed later).
- **Immune-mediated disease.** This is another form of chronic antigenic stimulation, but in this case, the antigen is, at least partially, a molecule or molecules that are native to the body. These antigens have been abnormally exposed to the body's immune system or combined with other substances (e.g., haptens) to be recognized as being foreign. The chronic antigenic stimulation occurring in these autoimmune diseases leads to a polyclonal gammopathy (discussed earlier).

- **Liver disease.** Especially when chronic, liver disease may lead to increased globulin production, which has been well-documented in horses but also occurs in other species. The globulins that are produced in association with liver disease often migrate in the beta or gamma region of an electrophoretogram. The increased globulin concentration in this region can obscure the border between the beta and gamma regions and is known as beta–gamma bridging. The mechanism leading to polyclonal gammopathy in liver disease is not known. A prevalent theory, however, is that enteric-derived antigens in the portal blood of animals with liver disease escape removal by Kupffer cells of the mononuclear phagocyte system. This system is responsible for removing and destroying antigens that are absorbed from the intestine and travel to the liver via the portal circulation. When these antigens escape the liver and pass into the remainder of the bloodstream, they come in contact with B lymphocytes, which mount an immune response. The result may be increased serum immunoglobulin concentrations. Because these antigens are heterogeneous, the immunoglobulins that are produced also are heterogeneous, and a polyclonal gammopathy results. If these immunoglobulins are IgM or IgA, they might migrate between the beta and gamma regions, and beta–gamma bridging is evident.
- **Lymphoma and lymphocytic leukemia.** Polyclonal gammopathy occasionally occurs with lymphoma and lymphocytic leukemia, sometimes because of increased production of heterogeneous immunoglobulins by proliferating, neoplastic lymphoid cells. Moreover, secondary infectious processes may stimulate immunoglobulin production in animals with lymphoma and lymphocytic leukemia. Monoclonal gammopathies also can result from lymphoma and lymphocytic leukemia (discussed later).

Monoclonal gammopathies. Hypoalbuminemia often accompanies monoclonal gammopathies, but the mechanism is unknown. Monoclonal gammopathies can occur with the following disorders:

- **Multiple myeloma.** This is a malignant, proliferative disease of plasma cells that involves the bone marrow at multiple sites and, often, other tissues (e.g., spleen, liver). Multiple myeloma results from the proliferation of a single clone of B lymphocytes, which often are differentiated to plasma cells. This clone produces a homogeneous type of protein that is referred to as paraprotein or M-component. This protein most commonly is IgA or IgG; IgM paraproteinemias occur with lymphoma and lymphocytic leukemia. The paraproteins can be composed of entire immunoglobulin molecules or of heavy or light chains of these molecules.

Monoclonal gammopathies that are composed of complete immunoglobulin molecules have been reported in dogs, cats, and horses. Heavy- and light-chain monoclonal gammopathies have been reported in dogs. Paraproteins typically are found as a monoclonal peak in the beta or gamma region and, more rarely, in the alpha region of the electrophoretogram. Light chains also may be detected in the urine and are referred to as Bence-Jones proteins (discussed later). The diagnosis of this disease is established on the basis of finding at least three of the following four features:

1. Monoclonal gammopathy.
2. Plasma cells accounting for more than 5% to 20% of nucleated cells on a bone marrow film. The percentage of plasma cells that is considered to be suggestive of myeloma varies with different authors. Chronic antigenic stimulation also can result in greater than 5% plasma cells on a bone marrow film. Other features that are suggestive of plasma cell neoplasia, such as the presence of plasma cell aggregates, poorly differentiated plasma cells, or both, are helpful in differentiating myeloma from antigenic stimulation in bone marrow films with increased numbers of plasma cell.
3. Radiographic evidence of osteolytic bone lesions.
4. Bence-Jones proteinuria. Bence-Jones proteins are light chains of immunoglobulins that are produced in some gammopathies. Because of their small size, these proteins readily pass the glomerulus. If the concentration of Bence-Jones proteins in the urine exceeds the tubular reabsorptive capacity, they are excreted in the urine. Bence-Jones proteins rarely are detected by urine dipstick tests for proteins, because dipsticks primarily detect albumin. Bence-Jones proteins can be detected by several techniques, including the heat precipitation test, electrophoresis,. and immunoelectrophoresis. The heat precipitation test can be performed in a practice laboratory, but this test is difficult and very unreliable. Bence-Jones proteins are detectable in approximately 30% of dogs and cats with multiple myelomas and have been reported in a horse with multiple myeloma. Bence-Jones proteins also have been reported in dogs with monoclonal gammopathies associated with chronic pyoderma, lymphocytic leukemia, and idiopathic monoclonal gammopathy.

■ **Extramedullary plasmacytoma.** Extramedullary plasmacytomas are proliferations of plasma cells originating from a site other than bone. They most commonly occur in dogs but have been reported in cats. Monoclonal gammopathies rarely occur in association with these tumors. A biclonal gammopathy has been reported in a cat with two extramedullary plasmacytomas. Biclonal gammopathies are rare, however, and likely result from the proliferation of two different plasma cell clones.

■ **Lymphoma and lymphocytic leukemia.** Monoclonal gammopathies can occur with lymphoma and lymphocytic leukemia in dogs. Approximately 5% of dogs with lymphoma and lymphocytic leukemia have monoclonal gammopathies. This incidence is higher in dogs with chronic lymphocytic leukemia, however, with the results of some studies indicating an incidence of greater than 50% in such cases. The immunoglobulin most commonly increased is IgM, especially in cases of chronic lymphocytic leukemia, but IgG and IgA monoclonal gammopathies also have been reported in dogs with chronic lymphocytic leukemia. Monoclonal gammopathies of the IgM type also are termed *macroglobulinemias*, and the term *primary macroglobulinemia* has been applied to IgM monoclonal gammopathies in which the proliferating cells are intermediate between small lymphocytes and plasma cells. This syndrome is analogous to Waldenström macroglobulinemia in humans. The distinction between Waldenström macroglobulinemia and other lymphomas that produce monoclonal IgM is confusing, however, and of questionable importance in dogs.

■ **Chronic pyoderma.** An IgG monoclonal gammopathy with Bence-Jones proteinuria has been reported in a dog with chronic pyoderma. Treatment and resolution of the pyoderma were followed by disappearance of the monoclonal gammopathy.

■ **Plasmacytic enterocolitis.** Monoclonal gammopathy has been reported in a dog with this disease. The monoclonal gammopathy disappeared after treatment and resolution of the inflammation.

■ **Canine ehrlichiosis.** Both monoclonal and, more commonly, polyclonal gammopathies can occur in *Ehrlichia canis*–infected dogs. Infrequently, polyclonal gammopathies progress to monoclonal gammopathies. Typically, these are composed of IgG and result from an unexplained proliferation of one plasma cell clone. Monoclonal spikes disappear after treatment for ehrlichiosis. The serum hyperviscosity syndrome (discussed later) has been reported in dogs with *Ehrlichia* sp.–associated, IgG monoclonal gammopathy.

■ **Visceral leishmaniasis (in dogs).** Most dogs with visceral leishmaniasis have polyclonal gammopathies. In a few such dogs, a single clone of plasma cells may proliferate and result in IgG monoclonal gammopathy.

■ **Lymphoplasmacytic stomatitis (in cats).** Monoclonal gammopathy with Bence-Jones proteinuria infrequently occurs in cats with this disease.

■ **Idiopathic monoclonal gammopathy.** Unexplained monoclonal gammopathies among animals in which known causes have been eliminated are termed *idiopathic*. These animals usually have stable production of the monoclonal immunoglobulin during a prolonged period of time (i.e., months) and, in some cases, even are reported to remain stable for years. Bence-Jones proteinuria occurs in some of these cases. These gammopathies may not be neoplastic in origin, and they may relate to antigenic stimulation of a B-lymphocyte clone. "Idiopathic" monoclonal gammopathy, however, may precede the onset of overt multiple myeloma.

Hyperviscosity of the blood can result from high concentrations of immunoglobulins, especially in association with monoclonal gammopathies. Hyperviscosity syndrome might cause the initial clinical signs observed in animals with monoclonal gammopathies. These signs include epistaxis, ocular abnormalities (e.g., visual impairment, distension and tortuosity of retinal veins, retinal hemorrhage, papilledema), cardiovascular abnormalities (e.g., gallop rhythm, left ventricular hypertrophy), and neurologic dysfunction. Whereas IgM molecules commonly cause this syndrome, smaller IgA molecules also may cause this syndrome, probably because of the formation of dimers and polymers. In addition, IgG monoclonal gammopathies can result in hyperviscosity syndrome, but this is not common.

Monoclonal cryoglobulinemia is a variation of monoclonal gammopathy in dogs. In this disorder, the monoclonal globulins are soluble at 37°C but become reversibly insoluble at lower temperatures, thereby causing the serum to gel. To demonstrate cryoglobulins, serum must be harvested from the blood at 37°C. If blood samples are stored at refrigerator temperature before harvesting the serum, the cryoglobulins are not harvested, and cryoglobulinemia is not detected. If cryoglobulins are present in serum harvested at 37°C, such serum gels or develops a precipitate at refrigerator temperatures, and it becomes liquid when the serum is rewarmed. Cryoglobulins usually are IgM, but they may be IgG.

Hyperfibrinogenemia

Hyperfibrinogenemia can occur in the following disorders:

- **Dehydration.** With dehydration, fibrinogen increases in proportion to other plasma proteins. To eliminate the effect of hydration status, a plasma protein : fibrinogen ratio (PP : Fib) can be calculated. The PP : Fib should not change with changes in hydration status, and it is calculated as follows:

$$PP/Fib = \frac{Plasma\ protein\ (g/dL)}{Plasma\ fibrinogen\ (mg/dL)/1000}$$

The PP/Fib is interpreted as follows: in horses, 15 or greater is normal and can occur with dehydration, but less than 15 is suggestive of a true increase in fibrinogen concentration; in ruminants, 15 or greater is normal and can occur with dehydration, less than 10 is suggestive of a true increase in fibrinogen concentration, and 10 to 14 is suggestive of a true increase in fibrinogen concentration but is higher than typical of most inflammatory processes in ruminants.

- **Inflammation.** Fibrinogen is an important component of the hemogram in ruminants, because this concentration is markedly increased with inflammation. Milder increases occur in horses and llamas with inflammatory diseases, and fibrinogen is diagnostically useful in these species as well. Increases are inconsistent with inflammation in dogs and cats, however, so fibrinogen is not very diagnostically useful in these species.
- **Renal disease.** Chronic nephritis, especially glomerulonephritis, can result in hyperfibrinogenemia in dogs. Hyperfibrinogenemia also occurs in cattle with renal disease.
- **Disseminated neoplastic disease.**
- **Terminal pregnancy (in cattle).**

SUGGESTED READINGS

Qualitative and Semiquantitative Determination of Immunoglobulin Concentrations
Calves
Hudgens KAR, Tyler JW, Besser TE, et al. Optimizing performance of a qualitative zinc sulfate turbidity test for passive transfer of immunoglobulin G in calves. Am J Vet Res 1996;57:1711–1713.
Naylor JM, Kronfeld DS, Bech-Nielsen S. Plasma total protein measurement for prediction of disease and mortality in calves. J Am Vet Med Assoc 1977;171:635–638.
O'Rourke KI, Satterfield WC. Glutaraldehyde coagulation test for detection of hypogammaglobulinemia in neonatal nondomestic ruminants. J Am Vet Med Assoc 1981;179:1144–1146.
Perino LJ, Sutherland RL, Woollen NE. Serum gamma-glutamyltransferase activity and protein concentration at birth and after suckling in calves with adequate and inadequate passive transfer of immunoglobulin G. Am J Vet Res 1993;54:56–59.
Perino LJ, Wittum TE, Ross GS. Effects of various risk factors on plasma protein and serum immunoglobulin concentrations of calves at post-partum hours 10 and 24. Am J Vet Res 1995;56:1144–1148.
Pfeiffer NE, McGuire TC. A sodium sulfite–precipitation test for assessment of colostral immunoglobulin transfer to calves. J Am Vet Med Assoc 1977;170:809–811.
Rea DE, Tyler JW, Hancock DD, et al. Prediction of calf mortality by use of tests for passive transfer of colostral immunoglobulin. J Am Vet Med Assoc 1996;208:2047–2049.
Tennant B, Baldwin BH, Braun RK, et al. Use of the glutaraldehyde coagulation test for detection of hypogammaglobulinemia in neonatal calves. J Am Vet Med Assoc 1979;174:848–853.
Tyler JW, Besser TE, Wilson L, et al. Evaluation of a whole blood glutaraldehyde coagulation test for the detection of failure of passive transfer in calves. J Vet Intern Med 1996;10:82–84.
Tyler JW, Hancock DD, Parish SM, et al. Evaluation of three assays for failure of passive transfer in calves. J Vet Intern Med 1996;10:304–307.

Foals

Bauer JE, Brooks TP. Immunoturbidimetric quantification of serum immunoglobulin G concentration in foals. Am J Vet Res 1990;51: 1211–1214.

Bertone JJ, Jones RL, Curtis CR. Evaluation of a test kit for determination of serum immunoglobulin G concentration in foals. J Vet Intern Med 1988;2:181–183.

Clabough DL, Conboy HS, Roberts MC. Comparison of four screening techniques for the diagnosis of equine neonatal hypogammaglobulinemia. J Am Vet Med Assoc 1989;194:1717–1720.

Rumbaugh GE, Ardans AA, Ginno D, et al. Measurement of neonatal equine immunoglobulins for assessment of colostral immunoglobulin transfer: comparison of single radial immunodiffusion with the zinc sulfate turbidity test, serum electrophoresis, refractometry for total serum protein, and the sodium sulfite precipitation test. J Am Vet Med Assoc 1978;172:321–325.

Hypoproteinemia

Breitschwerdt EB, Barta O, Waltman C, et al. Serum proteins in healthy Basenjis and Basenjis with chronic diarrhea. Am J Vet Res 1983;44: 326–328.

Couto CG, Rutgers HC, Sherding RG, et al. Gastrointestinal lymphoma in 20 dogs: a retrospective study. J Vet Intern Med 1989;3:73–78.

Jacobs G, Collins-Kelly L, Lappin M, et al. Lymphocytic-plasmacytic enteritis in 24 dogs. J Vet Intern Med 1990;4:45–53.

Kern MR, Stockham SL, Coates JR. Analysis of serum protein concentrations after severe thermal injury in a dog. Vet Clin Pathol 1992; 21:19–22.

Meuten DJ, Butler DG, Thomson GW, et al. Chronic enteritis associated with malabsorption and protein-losing enteropathy in the horse. J Am Vet Med Assoc 1978;172:324–333.

Olson NC, Zimmer J. Protein-losing enteropathy secondary to intestinal lymphangiectasia in a dog. J Am Vet Med Assoc 1978;173:271–274.

Hyperproteinemia

Polyclonal Gammopathies

Parraga ME, Carlson GP, Thurmond M. Serum protein concentrations in horses with severe liver disease: a retrospective study and review of the literature. J Vet Intern Med 1995;9:154–161.

Williams DA. Gammopathies. Comp Cont Educ 1981;3:815–822.

Monoclonal gammopathies

Breitschwerdt EB, Woody BJ, Zerbe CA, et al. Monoclonal gammopathy associated with naturally occurring canine ehrlichiosis. J Vet Intern Med 1987;1:2–9.

Burkhard MJ, Meyer DJ, Rosychuk RA, et al. Monoclonal gammopathy in a dog with chronic pyoderma. J Vet Intern Med 1995;9: 357–360.

Couto CG, Ruehl W, Muir S. Plasma cell leukemia and monoclonal (IgG) gammopathy in a dog. J Am Vet Med Assoc 1984;184:90–92.

Diehl KJ, Lappin MR, Jones RL, et al. Monoclonal gammopathy in a dog with plasmacytic gastroenterocolitis. J Am Vet Med Assoc 1992; 210:1233–1236.

Dorfman M, Dimski DS. Paraproteinemias in small animal medicine. Comp Cont Educ 1992;14:621–632.

Edwards DF, Parker JW, Wilkinson JE, et al. Plasma cell myeloma in the horse: a case report and literature review. J Vet Intern Med 1993;7: 169–176.

Font A, Closa JM, Mascort J. Monoclonal gammopathy in a dog with visceral leishmaniasis. J Vet Intern Med 1994;8:233–235.

Hammer AS, Couto CG. Complications of multiple myeloma. J Am Anim Hosp Assoc 1994;30:9–14.

Hoenig M. Multiple myeloma associated with the heavy chains of immunoglobulin A in a dog. J Am Vet Med Assoc 1987;190: 1191–1192.

Hoenig M, O'Brien JA. A benign hypergammaglobulinemia mimicking plasma cell myeloma. J Am Anim Hosp Assoc 1988;24:688–690.

Jackson MW, Helfand SC, Smedes SL, et al. Primary IgG secreting plasma cell tumor in the gastrointestinal tract of a dog. J Am Vet Med Assoc 1994;204:404–406.

Jacobs RM, Couto CG, Wellman ML. Biclonal gammopathy in a dog with myeloma and cutaneous lymphoma. Vet Pathol 1986;23: 211–213.

Mandel NS, Esplin DG. A retroperitoneal extramedullary plasmacytoma in a cat with a monoclonal gammopathy. J Am Anim Hosp Assoc 1994;30:603–608.

Matus RE, Leifer CE, MacEwen G, et al. Prognostic factors for multiple myeloma in the dog. J Am Vet Med Assoc 1986;188:1288–1292.

McEwen EG, Hurvitz AI, Hayes A. Hyperviscosity syndrome associated with lymphocytic leukemia in three dogs. J Am Vet Med Assoc 1977;170:1309–1312.

Larsen AE, Carpenter JL. Hepatic plasmacytoma and biclonal gammopathy in a cat. J Am Vet Med Assoc 1994;205:708–710.

Leifer CE, Matus RE. Chronic lymphocytic leukemia in the dog: 22 cases (1974–1984). J Am Vet Med Assoc 1986;189:214–217.

Lyon KF. Feline lymphoplasmacytic stomatitis associated with monoclonal gammopathy and Bence-Jones proteinuria. J Vet Dent 1994; 11:25–27.

Thrall MA. Lymphoproliferative disorders. Vet Clin North Am Sm Ani Prac 1981;11:321–347.

APPENDIX 26.1

SODIUM SULFITE PRECIPITATION TEST: APPLICATION IN RUMINANTS

1. Prepare three solutions of sodium sulfite (14%, 16%, and 18%) from anhydrous sulfite and distilled water.
2. Place 1.9 mL of sodium sulfite solution into each of three test tubes.
3. Add 0.1 mL of serum into each of the three tubes.

4. Mix immediately, and then incubate at room temperature for 1 hour.
5. After 1 hour, examine the tubes for evidence of precipitation.
6. Interpret as described in *Table 26A.1*.

TABLE 26A.1 INTERPRETATION OF SODIUM SULFITE PRECIPITATION TEST RESULTS

Immunoglabulin Concentration	Sodium Sulfite Concentration		
	14%	16%	18%
<500 mg/dL	−	−	+
500–1500 mg/dL	−	+	+
>1500 mg/dL	+	+	+

−, No precipitation after 1 hour (cloudiness without visible flakes is a negative test); +, flakes of precipitation after 1 hour. If flakes are noted, the result is considered to be positive regardless of the density of the flakes.

APPENDIX 26.2

ZINC SULFATE TURBIDITY TEST: APPLICATION IN RUMINANTS

1. Prepare a solution of zinc sulfate ($ZnSO_4 \cdot 7H_2O$) by mixing 350 mg of zinc sulfate in 1 L of distilled water that has been previously boiled to remove CO_2. Note that lower concentrations of zinc sulfate might be appropriate in some cases. Lower concentrations have a higher sensitivity but a lower specificity; higher concentrations (e.g., 350 mg/L) have a lower sensitivity and a higher specificity *(Table 26A.2)*.
2. The solution should be stored in an air-tight bottle that is connected to a CO_2 trap to prevent CO_2 absorption.
3. Add 0.1 mL of serum (hemolysis might interfere with the test) to a tube (13×100 mm) containing 6 mL of the zinc sulfate solution. Cap the tube, because absorption of CO_2 adds to turbidity.
4. Mix the contents of the tube, and then allow those contents to incubate at room temperature (23°C) for 1 hour.
5. After the incubation period, mix the contents of the tube, and then hold the tube in front of newsprint.
6. Cloudiness sufficient to make newsprint illegible when viewed through the tube is considered to be a positive reaction.
7. Interpret a negative reaction as being suggestive of the failure of passive transfer.

TABLE 26A.2 SENSITIVITY AND SPECIFICITY FOR DETECTING FPT IN RUMINANTS AT VARIOUS CONCENTRATIONS OF ZINC SULFATE

Zinc Sulfate Concentration	Sensitivity	Specificity
200 mg/L	100%	25%
250 mg/L	100%	42%
300 mg/L	98%	65%
350 mg/L	94%	76%
400 mg/L	83%	91%

Adapted from Hudgens KAR, Tyler JW, Besser TE, Krytenberg DS. Optimizing performance of a qualitative zinc sulfate turbidity test for passive transfer of immunoglobulin G in calves. Am J Vet Res 1996;57:1711–1713.

ZINC SULFATE TURBIDITY TEST:
APPLICATION IN HORSES

1. Prepare a solution of zinc sulfate ($ZnSO_4 \cdot 7H_2O$) by mixing 208 mg of zinc sulfate in 1 L of distilled water that has been previously boiled to remove CO_2.
2. The solution should be stored in an air-tight bottle that is connected to a CO_2 trap to prevent CO_2 absorption.
3. Add 0.1 mL of serum to a tube (13 × 100 mm) containing 6 mL of the zinc sulfate solution. Cap the tube, because absorption of CO_2 adds to turbidity.
4. Mix the contents of the tube, and then allow those contents to incubate at room temperature (23°C) for 1 hour.
5. After the incubation period, mix the contents of the tube, and then observe for turbidity.
6. Interpret as follows:
    A. Visible turbidity is indicative of less than 400 mg/dL of immunoglobulin.
    B. This test can be made semiquantitative by using a spectrophotometer and reading absorbance at 600 nm; this also requires the use of standards.

GLUTARALDEHYDE COAGULATION TEST:
APPLICATION IN RUMINANTS

1. Prepare a 10% solution of glutaraldehyde (usually prepared via dilution of a 25% solution to a 10% solution).
2. Place 0.5 mL of serum into a tube.
3. Add 50 µL (0.05 mL) of the 10% glutaraldehyde reagent to the tube.
4. Mix immediately, and then incubate at room temperature.
5. Examine the tube at intervals for as long as 1 hour, looking for evidence of coagulation.
6. Interpret as follows:
    A. Complete coagulation is indicative of more than 600 mg/dL of immunoglobulin.
    B. Semisolid clot is indicative of 400 to 600 mg/dL of immunoglobulin.
    C. No coagulation is indicative of less than 400 mg/dL of immunoglobulin.

GLUTARALDEHYDE COAGULATION TEST:
APPLICATION IN HORSES

1. Perform steps 1 through 4 as outlined in Appendix 26.4.
2. Examine the tube at 5, 10, 15, 20, 30, 45, and 60 minutes.
3. A positive reaction is solid coagulation (i.e., does not move when the tube is tilted).
4. Interpret as follows:
    A. Coagulation by 10 minutes or less is indicative of more than 800 mg/dL of immunoglobulin.
    B. Coagulation by 60 minutes is indicative of more 400 to 800 mg/dL of immunoglobulin.
    C. No coagulation by 60 minutes is indicative of less than 400 mg/dL of immunoglobulin.

HEAT PRECIPITATION METHOD FOR MEASURING
PLASMA FIBRINOGEN CONCENTRATIONS

1. Fill two microhematocrit tubes with ethylenediaminetetraacetic acid (EDTA)–anticoagulated blood.
2. Sediment blood in both tubes using a microhematocrit centrifuge.
3. Break one tube at the bottom of the plasma column, apply the plasma to a refractometer, and read the protein concentration.
4. Place the second microhematocrit tube in a waterbath at 56 to 58°C for 3 to 5 minutes, which denatures and precipitates the fibrinogen in the sample. Note that hot tap water frequently is in the 56 to 58°C range. If so (check with a thermometer), such tap water placed in a styrofoam container can replace the waterbath as an incubation chamber.
5. After incubation, recentrifuge the second microhematocrit tube in the microhematocrit centrifuge to sediment the precipitated fibrinogen.
6. Measure the protein concentration in the second tube using a refractometer.
7. Subtract the protein concentration of the second tube from that of the first tube. The difference is the estimate of the plasma fibrinogen concentration. For example, if the protein concentration in the first tube is 7.1 g/dL and that in the second tube is 6.7 g/dL, then the fibrinogen concentration is 0.4 g/dL.
8. Fibrinogen concentrations usually are converted to mg/dL (e.g., 0.4 g/dL = 400 mg/dL).

27

LABORATORY DETECTION

OF MUSCLE INJURY

Laboratory tests that evaluate muscle are primarily aimed at detecting muscle injury. These tests include assays that measure the serum activities of enzymes that leak from injured muscle cells and the urine concentrations of myoglobin, which also leaks from injured muscle cells and is excreted via glomerular filtration.

CREATINE KINASE

Creatine kinase (CK), which also is sometimes referred to as creatine phosphokinase, is an enzyme located in skeletal muscle, cardiac muscle, smooth muscle, brain, and nerves. Creatine kinase is found free in the cytoplasm of muscle cells and leaks from these cells when they are damaged. Creatine kinase is considered to be a muscle-specific leakage enzyme. Although CK is present in the brain and nerves, increased CK activity is not found in the serum after injury to the central nervous system. Such injury can result in increased CK activity in the cerebrospinal fluid, but the enzyme does not pass into the blood via the blood-brain barrier in quantities significant enough to alter the serum CK activity. A falsely increased serum CK activity can occur as a result of hemolysis, hyperbilirubinemia and muscle fluid contamination of the blood sample during a difficult venipuncture.

Increased serum CK activity results from:

- **Skeletal muscle injury:** The magnitude of increase does not necessarily correlate with the extent of muscle injury. Muscle necrosis and ischemia, intramuscular injection of irritating substances, strenuous exercise, and trauma during shipping can result in an increased serum CK activity as well.
- **Cardiac muscle injury:** As with skeletal muscle injury, the magnitude of increase does not necessarily correlate with the extent of injury.
- **Muscle catabolism:** Increased CK activity can occur in anorexic cats that have diseases not directly involving muscle. A median serum CK activity of 2529 IU/L, with some activities being greater than 10,000 IU/L (reference range = 10–100 IU/L), has been reported in such cats. Muscle catabolism to supply amino acids for protein synthesis and gluconeogenesis is theorized to result in the leakage of CK from muscle cells. The CK activities in these cats decreases rapidly after nutritional support is initiated.

Serum CK activity increases rapidly after muscle injury and decreases rapidly after the injury ceases (Fig. 27.1). Serum CK activity peaks at 6 to 12 hours after acute muscle injury, and it returns to normal within 24 to 48 hours

417

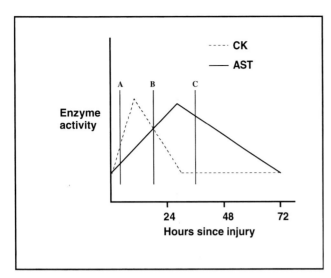

Figure 27.1 Serum activities of both AST and CK increase as a result of muscle injury, but these activities rise and fall at different rates. Various combinations of increased and normal CK and AST activities can help in the estimation of when a muscle injury occurred and whether such injury is still occurring. An increase in only the serum CK activity (line A) suggests very acute muscle injury. Increased serum activities of both AST and CK (line B) suggest active or recent muscle injury. An increase in only the serum AST activity (line C) suggests that muscle injury stopped more than 2 days earlier, and that the serum CK activity returned to normal as a result of the short half-life of CK. An increase in only the serum AST activity may also result from liver injury.

after the injury has stopped. The half-lives of CK in the blood of horses and cattle are less than 2 hours and 4 hours, respectively.

Extremely high serum CK activities (>10,000 IU/L) occasionally are detected in animals with muscle injuries. Technicians analyzing such serum for CK activity may have difficulty reaching an end point in the assay and must continue diluting the sample in an attempt to do so. These cases may represent extreme leakage of CK from injured muscle cells, but the dilution of serum may dilute endogenous inhibitors of CK. Therefore, serum CK activity continues to increase with serial dilution, and the effect of the inhibitors is progressively decreased. As a result, serum CK activity occasionally is reported as being greater than the highest activity measured at that point. In these cases, animals undoubtedly have increased serum CK activities and significant muscle injury; however, the exaggerated serum CK activities may be artifactually increased.

Creatine Kinase Isoenzymes

Enzymes with the same catalytic activity but differing in other chemical properties are termed *isoenzymes*. These isoenzymes may be produced in several different tissues, and they can be separated by testing chemical properties other than catalytic activity (e.g., electrophoretic mobil-

ity, thermal stability, resistance or susceptibility to chemical inactivation). Creatine kinase molecules are composed of two subunits: muscle (M) and brain (B). Three CK isoenzymes have been identified in animals and are designated as CK1, or BB (containing two brain subunits); CK2, or MB (containing one muscle and one brain subunit); and CK3, or MM (containing two muscle subunits). In most mammals, CK1 originates from the nervous tissue, and although present in the cerebrospinal fluid, it is not present in the serum of normal animals or of animals with neurologic disease. Although CK2 may be present in skeletal muscle, it originates primarily from cardiac muscle; CK3 originates in both skeletal and cardiac muscle. Cats do not have CK2 activity in their serum. Isolation and identification of CK isoenzymes is not practical in most clinical cases.

ASPARTATE AMINOTRANSFERASE

Aspartate aminotransferase (AST), which previously was known as serum glutamic oxaloacetic transaminase (SGOT), is present in the highest concentrations in hepatocytes as well as in skeletal and cardiac muscle cells. Aspartate aminotransferase is present in both the cytoplasm and the organelles of these cells. Increased serum AST activity results from hepatocyte (see Chapter 23) or muscle injury. Serum AST activity, however, increases more slowly than serum CK activity after muscle injury (Fig. 27.1). It peaks at approximately 24 to 36 hours after acute muscle injury, and it decreases more slowly than serum CK activity after the muscle injury ceases. The half-lives of AST in the blood of horses and dogs are approximately 50 hours and 12 hours, respectively.

The relative serum activities of both CK and AST can be used to estimate when muscle injury occurred—and whether active muscle injury is still occurring. These differences are diagrammed in Figure 27.1. An increase in only the serum CK activity (Fig. 27.1, line A) suggests very acute muscle injury (i.e., there has not been sufficient time since the injury occurred for the serum AST activity to increase). Increased serum activities of both AST and CK (Fig. 27.1, line B) suggest active or recent muscle injury. An increase in only the serum AST activity (Fig. 27.1, line C), however, suggests that muscle injury stopped more than 2 days earlier, and that the serum CK activity returned to normal as a result of the short half-life of CK. This latter combination of results also can occur with liver injury (i.e., if liver is the source of the AST, the CK activity would be normal).

ALANINE AMINOTRANSFERASE

Alanine aminotransferase (ALT) previously was known as serum glutamic pyruvic transaminase (SGPT). Previously, ALT was considered to be a liver-specific leakage enzyme, but increased serum ALT activity has been reported in dogs and cats with muscle damage but without apparent liver damage, thereby suggesting that muscle is a potential source of increased serum ALT activity. The ALT activities in skeletal and cardiac muscles are approximately 5% and 25%, respectively, of the liver ALT activity. Muscle, however, should be considered as a potential source of increased serum ALT activity, because the total mass of muscle is much greater than that of liver. Measuring the serum activity of an enzyme with greater muscle specificity (e.g., CK) is preferable for detecting muscle damage, because ALT is not specific for muscle. This enzyme is discussed in more detail in Chapter 23.

LACTATE DEHYDROGENASE

Lactate dehydrogenase (LDH) is located in the cytoplasm of most cells in the body. Injury to most tissues results in leakage of LDH into the extracellular space and the blood; therefore, LDH is a very nonspecific enzyme. Serum LDH activities increase as a result of muscle injury, but they also increase after injury to many other tissues. The serum LDH assay is not a useful test for the diagnosis of muscle injury.

Lactate Dehydrogenase Isoenzymes

Five LDH isoenzymes exist, and they can be identified by electrophoretic separation. Each isoenzyme is present in a limited number of tissues and, therefore, is more tissue specific than the serum total LDH activity. Lactate dehydrogenase molecules are composed of four components, which are either muscle (M) or heart (H) subunits. The five isoenzymes are LDH_1 (H_4), LDH_2 (MH_3), LDH_3 (M_2H_2), LDH_4 (M_3H), and LDH_5 (M_4). The designations H_4, MH_3, and so on refer to the number of each subunit (M or H) in the LDH isoenzyme molecule. The LDH_1 (H_4) isoenzyme is present predominantly in cardiac muscle, and the LDH_5 (M_4) isoenzyme is present predominantly in skeletal muscle. The remaining three isoenzymes are found in variable quantities in several different tissues. Analysis of LDH isoenzymes is, therefore, potentially useful for specifically detecting cardiac or skeletal muscle injury. Isoenzyme analysis is not practical in most situations, however, and rarely is performed in veterinary medicine.

MYOGLOBINEMIA AND MYOGLOBINURIA

Myoglobin is released from dead or dying muscle cells into the blood as a result of severe, usually acute muscle injury. Because myoglobin has a low molecular weight and is not significantly bound to proteins in the blood, it quickly passes through the glomerulus and is excreted in the urine. The urine will be brown to red-brown *(Fig. 27.2)* if the urinary myoglobin concentration is high enough. Myoglobin is detected as a positive reaction on the urine dipstick test for blood or hemoglobin because of its peroxidase activity. Therefore, myoglobinuria must be differentiated from hemoglobinuria, but this differentiation can be aided by observing the color of the serum. Hemoglobin is a larger molecule than myoglobin. The larger hemoglobin molecules do not pass through the glomerulus as readily as myoglobin molecules.

Hemoglobin released into the plasma because of hemolysis is quickly bound to a carrier protein, haptoglobin. Hemoglobin–haptoglobin complexes are even larger, and they also do not readily pass through the glomerulus. Therefore, hemoglobin tends to be retained in the serum after hemolysis and imparts a red color to the serum. Myoglobin, however, is readily excreted by the kidneys, tends not to be retained in the serum after muscle injury, and, therefore, does not readily cause a color change in the serum. Colorless to yellow serum in animals with a positive reaction for hemoglobin on a urine dipstick test suggests myoglobinuria; red serum in such animals is suggestive of hemolysis and, therefore, hemoglobinuria.

A screening test is available for differentiating hemoglobin from myoglobin in the urine. This test is based on the fact that hemoglobin precipitates in urine that is 80% saturated with ammonium sulfate, whereas myoglobin does not. This test can be used with urine that is positive on the hemoglobin portion of the urine dipstick test. Addition of ammonium sulfate to such urine in a quantity sufficient to produce an 80% concentration will cause hemoglobin to precipitate, and the resulting supernatant will react negatively on the dipstick test if the original

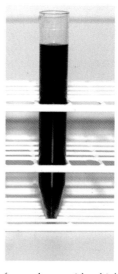

Figure 27.2 Urine from a horse with a high myoglobin concentration. High concentrations of myoglobin result in brown to red-brown urine.

cause of the positive reaction for hemoglobin was, in fact, hemoglobinuria (i.e., hemoglobin precipitated and was eliminated from the supernatant). Similar treatment of urine containing myoglobin rather than hemoglobin results in a supernatant that continues to react positively on the dipstick test (i.e., myoglobin does not precipitate and remains in the supernatant). This test is not completely accurate, however, and its results can suggest the presence of myoglobin in urine with an extremely high hemoglobin concentration because of incomplete precipitation of the hemoglobin. The presence or absence of laboratory evidence for hemolysis (e.g., anemia) or muscle damage (e.g., increased serum CK and/or AST activity) is helpful in differentiating hemoglobinuria from myoglobinuria.

SUGGESTED READINGS

Dow SW, LeCouteur RA, Fettman MJ, et al. Potassium depletion in cats: Hypokalemic polymyopathy. J Am Vet Med Assoc 1987;191:1563–1568.

Fascetti AJ, Mauldin GE, Mauldin GN. Correlation between serum creatine kinase activities and anorexia in cats. J Vet Int Med 1997;11:9–13.

Spier SJ, Carlson GP, Holliday TA, et al. Hyperkalemic periodic paralysis in horses. J Am Vet Med Assoc 1990;197:1009–1017.

Swenson CL, Graves TK. Absence of liver specificity for canine alanine aminotransferase (ALT). Vet Clin Pathol 1997;26:26–28.

Valentine BA, Blue JT, Shelley SM, et al. Increased serum alanine aminotransferase activity associated with muscle necrosis in the dog. J Vet Int Med 1990;4:140–143.

28

LABORATORY EVALUATION

OF LIPIDS

Lipids serve many important roles in the body. Compared to carbohydrates and protein, they provide a higher-caloric-density form of energy storage, which is necessary for survival during prolonged fasts and for effective function during extended aerobic activities. Lipids represent the principle component of cellular membranes and, as such, contribute to the structural integrity of cells and their organelles. The hydrophobic properties of lipids make them ideal as semipermeable barriers between fluid compartments and as insulation against undesired conduction of ions and electrical potentials. When deposited in appropriate amounts and locations, lipids provide a physical buffer against trauma and adverse, external thermal challenges. When in suspension in the body fluids, lipids serve as polar solvents that facilitate movement of fat-soluble chemicals, including vitamins and hormones. Lipids also serve as precursors for de novo synthesis of chemicals that are integral to normal metabolism, including steroid hormones and bile acids.

Abnormalities of lipid metabolism can result in life-threatening consequences. These abnormalities may result from factors as varied as excessive caloric intake to metabolic abnormalities that deter lipid transport and turnover. Abnormalities of lipid metabolism in domestic animals and methods for establishing the diagnosis of these abnormalities are discussed in this chapter. Before considering these abnormalities and their diagnosis, however, it is necessary to understand which lipids normally are present in the blood, the role they play in lipid metabolism, and the methods of measuring blood lipid concentrations.

LIPIDS NORMALLY PRESENT IN BLOOD

Lipids that normally are present in the blood include long-chain fatty acids (LCFAs), triglycerides, and cholesterol. These lipids are transported attached to proteins, and in the cases of triglycerides and cholesterol, the resulting lipid–protein complexes are termed *lipoproteins*.

Long-Chain Fatty Acids

Long-chain fatty acids are the building blocks of triglycerides. Three LCFA molecules combine with one glycerol molecule to form one triglyceride molecule *(Fig. 28.1)*. Long-chain fatty acids may be absorbed from the digestive tract, where they are incorporated into triglycerides by the intestinal epithelial cells; they do not enter the blood as single LCFA molecules *(Fig. 28.2)*. They also are synthesized in tissues such as the liver, adipose tissue, and mammary gland from glucose or acetate. Glucose is the most

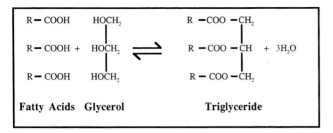

Figure 28.1 A triglyceride molecule is formed by the combination of three fatty acid molecules with one glycerol molecule.

important LCFA precursor in nonruminants, whereas acetate is the most important in ruminants. Synthesized LCFAs are combined with glycerol to form triglycerides; they do not directly enter the blood as LCFA molecules. Synthesis of LCFAs is promoted or inhibited by changes in hormone production. After a meal, increased insulin production and decreased glucagon production promote increased LCFA synthesis. In contrast, during food deprivation, decreased insulin production and increased glucagon production inhibit LCFA synthesis. During situations in which LCFAs are needed for energy, triglyceride molecules in adipose tissue are converted to LCFAs and glycerol. The resulting LCFAs then enter the blood and are transported to tissues that require them for energy. Because circulating LCFAs are not water soluble, they are attached to protein, primarily albumin. Tissues, primarily liver and striated muscle, derive energy from LCFAs

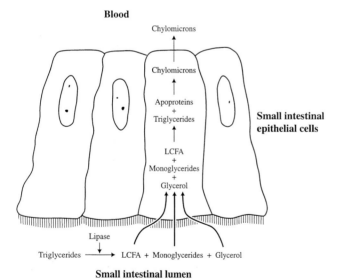

Figure 28.2 Triglycerides in ingested fat are hydrolyzed into long-chain fatty acids (LCFA), monoglycerides, and glycerol by lipase in the small intestine. These molecules are absorbed by intestinal epithelial cells and reassembled to form triglycerides. The triglycerides are combined with apoproteins to form chylomicrons, which then pass into the blood.

by β-oxidation. β-Oxidation results in production of two-carbon acetyl–coenzyme A (acetyl-CoA) units, which are oxidized via the citric acid cycle if adequate oxaloacetate is available to bind with them to form citrate. If oxaloacetate units are insufficient for this process, the acetyl–CoA molecules may be converted to ketones, which sometimes results in ketosis (discussed later).

Triglycerides (Triacylglycerols)

Triglycerides, which also are called triacylglycerols, are composed of three LCFA molecules attached to one glycerol molecule (Fig. 28.1). Triglyceride is the major lipid in adipose tissue; therefore, it also is the major storage form of fat in the body. Triglycerides are synthesized primarily in adipose tissue, liver, small intestine, and mammary gland. Circulating concentrations of triglycerides in normal animals reflect the balance among triglyceride absorption by the small intestine, synthesis/secretion by the hepatocytes, and uptake by the adipose tissue. This balance is affected by the concentration of fat in the diet and the production of hormones such as insulin and glucagon.

Triglycerides are synthesized by the small intestine as part of the digestive and absorptive process (Fig. 28.2). Ingested fat is digested to form LCFA and monoglycerides (monoacylglycerols) in the lumen of the small intestine under the influence of pancreatic lipase. These molecules are absorbed by the intestinal epithelial cells, which recombine them to form triglycerides. The triglycerides are coated with protein to form globular, water-soluble structures termed *chylomicrons*. The chylomicrons are secreted by the epithelial cells, enter the lymphatics of the small intestine, and eventually, enter the blood via the thoracic duct. Triglycerides in circulating chylomicrons are extracted by various tissues. The enzyme, lipoprotein lipase, that is located on the surface of the endothelial cells of tissues such as adipose tissue and muscle catalyzes this process.

The liver synthesizes triglycerides from LCFAs derived from adipose tissue. Most triglycerides that are synthesized in the liver enter the blood and then are removed from the circulation by the adipose tissue. Because triglycerides produced by the liver are not water soluble, they must be transported in the blood attached to proteins, and the resulting molecules are primarily very low-density lipoproteins (VLDL; discussed later).

The LCFAs that are incorporated into triglycerides in adipose tissue are either derived from circulating LCFAs or are synthesized de novo in the tissue from either glucose (most important in nonruminants) or acetate (most important in ruminants) *(Fig. 28.3)*. Synthesis of triglycerides in adipose tissue is hormone dependent. Insulin promotes the synthesis of triglycerides by increasing the concentration of lipoprotein lipase in adipose tissue. In turn, lipoprotein lipase converts the plasma triglycerides in chylo-

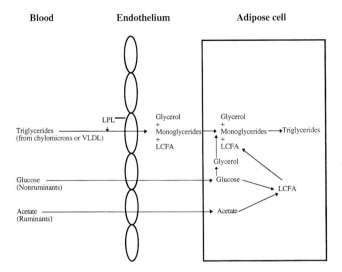

Figure 28.3 In adipose tissue, triglycerides are synthesized from glycerol or monoglycerides combined with long-chain fatty acids (LCFA). These molecules may be derived from triglyceride in the blood, which is incorporated into either chylomicrons or VLDL. Lipoprotein lipase (LPL) on the surface of endothelial cells of adipose tissue convert these triglycerides to glycerol, monoglycerides, and LCFA, which then can enter adipose cells. In nonruminants, both glycerol and LCFA also may be synthesized from glucose that has entered the adipose cell. In ruminants, LCFA may be synthesized from acetate that has entered the adipose cell as well.

microns and VLDL to LCFAs and glycerol. The resulting LCFA then can be used in the adipose tissue for triglyceride synthesis. Insulin also promotes the entry of glucose into adipose cells, where it can be converted to glycerol and LCFAs. Increased insulin secretion and decreased glucagon secretion, as occurs in recently fed animals, results in increased triglyceride production and increased adipose tissue. Glucagon, however, has effects opposite to those of insulin. Decreased insulin secretion and increased glucagon secretion in fasting animals, therefore, result in less production of triglycerides and decreased amounts of adipose tissue. In addition, decreased plasma insulin secretion and increased glucagon secretion cause the mobilization of fat stores via conversion of triglycerides to LCFAs and glycerol. The resulting LCFAs then enter the blood and are available for use by other tissues. Triglycerides produced in the mammary gland are secreted in the milk.

Cholesterol

Cholesterol is a specific form of lipid that is present only in animal tissues. Cholesterol may be synthesized or absorbed from the intestine if the diet contains animal tissue. The major site of cholesterol synthesis is the liver. Because cholesterol is not water soluble, it is transported in the blood attached to protein. This cholesterol–protein complex is a type of lipoprotein (discussed later). Choles-

terol is used by organs such as the adrenal cortex, ovary, and testis to produce steroid hormones. Cholesterol also is an important component of cell membranes. Cholesterol that is synthesized by the liver may be converted to bile acids or excreted unchanged into the bile. Therefore, the liver is a major site of cholesterol excretion and catabolism as well as cholesterol synthesis.

Lipoproteins

Lipoproteins are not a separate class of lipids but, rather, are molecules of protein combined with certain of the lipids discussed earlier. Because these lipids are not water soluble, they cannot be transported unless they are attached to a protein. Circulating triglyceride and cholesterol are attached to proteins called apoproteins. The combination of these lipids with apoproteins results in the formation of lipoproteins. Apoproteins play a role in uptake of the lipoprotein molecule at various sites of metabolism. Different classes of apoproteins are designated by the letters A through E, and subclasses are designated by a Roman or an Arabic number after these letters (e.g., A-IV, B48).

Lipoproteins can be separated and identified by several different methods, including electrophoresis (separation determined by net charge) and ultracentrifugation (separation determined by relative hydrated density). Lipoprotein classes as identified by electrophoresis are designated α-1, α-2, β-1, and β-2. Lipoprotein classes as identified by ultra-centrifugation are designated as very low-density lipoprotein (VLDL), low-density lipoprotein (LDL), intermediate-density lipoprotein (IDL), and high-density lipoprotein (HDL). Chylomicrons also are lipoproteins with a density lower than that of VLDL. Lipoprotein concentrations for several species as determined by density-gradient centrifugation have been reported *(Tables 28.1 and 28.2). High-density lipoprotein is reported to be the major lipoprotein in cats, and the lipoprotein triglyceride and cholesterol content has been quantitated for dogs and cats* (Table 28.3). *The relative proportions of lipid and protein* as well as of the specific apoproteins present in various lipoproteins varies. The percentage content of proteins and types of apoproteins present in different types of canine and feline lipoproteins are summarized in *Table 28.4.*

Digested fat is absorbed as fatty acids and monoglycerides, converted to triglycerides, and incorporated into chylomicrons within small intestinal epithelial cells. Chylomicrons enter the blood and deliver their triglycerides to peripheral tissues such as muscle and adipose tissue. Likewise, triglycerides synthesized in the liver are incorporated into VLDL, which enters the blood and can be cleared by muscle and adipose tissue *(Fig. 28.4)*. Lipoprotein lipase cleaves the triglycerides in chylomicrons and VLDL into monoglycerides and fatty acids, which then can enter myocytes and adipocytes. Chylomicrons have high apoprotein B48 content, and VLDL has a high apoprotein

TABLE 28.1 SERUM LIPOPROTEIN CONCENTRATIONS IN SEVERAL SPECIES

Species	VLDL (mg/dL)	LDL (mg/dL)	HDL (mg/dL)
Horse	33.3	47.7	231.7
Rabbit	38.1	39.8	149.8
Dog	45.3	118.6	693.0
Rat	45.2	27.2	205.4
Pig	43.5	110.3	177.3
Cow	10.0	188.4	208.6

Reprinted from Hollanders B, Mougin A, N'Diaye F, Hentz E, Aude X, Girard A. Comparison of the lipoprotein profiles obtained from rat, bovine, horse, dog, rabbit, and pig serum by a new two-step ultra-centrifugal gradient procedure. Comp Biochem Physiol B 1986;84:83–89.
HDL, high-density lipoprotein; LDL, low-density lipoprotein; VLDL, very low-density lipoprotein.

TABLE 28.2 SERUM LIPOPROTEIN CONCENTRATIONS AND CHOLESTEROL AS DISTRIBUTED IN VARIOUS LIPOPROTEINS

Species	VLDL (mg/dL)	LDL (mg/dL)	HDL (mg/dL)
Ponies[a]			
Fed	5.5	15.0	58.9
Fasted 72 h	367.3	50.8	32.0
Cows[b]			
2-wk postpartum	3.4	29.7	184.4
4-wk postpartum	4.1	133.2	280.0

HDL, high-density lipoprotein; LDL, low-density lipoprotein; VLDL, very low-density lipoprotein.
[a] Data from Freestone JF, Wolfsheimer KJ, Ford RB, Church G, Bessin R. Triglyceride, insulin, and cortisol responses of ponies to fasting and dexamethasone administration. J Vet Intern Med 1991;5:15–22.
[b] Data from Rayssiguier Y, Mazur A, Gueux E, Reid IM, Roberts CJ. Plasma lipoproteins and fatty liver in dairy cows. Res Vet Sci 1988;45:389–393.

TABLE 28.3 CONCENTRATIONS OF TRIGLYCERIDE AND CHOLESTEROL AS DISTRIBUTED IN VARIOUS LIPOPROTEINS

Species	VLDL (mg/dL)		LDL (mg/dL)		HDL (mg/dL)	
	TG	Chol	TG	Chol	TG	Chol
Cat[a]						
Nonobese	11	10	10	36	24	76
Obese	22	9.5	9	36	14	75
Dog[b]						
Normal	7.2	3.0	10.8	36.4	30.0	134.0
With lymphoma	29.7	24.0	21.6	42.7	30.0	134.0

Chol, cholesterol; HDL, high-density lipoprotein; LDL, low-density lipoprotein; TG, triglyceride; VLDL, very low-density lipoprotein.
[a] Data from Dimski DS, Buffington CA, Johnson SE, Sherding RG, Rosol TJ. Serum lipoprotein concentrations and hepatic lesions in obese cats undergoing weight loss. Am J Vet Res 1992;53:1259–1262.
[b] Data from Ogilvie GK, Ford RD, Vail DM, Walters LM, Babineau C, Fettman MJ. Alterations in lipoprotein profiles in dogs with lymphomas. J Vet Intern Med 1994;8:62–66.

TABLE 28.4   PROTEIN COMPOSITION AND MAJOR LIPOPROTEINS IN CANINE AND FELINE SERUM LIPOPROTEINS

Particle	Protein Composition (%)	Major Apoproteins
Chylomicron[a]	2	A, B48, C, E
VLDL[a]	12	B100, C, E
LDL[a]	27	B100
HDL₁[b]	23	A, C, E
HDL₂[c]	33	A, C, E
HDL₃[a]	35	A, C

Reprinted from Watson TDG, Barrie J. Lipoprotein metabolism and hyperlipidaemia in the dog and cat: A review. J Small Anim Pract 1993;34: 479–487. *HDL₁*, *HDL₂*, and *HDL₃*, are three separate high-density lipoprotein fractions.; *LDL*, low-density lipoprotein; *VLDL*, very low-density lipoprotein.
[a] Cat and dog.
[b] Dog.
[c] Cat.

B100 content. These apoproteins facilitate the removal of chylomicrons and VLDL from the circulation by their interaction with specific receptors on endothelial cells.

The remnants of triglyceride-rich lipoproteins (chylomicrons and VLDL) that have given up their lipids may be cleared by the liver or may undergo changes in protein content and accumulate cholesterol. The latter process

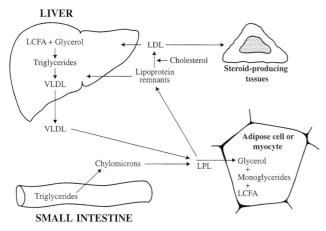

Figure 28.4   Both chylomicrons from the intestinal tract and very low-density lipoproteins (VLDL) from hepatocytes carry triglycerides in the blood, and both deliver these triglycerides to adipose cells and myocytes. This process is promoted by lipoprotein lipase (LPL) on the surface of endothelial cells in these tissues. After delivering their triglycerides, the remnants of chylomicrons and VLDL may be removed by hepatocytes, or they may accumulate cholesterol and become low-density lipoproteins (LDL). Low-density lipoproteins are preferentially cleared from the circulation by steroid-producing tissues, in which cholesterol is used for steroid synthesis. Low-density lipoproteins also may be removed by hepatocytes.

results in the formation of IDL and LDL. Low-density lipoproteins are preferentially cleared from the circulation by tissues such as the adrenal cortex and gonads, which use cholesterol in the synthesis of steroid hormones.

The liver and intestine also produce HDL, which contains little triglyceride. High-density lipoproteins bind cholesterol that has been released from extrahepatic tissues. This process is catalyzed by the enzyme lecithin–cholesterol acyltransferase. After binding to cholesterol, HDL is removed from the circulation by hepatocytes. Some poproteins from HDL are transferred to chylomicrons and VLDL during the course of normal metabolism, and these apoproteins facilitate the activation of lipoprotein lipase in peripheral tissues (e.g., apoprotein CII).

MEASUREMENT OF BLOOD LIPID CONCENTRATIONS

Although LCFAs are a normal constituent of the blood, their plasma concentrations typically are not measured. The most commonly measured blood lipids are triglycerides and cholesterol. Serum lipoprotein analysis is less commonly performed in veterinary medicine; as a result, changes in serum lipoprotein concentrations rarely are determined or interpreted.

Measurement of serum cholesterol concentration is a common component of serum biochemical profiles. Measurement of serum triglyceride concentration is less commonly performed in veterinary medicine. Both cholesterol and triglyceride concentrations can be determined spectrophotometrically. As noted earlier, serum lipoprotein concentrations can be measured by several different techniques, with electrophoresis and ultracentrifugation being the most commonly used methods of separating and measuring serum lipoprotein concentrations.

ABNORMALITIES OF LIPID METABOLISM

Disruption of normal lipid production or metabolism (or both) can result from a variety of diseases. Less commonly, it can be a primary disease process. Abnormalities of lipid metabolism that result in abnormal blood lipid concentrations are discussed here.

Hyperlipidemia

Hyperlipidemia (i.e., increased serum concentrations of triglycerides, cholesterol, or both) can result from physiologic or pathologic processes. Pathologic hyperlipidemia can be a primary disease process or be secondary to a variety of other diseases. Primary hyperlipidemias are caused by genetic abnormalities, whereas secondary hyperlipidemias accompany other primary diseases in which the pathophysiology includes some degree of interference with normal lipoprotein metabolism. The latter are commonly endocrine or metabolic disorders, but infectious and inflammatory diseases causing secondary metabolic anomalies also may result in altered lipid metabolism. An algorithm for the evaluation of animals with hyperlipidemias is presented in *Figure 28.5*.

Hyperlipidemia does not always result in lipemia, which refers to grossly cloudy and white to pink (lactescent) serum or plasma *(Fig. 28.6)*. Lipemia usually results from increased blood concentrations of chylomicrons or VLDL. If lipemia is caused by chylomicrons only, these often will float to the top of refrigerated serum within 10 hours of collection, resulting in a layer of cream-like material at the top and clear serum at the bottom. If lipemia is caused by VLDL only, no cream-like layer will develop, and the serum will remain cloudy. If lipemia is caused by both chylomicrons and VLDL, a cream-like layer will form, but the serum also will remain somewhat cloudy.

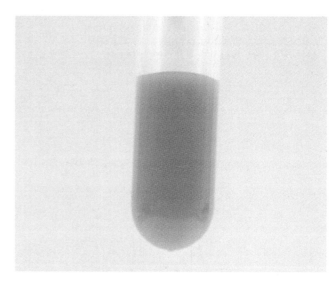

Figure 28.6 Lipemia in a serum sample. Lipemia may vary from a slight cloudiness to an opaque, white to pink (lactescent) appearance. The pink color is caused by mild hemolysis, which is common in lipemic serum.

Physiology Hyperlipidemia

In small animals, the most common cause of hyperlipidemia is postprandial hyperlipidemia caused by increased circulating chylomicron concentrations. Postprandial hyperlipidemia typically begins at 1 to 2 hours, peaks at 6 to 8 hours, and may persist for as long as 16 hours after the ingestion of a fat-containing meal. Postprandial hyperlipidemia causes the serum to be grossly cloudy and white to pink in appearance (i.e., lipemic). This lactescence may interfere with laboratory determination of several commonly analyzed components of serum. Triglycerides account for most of the hyperlipidemia, but the cholesterol concentration may be slightly increased as well. To prevent postprandial hyperlipidemia, nonruminants should be fasted for at least 12 hours before blood samples are obtained for lipid analysis. Because ruminants receive low-fat diets and absorb nutrients continuously, they need not be fasted before blood collection.

Equine Hyperlipidemia

Diseases such as starvation and chronic illness result in negative energy balance and cause markedly increased serum triglyceride concentrations in miniature horses, ponies, and donkeys. The hypertriglyceridemia appears to result from excessive release of triglycerides in the form of VLDL from the liver, pursuant to adipose-tissue lipid mobilization of LCFA and hepatic processing of these LCFA, rather than from reduced clearance of VLDL by peripheral tissues. The magnitude of these serum triglyc-

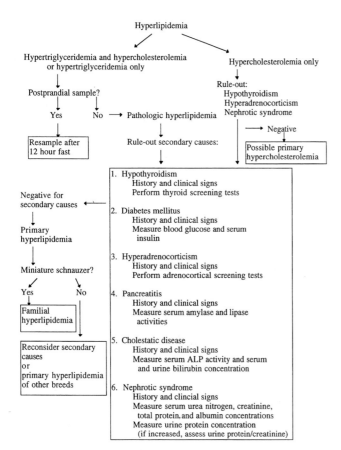

Figure 28.5 Algorithm for the evaluation of animals with hyperlipidemia.

eride concentrations is moderate in most miniature horses, ponies, and donkeys, but it can be marked (e.g., >20-fold increases) in some animals. The hyperlipidemia can result in severe hepatic lipid accumulation, which can lead to death. Affected animals also commonly have hyperlipemias. Fat animals and animals during late pregnancy appear to be most susceptible. Pre-existing hepatopathy, hyperadrenocorticism, or administration of exogenous glucocorticoids appears to predispose to development of this syndrome. Full-sized horses also may develop hypertriglyceridemia as a result of negative energy balance, but this rarely leads to the complications seen in small equids.

Pathologic Hyperlipidemia

This may be a primary disease process or may occur secondary to several diseases.

Primary Hyperlipidemia. Primary hyperlipidemia may occur in miniature schnauzers and probably results from an inherited defect in lipoprotein lipase or apoprotein CII, which is required for the activation of lipoprotein lipase by chylomicrons and VLDL. Affected animals typically are middle-aged or older. Increased serum triglyceride, cholesterol, and chylomicron concentrations occur in affected dogs. Chronic hyperlipidemia may result in secondary disorders, including pancreatitis and seizures. Primary hyperlipidemia with unknown inheritance has been reported in other canine breeds, including Brittany Spaniels and mixed-breed dogs.

Primary hyperlipidemia characterized by hypercholesterolemia and normal serum triglyceride concentration has been reported in Doberman pinschers and rottweilers. Dogs with hypercholesterolemia and normal serum triglyceride concentrations should always be evaluated for underlying diseases such as hypothyroidism, hyperadrenocorticism, and nephrotic syndrome.

Primary fasting hyperlipidemia, which is inherited in an autosomal recessive pattern, has been reported in cats. This disease results either from decreased lipoprotein lipase activity or from an inability of lipoprotein lipase to bind normally to capillary endothelium. The decreased lipoprotein lipase activity in peripheral tissues results in decreased removal of lipids from the blood. Affected cats have increased serum concentrations of triglycerides, cholesterol, and chylomicrons, and they display fasting hyperlipidemia, anemia, xanthomata (i.e., deposits of lipid in the skin or other tissues), peripheral nerve dysfunction associated with local displacement by xanthomas, and ocular disorders (e.g., lipemia retinalis, lipid in the anterior chamber, lipid keratopathy). Unlike in other species with fasting hyperlipidemia, however, recurrent pancreatitis has not been observed in affected cats.

Secondary Hyperlipidemia

Hypothyroidism. Serum cholesterol concentrations are increased in approximately two-thirds of hypothyroid dogs. Serum triglyceride concentrations are less commonly increased. The mechanism of these increases is not known.

Diabetes mellitus. Serum triglyceride concentrations commonly are increased in dogs and cats with uncontrolled diabetes mellitus. Serum cholesterol concentrations also may be increased in such dogs, and chylomicronemia is common. Decreased insulin production results in increased mobilization of LCFA from adipose tissue; these LCFAs are removed by the liver, converted to triglycerides, and returned to the blood in VLDL. Because synthesis of lipoprotein lipase depends partially on insulin, the activity of this enzyme decreases in peripheral tissue, thus resulting in decreased removal of triglycerides from the blood in both VLDL and chylomicrons.

Hyperadrenocorticism. Hypercholesterolemia may occur in dogs with hyperadrenocorticism. The mechanism of this hypercholesterolemia is not known.

Pancreatitis. Both serum triglyceride and cholesterol concentrations may be increased in animals with pancreatitis. The cause of hyperlipidemia in pancreatitis is not certain, but in some cases, it may be related to diabetes mellitus or cholestatic hepatic disease, which develop secondary to pancreatitis. In addition, hyperlipidemia may predispose to pancreatitis rather than resulting from pancreatitis. As blood with a high concentration of lipid passes through pancreatic capillaries, pancreatic lipase may hydrolyze this lipid and form LCFA. These LCFAs injure capillary endothelium or pancreatic acinar cells (or both), thereby resulting in increased release of pancreatic enzymes. In turn, these enzymes cause further pancreatic damage, which escalates into clinically recognizable, acute pancreatitis. This process could account for the association between onset of acute pancreatitis and ingestion of a high-fat meal.

Hepatic disease. Increased serum triglyceride and cholesterol concentrations may occur in animals with hepatic disease, especially cholestatic disorders. The liver is the major route of cholesterol excretion, and the hypercholesterolemia may be caused by decreased hepatic uptake from the blood and excretion of cholesterol into the bile. Affected livers also may possibly produce and secrete into the blood an abnormal lipoprotein that is rich in cholesterol. The mechanism of the hypertriglyceridemia is not known, but it may relate to abnormalities in hepatocellular apoprotein synthesis and subsequent abnormalities in lipoprotein metabolism.

Nephrotic syndrome. Hypercholesterolemia is a common finding in dogs and cats with protein-losing nephropathies. Such animals less commonly have increased serum triglyceride concentrations. The combination of hypoalbuminemia, proteinuria, hypercholesterolemia, and edema or ascites is referred to as nephrotic syndrome. The mechanism leading to increased serum lipid concentrations is not known. It is theorized, however, that loss of albumin or other factors that partially inhibit hepatic production of VLDL results in increased hepatic production of this lipid. Because VLDL is triglyceride-rich and cholesterol-poor, this theory could explain the increased serum triglyceride concentrations, but it does not explain the increased serum cholesterol concentrations. Abnormal lipoprotein metabolism related to pathologic urinary apoprotein excretion is another, more likely mechanism for the blood lipid abnormalities associated with this syndrome.

Therapy-related. Increases in serum triglyceride concentrations have been observed in canine lymphoma patients treated with doxorubicin.

Hypolipidemia

The most common form of hypolipidemia in animals is hypocholesterolemia. The liver is a major site of cholesterol synthesis, and hypocholesterolemia most commonly is associated with hepatic diseases such as chronic parenchymal disease or cirrhosis (or both) resulting in hepatic failure. In some forms of hepatic failure, decreased cholesterol synthesis can lead to decreased blood cholesterol concentrations (i.e., hypocholesterolemia). If, however, cholestasis also is a component of the disease, decreased cholesterol synthesis and decreased cholesterol excretion may balance each other, thereby resulting in a normal serum cholesterol concentration.

Maldigestion/malabsorption syndromes such as pancreatic acinar insufficiency or small intestinal inflammatory disease can result in hypotriglyceridemia. Inflammatory bowel disease with lymphangiectasia may lead not only to a protein-losing enteropathy but also to pathologic lipoprotein loss. Hypotriglyceridemia has been observed in dogs with experimentally induced portosystemic shunts, experimental carbon tetrachloride–induced hepatic necrosis, and experimental dimethylnitrosamine hepatotoxicosis.

Ketosis

During starvation, the rate of fat mobilization from peripheral adipose storage sites exceeds the metabolic capacity of the liver to oxidize this fat or to repackage triglycerides into lipoproteins for delivery to muscle. Deleterious pathways for handling the excess lipid may then be activated. Under normal circumstances, LCFAs removed from the blood by hepatocytes undergoes β-oxidation to form acetyl-CoA, much of which then is combined with oxaloacetate to form citrate *(Fig. 28.7).* In turn, citrate is metabolized via the tricarboxylic acid (TCA) cycle. If, through lipolysis, excessive amounts of acetyl-CoA (relative to the amounts of oxaloacetate) are produced, that acetyl-CoA may be shunted to triglceride resynthesis, de novo cholesterol synthesis, or ketogenesis.

Deficiencies of nutrients required as cofactors or coenzymes for oxidative metabolism can effectively block lipid metabolism. For instance, CoA and acyl carrier protein both derive from the vitamin pantothenic acid, which, if deficient, leads to widespread disorders of metabolism that particularly affect the liver and central nervous system. Cats have a particularly high dietary requirement for pantothenic acid, perhaps because of their evolutionary development as carnivores that must metabolize large amounts of lipids. If the level of niacin is inadequate, the

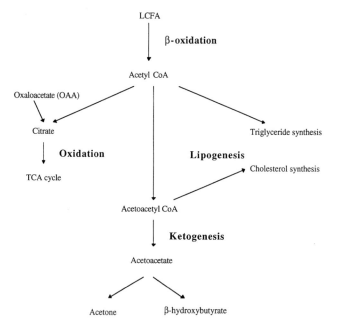

Figure 28.7 During periods of energy deficiency, increased mobilization of fat stores occurs, thus resulting in delivery of large amounts of long-chain fatty acids (LCFA) to the liver. Hepatocytes metabolize these LCFA via β-oxidation, thereby resulting in production of large amounts of acetyl–coenzyme A (acetyl-CoA), which can be metabolized in several different ways. A major route of metabolism is combining acetyl-CoA with oxaloacetate (OAA) to form citrate, which then can be oxidized for energy through the tricarboxylic acid (TCA) cycle. When overwhelming amounts of acetyl-CoA are produced, there may be insufficient OAA for this route of metabolism. The acetyl-CoA then must be metabolized through another route, one of which involves production of acetoacetate and subsequent production of acetone and β-hydroxybutyrate, all of which are ketones. This process can result in excessive ketone body production and increased blood concentrations of ketones (ketosis).

amount of nicotinomide adenine dinucleotide (NAD) produced may be inadequate to handle the reducing equivalents generated by acetyl-CoA oxidation. Cats cannot synthesize niacin from tryptophan; thus, they have a significant dietary requirement for this vitamin as well. Inadequate propionate or vitamin B_{12} (as a coenzyme for methylmalonyl CoA mutase) in ruminants may lead to deficiency of oxaloacetate and an inability to form citrate from acetyl-CoA. Deficiencies of so-called lipotropes, which are compounds necessary to process phospholipids for export from the liver, may lead to abnormal hepatic lipid accumulation. Nutritional deficiencies of choline (necessary for phosphatidylcholine synthesis), of methyl donors such as methionine (necessary for phosphatidyl-choline and phophatidyl-ethanolamine synthesis), or of folacin or vitamin B_{12} (necessary for methyl group transfer during choline and etholamine synthesis) also can lead to hepatic lipidosis.

Hepatic Lipidosis

Hepatic lipidosis may occur in many species because of alterations in fat metabolism, but it is most serious in lactating dairy cows, anorexic obese cats, and anorexic small equids such as miniature horses, ponies, and donkeys. Hepatic lipidosis occurs in cattle that are also at risk for ketosis because of high energy demands during the early stages of lactation. Because healthy cattle produce little hepatic VLDL and cattle with hepatic lipidosis typically have decreased serum triglyceride-rich lipoprotein concentrations, the disorder is thought to result from increased hepatocyte uptake of LCFA mobilized from adipose tissue in combination with impaired hepatocyte synthesis and secretion of triglyceride-rich lipoproteins. The net effect is accumulation of fat in hepatocytes. Large doses of niacin (6 g/d) appear to prevent hepatic lipidosis and ketosis in dairy cattle, and administration of glucogenic precursors is a highly effective treatment.

Hepatic lipidosis frequently is a significant complication in obese cats that become ill due to any cause and are anorexic for a period of more than 2 days. Over-zealous weight-reduction management in obese cats also may predispose to this disease. During fasting, affected cats appear to mobilize excessive amounts of LCFA from adipose tissue, thereby overwhelming the capacity of the liver to convert LCFA to triglycerides and to secrete triglyceride-rich lipoproteins.

SUGGESTED READINGS

Barrie J, Watson TDG, Stear MJ, Nash AS. Plasma cholesterol and lipoprotein concentrations in the dog: The effects of age, breed, gender, and endocrine disease. J Small Anim Pract 1993;34:507–512.

Center SA, Crawford MA, Guida L, Erb HN, King J. A retrospective study of 77 cats with severe hepatic lipidosis: 1975–1990. J Vet Intern Med 1993;7:349–359.

Dimski DS, Buffington CA, Johnson SE, Sherding RG, Rosol TJ. Serum lipoprotein concentrations and hepatic lesions in obese cats undergoing weight loss. Am J Vet Res 1992;53:1259–1262.

Ford RB. Idiopathic hyperchylomicronaemia in miniature schnauzers. J Small Anim Pract 1993;34:488–492.

Freestone JF, Wolfsheimer KJ, Ford RB, Church G, Bessin R. Triglyceride, insulin, and cortisol responses of ponies to fasting and dexamethasone administration. J Vet Intern Med 1991;5:15–22.

Hollanders B, Mougin A, N'Diaye F, Hentz E, Aude X, Girard A. Comparison of the lipoprotein profiles obtained from rat, bovine, horse, dog, rabbit, and pig serum by a new two-step ultracentrifugal gradient procedure. Comp Biochem Physiol B 1986;84:83–89.

Jones BR. Inherited hyperchylomicronaemia in the cat. J Small Anim Pract 1993;34:493–499.

Moggs TD, Palmer JE. Hyperlipidemia, hyperlipemia, and hepatic lipidosis in American Miniature Horses: 23 cases (1990–1994). J Am Vet Med Assoc 1995;207:604–607.

Ogilvie GK, Ford RD, Vail DM, Walters LM, Babineau C, Fettman MJ. Alterations in lipoprotein profiles in dogs with lymphomas. J Vet Intern Med 1994;8:62–66.

Rayssiguier Y, Mazur A, Gueux E, Reid IM, Roberts CJ. Plasma lipoproteins and fatty liver in dairy cows. Res Vet Sci 1988;45:389–393.

Rogers WA, Donovan EF, Kociba GJ. Idiopathic hyperlipoproteinemia in dogs. J Am Vet Med Assoc 1975;166:1087–1091.

Rogers WA, Donovan EF, Kociba GJ. Lipids and lipoproteins in normal dogs and in dogs with secondary hyperlipoproteinemia. J Am Vet Med Assoc 1975;166:1092–1100.

Watson TDG, Barrie J. Lipoprotein metabolism and hyperlipidaemia in the dog and cat: A review. J Small Anim Pract 1993;34:479–487.

Watson TDG, Love S. Equine hyperlipidemia. Comp Cont Educ Pract Vet 1994;16:89–98.

LABORATORY EVALUATION OF THE ENDOCRINE PANCREAS AND OF GLUCOSE METABOLISM

The islets of Langerhans contain the cells of the endocrine pancreas *(Fig. 29.1)*. The most common functional abnormalities of the endocrine pancreas involve the beta cells, which secrete insulin. Both deficient and excessive insulin production by these cells result in serious abnormalities of glucose metabolism. Many factors in addition to the endocrine pancreas, however, play key roles in glucose metabolism. This chapter reviews the major factors affecting glucose metabolism, discusses the causes of decreased blood glucose concentration (i.e., hypoglycemia) and increased blood glucose concentration (i.e., hyperglycemia), and describes a variety of tests for evaluating the status of glucose metabolism.

NORMAL GLUCOSE METABOLISM

Sources of Blood Glucose

Glucose in blood derives from three sources:

- **Intestinal absorption.** Intestinal absorption of glucose can increase blood glucose concentrations in simple-stomached animals for 2 to 4 hours after a meal.
- **Hepatic production.** Hepatic production of glucose results from gluconeogenesis and glycogenolysis. Gluconeogenesis is the formation of glucose from noncarbohydrate sources, primarily amino acids (from protein) and glycerol (from fat) in simple-stomached animals. Ruminants absorb volatile fatty acids rather than carbohydrates, and gluconeogenesis from propionic acid is a major source of blood glucose in ruminants. Glycogenolysis is the hydrolysis of glycogen stored in hepatocytes to glucose.
- **Kidney production.** Gluconeogenesis and glycogenolysis can occur in renal epithelial cells, but under normal circumstances, this activity is minor compared with that in the liver.

Regulation of Blood Glucose Concentration

Blood glucose concentrations are regulated by several interacting factors, including time since last meal, hormonal

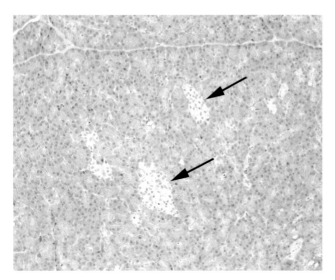

Figure 29.1   The islets of Langerhans (arrow) are the endocrine portion of the pancreas. Both deficient and excessive production of insulin by beta cells in the islets result in abnormalities of glucose metabolism.

influences, and use of glucose by peripheral tissues such as skeletal muscle. Time since the last meal is important only in simple-stomached animals, in which food ingestion is followed by an increase in the blood glucose concentration.

Hormones affect the blood glucose concentration by regulating hepatic production and peripheral use of glucose. Insulin is secreted by beta cells of the pancreatic islets. Insulin lowers blood glucose concentrations by promoting glucose uptake by liver, skeletal muscle, and fat; by inhibiting gluconeogenesis in the liver; and by promoting the formation and storage of liver glycogen. After a meal, approximately 50% of absorbed glucose is stored as glycogen within the liver, and approximately 50% is used as energy by other tissues. Insulin also accelerates the conversion of glucose to fat, accelerates glucose oxidation, and promotes protein and glycogen synthesis in muscle. The net effect of these actions is increased hepatic and peripheral uptake and use of glucose, with decreased hepatic synthesis of glucose.

Glucocorticoids increase blood glucose concentrations by promoting hepatic gluconeogenesis, inhibiting cellular insulin-receptor affinity, and exerting a postreceptor influence within cells that inhibits the action of insulin on glucose metabolism. The net effect of these actions is decreased peripheral use of glucose and increased hepatic synthesis of glucose.

Glucagon is secreted by alpha cells of the pancreatic islets. Glucagon increases blood glucose concentrations by stimulating hepatic gluconeogenesis and hepatic glycogenolysis, inhibiting cellular insulin-receptor affinity, and

exerting a postreceptor influence within cells that inhibits the action of insulin on glucose metabolism. The net effect of these actions is decreased peripheral use of glucose and increased hepatic synthesis of glucose.

Catecholamines (i.e., epinephrine and norepinephrine) increase blood glucose concentrations by increasing hepatic glycogenolysis, inhibiting insulin secretion, stimulating glucagon secretion, and exerting a postreceptor influence within cells that inhibits the action of insulin on glucose metabolism The net effect of these actions is decreased peripheral use of glucose and increased hepatic synthesis of glucose.

Growth hormone increases blood glucose concentrations by inhibiting insulin-mediated uptake of glucose by hepatocytes, muscle cells, and adipose cells; by increasing hepatic production of glucose; and by exerting a postreceptor influence within cells that inhibits the action of insulin on glucose metabolism. The net effect of these actions is decreased peripheral use of glucose and increased hepatic synthesis of glucose.

Extreme physical activity might result in a decreased blood glucose concentration because of increased use of glucose by tissues such as skeletal muscle. In normal animals, hormonal influences keep the blood glucose concentrations stable during most types of physical activity.

CAUSES OF HYPOGLYCEMIA

Conditions that can cause hypoglycemia are listed in *Table 29.1*.

TABLE 29.1   CAUSES OF HYPOGLYCEMIA
Decreased glucose absorption (starvation or malabsorption)
Increased insulin production (beta-cell tumors)
Therapeutic insulin overdose
Hypoadrenocorticism
Hypothyroidism
Growth hormone deficiency
Hepatic failure
Portosystemic shunt
Extreme exertion
Ketosis (in cattle)
Pregnancy toxemia (in sheep)
Sepsis
Glycogen storage diseases
Neonatal hypoglycemia
Juvenile hypoglycemia (in toy and miniature dogs)
Neoplasia (nonbeta-cell tumors)

Decreased Glucose Absorption From the Intestine

Decreased glucose absorption from the intestine is a rare cause of hypoglycemia. Potential underlying causes include starvation or malabsorption syndrome. Hypoglycemia only occurs after long-term starvation or malabsorption, because gluconeogenesis helps to maintain a normal blood glucose concentration at the expense of other substances, principally protein.

Increased Insulin Production or Therapeutic Insulin Overdose

Neoplasms of the beta cells of the pancreatic islets (i.e., beta-cell tumors/insulinomas) are the most common source of increased insulin production and have been reported in dogs, cats, and ferrets. Therapeutic insulin overdose can occur when treating diabetes mellitus. An increased insulin concentration decreases gluconeogenesis and glycogenolysis and increases cellular use of glucose.

Hypoadrenocorticism (Adrenocortical Insufficiency)

Hypoglycemia occurs inconsistently in dogs with hypoadrenocorticism, and many dogs with this syndrome have either normal or increased blood glucose concentrations. Hypoglycemia, when present, usually is mild and probably results from decreased gluconeogenesis and increased insulin-mediated uptake of glucose by muscle tissue.

Hypothyroidism

Although hypoglycemia is not common in hypothyroid animals, it may occur if hypothyroidism is a component of a more general syndrome of pituitary dysfunction (i.e., hypopituitarism).

Growth Hormone Deficiency

Hypoglycemia is uncommon in animals with growth hormone deficiency. It occurs most commonly if concurrent hypoadrenocorticism is present.

Hepatic Failure

Hepatic failure results in decreased hepatic gluconeogenesis and glycogenolysis. Hypoglycemia occurs only after a loss of more than 70% of functional capacity. Hepatic failure should be considered as a possible cause of hypoglycemia only if other clinical signs and laboratory abnormalities are suggestive of this problem (see Chapter 23).

Hyperglycemia occasionally can occur with liver failure resulting from a lack of hepatic uptake of glucose absorbed from the intestine.

Portosystemic Shunts

Hypoglycemia in patients with portosystemic shunts occurs only if hepatic dysfunction is severe.

Extreme Exertion

Extreme exertion occurs in hunting dogs and endurance horses. Possible underlying causes include depletion of glycogen stores, increased glucose use, and decreased epinephrine response to hypoglycemia.

Ketosis in Cattle

Negative energy balance in cattle during early lactation results in decreased blood glucose concentration, decreased liver glycogen stores, and increased fat mobilization. Increased production of ketone bodies ultimately occurs.

Pregnancy Toxemia in Sheep and Goats

Pregnancy toxemia in sheep and goats is a syndrome that results from negative energy balance during late pregnancy. Hypoglycemia is not a consistent finding.

Sepsis

Hypoglycemia occurs inconsistently with sepsis. Hyperglycemia is more common in animals with early sepsis, whereas hypoglycemia is more common in animals with advanced or later sepsis. The causes of hypoglycemia in association with sepsis are not completely understood. Possible causes include impaired gluconeogenesis and glycogenolysis and increased use of glucose by tissues, including leukocytes.

Glycogen Storage Diseases

Glycogen storage diseases are inherited defects in glycogenolysis and result in the accumulation of glycogen in cells of the liver, kidney, and myocardium. Type I (i.e., von Gierke's disease) and type II (i.e., Pompe's disease) glycogen storage diseases are associated with hypoglycemia in dogs.

Neonatal Hypoglycemia

Neonatal hypoglycemia is especially common in pigs, but it can occur in other species. It usually is associated with poor nursing secondary to diarrhea, dehydration, or hypothermia. Agalactia in the dam also can lead to this type of hypoglycemia. Hypoglycemia during periods of decreased food intake in neonates results from inadequate storage pools of glycogen and protein, which are substances that, if available, could be used to produce glucose during these times. Hepatic enzymes that are necessary for converting these substances to glucose also may be deficient in neonates.

Juvenile Hypoglycemia in Toy and Miniature Dog Breeds (Puppy Hypoglycemia)

Juvenile hypoglycemia is a syndrome that usually is seen in puppies younger than 6 months. Clinical signs often are triggered by stresses such as diarrhea, fasting, or parasitism. As in neonatal hypoglycemia, inadequate storage pools of glycogen and protein probably play an important role in this syndrome. Inadequate levels of hepatic enzymes for gluconeogenesis also may contribute.

Neoplasia Other Than Insulinoma

Hypoglycemia has been reported in association with lymphocytic leukemia, lymphoma, leiomyoma, leiomyosarcoma, hepatocellular carcinoma, mammary carcinoma, pulmonary carcinoma, hemangiosarcoma, hepatoma, plasma-cell tumor, malignant melanoma, and salivary adenocarcinoma. Possible causes of hypoglycemia in association with such neoplasms include excessive glucose use and secretion of insulin-like substances by the tumor. Secretion of an insulin-like molecule (i.e., insulin-like growth factor) appears to be involved in the pathogenesis of hypoglycemia associated with some types of tumors in humans.

CAUSES OF HYPERGLYCEMIA

Conditions that can cause hyperglycemia are listed in *Table 29.2*.

Postprandial Hyperglycemia

Postprandial hyperglycemia can occur in simple-stomached animals for 2 to 4 hours after eating a meal, but it does not occur in ruminants.

Diabetes Mellitus

Diabetes mellitus is caused by a deficiency of insulin production or an interference with the action of insulin in target tissues, thereby resulting in abnormal glucose metabolism. Altered protein and lipid metabolism also occurs in diabetes mellitus. Animals with diabetes mellitus usually

TABLE 29.2 CAUSES OF HYPERGLYCEMIA

Postprandial hyperglycemia (in simple-stomached animals)
Diabetes mellitus
Increased glucocorticoid concentrations
   Hyperadrenocorticism
   Stress
   Therapeutic corticosteroids
Catecholamine release
   Exertion
   Pain
   Excitement
   Pheochromocytoma
Increased growth hormone (growth hormone–producing tumor)
Increased glucagon (glucagon-producing tumor)
Increased progesterone production (diestrus in bitches)
Pancreatitis
Pituitary pars intermedia dysfunction (in horses)
Drugs
   Glucocorticoids
   Adrenocorticotrophic hormone
   Progesterone
   Xylazine
   Ketamine
   Morphine
   Phenothiazine
   Fluids with high glucose concentrations
Milk fever (in cattle)
Neurologic diseases (in cattle)
Proximal duodenal obstruction (in cattle)
Colic (in horses)
Hyperthyroidism
Moribund animals

have blood glucose concentrations greater than the renal threshold and, therefore, glucosuria. Glucosuria occurs less commonly with other causes of glucose intolerance.

Diabetes mellitus has been classified by its underlying causes as either type 1 or type 2 and by the dependence of the affected animal on insulin therapy as either insulin dependent and noninsulin dependent. These two classification schemes overlap, thereby resulting in confusion regarding the types of diabetes mellitus occurring in animals. Type 1 diabetes mellitus results from immune-mediated destruction of pancreatic beta cells by cellular and humoral mechanisms. Animals with type 1 diabetes mellitus are insulin dependent. Type 1 diabetes is the most frequent cause of diabetes in dogs, but it has not been well documented in cats. Type 2 diabetes mellitus results from impaired beta-cell function as a result of causes other than immune-mediated beta-cell destruction. Animals with type 2 diabetes mellitus may be either insulin or noninsulin dependent. This is the most common type of diabetes mellitus in cats, but it can occur in dogs as well. Approximately 50% to 70% of cats with type 2 diabetes mellitus are insulin dependent. A sluggish insulin response to hyperglycemia (i.e., decreased capacity to produce insulin) and a poor tissue response to insulin (i.e., insulin resistance) are the underlying features of type 2 of diabetes mellitus.

Deposition of amyloid in the pancreatic islets is found in most cats with type 2 diabetes mellitus. Amyloid deposition occurs before the onset of clinical diabetes mellitus, and the amount of amyloid found in the pancreatic islets of cats correlates directly with the degree of glucose intolerance that is present. Islet amyloid surrounding beta cells is theorized to prevent contact between these cells and blood constituents such as glucose. Because absorption of glucose by beta cells may play an important role in determining the appropriate secretion of insulin by these cells, this interference by islet amyloid may contribute to the sluggish insulin response associated with type 2 diabetes mellitus.

Deposition of amyloid in islets also results in death of beta cells. Islet amyloid primarily is composed of a pancreatic islet hormone, which is termed *amylin*, that synthesized in beta cells and cosecreted with insulin. Stimulation of insulin secretion also results in amylin secretion. Islet amyloid deposition is thought to occur when amylin of a molecular structure that is optimal for the formation of amyloid is secreted in excessive quantities. Cats secrete amylin with such a structure. Cats that develop islet amyloid deposits are theorized to initially secrete large quantities of insulin and amylin, and the amylin then forms amyloid deposits that result in impaired beta-cell function as well as destruction. Whether this increased production of amylin results from a beta-cell dysfunction or from overproduction of insulin and amylin as a result of peripheral insulin resistance is not known.

Circulating amylin inhibits insulin secretion and also causes peripheral insulin resistance by impairing glucose use by skeletal muscle. Amylin does not impair glucose use by adipose tissue, however, and increased blood amylin concentrations can shift the glucose deposition from skeletal muscle to fat, which can result in obesity. In turn, obesity causes reversible glucose intolerance through a variety of mechanisms that relate to impaired insulin secretion, abnormal responses by insulin receptors on cells, and abnormalities in glucose transport or use. Obesity is considered to be a major risk factor for diabetes mellitus in cats. The relationship of amylin production and obesity, however, is uncertain. Increased amylin secretion may result in obesity, but obesity also may lead to insulin resistance, which results in increased insulin and amylin production. Obesity-associated glucose intolerance and insulin resistance that has not yet become clinical diabetes mellitus probably occurs in all species and, given

the incidence of obesity, may be more common than clinical diabetes mellitus.

Increased Blood Glucocorticoid Concentration

An increased blood glucocorticoid concentration is the most common cause of hyperglycemia. Such increased concentrations can result from glucocorticoid treatment or from increased endogenous glucocorticoid production secondary to stress or hyperadrenocorticism. Hyperglycemia commonly occurs in cats, but only rarely in dogs, that are receiving long-term, anti-inflammatory doses of steroids. Blood glucose concentrations usually are less than the renal threshold, but higher concentrations can occur. Glucosuria has been reported in cats, dogs, and cattle with increased blood glucocorticoid concentrations. Prolonged increases in blood glucocorticoid concentrations produce impaired insulin secretion by beta cells and insulin resistance because of receptor or postreceptor defects. In turn, this can lead to beta-cell exhaustion atrophy and can result in insulin-dependent diabetes mellitus.

Increased Blood Catecholamine Concentrations

Catecholamines are released as a result of exertion, fear, or pain. Blood glucose concentrations as high as 400 mg/dL can occur in excited cats. Increased catecholamine production also occurs with certain tumors of the adrenal gland (i.e., pheochromocytomas). Blood glucose concentrations greater than the renal threshold and glucosuria also have been reported in dogs and cattle with increased blood catecholamine concentrations.

Increased Growth Hormone

Insulin-resistant diabetes mellitus has been reported in a dog and a cat with acidophilic pituitary adenomas that produce excess growth hormone. The insulin resistance resulting from excessive growth hormone in the dog might have led to alterations in beta cells of the islets of Langerhans and subsequent diabetes mellitus.

Glucagon-Producing Tumors

Glucagon-producing tumors in the pancreas have been reported in two dogs that were hyperglycemic. These dogs had blood glucose concentrations of greater than 300 mg/dL but were not ketoacidotic.

Increased Progesterone Production

Progesterone stimulates the secretion of growth hormone, which can result in hyperglycemia. Increased progesterone concentration and hyperglycemia can occur during diestrus in bitches. Increased serum progesterone concentrations during pregnancy can cause a preclinically diabetic bitch to become overtly diabetic. In bitches that are known to be diabetic, increased serum progesterone concentrations during pregnancy can cause difficulty in therapeutic regulation of blood glucose concentration.

Pancreatitis

Pancreatitis is thought to be a major predisposing factor to diabetes mellitus in dogs. Islet injury secondary to pancreatic inflammation with resultant decreased insulin production is the most likely cause.

Pituitary Pars Intermedia Dysfunction in Horses

Hyperplasia and, possibly, adenomas of the pars intermedia in horses result in the production of increased quantities of adrenocorticotrophic hormone (ACTH), melanocyte-stimulating hormone, and β-endorphin–related peptides. Adrenocorticotrophic hormone causes increased cortisol production by the adrenal gland. Melanocyte-stimulating hormone and β-endorphin–related peptides potentiate the actions of ACTH, thereby resulting in persistent hyperglycemia with glucosuria. Hirsutism, polyuria, and polydipsia also are common in this syndrome.

Drugs

A variety of drugs can cause hyperglycemia. These include:

- Glucocorticoids.
- ACTH, which stimulates production of glucocorticoids by the adrenal gland.
- Megestrol acetate, which can produce glucose intolerance and resulting hyperglycemia in cats.
- Xylazine.
- Ketamine (in cats).
- Morphine.
- Phenothiazine.
- Fluids containing high glucose concentrations.

Severe Disease or Stress in Sheep

Severe disease or stress in sheep may result in blood glucose concentrations greater than the renal threshold, with resulting glucosuria.

Milk Fever or Neurologic Diseases in Cattle

Hyperglycemia results from increased blood glucocorticoid and epinephrine concentrations, which occur during milk fever or neurologic diseases in cattle. Glucosuria also is possible in these diseases.

Proximal Duodenal Obstruction in Cattle

Cattle with proximal duodenal obstruction have blood glucose concentrations ranging from 250 to 1000 mg/dL. Insulin concentrations in these cattle are not decreased, however, and hyperglycemia is thought to result from a combination of stress and decreased peripheral glucose use secondary to shock and dehydration (e.g., decreased blood flow to the peripheral tissues). These extreme hyperglycemias can be helpful in distinguishing cattle with proximal duodenal obstructions from those with abomasal volvulus. Cattle with abomasal volvulus are hyperglycemic (100 to 200 mg/dL), but this most likely results from stress.

Colic in Horses

Hyperglycemia is not commonly associated with equine colic, but when present, it appears to have prognostic implications. Horses with blood glucose concentrations of greater than 200 mg/dL usually have serious underlying causes of colic, and horses with blood glucose concentrations of greater than 300 mg/dL have a poor prognosis. Stress and decreased peripheral use of glucose may play roles in these hyperglycemias. Concomitant causes of hyperglycemia that are unrelated to colic (e.g., pituitary pars intermedia dysfunction) also should be considered in such cases.

Hyperthyroidism

Hyperglycemia occurs in from 3% to 12% of cats with hyperthyroidism. In some of these cases, the hyperglycemia is attributable to causes other than hyperthyroidism (e.g., diabetes mellitus, stress).

Moribund Animals

Moribund animals, most commonly ruminants, may have blood glucose concentrations greater than the renal threshold, with resultant glucosuria. Hyperglycemia probably results from increased blood glucocorticoid and epinephrine concentrations and decreased peripheral use of glucose.

OTHER CAUSES OF GLUCOSE INTOLERANCE

Causes of glucose intolerance, in addition to the causes of hyperglycemia previously listed, can lead to abnormal results with oral or intravenous glucose tolerance tests. These causes include renal failure and acidosis. Renal failure causes increased serum glucagon concentrations and decreased numbers of insulin receptors on cells. Acidosis causes a decreased affinity of cellular receptors for insulin and disrupts intracellular glycolysis.

The serum insulin concentration frequently is increased in animals with decreased glucose tolerance for reasons other than insulin-dependent diabetes mellitus. Increased blood glucose concentrations and resultant exhaustion atrophy of the beta cells associated with these disorders can lead to insulin-dependent diabetes mellitus if the underlying problem is not corrected. Glucose intolerance resulting from one of these factors should be recognized and treated.

LABORATORY EVALUATION OF GLUCOSE METABOLISM

Differentiation of the previously listed causes of hypoglycemia and hyperglycemia requires an evaluation of the patient history and clinical signs in addition to laboratory testing. Common laboratory tests used to evaluate pancreatic function and glucose metabolism are discussed in this section.

Blood Glucose Analysis

Measurement of the blood glucose concentration is the initial step in evaluating glucose metabolism. After detection of either hyperglycemia or hypoglycemia, tests for more specific evaluation of glucose metabolism are performed. Analysis of blood glucose concentrations can be performed by a reference laboratory, but several inexpensive and accurate reflectance photometers are available for measuring these concentrations in practice laboratories. These latter instruments allow rapid and repeated measurements of blood glucose concentrations, which are important for monitoring insulin therapy in diabetics and for assessing critically ill animals that might be hyperglycemic or hypoglycemic.

Because blood glucose concentrations in simple-stomached animals are increased beyond the baseline value for 2 to 4 hours postprandially, glucose concentrations should be measured after fasting. Dogs and cats should be fasted for 12 hours before sampling to avoid postprandial influences. Potentially hypoglycemic animals should not be fasted before sampling, however, because severe hypoglycemia may result. Horses usually are not fasted before collecting blood samples for glucose analysis; however, blood glucose concentrations possibly could increase beyond baseline concentrations during a period of 2 to 4 hours after eating high-energy supplements. It is not necessary to fast ruminants before blood glucose analysis, because they primarily absorb volatile fatty acids rather than glucose from the gastrointestinal tract.

In diabetic animals receiving initial insulin therapy, measurement of blood glucose concentrations at 1- to 2-hour intervals during a period of 10 to 24 hours helps to assess the efficacy and appropriateness of the insulin dosage. These results, which are known as the serial glucose curve, then are analyzed to ensure that the insulin therapy has lowered the blood glucose concentrations, that the lowest glucose concentration after insulin treatment is in an appropriate range, and that the duration of the insulin effect is appropriate.

Serum or plasma to be analyzed for blood glucose concentration should be separated from erythrocytes within 30 minutes. Glycolysis in erythrocytes results in loss of 10% of glucose per hour if the serum or plasma remains in contact with erythrocytes. Sodium fluoride anticoagulant inhibits glycolysis and should be used if serum or plasma cannot be separated from cells within 30 minutes.

Blood glucose concentrations can be misleading in excited animals, because excitement results in high catecholamine concentrations that can cause hyperglycemia in otherwise euglycemic animals. Excited cats can have blood glucose concentrations as great as 400 mg/dL; thus, a blood sample for glucose analysis should not be obtained until the animal is calm.

Urine Glucose Analysis

Urine glucose measurement is discussed in Chapter 21. Glucosuria occurs when the blood glucose concentration exceeds the renal threshold for that species. Renal thresholds are between 180 and 220 mg/dL in the dog and cat, 180 mg/dL in the horse, and 100 mg/dL in cattle. Glucosuria can occur in animals with normal to slightly increased blood glucose concentrations but with decreased renal thresholds. Decreased renal thresholds usually result from proximal tubular abnormalities, which include primary renal glycosuria of Norwegian Elkhounds, Fanconi syndrome, amyloidosis in dogs (nearly 20% have glucosuria), and exposure to nephrotoxins, including aminoglycosides and amphotericin B. Animals with hypercalcemia and resulting proximal tubular damage also may have glucosuria resulting from a decreased renal threshold.

Oral Glucose Tolerance Test

The oral glucose tolerance test can be used to detect glucose intolerance in persistently hyperglycemic animals. Because it depends on the intestinal absorption of glucose, however, this test is inferior to the intravenous glucose tolerance test when used for this purpose. This test also can be used to evaluate intestinal absorptive capacity, but it is considered to be an inaccurate indicator of such capacity, especially in small animals. In addition, the oral glucose tolerance test can be used to detect increased glucose tolerance in animals with persistently low normal glucose concentrations, but measurement of concurrent serum insulin and glucose concentrations is preferred to the oral glucose tolerance test in such animals (discussed later).

Chemical restraining agents (e.g., ketamine, xylazine, thiopental, acetylpromazine, morphine) should be avoided when performing glucose tolerance tests. These agents tend to delay the disappearance of glucose (i.e., cause decreased glucose tolerance).

The oral glucose tolerance test in dogs is performed as follows:

- Fast the dog for 12 hours, but do not fast hypoglycemic animals. Blood glucose concentrations of potentially hypoglycemic dogs should be monitored during this period, and the fasting period should be ended if hypoglycemia is detected.
- Administer orally 1 g of glucose per each pound of body weight.
- Collect blood samples for glucose analysis before the administration of glucose and at 30-minute intervals for 3 to 4 hours thereafter.

A normal response and those responses that are suggestive of decreased and increased glucose tolerance in dogs are illustrated in *Figure 29.2*. The blood glucose concentration should reach a peak of approximately 160 mg/dL by 30 to 60 minutes and then return to baseline by 120 to 180 minutes (and, possibly, even go a bit below baseline at these times) in normal dogs. Failure to return to baseline within this time period implies decreased glucose tolerance.

The oral glucose tolerance test in horses and ponies is performed as follows:

- Fast the animal for 18 to 24 hours.
- Administer 1 g of glucose (10% solution or less) per 1 kg of body weight via a stomach tube.

- Collect blood samples for glucose analysis before the administration of glucose and at 30-minute intervals for 6 hours thereafter.

A normal response and those responses that are suggestive of decreased and increased glucose tolerance in horses are illustrated in *Figure 29.3*. The blood glucose concentration in horses should reach approximately 175 mg/dL, or approximately twofold the baseline value, by 120 minutes and then return to baseline by 360 minutes. Peak blood glucose concentration in ponies also occurs by approximately 120 minutes, but this concentration usually is lower than that in horses (~140 mg/dL, or 1.8-fold the baseline value), probably because of a more rapid insulin response. Failure to return to baseline within 6 hours implies decreased glucose tolerance.

Failure to attain the peak blood glucose concentrations noted previously or a more rapid return to baseline (or both) is suggestive of increased glucose tolerance. Increased glucose tolerance can occur with intestinal malabsorption, delayed gastric emptying, hypothyroidism, hypoadrenocorticism (i.e., adrenal insufficiency), hypopituitarism, and hyperinsulinism.

Intravenous Glucose Tolerance Test

The intravenous glucose tolerance test is superior to the oral glucose tolerance test, because it does not depend on the intestinal absorption of glucose and, therefore, is not affected by gastrointestinal factors. The intravenous glucose tolerance test is useful for detecting decreased glucose tolerance in persistently hyperglycemic animals. This test also can be used for detecting increased glucose tolerance in animals with persistently low normal glucose concentrations. Measurement of concurrent serum insulin and glucose concentrations is preferred to performing the intravenous glucose tolerance test in persistently hypoglycemic animals (discussed later).

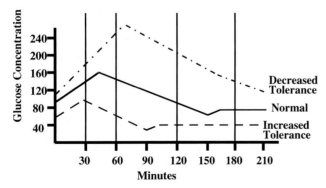

Figure 29.2 Normal and abnormal responses to the oral glucose tolerance test in dogs.

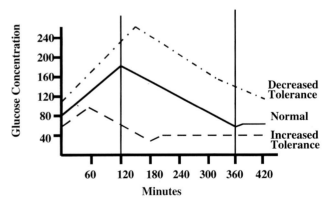

Figure 29.3 Normal and abnormal responses to the oral glucose tolerance test in horses.

Chemical restraining agents (e.g., ketamine, xylazine, thiopental, acetylpromazine, morphine) should be avoided when performing glucose tolerance tests. These agents tend to delay the disappearance of glucose (i.e., cause decreased glucose tolerance).

The intravenous glucose tolerance test in dogs and cats is performed as follows:

- Fast the animal for 12 to 24 hours, but do not fast hypoglycemic animals. Blood glucose concentrations of potentially hypoglycemic dogs should be monitored during this period, and the fasting period should be ended if hypoglycemia is detected.
- Administer intravenously 0.5 g of glucose (50% solution) per 1 kg of body weight during a 30-second period.
- Collect blood samples for glucose analysis before administration and at 5, 15, 25, 35, 45, and 60 minutes after administration.
- Plot the glucose concentrations (on log scale) versus time (on an arithmetic scale).
- Calculate the time for the blood glucose concentration to decrease by 50% ($t_{1/2}$).
- Calculate the fractional turnover rate or disappearance coefficient (k) for glucose as follows:

$$k(\%/min) = (0.063/t_{1/2}) \times 100$$

A normal response to the intravenous glucose tolerance test and a response that is suggestive of decreased glucose tolerance in dogs are illustrated in *Figure 29.4*. The normal $t_{1/2}$ in the dog is 17 to 33 minutes (others consider the normal $t_{1/2}$ in dogs to be <45 min). The normal $t_{1/2}$ in cats is 50 to 60 minutes. The normal k value in dogs is 1.85% to 3.67% per minute; the normal k value in cats is 1.4% to 2.6% per minute. The 5-minute peak is important to observe and is abnormally high in diabetic animals. The

60-minute value should have returned to normal in both dogs and cats. Marked variability in response to the intravenous glucose tolerance test has been reported within individual cats, but this is attributed to cats' tendency to release catecholamines when acutely stressed, as can occur during phlebotomy. The catecholamines affect glucose tolerance. Delayed glucose disappearance (i.e., longer $t_{1/2}$ and lower k) is suggestive of decreased glucose tolerance.

The intravenous glucose tolerance test in horses is performed according to the same procedure as that in dogs and cats. Blood glucose concentrations increase greater than 300% in normal horses by 15 minutes after intravenous glucose administration but then rapidly decrease to baseline. Horses with pars intermedia dysfunction have lower peak glucose concentrations and more gradual returns to baseline glucose concentrations after intravenous administration of glucose.

Increased glucose tolerance as detected by the intravenous glucose tolerance test (i.e., shorter $t_{1/2}$ and higher k) occurs with hypothyroidism, hypoadrenocorticism (i.e., adrenocortical insufficiency), hypopituitarism, and hyperinsulinism.

The intravenous glucose tolerance test also can be used in combination with insulin assays to classify diabetes mellitus as either insulin or noninsulin dependent (discussed later).

Serum Insulin Assay

Measurement of the serum insulin concentration is useful in evaluating both hyperglycemic and hypoglycemic disorders. Serum insulin concentrations are most useful diagnostically when compared with serum glucose concentrations. Serum insulin measurements are not species specific, but reference ranges may not be available for all species. Serum for insulin assay should be harvested from clotted blood within 30 minutes and then immediately assayed or frozen.

Serum Insulin Assay in Hypoglycemic Animals

If the animal being tested is sporadically hypoglycemic, serum insulin measurements should be done while the animal is hypoglycemic. A protocol for performing this comparison in hypoglycemic dogs is as follows:

- Withhold food early on the morning of the test day (7:00 to 8:00 AM).
- Monitor blood glucose concentrations on an hourly basis until the concentration is less than 60 mg/dL. In dogs with insulinomas, life-threatening hypoglycemia can develop during the fasting period; thus, careful monitoring is imperative. Most dogs with insulin-secreting tumors develop hypoglycemia 8 to 10 hours

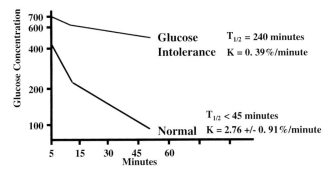

Figure 29.4 Normal and abnormal responses to the intravenous glucose tolerance test in dogs.

after a meal, but more than 24 hours of fasting are required in some dogs. An insulin-secreting tumor is not likely if a glucose concentration of less than 60 mg/dL is not induced by this process.

- When the blood glucose concentration is less than 60 mg/dL, obtain a serum sample for blood glucose and insulin analysis.

After these samples have been obtained, the dog should be fed several small meals before returning it to its previous feeding schedule.

In normal dogs, the serum insulin concentration should decrease with the blood glucose concentration. In normal fasted dogs, blood glucose concentrations typically are 70 to 100 mg/dL, and serum insulin concentrations typically are 5 to 20 μU/mL.

In fasted dogs with insulinomas, serum insulin concentrations will not decrease with glucose concentrations. If the blood glucose concentration is less than 60 mg/dL and the serum insulin concentration is increased, an insulin-secreting tumor is likely. If the blood glucose concentration is less than 60 mg/dL and the serum insulin concentration is in the middle to upper reference interval, an insulin-secreting tumor is a possibility; this occurs in approximately 25% of dogs with insulinomas. Repeating the test may yield results that are more strongly suggestive of an insulinoma. If the blood glucose concentration is less than 60 mg/dL and the serum insulin concentration is decreased, an insulin-secreting tumor is unlikely.

Calculated ratios such as the amended insulin:glucose ratio, insulin:glucose ratio, and glucose:insulin ratio result in a high number of false-positive results. Therefore, use of such ratios is not recommended in domestic animals.

Serum Insulin in Hyperglycemic Animals

Concurrent measurement of serum insulin and blood glucose concentrations during an intravenous glucose tolerance test can be used to confirm abnormalities of insulin secretion. The test is performed by administering glucose intravenously at the dosage recommend in the previous discussion of the intravenous glucose tolerance test. Serum insulin concentrations then are measured on samples obtained before and at 5, 15, 30, 60, and 120 minutes after the administration of glucose. These measurements may aid in characterizing diabetes mellitus as either insulin or noninsulin dependent. Application of this test in the evaluation of diabetics is limited, however, both because almost all nonobese diabetic dogs have insulin-dependent diabetes mellitus and because insulin secretion in cats with noninsulin-dependent diabetes mellitus is unpredictable.

Possible results of the combined intravenous glucose tolerance test and serum insulin assay in dogs and cats are diagrammed in *Figure 29.5*. In normal dogs, the serum

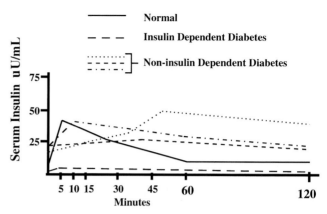

Figure 29.5 Serum insulin responses after intravenous administration of glucose. Measurement of this response can aid in verifying insulin-dependent diabetes mellitus and in differentiating insulin-dependent from potentially noninsulin-dependent diabetes mellitus. In animals with insulin-dependent diabetes mellitus, baseline plasma insulin concentrations are decreased, and insulin response after intravenous administration of glucose is minimal. In animals with diabetes mellitus that may be noninsulin dependent, baseline plasma insulin concentrations are normal to increased, and the insulin response after intravenous administration of glucose varies from minimal to normal to delayed.

insulin concentration increases by 5- to 10-fold at 5 minutes and then returns to baseline by 60 minutes after intravenous administration of glucose. In normal cats, the serum insulin concentration increases two- to threefold by 5 to 15 minutes and then returns to near the baseline concentration at 120 minutes after intravenous administration of glucose. A very low baseline serum insulin concentration, with little or no increase in serum insulin concentration, in response to intravenous glucose administration is suggestive of insulin-dependent diabetes mellitus. A normal to increased baseline serum insulin concentration with a response to intravenous glucose injection that varies from none to normal to delayed (e.g., less-than-normal increase in serum insulin concentration during the first hour but a normal to exaggerated increase by 2 hours after injection) is suggestive of noninsulin-dependent diabetes mellitus.

In horses, the serum insulin concentration normally increases by 600% to 700% at 15 to 30 minutes after intravenous administration of glucose. An increased baseline serum insulin concentration with little insulin response to intravenous administration of glucose is typical of pars intermedia dysfunction.

Serum or Plasma Fructosamine Concentration

Fructosamine is a general term that refers to any glycated protein (i.e., a protein with an attached carbohydrate). Glucose combines with the amine groups of albumin and other proteins in the blood, and through a series of chemical reactions, this results in the formation of stable compounds, which are called fructosamines. Fructosamine is formed in normal animals, but high blood glucose concentrations result in the formation of increased amounts. The serum or plasma fructosamine concentration is an indicator of blood glucose concentrations during the previous 1 to 2 weeks (based on the average life-span of the proteins involved in this complex). Fructosamine provides more reliable information regarding the long-term state of glucose metabolism than the blood glucose concentration, which only reveals the momentary situation. Fructosamine, therefore, has potential in establishing the diagnosis of diabetes mellitus and in monitoring therapy for diabetics. Increased fructosamine concentrations are suggestive of increased blood glucose concentrations and, in diabetic animals receiving insulin treatment, of a lack of therapeutic control of blood glucose concentrations during the previous 1 to 2 weeks.

Albumin is the protein that most frequently is incorporated into the fructosamine molecule. Hypoalbuminemia, therefore, can result in falsely decreased fructosamine concentrations. The following adjustment for albumin concentration has been suggested in dogs:

$$\text{Adjusted fructosamine (mmol/L)} = 2.82/\text{Albumin (g/dL)} \times \text{Fructosamine (mmol/L)}$$

Fructosamine also is useful in distinguishing excitement-induced hyperglycemia from diabetic hyperglycemia in cats. Fructosamine concentrations are within the reference ranges in cats with hyperglycemia caused by excitement, because this is a short-term change. Animals must be hyperglycemic for approximately four days before increased fructosamine concentrations are detected. Thus, fructosamine concentrations tend to be increased in diabetic cats because this hyperglycemia persists for a long period of time (specificity, 86%; sensitivity, 93%).

Fructosamine assays are available at a limited number of reference laboratories. Serum or plasma (with heparin or ethylenediaminetetraacetic acid [EDTA] but not with sodium fluoride) can be assayed. Fructosamine is stable at refrigerator temperatures for as long as 2 weeks and frozen for as long as 2 months. Lipemia does not interfere with this assay, but more than slight hemolysis does.

Blood Glycated Hemoglobin Concentration

Glycated hemoglobin (GHb) is formed in erythrocytes by an irreversible reaction between carbohydrates (especially glucose) and hemoglobin. Glycated hemoglobin forms continuously during the life span of an erythrocyte; therefore, older erythrocytes usually contain more GHb compared with younger erythrocytes. The amount of GHb that is formed is proportional to the blood glucose con-

centration during the life span of the erythrocyte. The blood GHb concentration reflects glucose status during a longer period of time than the serum fructosamine concentration, because erythrocytes have longer life spans than protein molecules. The period of time for which GHb reflects glucose status depends on the average life span of erythrocytes in different species. Increased GHb concentrations do not immediately return to normal after reestablishing more normal blood glucose concentrations, because this requires the removal of senescent erythrocytes with high GHb concentrations. Such decreases in GHb concentrations might be delayed for several weeks.

Glycated hemoglobin can be used in the same situations as fructosamine. The shorter time period gauged by fructosamine compared with GHb, however, might be an advantage, because this allows earlier recognition of the deteriorating control of hyperglycemia and of the return to adequate control of hyperglycemia.

OTHER LABORATORY ABNORMALITIES ASSOCIATED WITH DIABETES MELLITUS

Other laboratory abnormalities may be associated with diabetes mellitus.

Increased Packed Cell Volume and Plasma Protein Concentration

An increased packed cell volume or plasma protein concentration (or both) may result from dehydration.

Stress or Inflammatory Leukogram.

A leukogram that is indicative of stress or inflammation may occur.

Prerenal or Renal Azotemia

Glomerular lesions have been reported in diabetic dogs and cats, but the occurrence of clinical renal disease in such animals is not well documented. Urine specific gravity usually is low in animals with glucosuria, generally because of the osmotic effect of glucose rather than from a defect in the ability of the tubules to concentrate urine (discussed later). Low urine specific gravity in combination with azotemia, however, may be indicative of renal failure. The serum phosphorus concentration also may be increased in azotemic animals because of the decreased glomerular clearance of phosphorus. Some diabetic animals have hyperphosphatemia, but hypophosphatemia may occur in others (discussed later).

Decreased Urine Concentrating Ability

Glucosuria results in osmotic diuresis. Concentrating capacity is impaired by the solute concentration in the filtrate.

Pyuria, Hematuria, and Proteinuria

Urinary tract infection is common in diabetic animals. Such infection can result in increased numbers of leukocytes, erythrocytes, and bacteria in the urine as well as in an increased concentration of protein. Increased urine protein concentration without evidence of inflammation could result from glomerular damage, which commonly occurs in humans with diabetes but is not well documented in animals with diabetes mellitus.

Electrolyte Loss

Osmotic diuresis and ketonuria cause the loss of sodium, chloride, potassium, and phosphorus in the urine. Hyponatremia, hypochloremia, and less commonly, hypokalemia and hypophosphatemia may result. The serum potassium concentration may be normal or increased in diabetic animals, especially if the animals are acidotic, but the whole-body potassium concentration often is depleted. Potassium depletion results from hypoinsulinemia, which allows intracellular potassium to enter the blood; this potassium then is lost via the urine. Phosphorus depletion results from multiple factors, including increased renal excretion, increased tissue catabolism, and in animals treated with insulin, passage of phosphorus from the serum into cells. Serum phosphorus concentrations of less than 1.5 mg/dL may occur in diabetic dogs and cats, especially after the initiation of insulin therapy. Such hypophosphatemia potentially can result in hemolysis, leukocyte or platelet dysfunction, neurologic disorders, and abnormal muscle function.

Increased Hepatic and Pancreatic Enzyme Activities

Metabolic alterations in hepatocytes can lead to the leakage of enzymes. Fatty change in hepatocytes results from the increased liberation of fatty acids from adipose tissue, influx of these fatty acids into hepatocytes, and incorporation of fatty acids into triglycerides. Activities of induced enzymes also increase if these alterations result in hepatocyte swelling and cholestasis. Pancreatitis can cause diabetes mellitus as a result of islet damage, and if active pancreatitis is present, serum activities of amylase or lipase (or both) may be increased.

Increased Serum Bilirubin Concentrations

Cholestasis secondary to the hepatocyte swelling that is associated with fatty change may lead to hyperbilirubinemia. Moreover, hemolysis resulting from Heinz-body formation can occur in diabetic cats and result in increased serum bilirubin concentrations. Approximately one-third of diabetic cats have increased serum bilirubin concentrations.

Hyperlipidemia

Increased blood concentrations of several lipids, including triglycerides, cholesterol, and free fatty acids, result from decreased incorporation of triglycerides into fat deposits, decreased hepatic degradation of cholesterol, and increased hepatic production of very low-density lipoproteins. Increased concentrations of these proteins often result in visible lipemia.

Ketonemia and Ketonuria

Ketones include acetoacetate, β-hydroxybutyrate, and acetone. Deficient insulin production in diabetes mellitus results in decreased incorporation of fatty acids into triglycerides (i.e., decreased lipogenesis) *(Fig. 29.6)*. Fatty acids then are converted to acetyl–coenzyme A (acetyl-CoA). Almost all acetyl-CoA is converted to acetoacetate in animals with severe diabetes mellitus. Some of this acetoacetate then is converted to β-hydroxybutyrate and acetone. Increased blood ketone concentration (i.e., ketonemia) and, possibly, increased urine ketone concentration (i.e., ketonuria) can result. The nitroprusside reaction for detection of blood and urine ketones detects acetoacetate and acetone, but it does not detect

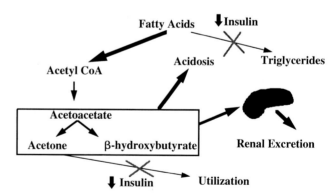

Figure 29.6 The pathogenesis of ketonemia and ketonuria in diabetes mellitus. Insulin deficiency causes decreased incorporation of fatty acids into triglycerides. Increased formation of acetyl-coenzyme A (acetyl-CoA) results. In turn, acetyl-CoA is converted to ketones. Insulin deficiency also decreases use of ketones; ketonemia and ketonuria result.

β-hydroxybutyrate. In some ketoacidotic patients, production of β-hydroxybutyrate can predominate, thereby resulting in failure to detect ketosis. Impaired peripheral use of ketones because of insulin deficiency also contributes to ketonemia and ketonuria in diabetes mellitus. The renal threshold for ketones is low, and ketonuria often precedes ketonemia. Causes of ketonemia and ketonuria, in addition to diabetes mellitus, include starvation, bovine ketosis, pregnancy toxemia in sheep, and hepatic lipidosis syndrome of cattle.

Metabolic Acidosis (Ketoacidosis)

Ketones are acidic, and increased concentrations lead to metabolic acidosis, which can be life threatening.

Increased Anion Gap

An increased anion gap primarily results from increased ketoacid concentration in the blood. Increased blood lactate concentration also can contribute to this gap.

Hyperosmolarity

Hyperosmolarity usually occurs in animals with extremely high blood glucose concentrations (>600 mg/dL). A serum osmolarity of greater than 350 mOsm/L can cause neurologic and gastrointestinal abnormalities. Approximately one-third of diabetic cats with ketoacidosis have a serum osmolarity of greater than 350 mOsm/L.

OTHER LABORATORY ABNORMALITIES ASSOCIATED WITH HYPERINSULINISM

In addition to hypoglycemia, the only laboratory abnormality that frequently is associated with hyperinsulinism is hypokalemia resulting from insulin-mediated passage of potassium into cells.

SUGGESTED READINGS

Akol KG, Waddle JR, Wilding P. Glycated hemoglobin and fructosamine in diabetic and nondiabetic cats. J Am Hosp Assoc 1992;28:227–231.

Bagley RS, Levy JK, Malarkey DE. Hypoglycemia associated with intra-abdominal leiomyoma and leiomyosarcoma in six dogs. J Am Vet Med Assoc 1996;208:69–71.

Beaudry D, Knapp DW, Montgomery T, et al. Hypoglycemia in four dogs with smooth muscle tumors. J Vet Intern Med 1995;9:415–418.

Biourge V, Nelson RW, Feldman EC, et al. Effect of weight gain and subsequent weight loss on glucose tolerance and insulin response in healthy cats. J Vet Intern Med 1997;11:86–91.

Breitschwerdt EB, Loar AS, Hribernik TN, et al. Hypoglycemia in four dogs with sepsis. J Am Vet Med Assoc 1981;178:1072–1076.

Caplan ER, Peterson ME, Mullen HS, et al. Diagnosis and treatment of insulin-secreting pancreatic islet cell tumors in ferrets: 57 cases (1986–1994). J Am Vet Med Assoc 1996;209:1741–1745.

Crenshaw KL, Peterson ME. Pretreatment clinical and laboratory evaluation of cats with diabetes mellitus: 104 cases (1992–1994). J Am Vet Med Assoc 1996;209:943–949.

Crenshaw KL, Peterson ME, Heeb LA, et al. Serum fructosamine concentration as an index of glycemia in cats with diabetes mellitus and stress hyperglycemia. J Vet Intern Med 1996;10:360–364.

Dennis JS. Glycosylated hemoglobins in dogs. Comp Cont Educ 1989;11:717–720,726.

Dybdal NO, Hargreaves KM, Madigan JE, et al. Diagnostic testing for pituitary pars intermedia dysfunction in horses. J Am Vet Med Assoc 1994;204:627–632.

Elie MS, Zerbe CA. Insulinoma in dogs, cats and ferrets. Comp Cont Educ 1995;17:51–59.

Elliott DA, Nelson RW, Feldman EC, Neal LA. Glycosylated hemoglobin concentration for assessment of glycemic control in diabetic cats. J Vet Intern Med 1997;11:161–165.

Elliott DA, Nelson RW, Feldman EC, Neal LA. Glycosylated hemoglobin concentrations in the blood of healthy dogs and dogs with naturally developing diabetes mellitus, pancreatic β-cell neoplasia, hyperadrenocorticism, and anemia. J Am Vet Med Assoc 1997;211:723–727.

Garry F, Hull BL, Rings DM, et al. Comparison of naturally occurring proximal duodenal obstruction and abomasal volvulus in dairy cattle. Vet Surg 1988;17:226–233.

Greco DS. Endocrine emergencies. Part I. Endocrine pancreatic disorders. Comp Cont Educ 1996;19:15–23,83.

Hawks D, Peterson ME, Hawkins KL, et al. Insulin-secreting pancreatic (islet cell) carcinoma in a cat. J Vet Intern Med 1992;6:193–196.

Hsu WH, Hembrough FB. Intravenous glucose tolerance test in cats: influenced by acetylpromazine, ketamine, morphine, thiopental, and xylazine. Am J Vet Res 1982;43:2060–2061.

Johnson KH, O'Brien TD, Betsholtz C, Westermark P. Islet amyloid, islet-amyloid polypeptide, and diabetes mellitus. N Engl J Med 1989;321:513–518.

Kaneko JJ, Kawamoto M, Heusner AA, et al. Evaluation of serum fructosamine concentration as an index of blood glucose control in cats with diabetes mellitus. Am J Vet Res 1992;53:1797–1801.

Kawamoto M, Kaneko JJ, Heusner AA, et al. Relation of fructosamine to serum protein, albumin, and glucose concentrations in healthy and diabetic dogs. Am J Vet Res 1992;53:851–855.

Kirk CA, Feldman EC, Nelson RW. Diagnosis of naturally acquired type-I and type-II diabetes mellitus in cats. Am J Vet Res 1993;54:463–467.

Levy JK. Hypoglycemic seizures attributable to hypoadrenocorticism in a dog. J Am Vet Med Assoc 1994;204:526–530.

Lutz TA, Rand JS. Pathogenesis of feline diabetes mellitus. Vet Clin North Am Small Anim Pract 1995;25:527–552.

Moore GE, Hoenig M. Effects of orally administered prednisone on glucose tolerance and insulin secretion in clinically normal dogs. Am J Vet Res 1993;54:126–129.

Reusch CE, Liehs MR, Hoyer M, et al. Fructosamine. J Vet Intern Med 1993;7:177–182.

Sparkes AH, Adams DT, Cripps PJ, et al. Inter- and intraindividual variability of the response to intravenous glucose tolerance testing in cats. Am J Vet Res 1996;57:1294–1298.

Steiner JM, Bruyette DS. Canine insulinoma. Comp Cont Educ 1996;18:13–24.

Walters PC, Drobatz KJ. Hypoglycemia. Comp Cont Educ 1992;14:1150–1158.

Van Keulen LJM, Wesdorp JL, Kooistra HS. Diabetes mellitus in a dog with a growth hormone-producing acidophilic adenoma of the adenohypophysis. Vet Pathol 1996;33:451–453.

LABORATORY EVALUATION OF THE THYROID, PARATHYROID, ADRENAL, AND PITUITARY GLANDS

DEBORAH S. GRECO

This chapter highlights some of the important laboratory features of small-animal endocrine disorders, and it emphasizes specific endocrine tests used by veterinary practitioners to establish the diagnosis of an endocrine disorder. The reader is referred to other portions of this textbook for specific disorders of the endocrine pancreas (e.g., diabetes mellitus and insulinoma). This chapter discusses the diagnosis of feline hyperthyroidism, canine hypothyroidism, hyperadrenocorticism, hypoadrenocorticism, hyperparathyroidism, hypoparathyroidism, diabetes insipidus (DI), and growth hormone (GH) disorders.

THYROID GLAND

The thyroid gland regulates basal metabolism. Two molecules, tyrosine and iodine, are important for thyroid hormone synthesis. Tyrosine is a part of a large molecule (molecular weight, 660,000) termed *thyroglobulin*, which is formed within the follicle cell and secreted into the lumen of the follicle. Iodine is converted to iodide in the intestinal tract and is then transported to the thyroid, where the follicle cells trap the iodide through an active-transport process. The tyrosyl ring can accommodate two iodide molecules. If one iodide molecule attaches, it is termed *monoiodotyrosine* (MIT); if two iodide molecules attach, it is called *diiodotyrosine* (DIT). The coupling of two iodinated tyrosines results in formation of the main thyroid hormones. Two DIT molecules form thyroxine (T_4), whereas one MIT coupled with one DIT molecule forms triiodothyronine (T_3). For thyroid hormones to be released from the thyroid gland, thyroglobulin (with its attached MIT, DIT, T_3, and T_4 molecules) must be translocated into the follicle cell, and the hormones must be cleaved from thyroglobulin. Thyrotropin, or thyroid-stimulating hormone (TSH), is the most important reg-

445

ulator of thyroid activity. Secretion of TSH is regulated by thyroid hormones via negative feedback inhibition of the synthesis of thyrotropin-releasing hormone (TRH) at the level of the hypothalamus and by inhibition of the activity of TSH at the level of the pituitary.

The major storage form of thyroid hormone is T_4, whereas the active form of the hormone is T_3. The majority of T_3 formation occurs outside the thyroid gland, by the deiodination of T_4. The enzyme that is involved in the removal of iodide from the outer phenolic ring of T_4 to form T_3 is termed *5'-monodeiodinase*. Another type of T_3 is formed when an iodide molecule is removed from the inner phenolic ring of T_4. This compound is called reverse T_3, and it has few of the biologic effects of thyroid hormones. Reverse T_3 increases in nonthyroidal illness and is responsible for the decrease in total T_4 seen in euthyroid sick syndrome. As with all lipid-soluble hormones that are transported in plasma, T_3 and T_4 are bound to plasma proteins. The amount of free thyroid hormone in plasma is remarkably low; for example, in dogs, the amount of free hormone is a little less than 1.0% for T_4 and slightly greater than 1.0% for T_3.

Canine Hypothyroidism

The usual cause of primary canine hypothyroidism is lymphocytic thyroiditis or idiopathic thyroid atrophy. Neoplasia accounts for fewer than 1% of cases. Congenital hypothyroidism may be caused by thyroid dysgenesis, dyshormonogenesis, T_4-transport defects, goitrogens, or rarely, iodine deficiency. Secondary hypothyroidism may be acquired, such as in German shepherds with a cystic Rathke pouch, or secondary to pituitary tumors, radiation therapy, or endogenous or exogenous glucocorticoids. Congenital causes of secondary hypothyroidism include hereditary TSH deficiency, as observed in the giant schnauzer breed. Tertiary hypothyroidism can be acquired, as in the case of hypothalamic tumors, or it can be congenital, as a result of TRH- or TRH-receptor defects.

The signalment of hypothyroid dogs carries a distinct breed predisposition, with high-risk breeds presenting as early as 2 to 3 years of age and low-risk breeds at 4 to 6 years of age. Breeds that are predisposed to hypothyroidism include golden retrievers, Doberman pinschers, dachshunds, Irish setters, miniature schnauzers, great danes, miniature poodles, boxers, Shetland sheepdogs, Newfoundlands, chow chows, English bulldogs, Airedales, cocker spaniels, Irish wolfhounds, giant schnauzers, Scottish deerhounds, and Afghan hounds.

Clinical signs of hypothyroidism are gradual and subtle in onset, with lethargy and obesity being the most common. Often, owners are not even aware of the onset of signs and think that their dog is just becoming "older." Dermatologic evidence of hypothyroidism is the most common clinical finding (other than lethargy and obesity). Symmetric truncal or tailhead alopecia is a classic finding in hypothyroid dogs. The skin is often thickened because of myxedematous accumulations in the dermis. In addition, common haircoat changes seen in hypothyroid dogs include dull and dry hair, the blond "frizzies," poor hair regrowth after clipping, and the presence or retention of a puppy hair. Hyperkeratosis, hyperpigmentation, secondary pyodermas, and demodicosis also are observed. Seborrhea, either sicca or oleosa, can be a clinical feature of canine hypothyroidism, and ceruminous otitis is common as well.

Cardiovascular signs of hypothyroidism include bradycardia, decreased cardiac contractility, and atherosclerosis, but these are uncommon presenting complaints. Neuromuscular signs, such as myopathies and megaesophagus, also are uncommon manifestations. Neuropathies, including bilateral or unilateral facial nerve paralysis, vestibular disease, and lower-motor-neuron disorders, occasionally are seen. Myxedema coma is an unusual finding in hypothyroid dogs, and it manifests as stupor and coma secondary to myxedematous fluid accumulations in the brain and severe hyponatremia. Less common signs of hypothyroidism include reproductive disorders in female dogs, such as prolonged interestrous intervals, silent heat, and weak or stillborn puppies. Corneal lipid deposits and gastrointestinal (GI) problems (e.g., constipation) are occasionally observed.

Clinicopathologic findings, such as normocytic normochromic anemia resulting from erythropoietin deficiency, decreased bone marrow activity, and decreased serum iron and iron-binding capacity, are observed in approximately 25%–30% of hypothyroid dogs. Hypercholesterolemia is seen in approximately 75% of hypothyroid dogs because of altered lipid metabolism, decreased fecal excretion of cholesterol, and decreased conversion of lipids to bile acids. Hyponatremia, which is a common finding in humans with hypothyroidism, was observed as a mild decrease in serum sodium in approximately 30% of hypothyroid dogs in one study. Hyponatremia is caused by an increase in total body water resulting from impaired renal excretion of water and from retention of water by hydrophilic deposits in tissues. An unusual clinicopathologic feature of hypothyroidism is increased serum creatine phosphokinase possibly as a result of hypothyroid myopathy.

The diagnosis is established based on measurement of serum basal total T_4 and T_3 concentrations, serum free T_4 and T_3 concentrations, endogenous canine serum TSH levels, and dynamic thyroid-function tests, including the TRH and TSH stimulation tests. Many variables affect T_4, including age, breed, environmental and body temperature, diurnal rhythm, obesity, and malnutrition. Specifically, greyhounds have approximately half the normal total and free T_4 concentrations compared with normal dogs. Obese dogs have mild increases in serum total T_4 concentrations. Puppies exhibit a serum total T_4 concentration two- to five-fold greater than that in adult dogs. Furthermore, an age-related decline occurs in serum total T_4 concentrations and response to TSH stimulation in dogs. Euthyroid sick syndrome is characterized by a decrease in serum total T_4 and an increase in reverse T_3 (discussed earlier). Concurrent illnesses, such as diabetes mellitus, chronic renal failure (CRF), hepatic insufficiency, and infections, can cause euthyroid sick syndrome, resulting in decreased serum total T_4 concentrations. Drugs such as anesthetics, phenobarbital, primidone, diazepam, trimethoprim-sulfas, quinidine, phenylbutazone, salicylates, and glucocorticoids can also decrease serum basal total T_4 concentrations.

Free thyroid hormone concentrations, or unbound T_3 and T_4, are used in human medicine to differentiate between euthyroid sick syndrome and true hypothyroidism. In humans, the diagnostic accuracy of a single free T_4 measurement is approximately 90%. Measurement of free T_4 concentrations is achieved by equilibrium dialysis (i.e., the gold standard) or analogue immunoassays. Theoretically, free T_4 is not subject to the spontaneous or drug-induced changes that affect total T_4. Early studies classifying dogs as hypothyroid based on TSH stimulation tests indicated that free T_4 measurement by equilibrium dialysis was 90% accurate, whereas other free T_4 assays (e.g., analogue assays) were no better than those for total T_4. Glucocorticoids will decrease both the free and total T_4 in dogs.

With the advent of the endogenous canine TSH assay, veterinarians now have a method of assessing the thyroid–pituitary axis in dogs without dynamic testing. With thyroid gland failure, decreases in serum free and total T_4 are sensed by the pituitary gland, resulting in an increased serum endogenous TSH concentration. Results of initial studies with experimentally induced hypothyroid dogs have been very encouraging. In humans, when both endogenous TSH and free T_4 are increased and decreased, respectively, the diagnostic accuracy for primary hypothyroidism approaches 100%. As the free T_4 concentration falls, a logarithmic increase occurs in the serum endogenous TSH concentration, making it the most sensitive test for detection of early hypothyroidism. Nonthyroidal disease, however, can affect endogenous TSH concentrations as well as free and total T_4 concentrations; therefore, use of endogenous TSH alone is not recommended for assessing thyroid function.

The antithyroglobulin autoantibody test also has recently become available and, based on initial studies, appears promising. The presence of antithyroglobulin antibodies theoretically presages the onset of hypothyroidism in dogs with autoimmune thyroiditis. Hopefully, this test will identify dogs with hereditary thyroid disease before

breeding; however, no large studies of dogs with naturally occurring thyroid disease have been performed to evaluate this assay.

For many years, the TSH stimulation test was considered to be the gold standard for diagnosis of hypothyroidism in dogs. Unfortunately, this test does not differentiate between early hypothyroid dogs and those with euthyroid sick syndrome, nor does it identify dogs with secondary or tertiary hypothyroidism. Furthermore, exogenous bovine TSH is no longer commercially available. Other thyroid function tests include the TRH stimulation test, thyroid scan, and thyroid biopsy, each of which, however, has the drawback of expense, inaccuracy, or invasiveness. Procedures for several thyroid function tests are listed in *Table 30.1*.

In summary, the diagnosis of hypothyroidism is based on signalment, historical findings, physical examination, clinicopathologic features, and confirmation with a battery of thyroid-function tests. I use total T_4, free T_4 (e.g., analogue, chemiluminescent), and endogenous thyroid stimulating hormone (eTSH). If all three test results are abnormal, the dog is hypothyroid. If two of the three test results are abnormal, secondary hypothyroidism (e.g., low free T_4, low TSH) or early primary hypothyroidism (e.g., high TSH, low free T_4) is possible. If only one of the tests is positive, then re-evaluate the dog in 3 to 6 months. An algorithm for the diagnosis of hypothyroidism in dogs is shown in *Figure 30.1*.

Feline Hyperthyroidism

Hyperthyroidism is the most common endocrinopathy of cats; however, it is rarely observed in dogs. The cause of hyperthyroidism in cats and dogs is adenomatous hyperplasia of the thyroid gland. Middle-aged and older cats typically are affected, and no breed or sex predilection has been observed. Hyperthyroidism is characterized by hypermetabolism; therefore, polyphagia, weight loss, polydipsia, and polyuria are the most prominent features of the disease. Activation of the sympathetic nervous system also is seen, with hyperactivity, tachycardia, pupillary dilatation, and behavioral changes also being characteristic of the disease in cats. Long-standing hyperthyroidism leads to hypertrophic cardiomyopathy, high-output heart failure, and cachexia, which may lead to death.

Clinicopathologic features of hyperthyroidism include erythrocytosis and an excitement leukogram (e.g., neutrophilia, lymphocytosis) caused by increased circulating catecholamine concentrations. Increased catabolism of muscle tissue in hyperthyroid cats may result in increased blood urea nitrogen (BUN), but not in increased creatinine. In fact, the glomerular filtration rate (GFR) is increased in hyperthyroid cats, which may mask an underlying renal insufficiency. Although hyperthyroidism increases

TABLE 30.1 SCREENING TESTS FOR HYPERTHYROIDISM AND HYPOTHYROIDISM

Serum Total T₄
Protocol: single serum sample, refrigerate or freeze, stable at room temperature
Reference range: canine, 1.4–4.0 μg/dL (18–52 nmol/L); feline, 1.2–4.8 μg/dL (15–62 nmol/L)

T₃ Suppression Test
Protocol: collect serum sample for T₃/T₄ analysis, then administer seven doses of Cytobin or Cytomel (synthetic T₃) at a dosage of 25 μg q8h. After the last dose (8 AM on Day 3), collect a sample for T₃/T₄ analysis 4 hours after the T₃ dose.
Reference range: 50% reduction in T₄; T₃ analysis to ensure compliance with administering T₃ medication

TRH Stimulation Test
Protocol: 0.1 mg/kg aqueous TRH IV, samples at 0 and 1 hour
Reference range: stimulation to at least double the baseline total T₄ value

TSH Stimulation Test
Protocol: 1 U bovine TSH IV, sample at 0 and 6 hours
Reference range: incremental increase in total T₄ of at least 2 μg/dL (26 nmol/L)

Free T₄ and T₃ by dialysis
Protocol: single serum sample
Reference range: 1.21–3.4 ng/dL (15.6–44 nmol/L)

Thyroid biopsy/scintigraphy
Protocol: mTch-99
Scan thyroid gland

Endogenous TSH
Protocol: single serum sample collected in red-top vacutainer, centrifuge, stable at room temperature
Reference range: 0.1–0.45 ng/mL (Immulite) or 0.01–0.65 ng/mL (RIA)

mTch-99, technesium 99 (isotopic); *RIA*, radioimmunoassay; *T₃*, triiodothyronine; *T₄*, tyroxine; *TRH*, thyrotropin-releasing hormones; *TSH*, thyroid-stimulating hormone.

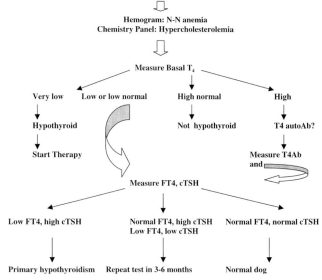

Figure 30.1 Diagnostic approach to canine hypothyroidism.

disease has become more common and now is being recognized during the early stages, serum free T₄ has recently been shown to be more diagnostic of early or "occult" hyperthyroidism. Free T₄, however, should be interpreted in light of the total T₄, because nonthyroidal illness (e.g., CRF) can result in spurious elevations of free T₄ as well. Establishing the diagnosis may be challenging in cats with occult hyperthyroidism that demonstrate clinical signs suggestive of hyperthyroidism (e.g., polyphagia, polydipsia, polyuria, weight loss, goiter) but who have normal (usually high-normal) total T₄ concentrations. In cases of suspected occult hyperthyroidism, dynamic endocrine testing using the T₃ suppression or TRH stimulation test may be beneficial. Procedures for both tests and an algorithm for establishing the diagnosis of feline hyperthyroidism are shown in Table 30.1 and *Figure 30.2*, respectively.

GFR, the effect of thyroid hormone excess on urinalysis is variable. Most cats, however, will have decreased urine specific gravity, particularly if they exhibit polyuria as a clinical sign. Increased metabolic rate results in liver hypermetabolism; therefore, serum activities of liver enzymes (e.g., alanine aminotransferase, aspartate aminotransferase) increase in 80%–90% of hyperthyroid cats. Serum cholesterol decreases, not as a result of decreased synthesis but, rather, as a result of increased hepatic clearance mediated by excess thyroid hormone.

The diagnosis of feline hyperthyroidism is established based on measurement of total serum T₄; total serum T₃ generally is noncontributory to a diagnosis. Because the

ADRENAL CORTEX

The adrenal cortex produces two major types of steroid hormones. The first type, mineralocorticoids, are produced by the zona glomerulosa and play an important role in electrolyte balance and the regulation of blood pressure. The major mineralocorticoid is aldosterone. The second type, glucocorticoids, are produced by the zona fasciculata and zona reticularis and are important in the regulation of all aspects of metabolism, either directly or indirectly (through interaction with other hormones). The major form of glucocorticoid is cortisol.

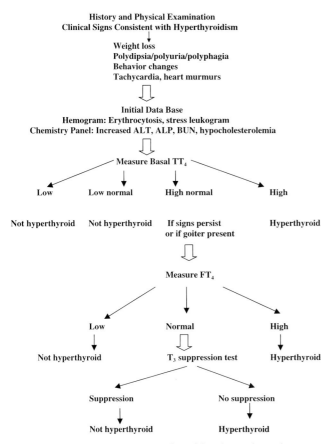

History and Physical Examination
Clinical Signs Consistent with Hyperthyroidism

Weight loss
Polydipsia/polyuria/polyphagia
Behavior changes
Tachycardia, heart murmurs

Initial Data Base
Hemogram: Erythrocytosis, stress leukogram
Chemistry Panel: Increased ALT, ALP, BUN, hypocholesterolemia

Measure Basal TT₄

Low — Not hyperthyroid
Low normal — Not hyperthyroid
High normal — If signs persist or if goiter present
High — Hyperthyroid

Measure FT₄

Low — Not hyperthyroid
Normal — T₃ suppression test
High — Hyperthyroid

Suppression — Not hyperthyroid
No suppression — Hyperthyroid

Figure 30.2   Diagnostic approach to feline hyperthyroidism.

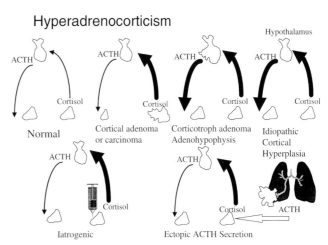

Hyperadrenocorticism

Figure 30.3   Pathogenesis of disorders resulting in hyperadreno-corticism.

The mechanism of action by adrenal hormones involves penetration of the cell membrane and interaction in the cytoplasm with specific cytosolic receptors. This complex is then transferred to the nucleus, with a resultant transcription of certain genes and synthesis of specific proteins that affect the biologic action of the adrenal hormones.

Secretion of glucocorticoids by the zona fasciculata and zona reticularis is controlled by adrenocorticotropic hormone (ACTH). A negative feedback system exists, whereby glucocorticoids inhibit the release of hypothalamic corticotropin-releasing hormone, which in turn results in decreased ACTH secretion by the pituitary.

Hyperadrenocorticism

Hyperadrenocorticism (i.e., Cushing syndrome) may be caused by a pituitary tumor, pituitary hyperplasia, adrenal tumors, adrenal hyperplasia, nonendocrine tumors (usually lung), or be iatrogenic (*Fig. 30.3*). Approximately 85% of dogs with hyperadrenocorticism have pituitary-dependent disease, whereas 15% exhibit adrenal tumors. Hyperadrenocorticism is a disease of middle-aged to older

dogs (7–12 years). Common breeds affected by pituitary-dependent hyperadrenocorticism include miniature poodles, dachshunds, boxers, Boston terriers, and beagles. Adrenal tumors are seen more frequently in large-breed dogs, and a gender predilection has been observed (female:male ratio, 3:1). Hyperadrenocorticism is a rare endocrine disorder of cats and, in that species, is usually pituitary in origin.

The most common clinical signs associated with canine hyperadrenocorticism are polydipsia, polyuria, polyphagia, heat intolerance, lethargy, abdominal enlargement or "pot belly," panting, obesity, muscle weakness, and recurrent urinary tract infections. Dermatologic manifestations of canine hyperadrenocorticism can include alopecia (especially truncal), thin skin, phlebectasias, comedones, bruising, cutaneous hyperpigmentation, calcinosis cutis, pyoderma, dermal atrophy (especially around scars), seborrhea, and secondary demodecosis. Thin skin is the hallmark of feline hyperadrenocorticism. Cats with Cushing syndrome develop such severe thinning of the epidermis that they may cause open wounds just by grooming themselves.

Establishing the diagnosis of hyperadrenocorticism can be challenging. Uncommon clinical manifestations of hyperadrenocorticism in dogs can include signs such as hypertension, congestive heart failure, bronchial calcification, pulmonary thromboembolism, polyneuropathy, polymyopathy, pseudomyotonia, behavioral changes, and blindness. Evidence of increased collagenase activity caused by hypercortisolemia may result in nonhealing corneal ulceration and bilateral cranial cruciate rupture (in small dogs). Unusual reproductive signs may include testicular atrophy, prostatomegaly (in castrated male dogs), clitoral hypertrophy, and perianal adenoma (in female or castrated male dogs).

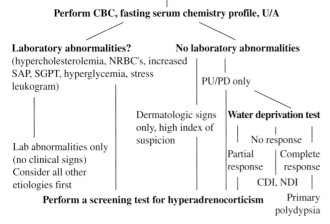

Diagnostic Algorithm for Hyperadrenocorticism

Clinical signs? (PU/PD, alopecia, panting, polyphagia, lethargy, calcinosis cutis, thin skin, recurrent UTI, anestrus, testicular atrophy, heat intolerance, comedones, cutaneous hyperpigmentation, cranial cruciate rupture, myotonia, hepatomegaly, clitoral hypertrophy, bruisability, etc.)

Perform CBC, fasting serum chemistry profile, U/A

Laboratory abnormalities?
(hypercholesterolemia, NRBC's, increased SAP, SGPT, hyperglycemia, stress leukogram)

No laboratory abnormalities

PU/PD only

Lab abnormalities only (no clinical signs) Consider all other etiologies first

Dermatologic signs only, high index of suspicion

Water deprivation test

No response

Partial response | Complete response

CDI, NDI

Perform a screening test for hyperadrenocorticism

Primary polydypsia

Figure 30.4 Diagnostic approach to hyperadrenocorticism.

Serum chemistry abnormalities associated with hypercortisolemia in dogs include increased serum activities of alkaline phosphatase (ALP) and alanine aminotransferase, hypercholesterolemia, hyperglycemia, and decreased BUN. The hemogram is often characterized by evidence of erythroid regeneration (e.g., nucleated red blood cells) and a classic "stress leukogram." Basophilia occasionally is observed. Many dogs with hyperadrenocorticism will also have evidence of urinary tract infection without

pyuria. Proteinuria resulting from glomerulosclerosis is common as well. Urine specific gravity is usually decreased, and urine may be hyposthenuric. Thyroid status often is affected in animals with hyperadrenocorticism, as evidenced by decreased total T_4 and total T_3, caused by euthyroid sick syndrome, and an attenuated response to TSH stimulation, caused by overcrowding of pituitary thyrotrophs by adrenocorticotrophs. Overt diabetes mellitus may result from the insulin antagonism caused by hypercortisolemia in approximately 15% of dogs with hyperadrenocorticism and 85% of cats with hyperadrenocorticism. Conversely, hyperadrenocorticism can cause insulin resistance and poor glycemic control in diabetic animals.

The diagnosis of hyperadrenocorticism should be established based on suggestive clinical signs followed by supporting minimum database abnormalities (e.g., high serum cholesterol, increased serum ALP activity) and confirmed via an appropriate screening test. If screening test results are inconclusive, test the dog again 3 to 6 months later rather than subject the animal to treatment without a definitive diagnosis. Diagnostic algorithms (*Figs. 30.4, 30.5, and 30.6*) point to special circumstances in which certain tests may not be accurate or a certain screening or differentiation test might be preferred. Protocols for the different diagnostic tests are listed in *Tables 30.2 and 30.3.*

Screening Tests

The urine cortisol:creatinine ratio is highly sensitive in separating normal dogs from those with hyperadrenocor-

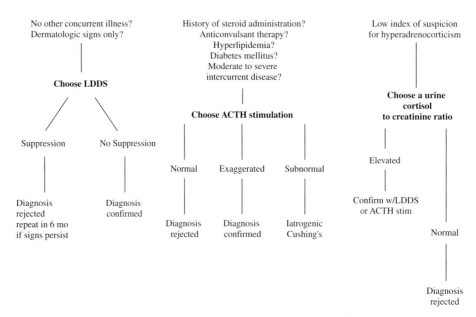

Figure 30.5 Diagnostic approach to choosing a screening test for hyperadrenocorticism.

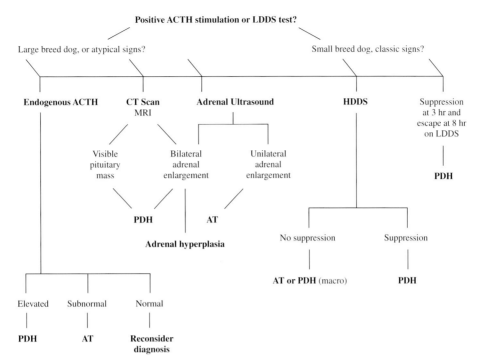

Figure 30.6 Diagnostic approach to choosing a differentiation test to determine if hyperadrenocorticism is of pituitary or adrenal origin.

ticism. The test is not highly specific for hyperadrenocorticism, however, because dogs with moderate to severe nonadrenal illness also exhibit increased ratios. An elevated ratio should always be confirmed with an ACTH stimulation or low-dose dexamethasone suppression (LDDS) test. The steroid-induced serum ALP isoenzyme (SIALP) is also available to practitioners. The advantages of SIALP measurement are wide availability and low cost; however, even small increases in serum cortisol, such as those occurring with exogenous steroid administration in ocular preparations, can induce SIALP. This test has a very low specificity (<44%), because it is affected by stress and nonadrenal disease. Another disadvantage is that it cannot differentiate between endogenous and iatrogenic hyperadrenocorticism.

Screening tests for hyperadrenocorticism, such as the LDDS and ACTH stimulation tests, work on the principle of suppression or stimulation of the pituitary–adrenal axis. With the LDDS test, dexamethasone is administered at a low dosage to cause negative feedback to the pituitary gland. In a normal animal, this negative feedback produces a decrease in endogenous ACTH secretion and a resultant decrease in circulating cortisol concentrations. Dexamethasone is the only synthetic corticosteroid that does not cross-react with the cortisol assay. The ACTH stimulation is used to determine the extent of adrenal enlargement; adrenal glands that are enlarged because of chronic pituitary stimulation by ACTH or that

are neoplastic will show an exaggerated response to exogenous ACTH.

LDDS test. The LDDS test has been the screening test of choice for canine hyperadrenocorticism in the past. It is sensitive (92%–95%), and only 5% to 8% of dogs with pituitary-dependent hyperadrenocorticism will exhibit suppressed cortisol concentrations at 8 hours (i.e., 5%–10% false-negative results). In addition, 30% of dogs with pituitary-dependent hyperadrenocorticism will exhibit suppression at 3 or 4 hours, followed by "escape" of suppression at 8 hours; this pattern is diagnostic for pituitary-dependent disease and makes further testing unnecessary. The major disadvantage of the LDDS test is the lack of specificity in dogs with nonadrenal illness. One recent report showed that more than 50% of dogs with nonadrenal illness have a positive LDDS test. Another study, which looked at the specificity of the LDDS versus the ACTH stimulation tests based on necropsy findings, showed that the LDDS test was much less specific than the ACTH stimulation test. Thus, a dog should be allowed to recover from the nonadrenal illness before undergoing an LDDS test for hyperadrenocorticism.

Corticotropin (ACTH) stimulation test. The corticotropin (ACTH) stimulation test is used to establish the diagnosis for a variety of adrenopathic disorders, including endogenous or iatrogenic hyperadrenocorticism and spontaneous

TABLE 30.2 PROTOCOLS FOR SCREENING AND DIFFERENTIATION TESTS FOR HYPERADRENOCORTICISM

Screening Tests

Low-Dose Dexamethasone Suppression Test
Protocol: 0.015 mg/kg IV or IM dexamethasone solution (Azium) or 0.01 mg/kg IV dexamethasone sodium phosphate; samples at 0, 3, and 8 hours
Reference range: pre, 1–4 mg/dL (28–110 mmol/L); 3 hours, <1.5 µg/dL (40 mmol/L); 8 hours, <1.5 µg/dL (40 mmol/L)

Corticotropin (ACTH) Stimulation Test
Protocol: 0.5 U/kg aqueous corticotropin IV, samples at 0 and 1 hour; 2.2 U/kg corticotropin gel IM (max, 20 U/dog), samples at 0 and 2 hours
Reference range: pre, 1–4 µg/dL (28–110 mmol/L), post, >20 µg/dL (550 mmol/L)

Urine Cortisol:Creatinine Ratio
Protocol: single urine sample, voided or collected by cystocentesis
Reference range: dependent upon laboratory

Alkaline Phosphatase Isoenzyme
Protocol: single serum sample, should be at least two- or threefold greater than normal
Reference range: <150 U/L

Combined ACTH Stimulation/High-Dose Dexamethasone Suppression Test
Protocol: 0.1 mg/kg dexamethasone IM; 2 hours later, inject 0.5 U/kg cosyntropin IV; collect samples at baseline, 2 hours (before ACTH), and 3 hours (1 hour after ACTH)
Reference range: 2 hours, <1.0 µg/dL (28 mmol/L); 3 hours, >20 µg/dL (550 mmol/L)

Differentiation Tests

High-Dose Dexamethasone Suppression Test
Protocol: 1 mg/kg IV dexamethasone, samples at 0 and 8 hours
Reference range: suppression to <1.5 µg/dL (40 mmol/L) at 8 hours

Combined ACTH Stimulation/High-Dose Dexamethasone Suppression Test
Protocol: 0.1 mg/kg dexamethasone IM; 2 hours later, inject 0.5 U/kg cosyntropin IV; collect samples at baseline, 2 hours (before ACTH), and 3 hours (1 hour after ACTH)
Reference range: suppression <1.0 µg/dL (28 mmol/L) at 2 hours; post-ACTH, stimulation > 20 µg/dL (550 mmol/L)

Endogenous ACTH
Protocol: single plasma sample (may be collected before screening test and frozen for later analysis); collect in EDTA vacutainer (with aprotinin), centrifuge and store in plastic, ship at 4°C (or frozen if not collected in aprotinin)
Reference range: 20–80 pg/mL (4.4–8.8 pmol/L)

ACTH, adrenocorticotropic hormone; *EDTA*, ethylenediaminetetraacetic acid.

hypoadrenocorticism. As a screening test for the diagnosis of naturally occurring hyperadrenocorticism, it has a diagnostic sensitivity of approximately 95% and a higher specificity than the LDDS test. In one study, only 15% of dogs with nonadrenal disease exhibited an exaggerated response to ACTH stimulation.

Differentiation Tests

Once the diagnosis of hyperadrenocorticism has been confirmed, differentiation of pituitary- versus adrenal-dependent disease may be necessary. Most dogs with hyperadrenocorticism suffer from pituitary-dependent disease, but certain atypical typicals (e.g., an anorexic dog with hyperadrenocorticism) should alert clinicians that a differentiation test is appropriate (*Table 30.4*). In particular, differentiation of pituitary macroadenomas from adrenal tumors is often necessary in large-breed dogs.

High-dose dexamethasone suppression test. The high-dose dexamethasone suppression test works on the principle that ACTH secretion has already been suppressed maximally in dogs with functioning adrenal tumors; therefore, administration of dexamethasone, no matter how high

TABLE 30.3   COMPARISON OF SCREENING TESTS FOR HYPERADRENOCORTICISM

Advantages	Disadvantages
LDDS Test	
Easy to perform	Lower specificity than ACTH stimulation in stressed dogs (56% false-positive rate)
Reliable	
High sensitivity (92%–95%)	Requires hospitalization
May be diagnostic for PDH, if suppression and escape are noted	Requires 8 hours of testing
	Less economical than ACTH stimulation
	Three samples required
Corticotropin Stimulation Test	
Easy to perform, reliable	Lower sensitivity overall than LDDS (85%), especially for adrenal tumors (50%–60%)
Higher specificity than LDDS (85%)	
Fewer serum samples required	Laboratory variation in normal range
Hospitalization not required	Will not differentiate PDH from adrenal tumors
1- or 2-Hour test	
Differentiates iatrogenic vs. endogenous hyperadrenocorticism	
Provides baseline for monitoring therapy	
Urine Cortisol : Creatinine Ratio	
Highly sensitive (no false-negative results)	Low specificity (24%)
Single voided urine sample	Must confirm a positive result with an LDDS or ACTH stimulation test
Increased convenience to owner	
Decreased cost (single sample)	
Steroid-Induced Alkaline Phosphatase Isoenzyme	
Widely available	Not diagnostic for iatrogenic hyperadrenocorticism
Inexpensive	Affected by stress
Requires only a single serum sample	Affected by nonadrenal disease
Predictive value of a negative test (100%)	Must confirm with LDDS or ACTH stimulation
Combined Corticotropin Stimulation and High-Dose Dexamethasone Suppression Test	
Combines a screening/differentiation test	Requires at least three cortisol samples
Single hospital visit	ACTH stimulation portion of test less reliable than ACTH stimulation test alone
Shorter duration than LDDS or HDDS	
May provide information about the clinical stage of hyperadrenocorticism	Difficult to interpret

ACTH, adrenocorticotropic hormone; *LDDS*; low-dose dexamethasone suppression; *PDH*, pituitary-dependent hyperadrenocorticism.

the dose, will not suppress the serum cortisol concentrations. In dogs with pituitary-dependent disease, however, high doses of dexamethasone suppress ACTH and, hence, cortisol secretion. One caveat is that dogs with pituitary macroadenomas (25%–50% of dogs with pituitary-dependent disease) fail to exhibit suppression.

Endogenous plasma ACTH concentrations. Measurement of endogenous plasma ACTH concentrations is the most reliable method of discriminating between pituitary-dependent hyperadrenocorticism and adrenal tumors. Dogs with adrenal tumors have low to undetectable ACTH concentrations. In contrast, dogs with pituitary-dependent hyperadrenocorticism exhibit normal to increased ACTH concentrations. The addition of the protease inhibitor

aprotinin to whole blood in ethylenediaminetetraacetic acid (EDTA) tubes will inhibit the degradation of ACTH.

Hypoadrenocorticism

Mineralocorticoids are produced in the outer zone (i.e., zona glomerulosa) of the adrenal cortex. Electrolyte balance and blood pressure homeostasis are the main physiologic effects of mineralocorticoids, and these actions are carried out at the level of the distal tubules in the kidney. The effect of mineralocorticoids is to promote retention of sodium and secretion of potassium and hydrogen. In the case of mineralocorticoids, the main controlling factors are produced in the target organ: the kidney. Cells in the juxtaglomerular apparatus of the kidney produce an en-

TABLE 30.4 COMPARISON OF TESTS AND TECHNIQUES FOR DIFFERENTIATION OF PITUITARY VERSUS ADRENAL HYPERADRENOCORTICISM

Advantages	Disadvantages
HDDS Test	
Does not require special facilities	Requires hospitalization
Inexpensive	Expensive
	Inconvenient
	8-Hour sampling period
	Pituitary macroadenomas may not suppress
Endogenous Adrenocorticotropin Measurement	
Single plasma sample	Expensive
May be collected before screening test and frozen for later analysis	Analysis restricted to certain laboratories
More reliable than HDDS	Special handling required
Ultrasonography of Adrenals	
Will differentiate AT from PDH	Requires sophisticated instrumentation
Noninvasive	Requires skilled ultrasonographer
Relatively inexpensive and widely available	
Computed Tomograph	
Noninvasive	Expensive
Localizes pituitary tumor	Requires sophisticated instrumentation
Estimates size of tumor	Not widely available
Magnetic Resonance Imaging	
Noninvasive	Expensive
Localizes pituitary tumor	Requires sophisticated instrumentation
Estimates size of tumor	Not widely available

AT, adrenal tumor; HDDS, high-dose dexamethasone suppression; PDH, pituitary-dependent hyperadrenocorticism.

zyme, termed *renin*, in response to decreases in blood pressure. This enzyme acts on angiotensinogen and results in the production of angiotensin I, which is further hydrolyzed to angiotensin II by angiotensin-converting enzyme. Angiotensin II stimulates the zona glomerulosa to produce mineralocorticoids and increases peripheral resistance of the blood vascular system by causing vasoconstriction of the smooth muscle of blood vessels. Another major regulatory factor in the control of mineralocorticoid secretion is blood potassium concentration. An increase in the potassium concentration stimulates the zona glomerulosa to secrete mineralocorticoids; a decrease in this concentration has the opposite effect.

One of the most well-recognized endocrine emergencies is the classic addisonian crisis. Caused by a deficiency in adrenocortical steroids, an addisonian crisis manifests as severe, profound shock. Although most dogs and cats are presented in severe cardiovascular collapse, there often is recent history of vague, waxing-and-waning symptoms that precedes the onset of collapse. Hypoadrenocorticism is most commonly diagnosed in young female dogs and usually has an immune-mediated cause. Certain breeds, such as Leonbergers, standard poodles, and Portuguese water dogs, are at increased risk for the disease; however,

hypoadrenocorticism may be diagnosed in any breed. Historical findings compatible with the diagnosis of hypoadrencorticism include intermittent vomiting, diarrhea, weight loss, lethargy, anorexia, and weakness. These symptoms often resolve with fluid therapy, corticosteroid treatment, or both. Physical examination of animals during an acute hypoadrenal crisis reveals weak pulse, bradycardia, prolonged capillary refill time, severe mental depression, and profound muscle weakness. Clinical features of hypoadrenocorticism that should heighten the index of suspicion include a normal or slow heart rate in the face of circulatory shock and the waxing-and-waning course of disease before collapse.

Electrolyte abnormalities consisting of severe hyponatremia and hypochloremia associated with hyperkalemia are the hallmarks of hypoadrenocorticism. A serum sodium : potassium ratio of less than 27 : 1 is considered to be suggestive of hypoadrenocorticism, but it is not pathognomonic. Gastrointestinal disease, acute renal failure, and postrenal azotemia also may cause a low sodium : potassium ratio. Furthermore, some patients with hypoadrenocorticism, particularly those with glucocorticoid deficiency only, will not show classic electrolyte imbalances. Azotemia and hyperphosphatemia also attend primary hypoadrenocorticism, making it difficult to differentiate from acute renal failure. Azotemia may be prerenal, as a result of dehydration and hypovolemia, or caused by GI hemorrhage. Hematologic abnormalities consist of eosinophilia and lymphocytosis or of normal eosinophil and lymphocyte counts in the face of severe metabolic stress. The anemia of hypoadrenocorticism classically has been attributed to a lack of glucocorticoid effects on the bone marrow. Recent studies, however, suggest that hemorrhagic gastroenteritis contributes significantly to the anemia. Hypoglycemia is more common with secondary or atypical hypoadrenocorticism and rarely is seen with typical hypoadrenocorticism.

Urine specific gravity frequently is low and attributed to medullary washout (i.e., inadequate medullary gradient caused by sodium depletion) and decreased medullary blood flow. Dilute urine in the face of azotemia and hyperkalemia may be easily mistaken for acute renal failure. Hormonal assays are required to confirm the presence or absence of adrenal disease and to differentiate between hypoadrenocorticism and renal failure.

Diagnostic Testing

The diagnosis of primary hypoadrenocorticism is established based on clinical signs, classic electrolyte imbalances, and confirmation with an ACTH response test. The baseline cortisol sample should be collected with the initial blood work, and synthetic ACTH (Cortrosyn, 0.25 mg) should be administered intravenously during the initial fluid therapy. A 1-hour post-ACTH sample may then be drawn, and glucocorticoids may be administered after the 1-hour sample is taken. Intramuscular injection of ACTH (gel or synthetic) may not be absorbed in animals experiencing circulatory shock; therefore, intravenous administration of synthetic ACTH is preferred. If glucocorticoids must be administered before the measurement of cortisol, dexamethasone sodium phosphate is preferred, because dexamethasone will not interfere with the cortisol assay. Endogenous plasma ACTH may be measured to determine if the hypoadrenocorticism is primary or secondary. This specimen must be collected in an EDTA tube, spun within 1 hour of sampling, and stored in plastic before the administration of any corticosteroids.

Dogs and cats with primary hypoadrenocorticism will exhibit a subnormal response to ACTH administration. The baseline cortisol concentration usually is low or undetectable, and the post-ACTH cortisol concentration also is low or undetectable. Endogenous plasma ACTH concentrations are dramatically increased in animals with primary hypoadrenocorticism as a result of the loss of negative feedback to the pituitary caused by decreased serum cortisol concentrations. In the case of secondary hypoadrenocorticism, which is caused by a pituitary deficiency of ACTH, endogenous ACTH concentrations typically are decreased (<20 pg/mL). The response to exogenous ACTH is diminished, but not as dramatically as that in primary hypoadrenocorticism. Baseline as well as post-ACTH cortisol concentrations may be in the normal range.

CALCIUM AND PHOSPHATE METABOLISM

The control of calcium and phosphate metabolism is important, because these ions play important roles in physiologic processes. Calcium is necessary for several intracellular reactions, including muscle contraction, nerve-cell activity, release of hormones through exocytosis, and activation of a number of enzymes. Inorganic phosphate also functions as an important hydrogen ion–buffering system in blood. Organic phosphate is an important part of the cell, including the plasma membrane and the intracellular components, such as nucleic acids, adenosine triphosphate, and adenosine monophosphate. The regulation of calcium involves control of the movement of calcium between the extracellular fluid and three body organs: bone, GI tract, and kidneys.

Parathyroid Hormone

The main endocrine organ involved in the control of calcium and phosphate metabolism is the parathyroid gland. The synthesis of parathyroid hormone (PTH) is similar to that of other protein hormones. Briefly, preproPTH is synthesized in the rough endoplasmic reticulum and then is cleaved to form proPTH. Next, a six–amino acid proportion is removed, resulting in PTH, which is secreted by the process of exocytosis. Parathyroid hormone is rapidly metabolized by the liver and kidneys, and it has a relatively short half-life (5–10 minutes in blood).

The effect of PTH is to increase calcium and decrease phosphate concentrations in extracellular fluids. Parathyroid hormone has direct effects on bone and kidney metabolism of calcium and indirect effects on GI metabolism of calcium. The initial effect of PTH on bone is to promote the transfer of calcium across the osteoblast–osteocyte membrane. It acts on the distal convoluted tubules of the kidneys to increase absorption of calcium and decrease renal reabsorption of phosphate through an effect on the proximal tubules, and it also is involved in activation of vitamin D at the kidney level. Parathyroid hormone mediates indirectly absorption of calcium from the gut through its effect on vitamin D. Secretion of PTH is controlled by free (i.e., ionized) calcium concentrations in blood. Decreases in calcium stimulate PTH secretion, and increases in calcium partially inhibit PTH secretion.

Hyperparathyroidism

Hypercalcemia can result from a variety of causes, including hypercalcemia of malignancy, hyperparathyroidism, fungal disease, osteoporosis, hypoadrenocorticism, chronic renal disease, and hypervitaminosis D. The initial signs of hypercalcemia are polydipsia and polyuria resulting from impaired response of the distal renal tubules to antidiuretic hormone (ADH). Listlessness, depression, and muscle weakness result from depressed excitability of neuromuscular tissue. Mild GI signs of hypercalcemia include inappetence, vomiting, and constipation. Persistent mild elevations in serum calcium (12–14 mg/dL) can cause uroliths and signs of urinary tract disease, such as hematuria and stranguria. On the other hand, severe hypercalcemia (>14 mg/dL) can progress rapidly to acute renal failure when the calcium–phosphorus product (Ca [mg/dL] × PO$_4$[mg/dL] exceeds 60 to 80 because of renal tissue mineralization.

The diagnostic approach to hypercalcemia consists of ruling out the most common cause of hypercalcemia, which is hypercalcemia of malignancy. A thorough patient history and physical examination, including lymph node and rectal examination (anal sac adenocarcinoma), complete blood count, urinalysis, serum chemistry profile, and chest/abdominal radiographs, are necessary to search for underlying neoplastic processes. If lymphoma is not detected on the minimum database, a bone marrow examination and skeletal radiographic survey may be necessary.

Once a diagnosis of neoplasia has been excluded, the next primary differential for hypercalcemia is chronic renal failure. This is the most difficult differential to exclude, because other causes of hypercalcemia may result in renal damage from soft-tissue mineralization of the kidneys. Therefore, an animal with hypercalcemia, azotemia, and hyperphosphatemia could suffer from primary hyperparathyroidism, primary renal failure with secondary renal hyperparathyroidism, or Vitamin D intoxication. Furthermore, patients with hypercalcemia secondary to renal disease also may exhibit elevations in the level of intact PTH.

The diagnosis of primary hyperparathyroidism is established based on the findings of hypercalcemia (preferably ionized), hypophosphatemia (unless azotemic), high-normal to elevated serum PTH concentrations, and a mass in the cervical region. Intact PTH, using a sandwich assay validated for use in dogs and cats, should be measured. A normal PTH concentration in the face of elevated total or ionized calcium is "inappropriate" for the calcium level, and this should be considered as diagnostic for primary hyperparathyroidism. For suspected hypercalcemia of malignancy in which the diagnostic approach has failed to identify a neoplastic process, PTH-related protein concentrations may be measured.

Hypoparathyroidism

The classic biochemical findings in animals with hypoparathyroidism are hypocalcemia (both total and ionized)

and hyperphosphatemia. Other causes of hypocalcemia include iatrogenic (i.e., postthyroidectomy) hypoparathyroidism, chronic and acute renal failure, acute pancreatitis, hypoalbuminemia, puerperal tetany (i.e., eclampsia), ethylene glycol intoxication, intestinal malabsorption, and nutritional secondary hyperparathyroidism. Early signs of hypocalcemia are nonspecific and include anorexia, facial rubbing, nervousness, and a stiff and stilted gait. Later signs progress to parathesias, hyperventilation, and finally, generalized tetany, seizures, or both.

The diagnosis of primary hypoparathyroidism is established based on results of an intact PTH assay. Serum or plasma PTH concentrations should be measured using a freshly drawn. morning sample from a fasted animal. Sample handling is crucial to establishing an appropriate diagnosis, because PTH may degrade if subjected to warm temperatures. Intact PTH refers to the entire 85–amino acid sequence of PTH; this is measured in a double-antibody "sandwich" assay in most endocrine laboratories that offer PTH measurement. For the diagnosis of primary hypoparathyroidism, the sample should be analyzed for both ionized calcium and intact PTH. Low ionized calcium and undetectable intact PTH concentrations are diagnostic for hypoparathyroidism.

PITUITARY GLAND

The pituitary gland is composed of the adenohypophysis (i.e., pars distalis or anterior lobe), neurohypophysis (i.e., pars nervosa or posterior lobe), pars intermedia (i.e., intermediate lobe), and pars tuberalis. The adenohypophysis is formed from an area of the roof of the embryonic oral ectoderm called the Rathke pouch, which extends upward to meet the neurohypophysis, which extends downward from the floor of the third ventricle. The neurohypophysis is composed of axons that originate within the supraoptic and paraventricular nuclei of the hypothalamus. The main activity of vasopressin, which is produced by the neurohypophysis, is the enhancement of water retention by the kidney. As a consequence, this hormone is often termed *antidiuretic hormone*, or ADH. Vasopressin is the most important hormone for the control of water balance. Control of vasopressin secretion is a result of changes in plasma osmolality. Increased osmolality activates cells in the hypothalamus that synthesize vasopressin.

Pituitary Disorders

Central DI

Diabetes insipidus is a disorder of water metabolism that is characterized by polyuria, urine with low specific gravity or osmolality, and polydipsia. It results from defective

---

TABLE 30.5 PROCEDURES FOR THE MODIFIED WATER DEPRIVATION TEST AND ADH SUPPLEMENTATION TEST

Modified Water-Deprivation Test

1. The animal is confined to a cage with no food or water and is weighed at 1- to 2-hour intervals after emptying the urinary bladder and measuring an initial body weight.
2. When >5% of body weight has been lost, the urinary bladder should be completely emptied and the urine checked for specific gravity or osmolality.
3. A urine specific gravity > 1.025 or urine osmolality > 900 mOsm/L is generally considered an adequate response to water deprivation.
4. Failure to concentrate urine to this degree in the absence of renal disease indicates central or nephrogenic DI or medullary washout.
5. Immediately after water deprivation, if the animal fails to concentrate urine adequately after losing 5% or more of its body weight, an ADH response test is performed.
6. A synthetic form of ADH (DDAVP) may be given SC or IV, or 20 μg of DDAVP (≈4 drops of the 100 μg/mL of intranasal preparation) can be administered as intranasal or conjunctival drops.
7. Urine concentrating ability is then monitored every 2 hours for 6–10 hours.
8. Increases in urine specific gravity > 1.025 or urine osmolality > 900 mosm/L after administration of aqueous vasopressin or DDAVP is suggestive of central DI.
9. An inability to concentrate urine after ADH administration indicates nephrogenic DI or severe medullary washout.
10. Frequent patient monitoring is essential, because severe dehydration, possible neurologic complications, and even death can ensue.

DDAVP Therapeutic Trial

1. The owner should measure the animal's 24-hour water intake 2–3 days before the therapeutic trial with DDAVP is initiated, allowing free-choice water intake.
2. The intranasal preparation of DDAVP is administered in the conjunctival sac (1–4 drops every 12 hours) for 3–5 days.
3. A dramatic reduction in water intake (> 50%) during the first few treatment days strongly suggests an ADH deficiency.
4. When the polyuria is from other causes, the decrease is seldom >30%.

ADH, antidiuretic hormone; *DDAVP*, desmopressin acetate; *DI*, diabetes insipidus.

---

secretion of ADH (i.e., central DI) or inability of the renal tubule to respond to ADH (i.e., nephrogenic DI). Deficiency of ADH (or vasopressin) can be partial or complete. Central DI is characterized by an absolute or relative lack of circulating ADH and is classified as primary (i.e., idiopathic and congenital) or secondary. Secondary central DI usually results from head trauma or neoplasia. In dogs and cats, both central and nephrogenic DI are extremely rare.

Central DI may appear at any age, in any breed, and in either gender, but young adults (6 months of age) are most commonly affected. The major clinical signs of DI are profound polyuria and polydipsia (>100 mL/kg per day; normal, 40–70 mL/kg per day), nocturia, and incontinence (usually of several months' duration). The severity of clinical signs varies, because DI may result from a partial or a complete defect in ADH secretion or action. Other, less-consistent signs include weight loss (because these animals are constantly seeking water) and dehydration.

Routine complete blood count as well as serum biochemical and electrolyte profiles usually are normal in animals with DI. Plasma osmolality often will be high (>310 mOsm/L) in central or nephrogenic DI as a result of dehydration. Animals with primary polydipsia often exhibit low plasma osmolality (<290 mOsm/L) as a result of overhydration. When abnormalities such as slightly increased hematocrit or hypernatremia are present at the initial evaluation, they usually are secondary to dehydration from water restriction by the pet owner. In DI, urinalysis is unremarkable, except for the finding of a persistently dilute urine (urine specific gravity, 1.004–1.012).

Diagnostic tests to confirm and differentiate central DI, nephrogenic DI, and psychogenic polydipsia include the modified water-deprivation test or response to ADH supplementation (*Table 30.5*). The modified water-deprivation test is designed to determine whether endogenous ADH is released in response to dehydration and whether the kidneys can respond to ADH. The more common causes of polyuria and polydipsia, however, should be ruled out before this procedure is performed. Failure to recognize renal failure before water deprivation may lead to an incorrect or inconclusive diagnosis or even cause significant patient morbidity.

Anterior Pituitary

The adenohypophysis is comprised of the pars distalis and pars intermedia. The major hormones produced by the anterior pituitary include GH or somatotropin, prolactin, TSH, follicle-stimulating hormone (FSH), luteinizing hormone (LH); and ACTH. Growth hormone is produced by acidophilic somatotropes. It is a single-chain protein that contains two disulfide bonds, and it is uniquely species-specific in its activity.

Pituitary Dwarfism

Pituitary dwarfism results from destruction of the pituitary gland via a neoplastic, degenerative, or anomalous process. It may be associated with decreased production of other pituitary hormones, including TSH, ACTH, LH, FSH, and GH. Pituitary dwarfism is most common in German shepherds from 2 to 6 months of age. Other affected breeds include carnelian bear dogs, spitz, toy pinschers, and weimaraners. The disease is inherited as a simple, autosomal-recessive trait in German shepherds and results from a cystic Rathke pouch. The first observable clinical signs of pituitary dwarfism are slow growth noticed during the first 2 or 3 months of life as well as mental retardation, which usually manifests as difficulty in house-training. Physical examination findings may include proportionate dwarfism, retained puppy haircoat, hypotonic skin, truncal alopecia, cutaneous hyperpigmentation, infantile genitalia, and delayed dental eruption. Clinicopathologic features include eosinophilia, lymphocytosis, mild normocytic normochromic anemia, hypophosphatemia, and occasionally, hypoglycemia resulting from secondary adrenal insufficiency. Differential diagnoses include other causes of stunted growth, such as hypothyroid dwarfism, portosystemic shunt, diabetes mellitus, hyperadrenocorticism, malnutrition, and parasitism. The diagnosis is established based on measuring serum GH concentrations (no longer commercially available) or serum somatomedin C (i.e., insulin-like growth factor [IGF]-1). The advantage of IGF-1 is that it is not species-specific. A subnormal response to exogenous TSH and ACTH stimulation tests usually is found; furthermore, endogenous TSH and ACTH are decreased in affected dogs as a result of panhypopituitarism.

Hypersomatotropism (Acromegaly)

Acromegaly, or hypersomatotropism, results from chronic excessive GH secretion in adult animals. Canine acromegaly is an extremely rare disorder that is observed after administration of progestational compounds for suppression of estrus in intact female dogs. The disease is caused by excessive secretion of GH from mammary cells under the influence of exogenous progesterone. Acromegaly in cats, as in humans, results from a GH-secreting tumor of the anterior pituitary. Such GH-producing pituitary tumors in cats grow slowly and may be present for a long period of time before the onset of clinical signs. Feline acromegaly occurs in older cats (8–14 years of age) and occurs more commonly in males. Canine acromegaly occurs in intact female dogs given progestational compounds for estrus prevention.

Clinical signs of uncontrolled diabetes mellitus often are observed as the first sign of acromegaly; therefore, polydipsia, polyuria, and polyphagia are the most common presenting signs. Net weight gain of lean body mass in animals suffering from uncontrolled diabetes mellitus is a key sign of acromegaly. Organomegaly, including renomegaly, hepatomegaly, and enlargement of endocrine organs, also is observed. Some dogs and cats will show the classic enlargement of extremities, body size, jaw, tongue, and forehead that is characteristic of acromegaly in humans. Some of the most striking manifestations of acromegaly, however, occur in the musculoskeletal system, and these include increased muscle mass and growth of the acral segments of the body, including the paws, chin, and skull. Cardiovascular abnormalities, such as cardiomegaly (as determined radiographically and echocardiographically), systolic murmurs, and congestive heart failure, develop late in the course of disease. Renomegaly is observed in both cats and humans suffering from acromegaly. Azotemia develops late in the course of disease in approximately 50% of acromegalic cats. Neurologic signs of acromegaly in humans, such as peripheral neuropathies (e.g., paresthesias, carpal tunnel syndrome, sensory and motor defects), and parasellar manifestations (e.g., headache and visual field defects) generally are not detected in acromegalic small animals.

Impaired glucose tolerance and insulin resistance resulting in diabetes mellitus are observed in all cats and most dogs with acromegaly. Measurement of endogenous insulin reveals dramatically increased serum insulin concentrations. Despite severe insulin resistance and hyperglycemia, ketosis is rare in acromegalics. Feline acromegaly should be suspected in any diabetic cat (especially males) with severe insulin resistance (insulin requirement, >20 U/day). Hypercholesterolemia and mild increases in serum activities of liver enzymes are attributed to the diabetic state. Hyperphosphatemia without azotemia also is a common clinicopathologic finding, perhaps because of GH-stimulated bone growth. Urinalysis is unremarkable, except for persistent proteinuria, probably because of systemic hypertension and glomerulosclerosis.

Establishing a definitive diagnosis of acromegaly requires documentation of increased plasma GH or somatomedin C concentrations. Unfortunately, feline and canine GH assays no longer are commercially available. Serum IGF-1 or somatomedin C concentrations usually are dramatically increased in acromegalic animals; furthermore, IGF-1 is not a species-specific assay. Caution should be used when measuring IGF-1 in diabetic cats with insulin resistance. Administration of large doses of insulin, particularly in poorly perfused sites such as the back of the neck, can cause cross-reaction with the IGF-1 assay. Therefore, other causes of insulin resistance (e.g., poor injection technique, Cushing syndrome, hyperthyroidism) should be ruled out before levels of this hormone are measured. At this time, the most definitive test for the diagnosis of acromegaly in cats is computed tomography of the pituitary region. Coupled with the exclusion of other disorders that cause insulin resistance (e.g., hyperthyroidism, hyperadrenocorticism) in cats that exhibit clinical signs of acromegaly, computed tomography should lead the clinician to a diagnosis of acromegaly.

SUGGESTED READINGS

Bruyette DS. Polyuria and polydipsia. In: August JR, ed. Consultations in feline internal medicine. Philadelphia: WB Saunders, 1991:227–236.

Burns MG, Kelly AB, Hornof WJ, et al. Pulmonary artery thrombosis in three dogs with hyperadrenocorticism. J Am Vet Med Assoc 1981;178:388–393.

Campbell KL. Growth hormone-related disorders in dogs. Compend Contin Educ Pract 1988;10:477–482.

Chastain CB, Franklin RT, Granham VK, et al. Evaluation of the hypothalamic pituitary–adrenal axis in clinically stressed dogs. J Am Anim Hosp Assoc 1986;22:435–441.

Chew DJ, Meuten DJ. Disorders of calcium and phosphorus metabolism Vet Clin North Am Small Anim Pract 1982;12:411–438.

Contreras LN, Hane S, Tyrrell JB. Urinary cortisol in the assessment of pituitary–adrenal function: utility of 24-hour and spot determinations. J Clin Endocrinol Metab 1986;65:965–969.

Dibartola SP. Disorders of sodium and water: hypernatremia and hyponatremia. In: Dibartola SP, ed. Fluid therapy in small animal practice. Philadelphia: WB Saunders,1992:57.

Dorner JL, Hoffman WE, Long GB. Corticosteroid induction of an isoenzyme of alkaline phosphatase in the dog. Am J Vet Res 1974;35:1457–1458.

Feldman BF, Feldman EC. Routine laboratory abnormalities in endocrine disease. Vet Clin North Am Small Anim Pract 1977;7:433–464.

Feldman EC. Comparison of ACTH response and dexamethasone suppression as screening tests in canine hyperadrenocorticism. J Am Vet Med Assoc 1983;182:505–510.

Feldman EC. Distinguishing dogs with functioning adrenocortical tumors from dogs with pituitary-dependent hyperadrenocorticism: J Am Vet Med Assoc 1983;183:195–200.

Feldman EC, Mark RE. Urine cortisol:creatinine ratio as a screening test for hyperadrenocorticism in the dog. J Am Vet Med Assoc 1992;200:1637–1641.

Feldman EC, Nelson RW. Hypercalcemia and primary hyperparathyroidism. In: Feldman EC, Nelson RW, eds. Canine and feline endocrinology and reproduction. Philadelphia: WB Saunders, 1996:455–496.

Feldman EC, Nelson RW. Hypocalcemia and primary hypoparathyroidism. In: Feldman EC, Nelson RW, eds. Canine and feline endocrinology and reproduction. Philadelphia: WB Saunders, 1996:497–516.

Graves T. Complications of treatment and concurrent illness associated with hyperthyroidism in cats. In: Kirk RW, Bonagura JA, eds. Current veterinary therapy XII. Philadelphia: WB Saunders, 1994:369–372.

Greco DS. Feline acromegaly. In: August JR, ed. Consultations in feline medicine II. Philadelphia: WB Saunders, 1994:169–176.

Kaplan AJ, Peterson ME, Kemppainen RJ: Effects of nonadrenal disease on the results of diagnostic tests for hyperadrenocorticism in dogs (abstract). J Vet Intern Med 1994;8:161.

Katherman KA, O'Leary TP, Richardson RC. Hyperadrenocorticism and diabetes in the dog. J Am Anim Hosp Assoc 1980;16:705–717.

Kemppainen RJ, Clark TP, Peterson ME. Aprotinin preserves immunoreactive adrenocorticotropin in canine plasma (abstract). J Vet Intern Med 1984;8:163.

Kidney BA, Jackson ML. Diagnostic value of alkaline phosphatase isoenzyme separation by affinity electrophoresis in the dog. Can J Vet Res 1988;52:106–110.

Kornegay JN. Hypocalcemia in dogs. Compend Contin Educ Small Anim Pract 1982;4:103–110.

Krause KH. The use of desmopressin in diagnosis and treatment of diabetes insipidus in cats. Compend Contin Educ Pract Vet 1987;9:752–758.

Mack RE, Feldman EC, Wilson SM. Diagnosis of hyperadrenocorticism in dogs. J Contin Educ Pract 1994;16:311–328.

Mark RE, Feldman EC. Comparison of two low-dose dexamethasone suppression protocols as screening and discrimination tests in dogs with hyperadrenocorticism. J Am Vet Med Assoc 1990;197:1603–1606.

Meric SM. Diagnosis and management of feline hyperthyroidism. Compend Contin Educ Pract 1989;11:1053–1060.

Nichols CE. Endocrine and metabolic causes of polyuria and polydipsia. In: Kirk RW, Bonagura JD, eds. Current veterinary therapy XI. Philadelphia: WB Saunders, 1992:293–301.

Nichols R. Diabetes insipidus. In: Kirk RW, ed. Current veterinary therapy X. Philadelphia: WB Saunders, 1989:973–978.

Owens JM, Drucker WD. Hyperadrenocorticism in the dog: canine Cushing's syndrome. Vet Clin North Am Small Anim Pract 1977;7:583–602.

Peterson M. Hyperadrenocorticism. Vet Clin North Am Small Anim Pract 1984;14:731–749.

Peterson ME. Feline hyperthyroidism. Vet Clin North Am 1984;14:809–825.

Peterson ME. Feline hyperthyroidism: pretreatment clinical and laboratory evaluation of 131 cases. J Am Vet Med Assoc 1983;183:103–110.

Peterson ME. Hypoparathyroidism and other causes of hypocalcemia in cats. In: Kirk RW, Bonagura JA, eds. Current veterinary therapy XI. Philadelphia: WB Saunders, 1992:376–379.

Peterson ME, Gilbertson SR, Drucker WD. Plasma cortisol response to exogenous ACTH in 22 dogs with hyperadrenocorticism caused by adrenocortical neoplasia. J Am Vet Med Assoc 1982;180:542–544.

Peterson ME, Graves TK, Gamble DA. Triiodothyronine (T₃) suppression test: an aid in the diagnosis of mild hyperthyroidism in cats. J Vet Intern Med 1990;4:233–238.

Peterson ME, Kintzer PP. Challenges in the diagnosis of canine hyperadrenocorticism (Cushing's disease). Proc ACVIM Forum 1994;12:162–164.

Peterson ME, Taylor RS, Greco DS, et al. Acromegaly in fourteen cats. J Vet Intern Med 1990;4:192–201.

Reimers TJ. Radioimmunoassays and diagnostic tests for thyroid and adrenal disorders. Compend Contin Educ Pract 1982;4:65–75.

Rijnberk A, Van Wees A, Mol JA. Assessment of two tests for the diagnosis of canine hyperadrenocorticism. Vet Rec 1988;122:178–180.

Schick MP. Calcinosis cutis secondary to percutaneous penetration of calcium chloride in dogs. J Am Vet Med Assoc 1987;191:207–211.

Smiley LE, Peterson ME. Evaluation of a urine cortisol:creatinine ratio as a screening test for hyperadrenocorticism in dogs. J Vet Intern Med 1993;7:163–168.

White SD, Ceragioli KL, Bullock LP, et al. Cutaneous markers of canine hyperadrenocorticism. Compend Contin Educ Pract 1989;4:446–465.

Wilson SM, Feldman EC. Diagnostic value of the steroid-induced isoenzyme of alkaline phosphatase in the dog. J Am Anim Hosp Assoc 1992;28:245–250.

FIVE

Clinical Chemistry

of Common Nondomestic

Mammals, Birds, Reptiles,

Fish, and Amphibians

31

CLINICAL CHEMISTRY OF MAMMALS: LABORATORY ANIMALS AND MISCELLANEOUS SPECIES

Blood biochemistry profiles are commonly used to assess the health of nondomestic, mammalian patients. Biomedical research involves use of laboratory animals such as mice, rats, and rabbits, resulting in a large amount of information concerning the interpretation of biochemical profiles in these species. Fewer clinical chemistry studies, however, have been performed on other nondomestic mammals, such as ferrets, llamas, minipigs, and deer. In general, interpretation of clinical chemistry results in nondomestic mammals is the same as that described for domestic species.

Many variables, such as age, gender, hydration, and nutritional status, affect biochemical test results. Environmental conditions such as photoperiod, temperature, and husbandry as well as the sampling and analytic methods and the instrumentation used are other sources of variation. Sampling variables include restraint methods, type of anesthetic used, time of day when sampled, anticoag-

ulant used, site of sample collection, and sample processing and storage. A 16- to 18-hour fast is required in rats to obtain nonlipemic plasma samples, whereas a 16-hour fast in rabbits results in decreased plasma glucose and insulin concentrations but increased glucagon and fatty acid concentrations. Release of epinephrine related to excitement of transportation and blood collection in rabbits results in increased plasma glucose and free fatty acid concentrations. Blood collected by cardiocentesis may be contaminated with muscle enzymes such as creatine kinase (CK), aspartate aminotransferase (AST), lactate dehydrogenase (LD), and alanine aminotransferase (ALT), which are found at high concentrations in cardiac muscle. In mice, plasma calcium concentrations tend to be greater in samples obtained from the orbital sinus compared with concentrations in those obtained by cardiocentesis. Results of clinical chemistry analyses performed on identical serum or plasma samples often vary significantly among laboratories; thus, published reference values exhibit considerable variation for many analytes *(Tables 31.1).*

Blood samples for biochemical studies can be collected using the same techniques as those described for hematologic studies (see Chapter 16). Many modern analyzers can perform as many as 20 tests on as little as 50 μL of serum or plasma. Heparinized plasma is routinely used for clinical chemistry evaluations in small rodents such as mice, hamsters, and gerbils, because collection of serum commonly results in hemolysis and a larger sample volume can be obtained with plasma than with serum. The aqueous form of lithium heparin is the preferred anticoagulant for plasma biochemical analysis. As a general guideline, a blood sample volume comprising 10% or less of the total-body blood volume (or 1% of the body weight) can be safely taken from a healthy mammal.

Hemolysis or prolonged contact between serum and blood cells produces changes in the analyte concentrations. Increases in the potassium, phosphorus, LD, and bilirubin concentrations as well as decreases in the glucose concentration may be observed. Serum samples from guinea pigs have greater LD and γ-glutamyltransferase (GGT) activity compared with that in plasma samples produced by leakage of these enzymes from erythrocytes during the clotting process. In mice, serum CK activity decreases with freezing. Because of the cryoprecipitation of some proteins in serum or plasma samples from rats,

apparent protein concentrations may decrease during freezing.

Plasma biochemical analyte reference ranges for common laboratory rodents and rabbits, ferrets, primates, minipigs, llamas, and deer are provided in *Tables 31.1, 31.4, 31.5, 31.7, and 31.8,* respectively. Hormone concentrations also may vary between serum and plasma. *Tables 31.2, 31.3, and 31.6* compare serum or plasma hormone concentrations of rodents, rabbits, and common nonhuman primates, respectively.

RODENTS: MICE, RATS, GUINEA PIGS, HAMSTERS, AND GERBILS

Laboratory Evaluation of the Kidneys

Laboratory evaluation of rodent kidneys is the same as that for domestic mammals, and it involves evaluation of blood parameters, such as urea nitrogen, creatinine, and electrolytes, and urinalysis. The plasma urea nitrogen is influenced by diet, liver function, gastrointestinal absorption, and hydration. Increases in plasma urea nitrogen and creatinine concentrations only occur when more than 75% of renal function is compromised; therefore, these tests lack sensitivity for renal disease. Common causes of renal azotemia in rodents, especially mice, include amyloidosis, immune complex diseases, and polycystic disease.

TABLE 31.1   PLASMA BIOCHEMICAL VALUES IN COMMON LABORATORY ANIMALS

	Mice	Rats	Guinea Pigs	Hamsters	Rabbits
Glucose (mg/dL)	196–278	114–143[a]	89–95	65–144	89–144
Urea nitrogen (mg/dL)	21–26	16–19[a]	22–25	14–30	14–23
Creatinine (mg/dL)	0.5	0.5–1.4	1.4	0.5–0.6	0.8–2.9
Uric acid (mg/dL)	—	1.3–2.8	—	1.3–5.1	1.1–1.2
Total protein (g/dL)	5.0–7.0	6.4–8.5[a]	4.8–5.6	1.3–5.1	5.0–8.5
Albumin (g/dL)	3.0–4.0	4.1–5.4[a]	2.4–2.7	3.2–4.3	3.0–3.4
Calcium (mg/dL)	7.9–10.5	10.5–13.0	9.6–10.7	10.4–12.4	13.0–15.0
Phosphorus (mg/dL)	5.6–9.2	5.0–13.0	5.0	5.0–8.0	5.6–9.2
Sodium (mEq/L)	138–186	143–150	122–125	128–145	114–156
Potassium (mEq/L)	5.3–6.3	5.3–7.5	4.9–5.1	4.7–5.3	4.4–7.4
Chloride (mEq/L)	99–108	85–102	92–97	94–99	89–120
Cholesterol (mg/dL)	—	36–100	—	94–237	22–69
Total bilirubin (mg/dL)	—	0.0–0.6	0.0–0.9	0.2–0.5	0.0–0.7
Alkaline phosphatase (IU/L)	66–262	70–132[a]	66–74	8–202	<120
Alanine aminotransferase (IU/L)	40–189	26–37[a]	39–45	28–107	<100
Aspartate aminotransferase (IU/L)	77–383	40–53[a]	46–48	53–202	<100
Lactate dehydrogenase (IU/L)	—	63–573	—	94–237	<200
Creatine kinase (IU/L)	—	6–309	—	469–1553	<275

Data compiled from the ranges of mean values without consideration of strain, age, gender, and method of blood collection as published in Loeb WF, Quimby FW, eds. The clinical chemistry of laboratory animals. New York: Pergamon Press, 1989:417—509.
[a] Values obtained from samples collected via the orbital sinus of Sprague-Dawley rats.

TABLE 31.2 PLASMA CONCENTRATIONS OF THE MAJOR HORMONES IN RODENTS

	Rats	Mice	Hamsters	Guinea Pigs
Triiodothyronine (ng/dL)	30–100	30–100	30–80	20–60
Free triiodothyronine (ng/dL)	—	—	—	0.20–0.32
Thyroxine (μg/dL)	3–7	3–7	3–7	2–4
Free thyroxine (μg/dL)	—	—	—	0.9–2.0
Thyroid-stimulating hormone (ng/mL)	400–600	300	300	40–100
Adrenocorticotropic hormone (pg/dL)	30–100	2.6–5.5	40[a]	23[a]
Corticosterone (μg/dL)	15–23[d] 1–6[e]	9[a,b] (males) 40[a,b] (females) 5[a,c] (males) 13.5[a,c] (females)	2.75[c] (males) 0.33[c] (females)	—
Cortisol (μg/dL)	—	—	—	5–30
Free cortisol (μg/dL)	—	—	—	0.6–5.8
Parathormone (pg/mL)	70–700 (males) 0–400 (females)			
Calcitonin (pg/mL)	200–500 (6–8-mo-old males) 450–1100 (6–8-mo-old females) 400–900 (12–14-mo-old males) 700–1800 (12–14-mo-old females)			
1,25-dihydroxy-vitamin D (pg/mL)	72–86 (males) 79–113 (females)			

[a] Average concentration.
[b] Start of dark period.
[c] End of dark period.
[d] Mean maximum values.
[e] Mean minimum values.

Serum or plasma urea nitrogen concentrations increase with high protein diets because of increased nitrogen metabolism rather than renal disease. Age should be considered when evaluating plasma urea nitrogen in rodents; aged hamsters demonstrate increased plasma urea nitrogen concentrations. Other laboratory abnormalities that may be associated with renal disease are hyperphosphatemia, resulting from decreased glomerular filtration, and hypoproteinemia, resulting from glomerular disease and urinary protein loss.

γ-Glutamyltransferase N-acetyl-β-D-glucosaminidase, and alkaline phosphatase (AP) have high tissue activity in the kidney, and measurement of these enzymes in urine may improve the sensitivity of clinical chemical testing for renal disease in rodents. Testing of endogenous creatinine clearance may provide a specific and sensitive test for decreased glomerular filtration before plasma urea nitrogen and creatinine concentrations are increased.

Urine may contain artifacts if proper attention is not paid to the collection technique. The urine should be collected on a clean, dry surface. Without use of commercially available metabolism cages, urine commonly is contaminated with feces, food, hair, bedding, or drinking water. Rodents often spontaneously urinate when handled, thereby providing a clean sample for those who are prepared to collect this urine. Cystocentesis eliminates much of the artifact associated with voided urine but may result in blood contamination. Urinalysis should be performed within 2 hours of collection; otherwise, urine may be refrigerated at 4°C for as long as 48 hours. Refrigerated urine should be warmed to room temperature before testing.

The urine of normal rodents usually is yellow, but it may vary in both shade and transparency depending on the hydration status of the animal. Urinary pH is influenced by diet. Diets that are high in animal proteins contain high concentrations of sulfates and phosphate precursors, which produce more acid urine; cereal protein–based diets tend to produce a neutral to slightly alkaline urine. Rodents tend to have alkaline urine because of the bacterial conversion of urea to ammonia. The urine pH is helpful in determining the acid-base status of the animal. Rodents suffering from catabolic conditions such as starvation, ketosis, or fever commonly have acidic urine.

Urine specific gravity and osmolality are used to evaluate the ability of the kidneys to concentrate or dilute urine. A water-deprivation test for detecting renal disease in rodents can be conducted by withholding water for 24 hours, after which the urinary specific gravity is determined. Those animals that are unable to concentrate their urine to a specific gravity greater than 1.030 either have significant renal disease and are unable to concentrate their urine or suffer from diabetes insipidus. The urine specific gravity value obtained from a refractometer will be erroneous if the urine contains significant quantities of glucose, protein, or other metabolites that normally are not found in urine. Urine osmolality is the definitive method for measuring the concentrating ability of the kidneys; it depends on the number of particles in solution and is not affected by the degree of ionization or the mass of molecules and ions that are present. The normal urine osmolality of rats and hamsters ranges from 331 to 445 and 307 to 355 mOsm/Kg, respectively.

The urine of normal rodents may contain a trace amount of glucose. Large amounts of ascorbic acid normally are found in mouse urine and may interfere with urine chemical strips that use glucose oxidase, thus resulting in a false-negative glucose determination.

Proteinuria is common in normal mice and rats. The semiquantitative urine chemical strips detect large-molecular-weight proteins such as albumin, but not the low-molecular-weight glycoproteins of renal origin that are found in the urine of rodents. The normal proteinuria of rodents is associated with a variety of urinary proteins, which include α- and β-globulins, uromucoid protein, and prealbumin. The degree of proteinuria increases with age, and male mice tend to be more proteinuric than female mice.

Rodent urine sediment normally contains fewer than five erythrocytes and leukocytes per high-power field. Increases in the concentration of these cells are suggestive of urinary tract inflammation, calculi, or neoplasia. If urinary casts containing erythrocytes and leukocytes are concurrently present, cells are likely of renal origin, whereas increased numbers of cells without casts are suggestive of lower urinary tract inflammation, such as cystitis and urethritis. Interpretation of rodent urine sediment findings is the same as that described for domestic mammals.

Electrolytes and Acid-Base

Interpretation of serum or plasma electrolyte and acid-base changes in rodents is the same as that described in domestic mammals. Normal serum and plasma sodium concentrations in mice (174 ± 23 mEq/L) tend to be slightly greater than those reported for other mammals. Hypernatremia resulting from neurogenic diabetes insipidus occurs as a hereditary disorder in some strains of rat. Nephrogenic diabetes insipidus, which usually is associated with renal amyloidosis, frequently occurs in certain strains of mice and aged Syrian hamsters. Chronic nephropathies causing abnormal retention of sodium in rats may cause hypernatremia, which in turn results in myocarditis. Renal amyloidosis alters the renal tubular permeability to water, thereby resulting in hyperchloremia. Increased serum and plasma phosphorus concentrations occur in younger rodents compared with concentrations in adults. Serum or plasma magnesium concentrations increase in hamsters during hibernation.

Laboratory Evaluation of the Liver

Serum or plasma enzymes commonly used to detect liver disease in rodents include AP, GGT, AST, ALT, LD, and sorbitol dehydrogenase. Serum or plasma concentrations of these enzymes increase with increased production, increased release, or decreased clearance. Other biochemical tests to detect liver disease in rodents include serum or plasma total bilirubin, bile acid, and cholesterol concentrations.

Alkaline phosphatase is a membrane-bound enzyme with highest activity in osteoblasts, biliary epithelium, and epithelial cells of the kidneys and intestines. Young rodents have higher plasma AP activity than adults because of osteoblastic activity, and male rats tend to have higher plasma AP activities than female rats. Hepatic AP of rodents is heat labile at 56°C and sensitive to levamisole inhibition. Significant increases in serum or plasma AP activity occur in rodents with hepatic cholestasis. Ligation of the bile duct in rats produces elevation of both hepatic and intestinal AP isoenzymes. Plasma or serum AP activity is a more sensitive test than bilirubin or ALT for detection of hepatic disease in hamsters. Drugs that increase AP synthesis and plasma activity in rats include cortisol, phenobarbital, and theophylline. Increased plasma AP activity occurs in zinc- and manganese-deficient guinea pigs.

Plasma GGT activity is significantly increased in hamsters and rats with experimentally induced hepatic injury resulting in cholestasis. Guinea pigs have higher hepatic GGT activity than rats and demonstrate higher plasma GGT activities with cholestasis. Serum GGT activity is increased in guinea pigs after in vitro blood clot formation, which can be avoided with use of plasma for enzyme testing. The kidneys of rodents have the highest GGT activity, but the enzyme is nondetectable in the plasma or serum of most rodents. The kidneys of rats have 200- to 300-fold the GGT activity of the liver.

Aspartate aminotransferase is a mitochondrial and cytosolic enzyme with high activity in the liver, heart, skeletal muscle, and kidney and low activity in the intestines, brain, lung, and testes. Increases in plasma or serum AST activity usually are associated with hepatic, cardiac muscle, or skeletal muscle injury.

In rats and mice, the activity of ALT, which is a cytosolic and mitochondrial isoenzyme, is highest in the liver. The ratio of the cytosolic to mitochondrial ALT isoenzymes in the liver and heart muscle of rats is 5:1 and 50:1, respectively. In rodents, the intestines, kidneys, heart, skeletal muscle, brain, skin, and pancreas also have ALT activity. In guinea pigs, ALT activity in the heart is almost equal to that in the liver. Plasma and serum ALT activity increases with hepatocellular damage in most rodents, and the enzyme appears to be liver specific in rats and mice. Plasma ALT, however, does not appear to have diagnostic value for hepatic disease in guinea pigs, which have only half the hepatic ALT activity of rats and mice. Increases in serum ALT activity correlate with the degree of hepatic necrosis in rats. A threefold increase in plasma ALT activity occurs in mice that are restrained by holding the body compared with those that are restrained by the tail.

Lactate dehydrogenase is a cytosolic enzyme with the highest activity in skeletal muscle, followed by cardiac muscle, liver, kidney, and intestines, respectively. In the mouse, LD is characterized by five isoenzymes: LD-1 and LD-2 are found in cardiac muscle, LD-5 in the liver and skeletal muscle, and LD-3 in most other tissues. Serum or plasma LD activity elevates with hepatocellular disease in rodents; however, normal values are highly variable and depend on the analytic method used.

Sorbitol dehydrogenase is a cytosolic enzyme that is found in the liver, kidney, and seminal vesicles of mice but is liver specific in rats. Increases in serum or plasma sorbitol dehydrogenase activity occurs with hepatic disease in rodents and is a more sensitive test than ALT for detection of hepatocellular disease in rats. Sorbitol dehydrogenase assays usually are not performed by veterinary laboratories.

Serum and plasma total bilirubin concentration increases in rodents with primary hepatobiliary disease, extrahepatic biliary obstruction, or hemolysis. Increases in plasma or serum total bilirubin concentration should be evaluated by determining the erythrocyte mass and performing other tests that evaluate the liver or biliary system.

The total serum and plasma bile acid concentration is a sensitive and specific test for hepatobiliary disease and disorders of the enterohepatic circulation. Plasma bile acid concentration has an excellent potential for detecting hepatobiliary disease in rodents, especially rats with a high concentration of circulating bile acids.

The plasma cholesterol concentration may increase in rodents with extrahepatic biliary obstruction. Normal plasma cholesterol concentration varies between strains of mice. Hypercholesterolemia often is associated with fatty infiltration of many tissues. In guinea pigs, the intestine, rather than the liver, is the primary site of cholesterol production. Normal plasma cholesterol concentration (112–210 mg/dL) of hamsters is higher than that of other rodents and decreases during short photoperiods but increases with cold temperatures.

Laboratory Evaluation of Proteins

The normal plasma protein concentration in mice varies among strains. In mice, hyperproteinemia often is associated with severe dehydration and often occurs with loss of urinary protein from renal disease. The major classes of serum or plasma proteins in rodents are evaluated using electrophoresis. The major globulins of rats are α_1- and β-globulins, with lower concentrations of α_2- and γ-globulins. In hamsters, albumin concentrations decrease during the first year of life, α_2-globulins increase during the first 6 months of age, and β-globulins decrease at 8 weeks of age. Fibrinogen migrates into the γ-globulin peaks in hamster protein electrophoretic scans. Amyloidosis is a common disease of hamsters older than 18 months and results in hypoalbuminemia and hyperglobulinemia.

Laboratory Evaluation of Glucose Metabolism

Cells must be quickly separated from the serum or plasma of rodents, or fluoride added to the collection tube, to prevent decreased glucose concentration because of in vitro glycolysis. The plasma glucose concentration in rats and mice decreases with age, with an average decrease of 2 mg/dL per month in the latter.

Many strains of mice are used as animal models for diabetes mellitus; therefore, glucose tolerance tests have been developed for mice. A 1-hour glucose tolerance test compares the preinjection plasma glucose concentration to the glucose concentration obtained 1 hour after an intraperitoneal injection of glucose at a dose of 2 mg/g body weight. A 4-hour oral glucose tolerance test compares the baseline plasma glucose concentration with a plasma glucose concentration obtained 4 hours after the oral administration of a 10% glucose solution at a dose of 10 mL/kg. Certain strains of rodents, such as *ob/ob* obese mice, Zucker fatty rat (*fa/fa*), and the LA/N corpulent rat, are used as animal models for noninsulin-dependent diabetes mellitus. The Chinese hamster and Wistar BB rat are animal models for insulin-dependent diabetes mellitus. Insulin-dependent diabetes may result in guinea pigs from an infectious agent that causes fatty degeneration of the pancreas and affects both exocrine and endocrine pancreatic functions; affected guinea pigs have hyperglycemia, glucosuria, ketonuria, and beta-cell hypoplasia. Immunoassays for the determination of insulin in rats can be calibrated to measure plasma insulin in mice, but guinea pig insulin is immunologically different and cannot be determined using rat antibodies. Rat glucagon is measured using human immunoassay techniques; however, guinea pig glucagon, like insulin, is immunologically different and cannot be determined with human antibodies.

Laboratory Detection of Muscle Injury

Creatine kinase is a dimeric cytosolic enzyme that is composed of M and B subunits. Skeletal muscle contains MM subunits, and cardiac muscle contains MM, MB, and BB subunits. Brain contains BB subunits. As in domestic mammals, plasma CK activity is a useful marker for muscle injury in rodents. Nutritional myopathies, such as those resulting from hypovitaminosis E and selenium deficiency, cause increased plasma CK activity in rats and mice.

Laboratory Evaluation of Endocrine Disorders

The major hormones of rodents are secreted into the peripheral blood in a circadian rhythm that may vary among species. Hormonal secretion also is influenced by environmental factors, such as light-dark cycle. An ultradian rhythm, in which hormones are secreted in an episodic or pulsatile manner with a periodicity of less than 24 hours, can be superimposed on the normal circadian secretion of a hormone. Suggested ranges for the major plasma hormones in rodents are provided in Table 31.2.

Normal male rats have higher plasma thyroid-stimulating hormone (TSH) concentrations with use of reference preparation-1 standard from the National Hormone and Pituitary Program compared with normal female rats. Plasma TSH concentrations of normal female rats peak at the onset of the light cycle. Mice and hamsters have lower normal plasma TSH concentrations compared with rats (according to the same assay method used for rats). A bioassay method using radiolabeled iodine also can be used to obtain plasma TSH concentrations in rodents.

Plasma or serum thyroxine (T_4) and triiodothyronine (T_3) concentrations in rodents can be measured by radioimmunoassay. Transport proteins and binding affinity for T_4 and T_3 vary among species. In rats and mice, approximately 80% of the bound T_3 and T_4 are bound to albumin and 20% to T_4-binding prealbumin. Approximately 0.05% of plasma T_4 and 0.25% of T_3 in rats is the free, physiologically active form. Normal plasma total T_4 and T_3 concentrations in rats and mice vary between different strains but generally range between 3 to 7 μg/dL and 30 to 100 ng/dL, respectively. Plasma T_4 and T_3 concentrations exhibit a diurnal rhythm, in which peak concentrations occur during the light phase and minimum concentrations during the dark phase.

Normal plasma adrenocorticotropic hormone (ACTH) concentrations in rodents have been determined using either radioimmunoassay or bioassay techniques. The plasma ACTH concentration in normal mice exhibits a normal circadian rhythm, in which minimal concentrations occur during the morning and peak concentrations during the afternoon.

Corticosterone, which is the primary glucocorticoid in the plasma of mice and rats, exhibits a marked diurnal variation that is affected by the light cycle. In mice, maximum plasma corticosterone concentrations occur at the start of the dark period and minimum concentrations at the end of the dark period. Male mice have lower plasma corticosterone concentrations compared with female mice. Maximum plasma corticosterone concentrations occur late during the light period in rats, and minimum concentrations occur during the end of the dark period. In rats, approximately 80% of plasma corticosterone is bound to transcortin and 10% to albumin, thereby leaving 10% or less in the free, unbound state. Both corticosterone and cortisol are found in the plasma of normal hamsters. The total plasma glucocorticoid concentration 5.5 hours after onset of the light period in hamsters averages 1.8 μg/dL, with an average corticosterone : cortisol ratio of 3.5. The plasma corticosterone concentration is greater in male hamsters than in female hamsters. Cortisol is the primary glucocorticoid in the plasma of normal guinea pigs. Guinea pigs demonstrate maximum plasma cortisol concentrations late in the light period and, again, late in the dark period. Minimum concentrations occur early during the light period and, again, during the middle of the dark period. The stress of restraint or removal of a cagemate significantly increases plasma glucocorticoid concentrations. A twofold increase in plasma corticosterone concentration occurs in rats with 2 minutes of restraint, and a 12-fold increase results after 20 minutes of restraint.

In rodents, plasma concentrations of the calcium-regulating hormones parathormone, calcitonin, and 1,25-dihydroxyvitamin D_3 are influenced by dietary calcium, age, gender, photoperiod, and strain. Using radioimmunoassay techniques, the normal plasma parathormone concentration in male rats tends to be greater than that in female rats.

Normal plasma calcitonin concentrations of rats are extremely variable because of age, stage of light cycle, strain, and gender. Plasma calcitonin concentrations also are influenced by the stage of estrus in females, in which maximum concentrations occur during proestrus. Six- to eight-month-old male Wistar rats have lower plasma calcitonin concentrations compared with 12- to 14-month-old Wistar rats. Male Wistar rats also have lower plasma calcitonin concentrations than female rats. Plasma concentrations of 1,25-dihydroxyvitamin D vary in rats with strain, gender, and dietary calcium intake. Normal male Wistar rats have lower plasma 1,25-dihydroxyvitamin D concentrations than females.

RABBITS (ORYCTOLAGUS CUNICULUS)

Laboratory Evaluation of the Kidneys

Laboratory evaluation of the kidneys in rabbits is the same as that for rodents and domestic mammals. Plasma urea nitrogen and creatinine commonly are used as markers for renal function in rabbits. The normal plasma urea nitrogen of rabbits is influenced by breed, strain, and gender. Protein catabolism associated with high dietary protein intake, vigorous exercise, or disease increases plasma urea nitrogen concentration. The time of day when the blood sample is taken also influences the plasma urea nitrogen concentration in rabbits, in which peak concentrations occur between 4:00 and 8:00 PM. Plasma urea nitrogen and creatinine are insensitive tests for renal disease in rabbits, however, requiring a 50% to 75% loss of function before plasma concentrations increase.

Electrolytes and Acid-Base

The normal plasma calcium concentration of 13 to 15 mg/dL of rabbits is higher than that of most other mammals. The mean urinary fractional calcium excretion of rabbits is approximately 45%, compared with less than 2% in other mammals. Normal plasma electrolyte concentrations of rabbits vary with the breed and strain. Normal plasma magnesium concentrations of most rabbits are between 2.0 and 4.5 mg/dL. The serum iron- and total iron-binding capacity of normal rabbits vary with the time of day when the blood was collected, with the lowest concentrations occurring at 8:00 AM and the highest at 8:00 PM. Serum iron concentrations of normal rabbits range between 165 and 250 mg/dL.

Laboratory Evaluation of the Liver

Plasma enzymes used to detect liver disease in rabbits include ALT, AST, LD, glutamate dehydrogenase, AP, and GGT. In rabbits, ALT activity is equal in the liver and cardiac muscle; however, increased plasma ALT activity is considered to be a specific indicator of liver disease in rabbits. The degree of hepatic necrosis correlates positively with the increase in plasma ALT activity. Interestingly, the rabbit liver ALT activity is less than half that of the dog. Significant AST activity occurs in the liver, heart, skeletal muscle, kidney, and pancreas of rabbits. Therefore, increases in plasma AST activity are suggestive of injury to one or more of these tissues. Increases in plasma AST activity may be associated with cardiac or skeletal muscle injury during blood collection by cardiocentesis or use of restraint methods that cause exertion. Lactate dehydrogenase activity is present in a wide variety of tissues, with each demonstrating a different isoenzyme composition that corresponds with isoenzymes 1 through 5 in humans. Isoenzyme LD-1 and LD-2 predominate in the liver and skeletal muscle. Because erythrocytes have high LD activity, hemolysis may result in high plasma LD activity. The plasma LD activity can be used to detect liver disease in rabbits, but because of its wide tissue distribution and the effect of handling and hemolysis on plasma activity, it is not commonly used. Plasma glutamate dehydrogenase activity (range, 5.5–7.0 IU/L), although not commonly measured in veterinary laboratories, may be useful in the evaluation of hepatocellular injury in rabbits. Normal plasma AP activity of rabbits varies with age, breed, and strain.

Rabbits are unique in having three AP isoenzymes. Rabbits have an intestinal and two liver/kidney forms, compared with the intestinal and liver/kidney/bone forms found in mammals other than primates. The predominant liver/kidney isoenzyme of rabbits is similar to the intestinal form and the minor liver/kidney isoenzyme to the liver/kidney/bone isoenzyme of other mammals. The predominant liver AP isoenzyme is not inhibited by levamisole or heating to 56°F, as the hepatic AP isoenzyme of other mammals is. The plasma GGT activity of normal rabbits is less than 8 IU/L, is derived primarily from bile duct epithelial cells, and increases significantly in rabbits with hepatobiliary obstruction.

Rabbit bile contains approximately 70% biliverdin and 30% bilirubin, of which 90% is conjugated as a monoconjugate. Normal rabbit plasma lacks biliverdin, however, and the normal bilirubin concentration is low. A marked increase in plasma bilirubin concentration is expected in rabbits with biliary obstruction.

The normal plasma cholesterol concentration of rabbits varies with age, breed, strain, and gender. At birth, the plasma cholesterol concentration is approximately that of adults, increases by 25 days of age, and then returns to the adult concentrations by 60 to 80 days of age. Normal adult male rabbits have twice the plasma cholesterol concentration of adult female rabbits. A diurnal variation in plasma cholesterol occurs as well, with peak concentrations being seen between 4:00 and 8:00 PM. The plasma cholesterol concentration may increase in rabbits with extrahepatic biliary obstruction. Rabbits are used extensively as animal models for cholesterol metabolism studies because of their ability to rapidly develop cholesterolemia with high-cholesterol diets. Daily feeding of 1 g of cholesterol increases the serum cholesterol concentration to greater than 1000 mg/dL. The Watanabe heritable hyperlipemic rabbit, which primarily exhibits low-density lipoprotein (LDL) cholesterol, is an animal model for familial hypercholesterolemia in humans. The normal serum lipoprotein distributions of adult female rabbits are 46% to 58% high-density lipoprotein, which transports approximately two-thirds of the total cholesterol; 9% to 15 % pre- or intermediate-density lipoprotein or very LDL (VLDL); and 30% to 42 % LDL. High-cholesterol diets fed to rabbits lead to a 20- to 40-fold increase in VLDL and a four-to five-fold increase in LDL.

Liver function tests that evaluate plasma disappearance and biliary excretion of dyes, such as sulfobromophthalein (BSP) and indocyanine green (ICG), have been characterized for rabbits. The overall rate of BSP clearance for rabbits has been reported as 1.8 mg/min per kg, in which 75 % of the BSP is excreted in the conjugated form. Intravenous BSP dosages of 30, 60, and 120 mg/kg result in 32-minute plasma concentrations of 1, 2, and 20 mg/dL, respectively. Indocyanine green is excreted in the bile in the unconjugated form. Rabbits have a curvilinear plasma ICG clearance curve, with a greater capacity to remove ICG from the circulation than either dogs or rats. Rabbits that are given intravenous ICG dosages of 8, 16, and 32 mg/kg demonstrate disappearance rates of 46%, 20%, and 10% per minute, respectively.

Laboratory Evaluation of Proteins

The normal plasma total protein concentration in rabbits varies slightly with breed, strain, and gender. Approximately 40% to 60 % of the total plasma protein is albumin. The normal protein electrophoretic components of rabbit serum also include 5% to 10% α_1-globulin, 5% to 10% α_2-globulin, 5% to 15% β-globulin, and 5% to 15% γ-globulin. The normal albumin to globulin ratio ranges between 0.5 and 1.2. Female rabbits tend to have higher plasma albumin concentrations than male rabbits. Severe renal and hepatic diseases are responsible for most disorders that result in hypoproteinemia and hypoalbuminemia in rabbits. Hyperproteinemia commonly occurs with dehydration, shock, and hyperthermia.

Laboratory Evaluation of Glucose Metabolism

The normal plasma glucose concentration of rabbits is influenced by genetics, age, and diet. Pre- and postprandial plasma glucose variation occurs, in which the lowest plasma glucose concentrations are found 1 hour before feeding and the highest 3 hours after a meal. Healthy rabbits can maintain normal plasma glucose concentrations during short periods of fasting (e.g., <16 hours). Extreme hyperglycemia occurs with diabetes mellitus. Hyperglycemia and increased plasma urea nitrogen concentration occur with the increased protein catabolism associated with hyperthermia. Hyperglycemia resulting from glycogenolysis because of stress occurs early in the course of mucoid enteropathy. This common digestive tract dis-

order of rabbits causes anorexia, and when glycogen stores become depleted, the rabbit develops hypoglycemia.

Laboratory Detection of Muscle Injury

Laboratory detection of muscle injury in rabbits follows the same methods as that in rodents and domestic mammals, in which plasma CK, AST, and LD activities are sensitive to muscle injury. Blood collected by cardiocentesis contains CK-MB isoenzyme activity that is not found in serum collected from the ear vein. Blood collected by jugular venipuncture also contains CK-MB activity. Plasma CK activity, primarily the CK-MM isoenzyme, is a rapid, sensitive, and specific indicator of muscle disease in rabbits, and it increases more rapidly than AST and LD activities after muscle injury. Nutritional-related myopathies, such as those caused by hypovitaminosis E and selenium deficiency, result in increased plasma CK activity.

Laboratory Evaluation of Endocrine Disorders

Laboratory evaluation of endocrine disorders in rabbits follows the same methods as that in rodents and domestic mammals. The TSH concentration in rabbit serum can be obtained using a bioassay method that measures the percentage increase in blood levels of radiolabeled iodine. Serum T_4 and T_3 concentrations from normal rabbits are listed in *Table 31.3*. The serum protein-bound iodine concentration, as an indicator of thyroid function in rabbits, increases by 20 days of age before decreasing to adult concentrations by 60 days of age. The serum protein-bound iodine concentration varies with strain, gender, and time of day. The plasma ACTH concentration of rabbits as determined by bioassay is subject to circadian variation.

TABLE 31.3 PLASMA CONCENTRATIONS OF THE MAJOR HORMONES IN RABBITS

Triiodothyronine (ng/dL)	130–143
Thyroxine (µg/dL)	1.7–2.4
Thyroid-stimulating hormone (µU/mL)	40–100
Protein-bound iodine (nmol/L)	400 (adults)
Adrenocorticotropic hormone (pg/dL)	25[a]
Cortisol (µg/dL)	2.6–3.8 (early morning)
Aldosterone (ng/dL)	20[a] (early morning) 50[a] (late afternoon)
Calcitonin (pg/mL)	1125–1200
1,25-dihydroxy-vitamin D (pg/mL)	27–47

[a] Average concentration.

The major plasma glucocorticoid of rabbits is cortisol. Evidence is suggestive that genetics and circadian rhythms influence the plasma aldosterone concentration of rabbits, but little information is available regarding the plasma concentration of parathyroid hormone in rabbits.

FERRETS (MUSTELA PUTORIUS FURO)

Laboratory Evaluation of the Kidneys

Laboratory evaluation of renal function in ferrets involves blood biochemical tests, such as plasma urea nitrogen, creatinine, protein, bicarbonate, and electrolyte concentrations, and urinalysis. Interpretive considerations for the biochemical tests used to evaluate the kidneys are the same as those in domestic carnivorous mammals such as cats and dogs. In normal and azotemic ferrets, the plasma creatinine concentration is lower than that in dogs and cats. Insulin and exogenous creatinine clearance are sensitive tests for measuring glomerular filtration in ferrets; however, delayed clearance may occur before significant increases in plasma urea nitrogen or creatinine concentrations. *Table 31.4* lists reference ranges for various serum biochemical values in ferrets.

Electrolytes and Acid-Base

Interpretations of plasma electrolyte and acid-base disturbances in ferrets are the same as those in dogs and cats. Disorders that commonly result in electrolyte disturbances in dogs and cats, such as hypoadrenocorticism, hyper-

TABLE 31.4 REFERENCE RANGES FOR SERUM BIOCHEMICAL VALUES IN FERRETS

Glucose (mg/dL)	67–124
Urea nitrogen (mg/dL)	17–32
Creatinine (mg/dL)	0.2–0.6
Total protein (g/dL)	5.3–7.2
Albumin (g/dL)	3.3–4.1
Calcium (mg/dL)	8.5–11.0
Phosphorus (mg/dL)	3.3–7.8
Sodium (mEq/L)	146–160
Potassium (mEq/L)	3.7–5.4
Chloride (mEq/L)	112–129
Cholesterol (mg/dL)	60–220
Total bilirubin (mg/dL)	0.0–0.3
Total CO$_2$ (mmol/L)	17–23
Alkaline phosphatase (IU/L)	30–120
Alanine aminotransferase (IU/L)	30–100
Aspartate aminotransferase (IU/L)	15–40
Creatine kinase (IU/L)	60–300

aldosteronism, primary hyperparathyroidism, pseudo-hyperparathyroidism, hypoparathyroidism, and hypercalcitonism, have been poorly documented in ferrets.

Laboratory Evaluation of the Liver

Evaluation of the livers in ferrets by laboratory testing is the same as that for those in dogs and cats. The ferret liver has three- to 10-fold more ALT activity than any other tissue, and the plasma ALT activity is a sensitive and specific test for hepatocellular disease in ferrets. Ferrets with hepatocellular disease commonly have increased AST and LD activities as well. Those with cholestasis likely have increased plasma AP and GGT activities. Ferrets rarely become icteric or have plasma bilirubin concentrations greater than 2.0 mg/dL, even when hepatobiliary disease is severe.

Laboratory Evaluation of Proteins

The causes of hypoproteinemia and hyperproteinemia in ferrets are the same as those in dogs and cats. Ferrets with Aleutian disease typically demonstrate hypoalbuminemia and hyperglobulinemia, in which more than 20% of the total protein is γ-globulins.

Laboratory Evaluation of Glucose Metabolism

A high incidence of insulin-secreting pancreatic neoplasms (i.e., insulinomas) resulting in hypoglycemia occurs among domestic ferrets in North America. The normal plasma glucose concentration of ferrets varies with the genetic type. A 4- to 5-hour fasting plasma glucose level often is used to screen ferrets for insulinomas. Fasting plasma glucose concentrations less than 60 mg/dL are supportive of a presumptive diagnosis of insulinoma, whereas concentrations between 60 and 90 mg/dL merely are suggestive of an insulinoma. Concentrations greater than 90 mg/dL usually are considered to be normal. Normal serum reference ranges for serum immunoreactive insulin and the insulin:glucose ratio have been reported as being 4.6 to 43.3 μU/mL (SI units, 33–311 pmol/L) and 3.6 to 34.1 μUmg (SI units, 4.6–44.2 pmol/mmol), respectively. To compare immunoreactive insulin and the insulin:glucose ratio results from other laboratories using different radioimmunoassay kits to these reference intervals, however, one must validate the results by demonstrating a high correlation between the two assay methods. Calculation of an amended insulin:glucose ratio (AIGR) using the following formula may aid in establishing the diagnosis of hyperinsulinism:

$$\text{AIGR} = \text{insulin (μU/mL)} \times 100/\text{fasting glucose (mg/dL)} - 30$$

in which AIGR values greater than 30 are suggestive of hyperinsulinism. Other occasional causes for hypoglycemia in ferrets include delayed separation of plasma from erythrocytes, starvation, chronic hepatic disease, septicemia, and endotoxemia.

Other than a postprandial increase in plasma glucose concentration, hyperglycemia in ferrets may result from glucocorticoid excess (e.g., stress induced, exogenous corticoids, and hyperadrenocorticism), epinephrine release related to exertion, and diabetes mellitus. Diabetes mellitus in ferrets usually is iatrogenic and associated with surgical removal of pancreatic insulin-secreting neoplasms or with drugs, such as megestrol acetate, that affect insulin production and secretion.

Laboratory Detection of Muscle Injury

Detection of muscle injury in ferrets follows the same methods as those described in dogs and cats. Increases in the nonspecific plasma enzymes AST and LD and in the specific muscle enzyme CK are to be expected with muscle injury.

Laboratory Evaluation of Endocrine Disorders

The mean basal plasma T_4 concentration as reported for ferrets ranges between 0.99 and 2.63 µg/dL. A thyroid function test using 1 IU of TSH given intravenously to a ferret and measuring changes in the plasma T_4 concentration is preferable to use of thyrotropin-releasing hormone and measuring changes in the plasma T_3 concentration. The plasma T_4 concentration increases significantly as early as 2 hours after TSH stimulation in normal ferrets, whereas no increase in the plasma T_3 concentration is observed. Plasma T_4 concentration should at least double after TSH stimulation; failure to do so is suggestive of hypothyroidism.

Cortisol is the predominant circulating glucocorticoid in ferrets. The mean basal plasma cortisol concentration as reported for ferrets ranges between 0.45 and 2.13 µg/dL. Intravenous or intramuscular injection of ACTH at a dose of 0.5 to 1.0 µg/kg to a normal ferret results in a three- to fourfold increase in plasma cortisol by 30 minutes that persists for as long as 1 hour. A threefold decrease in plasma cortisol concentration occurs in normal ferrets after intravenous injection of 0.2 mg of dexamethasone. This dexamethasone suppression continues even after 5 hours, when plasma cortisol concentrations demonstrate a four- to fivefold decrease.

Domestic ferrets in North America experience a high incidence of adrenal gland neoplasms that produce a number of hormones. Excessive production of estradiol is a common occurrence with adrenal gland neoplasms of ferrets, but excessive cortisol production also can occur.

The ACTH stimulation and dexamethasone suppression tests have not been useful in establishing the diagnosis of hyperadrenocorticism associated with adrenal neoplasia in domestic ferrets.

PRIMATES

Laboratory Evaluation of the Kidneys

Serum and plasma urea nitrogen and creatinine concentrations are widely used to assess renal function in primates; *Table 31.5* compares such common serum biochemical values in nonhuman primates. Assessment of the kidneys in primates using serum or plasma biochemical testing and urinalysis follows the same methods as those described in domestic mammals. Uric acid is the end product of purine metabolism in primates, and plasma uric acid concentration can be an insensitive indicator of renal disease. Uricase in the hepatocytes of most mammals and prosimians (e.g., *Tupaia* sp., *Galago* sp., and *Nycticebus* sp.) converts uric acid to allantoin; therefore, the plasma uric acid concentration is increased in primates with hepatocellular disease and can be considered to be an insensitive hepatic function test. New World monkeys (e.g. *Cebus* sp., *Lagothrix* sp., and *Saguinus* sp.), great apes, and humans have little hepatic uricase and relatively high serum uric acid concentrations. Old World species, such as *Papio* and *Macaca* monkeys, have a distinct uricase that differs from those of nonprimate mammals and low serum uric acid concentrations.

Electrolytes and Acid-Base

Laboratory evaluation of electrolyte and acid-base disturbances in primates follows the same methods as those in domestic mammals. Diarrhea is a common disorder of primates and often leads to hyponatremia, hypochloremia, and metabolic acidosis. The metabolic acidosis often is associated with high anion gap values because of the presence of unmeasured ions such as lactate and phosphates that result from hypovolemic shock and renal retention, respectively.

Laboratory Evaluation of the Liver

Serum or plasma hepatic injury enzymes, such as ALT, AST, and LD, and enzymes that increase with cholestasis or drug induction, such as AP and GGT, commonly are used to detect hepatic abnormalities in primates. Other analytes, such as serum bilirubin, fasting bile acid, and cholesterol concentrations, along with serum concentrations of hepatic products, such as albumin, urea, glucose, and coagulation factors, also are used to evaluate the liver

TABLE 31.5 COMPARISON OF SERUM BIOCHEMICAL VALUES IN COMMON NONHUMAN PRIMATES

	Rhesus monkey (*Macaca mulatta*)	African Green Monkey (*Cercopithicus aethiops*)	Squirrel Monkey (*Saimiri sciureus*)	Chimpanzee (*Pan troglodytes*)
Glucose (mg/dL)	70 ± 17[a]	104 ± 23.6	80 ± 28	78 ± 16.3
Urea nitrogen (mg/dL)	16.9 ± 2.7	21 ± 5.6	31 ± 8	14.2 ± 4.8
Creatinine (mg/dL)	1.5 ± 0.9	—	—	—
Uric acid (mg/dL)	0.66 ± 0.11	—	—	—
Total protein (g/dL)	6.6 ± 0.5	7.6 ± 0.8	7.5 ± 0.6	7.4 ± 0.7
Albumin (g/dL)	4.4 ± 0.9	3.7 ± 1.0	4.1 ± 0.6	3.7 ± 0.4
Calcium (mg/dL)	9.7 ± 1.6	10.1 ± 0.8	9.0 ± 0.7	9.3 ± 0.9
Phosphorus (mg/dL)	5.0 ± 0.9	5.1 ± 1.4	4.5 ± 2.2	4.8 ± 1.2
Sodium (mEq/L)	158 ± 13	154 ± 4.6	149 ± 6.0	139 ± 3.6
Potassium (mEq/L)	4.7 ± 0.8	4.8 ± 0.7	4.4 ± 0.9	3.7 ± 0.5
Chloride (mEq/L)	114 ± 9	107.5 ± 4.0	114 ± 6.0	100 ± 4.1
Cholesterol (mg/dL)	128 ± 34	141 ± 28.2	167 ± 40.0	209 ± 48
Total bilirubin (mg/dL)	0.4 ± 0.3	0.3 ± 0.1	0.3 ± 0.2	0.2 ± 0.1
Alanine aminotransferase (IU/L)	42.1 ± 21.2	14.5 ± 8.3	83.5 ± 25.4	5.7 ± 4.3
Aspartate aminotransferase (IU/L)	27.0 ± 6.5	26.1 ± 9.4	87.0 ± 31.0	8.7 ± 4.7
Lactate dehydrogenase (IU/L)	186.9 ± 68.4	—	—	—

Data compiled from Loeb WF, Quimby FW, eds. The clinical chemistry of laboratory animals. New York: Pergamon Press, 1989:417–509.
[a] All values are mean ± standard deviation.

of primates. Increased serum ALT activity is a nonspecific, but sensitive, indicator of hepatic disease in primates. The ALT activity is high in the liver tissue of primates, but such activity also is found in the heart muscle and kidneys. Serum ALT activity is thought to increase with cell injury alone, whereas serum AST activity is thought to increase only when cell death occurs. The highest AST activity occurs in heart muscle; however, AST activity also occurs in the liver, skeletal muscle, kidney, and brain. Brain injury is an unlikely cause of increased serum AST activity, because AST does not cross the blood-brain barrier. Serum LD activity is a nonspecific test for hepatic disease in primates; an LD isoenzyme profile is needed to evaluate the cause of increased serum activity. Spontaneous cardiac infarcts occur in primates and should be considered when the serum LD activity is increased. Biliary and osteoblastic AP are the primary sources of serum AST activity. Male rhesus monkeys have 33 % greater serum AP activity than female rhesus monkeys; however, in other species, such as squirrel monkeys, female monkeys have greater serum AP activity. Young, growing primates have greater serum AP activities compared with adults because of the increased osteoblastic activity associated with growth. Increases in the serum AP activity of adult primates most often results from cholestasis. Disorders that affect the serum bilirubin concentration in nonhuman pri-

mates, such as hemolytic, hepatic, and obstructive jaundice, resemble those in humans. The serum bilirubin concentration in nonhuman primates is approximately 25% less than that in humans; therefore, significant serum bilirubin increases in these animals may be within the reference range for humans. Extensive lipid and lipoprotein studies have been performed using nonhuman primates as an animal model for human atherosclerosis. As in both humans and rats, serum cholesterol and triglyceride concentrations tend to increase with age in primates.

Laboratory Evaluation of Proteins

Laboratory evaluation of serum proteins of primates follows the same methods as those described in domestic mammals and humans. A significant decrease in serum total protein and albumin concentrations occurs when ketamine hydrochloride anesthesia is used for restraint during blood collection, and this decrease results either from an increase in plasma volume or from a loss of protein in the vascular compartment.

Laboratory Evaluation of Glucose Metabolism

A fasting plasma glucose concentration greater than 115 mg/dL is suggestive of impaired glucose metabolism, and concentrations greater than 140 mg/dL are suggestive of diabetes mellitus. Hypoglycemia in nonhuman primates is indicated by serum glucose concentrations less than 50 mg/dL.

The intravenous glucose tolerance test (IVGTT) is used more frequently than the oral glucose tolerance test, and it is indicated for use in primates that are mildly hyperglycemic. A diet that includes 2 to 4 g of carbohydrate per kilogram of body weight should be fed daily for at least 3 days and then followed by 16- to 18-hour food deprivation before IVGTT. The IVGTT can be performed on awake monkeys; however, the stress of handling and restraint can affect the clearance of glucose. Ketamine hydrochloride is the anesthetic agent of choice, because it has the least impact on glucose clearance. Barbiturates and atropine impair insulin secretion and, therefore, create a false glucose intolerance. To perform the IVGTT, a glucose load of 0.5 g/kg is given intravenously during a 30-minute period. Blood samples are taken immediately after infusion and at 5- to 15-minute intervals for 1 hour. The rapidity of glucose clearance is computed as

$$K \, (\%/\text{min}) = 0.693/T_{1/2} \times 100$$

in which $T_{1/2}$ is the time interval during which the serum glucose falls to half the initial glucose concentration (i.e., the half-life). Most K values for nondiabetic primates range between 2% and 3% per minute. Typical results for rhesus (*Macaca mulatta*) and squirrel monkeys (*Saimiri sciureus*) demonstrate serum glucose concentrations of 150 to 250 mg/dL at 5 to 10 minutes, less than 100 mg/dL within 20 minutes, and a return to fasting levels by 60 minutes. Prediabetic primates have prolonged hyperglycemia after administration of glucose. In humans, K values of less than 1 are diagnostic for diabetes mellitus. Decreased insulin response and glucose intolerance can occur with hemorrhage, stress, pregnancy, and use of certain pharmacological agents, such as atropine and barbiturates.

Laboratory Detection of Muscle Injury

As in domestic mammals, increased serum or plasma AST, LD, and CK activities occur with muscle injury in primates. The serum CK activity increases because of muscle exertion during capture and restraint. Because an increased serum CK activity precedes those of AST and LD after acute muscle injury, use of a muscle irritant, such as ketamine hydrochloride anesthesia, typically results in increased serum CK but not AST or LD activity. In primates, increased serum LD activity should be evaluated using an LD isoenzyme profile to rule out myocardial injury.

Laboratory Evaluation of Endocrine Disorders

The circulating TSH concentration of male rhesus monkeys lacks the circadian rhythm as found in other mammals. Serum T_4 and T_3 concentrations of primates are assayed using the standard radioimmunoassay methods for humans. Serum or plasma T_4 and T_3 concentrations for a few primate species are provided in *Table 31.6*.

Cortisol is the major glucocorticosteroid of primates and is influenced by diurnal variation. The diurnal secretion of cortisol in male rhesus monkeys results in the highest concentrations (15–35 µg/dL) occurring at the beginning of the light period and the lowest (6–20 µg/dL) at the start of the dark period. The lowest serum cortisol concentration of squirrel monkeys occurs 4 hours after onset of the dark period. The normal plasma cortisol concentration of male cynomolgus monkeys (*M. mulatta*) ranges between 10 and 40 µg/dL. Morning plasma cortisol concentrations of healthy squirrel monkeys range between 100 and 200 µg/dL in male monkeys and 25 to 125 µg/dL in female monkeys. Early morning serum cortisol concentrations of female chimpanzees during the early follicular phase of the menstrual cycle range between 25 and 35 µg/dL. Serum cortisol concentration in primates increases with stress, such as occurs with capture and restraint.

TABLE 31.6   SERUM OR PLASMA THYROXINE AND TRIIODOTHYRONINE CONCENTRATIONS IN SELECTED NONHUMAN PRIMATES

	Thyroxine (µg/dL)		Triiodothyronine (ng/dL)	
	Male	**Female**	**Male**	**Female**
Rhesus monkey (*Macaca mulatta*)	0.8–6.6	1.3–7.6	54–115	65–295
African Green monkey (*Cercopithicus aethiops*)	3.9–5.7	3.0–8.4	91–178	94–350
Squirrel monkey (*Saimiri sciureus*)	1.7–5.1	1.0–7.3	21–92	20–168
Chimpanzee (*Pan troglodytes*)	3.7–5.9	—	87–135	—

Data compiled from Depaolo LV, Masoro EJ. Endocrine hormones in laboratory animals. In: Loeb WF, Quimby FW, eds. The clinical chemistry of laboratory animals. New York; Pergamon Press, 1989;289.

Plasma aldosterone concentrations of normal male rhesus monkeys range between 2 and 30 ng/dL. A diurnal pattern of plasma aldosterone concentration occurs in rhesus monkeys, with the lowest concentrations occurring at the beginning of the light cycle.

MINIPIGS

The clinical chemistry interpretation of minipigs does not appear to be different from that in other breeds of swine *(Table 31.7)*. Minipigs have been used as animal models for human atherosclerosis. Their normal serum cholesterol and triglyceride concentrations typically range from 89 to 133 mg/dL and 20 to 154 mg/dL, respectively. The serum lipoproteins of minipigs contain high amounts of cholesterol compared with humans, and the composition of their β-VLDL resembles that of the dog.

LLAMAS (LAMA GLAMA)

The serum clinical chemistries of llamas are similar to those of cattle and horses *(Table 31.8)*. Normal serum glucose concentrations tend to be higher than those of cattle, however, and range between 82 and 160 mg/dL.

Compared with domestic mammals, llamas have higher serum T_4 and T_3 concentrations, ranging from 9.8 to 30 μg/dL and 48 to 468 ng/dL, respectively. Whether llamas have carrier proteins for thyroid hormones is not known. Normal llamas respond to TSH stimulation (3 IU per 44 kg) with a 2.5- and 2.0-fold increase in serum T_3 and T_4 concentrations, respectively. A diagnosis of hypothyroidism is established based on low basal serum T_3 and T_4 concentrations and inadequate response to TSH stimulation.

DEER

Most serum and plasma biochemical values of deer are similar to those of other ruminants, such as cattle and llamas (Table 31.8). Some of the serum biochemical profile analytes vary with age, gender, and handling. Serum activities of enzymes such as CK and AST, which increase with increased muscle exertion, usually are greater in deer than in domestic ruminants because of the fear and excitement of handling. Deer adapted to regular handling exhibit less increase in serum CK and AST activities. Greater increases in the serum concentrations of CK and AST occur in stags than in hinds, because of their greater muscle mass. Although serum LD and ALT activities also

TABLE 31.7 SERUM BIOCHEMICAL VALUES IN YUCATAN MINIATURE SWINE (*SUS SCROFA*)

	Mean	Reference Range[a]	Observed Range
Glucose (mg/dL)	79.8	36.4–123.2	56.0–153.0
Urea nitrogen (mg/dL)	19.2	9.2–29.2	10.0–29.0
Creatinine (mg/dL)	1.6	1.2–2.0	1.2–2.0
Total protein (g/dL)	7.5	6.1–8.9	6.3–9.4
Albumin (g/dL)	4.7	3.9–5.5	4.1–5.6
Globulin (g/dL)	2.8	1.6–4.0	1.4–3.6
Albumin : globulin ratio	1.8	0.8–2.8	1.11–3.49
Calcium (mg/dL)	10.6	9.6–11.6	9.3–11.6
Phosphorus (mg/dL)	6.9	5.1–8.1	5.0–8.3
Sodium (mEq/L)	147.0	144–152.6	142.0–153.0
Potassium (mEq/L)	4.6	4.0–5.2	3.9–5.2
Chloride (mEq/L)	104.2	94.4–114.0	95.0–114.0
Cholesterol (mg/dL)	101.8	38.4–165.2	47.3–173.0
Total bilirubin (mg/dL)	0.1	0.0–0.3	0.0–0.3
Alanine aminotransferase (IU/L)	33.6	20.4–46.8	20.0–48.0
Aspartate aminotransferase (IU/L)	28.2	10.4–56.0	15.0–53.0
Creatine kinase (IU/L)	168.0	48.0–288.0	37.0–270.0

[a] Adapted from Radin MJ, Weiser MG, Fettman MJ. Hematologic and serum biochemical values for Yucatan miniature swine. Lab Anim Sci 1986;36:425–427.

TABLE 31.8   COMPARISON OF SELECTED SERUM BIOCHEMICAL VALUES FOR LLAMAS AND DEER

	Llamas (*Lama glama*)	White-tailed deer (*Odocoileus virginianus*)	Mule deer (*Odocoileus hemionus*)
Glucose (mg/dL)	82–160	73–103	124–236
Urea nitrogen (mg/dL)	9–33	20–40	21–41
Creatinine (mg/dL)	1.1–3.2	1.9–3.1	1.0–1.8
Total protein (g/dL)	4.7–7.3	7.4–8.6	4.1–6.5
Albumin (g/dL)	3.1–5.2	2.1–3.3	2.3–3.5
Calcium (mg/dL)	7.9–10.9	10.5–12.5	—
Phosphorus (mg/dL)	2.8–10.0	10.0–13.6	—
Sodium (mEq/L)	148–158	151–167	—
Potassium (mEq/L)	3.7–6.2	5.0–7.8	—
Chloride (mEq/L)	100–120	105–117	—
Total CO_2 (mm/L)	13–31	—	—
Cholesterol (mg/dL)	22–176	60–176	20–92
Total bilirubin (mg/dL)	0.0–0.2	0.2–0.6	0.2–0.3
Alkaline phosphatase (IU/L)	31–779	—	—
Alanine aminotransferase (IU/L)	1–15	—	—
Aspartate aminotransferase (IU/L)	163–400	—	—
γ-Glutamyltransferase (IU/L)	6–29	—	—
Sorbitol dehydrogenase (IU/L)	1–15	—	—
Lactate dehydrogenase (IU/L)	87–741	—	—
Creatine kinase (IU/L)	8–89	—	—

Data compiled from Fowler ME, Zinkl JG. Reference ranges for hematologic and serum biochemical values in llamas (*Lama glama*). Am J Vet Res 1989;50:2049–2053; and Kitchen H. Hematological values and blood chemistries for a variety of artiodactylids. In: Fowler ME, ed. Zoo and wild animal medicine. Philadelphia: WB Saunders, 1986:1003–1017.

may increase with muscle exertion, serum CK and AST are more sensitive indicators of muscle injury.

Excitement of capture and restraint increases serum glucose concentrations. Deer that have adapted to handling and restraint demonstrate lower serum glucose concentrations than those not used to handling. The serum AP activity increases in stags during the annual active antler growth period and peaks before calcification of the antlers. The increased serum AP activity is derived from the proliferation of osteoblasts involved with antler growth. The serum total protein concentration of deer increases with age; adult concentrations are reached at approximately 10 months.

SUGGESTED READINGS

Rodents: Mice, Rats, Guinea Pigs, Hamsters, and Gerbils
Baker HJ, Lindsey JR, Weisbroth SH, eds. The laboratory rat. Vol 1: biology and diseases. New York: Academic Press, 1979.
Caisey JD, King DJ. Clinical chemical values for some common laboratory animals. Clin Chem 1980;26:1877–1879.
Camus M-C, Chapman MJ, Forgez P, et al. Distribution and characterization of the serum lipoproteins and apoproteins in the mouse, *Mus musculus*. J Lipid Res 1983;24:1210–1229.

Coleman D. Diabetes-obesity syndromes. In: Foster HL, Small JD, Fox JG, eds. The mouse in biomedical research. New York: Academic Press, 1982;4:126–132.
Dent NJ. The use of the Syrian hamster to establish its clinical chemistry and hematology profile. In: Duncan WA, Leonard BJ, eds. Clinical toxicology, XVIII. Amsterdam-Oxford: Excerpta Medica, 1977:321–323.
Falk HB, Schroer RA, Novak JJ, et al. The effect of freezing on various serum chemistry parameters from common lab animals. Clin Chem 1981;27:1039.
Foster HL, Small, JD, Fox JG, eds. The mouse in biomedical research. Vol 1. New York: Academic Press, 1981.
Loeb WF. Clinical chemistry of laboratory rodents and rabbits. In: Kaneko JJ, ed. Clinical chemistry of domestic animals. San Diego: Academic Press, 1989:869.
Maxwell KO, Wish C, Murphy JC, et al. Serum chemistry reference values in two strains of Syrian hamsters. Lab Anim Sci 1985;35:67–70.
Ottenweller JE, Tapp WN, Burke JM, et al. Plasma cortisol and corticosterone concentrations in the golden hamster (*Mesocritus auratus*). Life Sci 1985;37:1551–1558.
Rowlands I, Weir B, eds. The biology of hystricomorph rodents. London: Academic Press, 1974.
Seetharam S, Sussman NL, Komoda T, et al. The mechanism of elevated alkaline phosphatase activity after bile duct ligation in the rat. Hepatology 1986;6:374–380.
Suber RL, Kodell RL. The effect of three phlebotomy techniques on hematological and clinical chemical evaluation in Sprague-Dawley rats. Vet Clin Pathol 1985;14:23–30.
Van Hoosier GL, Ladiges WC. Biology and diseases of hamsters. In: Fox JG, Cohen BJ, Loew FM, eds. Laboratory animal medicine:

American College of Laboratory Animal Medicine series. New York: Academic Press, 1984:123–147.

Wagner J, Manning P, eds. The biology of the guinea pig. New York: Academic Press, 1976.

Waner T, Nyska A. The influence of fasting on blood glucose, triglycerides, cholesterol, and alkaline phosphatase in rats. Vet Clin Pathol 1994;23:78–81.

Wolford ST, Schroer RA, Gohs FX, et al. Reference range data base for serum chemistry and hematology values in laboratory animals. J Toxicol Environ Health 1986;18:161–188.

Wriston JC Jr. Comparative biochemistry of the guinea pig: a partial checklist. Comp Biochem Physiol B 1984;77:253–278.

Rabbits

Loeb WF. Clinical chemistry of laboratory rodents and rabbits. In: Kaneko JJ, ed. Clinical chemistry of domestic animals. San Diego: Academic Press, 1989:869.

Manning PJ, Ringer DH, Newcomer CE, eds. The biology of the laboratory rabbit. San Diego: Academic Press, 1994.

Ferrets

Esteves JI, Marini RP, Ryden EB, et al. Estimation of glomerular filtration rate and evaluation of renal function in ferrets (Mustela putorius furo). Am J Vet Res 1994;55:166–172.

Fox JG, ed. Biology and diseases of the ferret. Philadelphia: Lea & Febiger, 1988.

Fox JG, Hotaling L, Ackerman BP, et al. Serum chemistry and hematology reference values in the ferret (Mustela putorius furo). Lab Anim Sci 1986;36:583.

Gould WJ, Reimers TJ, Bell JA, et al. Evaluation of urinary cortisol:creatinine ratios for the diagnosis of hyperadrenocorticism associated with adrenal gland tumors in ferrets. J Am Vet Med Assoc 1995;206:42–46.

Heard DJ, Collins B, Chen DL, et al. Thyroid and adrenal function test in adult male ferrets. Am J Vet Res 1990;51:33–35.

Lee EJ, Moore WE, Fryer HC, et al. Haematological and serum chemistry profiles of ferrets (Mustela putorius furo). Lab Anim Sci 1982;16:133–137.

Mann FA, Stockham SL, Freeman MB, et al. Reference intervals for insulin concentrations and insulin:glucose ratios in the serum of ferrets. J Small Exotic Anim Med 1993;2:79–83.

Rosenthal KL, Peterson ME, Quesenberry KE. Evaluation of plasma cortisol and corticosterone responses to synthetic adrenocorticotropic hormone administration in ferrets. Am J Vet Res 1993;54:29–31.

Primates

Bennett JS, Gossett KA, McCarthy MP, et al. Effects of ketamine hydrochloride on serum biochemical and hematologic variables in rhesus monkeys (Macaca mulatta). Vet Clin Pathol 1992;21:15–18.

DiGiacomo RF, McDonash BF, Gibbs CJ Jr. The progression and evaluation of hematologic and serum biochemical values in the chimpanzee. J Med Primatol 1975;4:188–203.

Fulmer R, Loeb WF, Martin DP, et al. Effects of three methods of restraint on intravenous glucose tolerance testing in rhesus and African Green monkeys. Vet Clin Pathol 1984;13:19–25.

George JW, Lerche NW: Electrolyte abnormalities associated with diarrhea in rhesus monkeys: 100 cases (1986–1987). J Am Vet Med Assoc 1990;196:1654–1658.

Holmberg CA, Leininger R, Wheeldon E, et al. Clinicopathological studies of gastrointestinal disease in macaques. Vet Pathol 1982;19:163–170.

Howard CF. Nonhuman primates as models for the study of human diabetes mellitus. Diabetes 1982;31:37–42.

Kaack B, Walker L, Brizzee KR, et al. Comparative normal levels of serum triiodothyronine and thyroxine in non-human primates. Lab Anim Sci 1979;29:191–194.

Kessler MJ, Rawlins RG, London WT. The hemogram, serum biochemistry, and electrolyte profile of aged rhesus monkeys (Macaca mulatta). J Med Primatol 1983;12:184–191.

McClure HN, Keeling ME, Guilloud NB. Hematologic and blood chemistry data for the chimpanzee (Pan troglodytes). Folio Primatol 1972;18:444–462.

McClure HN, Keeling ME, Guilloud NB. Hematologic and blood chemistry data for the gorilla (Gorilla gorilla). Folio Primatol 1972;18:300–316.

McClure HN, Keeling ME, Guilloud NB. Hematologic and blood chemistry data for the orangutang (Pongo pygmaeus). Folio Primatol 1972;18:284–299.

Porter WP. Hematologic and other effects of ketamine and ketamine-acepromazine in rhesus monkeys (Macaca mulatta). Lab Anim Sci 1982;32:373–375.

Vondruska JF. Certain hematologic and blood chemical values in adult stump-tailed macaques (Macaca arctoides). Lab Anim Care 1970;20:97–200.

Minipigs

Parsons AH, Wells RE. Serum biochemistry of healthy Yucatan miniature pigs. Lab Anim Sci 1986;36:428–430.

Radin MJ, Weiser MG, Fettman MJ. Hematologic and serum biochemical values for Yucatan miniature swine. Lab Anim Sci 1986;36:425–427.

Llamas

Fowler ME, Zinkl JG. Reference ranges for hematologic and serum biochemical values in llamas (Lama glama). Am J Vet Res 1989;50:2049–2053.

Garry F. Clinical pathology of llamas. Vet Clin North Am Food Anim Pract 1989;5:55–70.

Lassen ED, Pearson EG, Long P, et al. Clinical biochemical values of llamas: reference values. Am J Vet Res 1986;47:2278–2280.

Smith BB, Pearson EG, Leon JL. Evaluation of normal triiodothyronine and tetraiodothyronine concentrations in llamas (Lama glama). Am J Vet Res 1989;50:1215–1219.

Deer

Chapple RS, English AW, Mulley RC, et al. Haematology and serum biochemistry of captive unsedated chital deer (Axis axis) in Australia. J Wildl Dis 1991;27:396–406.

English AW, Lepherd EE. The haematology and serum biochemistry of wild fallow deer (Dama dama) in New South Wales. J Wildl Dis 1981;17:289–295.

Kitchen H. Hematological values and blood chemistries for a variety of artiodactylids. In: Fowler ME, ed. Zoo and wild animal medicine. Philadelphia: WB Saunders, 1986:1003–1017.

Morris JM, Bubenik GA. Seasonal levels of minerals, enzymes, nutrients and metabolic products in plasma of intact and castrated adult male white-tailed deer (Odocoileus virginianus). Comp Biochem Physiol A 1983;74:21–28.

General References

Clampitt RB, Hart RJ. The tissue activities of some diagnostic enzymes in ten mammalian species. J Comp Pathol 1978;88:607–621.

Kaneko JJ, Harvey JW, Bruss ML, eds. Clinical biochemistry of domestic animals. San Diego: Academic Press, 1997.

Ladenson JH, Tsai LM, Michael JM, et al. Serum versus heparinized plasma for 18 common chemistry tests. Am J Clin Pathol 1974;62:545–552.

Loeb WF, Quimby FW, eds. The clinical chemistry of laboratory animals. New York: Pergamon Press, 1989.

Mitruka BM, Rawnsley HM. Clinical biochemical and hematological reference values in normal experimental animals and normal humans. 2nd ed. New York: Masson Publishing, 1981.

32

CLINICAL CHEMISTRY

OF BIRDS

SAMPLE COLLECTION
AND HANDLING

Most chemical analyses are conducted on plasma or serum. Because the collection of serum from birds frequently yields a very small sample size and the serum sample may clot, thereby creating difficulty in analysis, plasma is preferred for routine blood biochemical evaluations of birds. Lithium heparin is the anticoagulant of choice.

The method by which blood samples are collected and handled during processing has a significant effect on the test results. To prevent clotting when blood is collected into a syringe and then transferred into an anticoagulant, the blood should be rapidly collected and then immediately transferred and mixed with an anticoagulant. Hemolysis of the sample during handling should be avoided. Hemolysis results if blood is placed into tubes too quickly, agitated too vigorously while mixing with an anticoagulant, or improperly stored. Blood that is stored at room temperature for a prolonged period of time, kept at too high a temperature, or frozen will hemolyze.

Lipemia in the sample also interferes with many tests. Fasting samples often are not obtained from birds, because withholding food from birds that are sick is not advisable. Also, considering the nature of their digestive physiology and anatomy, a fasting state may be difficult to achieve safely.

REFERENCE INTERVALS
AND DECISION LEVELS

Reference intervals traditionally are established to produce a 95% confidence interval for each analyte. Establishment of normal reference intervals for a given species of bird depends on many factors, including age, state of health, and nutrition. It often is difficult to guarantee that a given bird is free of disease, and because the nutritional requirements for most birds are unknown, it also is difficult to determine if their nutritional needs are being met. Both environmental factors and the physiologic status of the birds should be considered when establishing reference values. Factors such as temperature, humidity, photoperiod, season of the year, and time of day may significantly influence a particular analyte. Also, methodology often varies among veterinary laboratories, which can create difficulty when comparing laboratory data obtained from one center with reference values provided by another. For these reasons, reference values should be established for an individual bird during health, and the same laboratory should be used so that subtle changes in the blood biochemistries can be detected.

Because of the difficulty in obtaining meaningful reference intervals for each species of bird that may be presented to a veterinary hospital, many avian clinicians use decision levels when assessing avian biochemical profiles. Decision levels are threshold values above or below which a decision is made to respond to a value of an analyte. The response may vary from repeating the test or ordering additional tests to treatment of the patient. Decision levels may be obtained by using published reference intervals and by applying these values to those obtained by the laboratory. Decision levels may vary among avian clinicians depending on their experience and the laboratory results. Values suggested in this text for each analyte in the avian blood profile are simply guidelines that can be used as decision levels. Obtaining a set of normal values from the bird when it is healthy and housed in a stable environment with a consistent husbandry protocol can refine the process of evaluating the avian patient. Therefore, when the bird becomes ill, it has its own set of normal reference values for comparison.

LABORATORY EVALUATION OF THE AVIAN KIDNEY

Normal Anatomy and Physiology of the Avian Kidney

The avian urinary system consists of paired kidneys that are located in the renal fossa of the synsarcum and of ureters that transport urine to the urodeum of the cloaca. Unlike mammals, birds lack a renal pelvis and a urinary bladder. Each kidney is composed of three divisions: cranial, middle, and caudal. In turn, each division is composed of lobules that contain poorly demarcated, large cortical areas and smaller medullary areas.

Birds have two types of nephrons. The superficial cortical or reptilian nephron has a glomerulus with a tubular system that is devoid of loops of Henle and is located entirely in the cortex. Cortical nephrons radiate around the central efferent veins to form lobules, and they empty at right angles to the collecting ducts. These nephrons are uricotelic and receive blood from the renal portal system. The deeper medullary or mammalian nephron has a glomerulus with a tubular system that contains loops of Henle. Therefore, medullary nephrons are involved in the countercurrent multiplier and osmotic gradient process to form urine as in mammalian kidneys. The glomeruli of birds appear to be smaller than those of mammals, however. The loops of Henle and the collecting ducts that drain both types of nephrons are bound by connective tissue to form a medullary cone, and each cone ends as a branch of the ureter.

Birds have a juxtaglomerular apparatus but only a rudimentary macula densa. The juxtaglomerular apparatus consists of an afferent arteriole, secretory juxtaglomerular cells that produce renin, and extraglomerular mesangial cells. Renin leads to the formation of angiotensin I and II, which are vasoconstrictors that stimulate the release of aldosterone. In turn, aldosterone stimulates NaCl and water reabsorption by the distal convoluted tubules and collecting ducts.

Blood is supplied to the kidney by the renal arteries, which eventually supply the afferent glomerular arterioles. Avian kidneys also receive blood from a renal portal system, in which the renal veins behave as arteries and supply approximately two-thirds of the blood to the kidney tubules. The cranial and caudal portal veins, which receive blood from the pelvic limbs, intestines, and oviduct, form a vascular ring around the kidney. Valves at the junction of the iliac and renal veins control the renal portal blood supply; these valves can be opened with cholinergic agents such as epinephrine and closed with adrenergic agents such as acetylcholine. The renal portal system aids in the secretion of urates by supplying blood to the peritubular capillary plexus, which supplies the cortical nephron and the proximal and distal tubules of the medullary nephron.

The kidney plays a major role in osmoregulation by maintaining water homeostasis and electrolyte balance. The medullary nephron concentrates urine by the countercurrent multiplier mechanism; however, it is less efficient than mammalian kidneys, perhaps because urea does not play a role in medullary hypertonicity among birds. Filtration occurs in the glomeruli, in which crystalloids and substances of small and medium molecular size pass into the glomerular filtrate. Electrolytes, glucose, uric acid, urea, and creatinine are a few of the substances that are removed from blood by glomerular filtration. Some filtrates (e.g., glucose) are reabsorbed by the tubules. The glomerular filtration rate (GFR) of birds is more variable than that of mammals because of intermittent filtration by avian glomeruli. The GFR, as measured by inulin clearance, varies between 1.2 and 4.6 ml/kg per minute and is affected by the state of hydration. Arginine vasotocin, like mammalian vasopressin, decreases the GFR and increases water reabsorption in response to dehydration or increases in plasma osmolality. Other important functions of the avian kidneys include excretion of metabolic wastes and toxins, metabolism of vitamin D, and production of erythropoietin.

Blood Chemistry Evaluation

Uric acid is the major end product of nitrogen metabolism in birds, and it is produced by the liver and kidney. Uric acid is excreted primarily by tubular secretion and largely independent of tubular water resorption. The principal site of uric acid secretion appears to be in the proximal tubules of the cortical nephrons. Approximately 90% of blood uric acid is removed by the kidneys. Therefore, evaluation of the serum or plasma uric acid concentration has been widely used to detect kidney disease in birds. In general, a blood uric acid concentration greater than 15 mg/dL is suggestive of impaired renal function from a variety of causes, including nephrotoxins such as lead or aminoglycoside antibiotics, urinary obstruction, nephritis, nephrocalcinosis, and nephropathy associated with hypovitaminosis A. The blood uric acid concentration is influenced by species, age, and diet. Juvenile birds tend to have lower blood uric acid values than adults, and carnivorous birds tend to have higher concentrations than granivorous birds. Increases in blood uric acid may be observed in birds shortly after consumption of a high-protein meal. This is especially apparent among raptors, in which 24-hour fasting is required to avoid postprandial increases in plasma uric acid concentration. The uric acid concentration also may increase with severe tissue necrosis or starvation because of increased catabolism of nitrogenous compounds such as proteins and nucleic acids.

When the plasma uric acid concentration exceeds the solubility of sodium urate, uric acid (in the form of monosodium urate monohydrate crystals) precipitates in tissues, which is a condition known as gout. Birds with gout exhibit precipitation of urate crystals especially in the synovial joints and on the visceral surfaces. Blood uric acid concentrations are extremely increased (e.g., fivefold greater than normal) in birds with gout and result from severe renal dysfunction.

Uric acid is not a sensitive test for renal disease in birds, because a loss of approximately 75% of renal function is required to increase the blood concentrations. Uric acid also is not a specific test for renal disease, because increases can occur after ingestion of a high-protein meal, during starvation, or with severe tissue necrosis. Therefore, whereas the blood uric acid can be used as an indicator of renal function in birds, it does not provide a diagnosis, nor do normal values guarantee an absence of renal disease. The blood uric acid concentration can be useful in monitoring treatment or progress of disease, however, when used as a sequential evaluation.

Because birds are uricotelic, small quantities of urea are present in plasma. Urea is formed in the liver as a product of protein catabolism, and higher amounts are present in carnivorous than in granivorous birds. The normal blood urea nitrogen (BUN) concentration of normal, noncarnivorous birds ranges between 0 and 5 mg/dL. Urea generally is considered to have limited diagnostic value in the detection of renal disease in birds compared with that of uric acid. Unlike uric acid, however, which is excreted independently of hydration, BUN may be a sensitive test for prerenal azotemia in some species, because it is eliminated by glomerular filtration, which de-

pends on the hydration status of the bird. Therefore, an increased BUN concentration may be useful in the detection of reduced renal arterial perfusion in some birds. Like the uric acid concentration, the plasma urea nitrogen concentration increases in birds, especially raptors, after ingestion of a high-protein meal.

Potassium is filtered and actively excreted by the kidneys. Birds with severe renal disease may retain potassium and develop hyperkalemia.

Sodium is filtered by the glomerulus and, depending on the osmotic needs, may be resorbed into the plasma or secreted by the kidney tubules for elimination. Birds with chronic renal disease may lose the ability to retain sodium, thereby resulting in hyponatremia.

Hyperphosphatemia can occur in birds with severe renal disease. It is not a consistent finding, however, with decreased GFR.

Severe renal disease may result in an increased plasma creatinine concentration. Creatinine usually is considered to have poor diagnostic value, however, because in birds, creatine is excreted by the kidney before it is converted to creatinine. Therefore, the plasma creatine rather than the creatinine concentration may better detect a decreased GFR in birds. Unfortunately, veterinary laboratories do not routinely provide analysis for creatine.

Urinalysis

A urinalysis, which routinely is applied to mammalian urine, also can be performed on avian urine. Therefore, the urine analysis includes notation of the gross appearance, measurement of the specific gravity or osmolality, chemical evaluation, and microscopic examination. Urine is not routinely analyzed in birds, however. Urinalysis usually is reserved for birds exhibiting polyuria, in which the urinary component of the droppings can be more easily separated from the fecal component. The liquid part of the dropping is aspirated into a pipette or syringe once the dropping has been deposited onto a nonabsorbable surface (e.g., aluminum foil or wax paper). Aspiration of fecal material or urates along with the liquid urine should be avoided. Ureteral urine enters the cloaca and is forced into the colorectum by antiperistaltic activity, thereby allowing reabsorption of water and electrolytes to occur. Exposure of urine to cloacal membranes and the large intestine cannot be prevented; however, this exposure is presumed to be minimal when urine is produced at moderate to high rates.

Avian urine typically is a thick, mucoid, cream-colored material containing insoluble sodium and potassium urates. Generally, avian urine is hyperosmotic to plasma (362–2000 mOsmol/L), especially in birds that have adapted to arid environments. The normal specific gravity of avian urine ranges from 1.005 to 1.020 depending on the species, hydration status, and osmolality. Osmolality is a direct measure of the number of solute particles in the urine, whereas the specific gravity is a crude index of renal tubule function and is affected by the number, size, and weight of solute particles in the urine. The two determinations are related, however, and both can be used to determine the loss of concentrating ability in birds with renal disease. A urine osmolality of 450 mOsmol/kg represents the normal renal concentrating ability in the pigeon (*Columbia livia*) and can be used as a guide for water-deprivation studies in that species.

Dietary pigments that stain the urine as dropping is held in the cloaca can affect the color of the urine in avian droppings. Even so, the color of urine can be helpful in detection of certain diseases. For example, a biliverdinuria represented by green urine is suggestive of severe liver disease in birds. Yellow urine is observed in some species such as macaws with liver disease, and this most likely represents bilirubinuria. Hematuria or hemoglobinuria is represented by red urine that changes to brown on standing. Polyuric birds produce liquid urine that may appear to be cloudy if contaminated with urates or containing large concentrations of cells, mucus, fat, or bacteria. Microscopic examination can determine the cause of the cloudy appearance.

Compared with those of mammalian urine, the principle difference in the nitrogenous components of avian urine is the large amount of uric acid and creatine. Commercially available test strips for biochemical examination of mammalian urine can be used for avian urine as well. These test strips usually indicate a trace amount of protein in the urine of normal birds. Alkaline urine (pH, >8) can produce a false-positive reading in the protein portion of the test strip. Therefore, other methods for testing urine protein should be employed with alkaline urine. Postrenal proteinuria is associated with inflammation of the lower urinary tract and cloaca. Detection of significant proteinuria in the absence of hematuria or hemoglobinuria is indicative of the renal proteinuria that occurs with abnormal glomerular permeability, such as that which occurs with glomerulonephritis.

The pH of avian urine varies from 4.7 to 8.0 and depends primarily on the diet. Carnivorous birds that ingest large amounts of animal protein have acidic urine, whereas granivorous birds have more alkaline urine. Increased urine acidity (pH, <5.0) may result from acidosis or increased protein catabolism, such as that which occurs during starvation. Increased urine alkalinity (pH, >8.0) may be associated with alkalosis. The urine pH also can vary with physiologic state. For example, in poultry, acidic urine is observed in laying hens that are depositing calcium into developing egg shells.

Urine from normal birds contains no glucose, because glucose is completely reabsorbed by the tubules after glomerular filtration. Glucosuria occurs when the renal threshold for glucose is exceeded. In most birds, this threshold is approximately 600 mg/dL. Birds suffering from diabetes mellitus, however, often exhibit blood a glucose concentration of greater than 800 mg/dL and significant glucosuria.

Normal avian urine is devoid of ketones. Excessive ketone formation and ketonuria occurs with increased oxidation of fatty acids as an energy source. Ketonuria may be expected with severe malnutrition or diabetes mellitus, but this has been poorly documented in birds. If the predominant ketone produced is γ-hydroxybutyrate, the urine test strip, which is insensitive to that ketone, will be negative.

Biliverdin is the major bile pigment of birds; therefore, bilirubin is not normally present in the urine. Biliverdin does not react with the bilirubin portion of the urine test strip. Biliverdinuria is indicated by a green coloration of the urine and is suggestive of hepatobiliary disease in birds. The normal urinary urobilinogen concentration in birds ranges from 0 to 0.1 u/dL. In general, this test has limited diagnostic value in birds.

Occult blood in the urine of normal birds is negative to trace. A positive occult blood reaction is suggestive of erythrocytes, free hemoglobin, or myoglobin in the urine. Microscopic examination of the urine sediment can determine the presence of erythrocytes. A positive test of the supernatant after centrifugation is suggestive of hemoglobinuria, and high plasma creatine kinase (CK) values may be supportive of myoglobinuria. Hematuria is indicative of hemorrhage originating from either the urinary, reproductive, or gastrointestinal tracts or the cloaca. Hemoglobinuria is suggestive of the intravascular destruction of erythrocytes or, perhaps, the lysis of erythrocytes in hypotonic urine.

Urinary nitrite tests are designed to detect bacteriuria. This test has limited diagnostic value, however, in the urine of birds.

Microscopic examination of urine sediment is an important part of urinalysis. Whereas 5 mL of urine is suggested to provide a uniform semiquantitation in mammalian urine, this amount rarely is achieved in most avian samples. Microscopic examination, however, can still provide valuable information.

Normal avian urine contains few cells. As many as three erythrocytes and three leukocytes per high-power field are considered to be normal. Epithelial cells are rare in normal avian urine samples. Increased cell numbers are a cause for concern, but epithelial cells can originate from the urinary tract, gastrointestinal tract, reproductive tract, or cloaca.

Casts in the urine of birds is indicative of renal disease, because casts are formed within the renal tubules. Granular casts are the most common and are suggestive of renal tubular epithelial cell degeneration (i.e., tubular nephrosis). Cellular casts also may be present, and the types of cells that are observed reflect the renal pathology. Casts containing epithelial cells are suggestive of acute tubular damage that results in sloughing of the cells that line the tubules. Leukocytes in the casts are indicative of renal inflammation (e.g., nephritis). Erythrocytes within the casts are indicative of renal hemorrhage and, typically, occur after trauma to the kidneys.

Crystals in avian urine sediment are primarily sodium and potassium urates. These are round crystals with a spokelike appearance that are refractile under polarized light. Urinalysis usually can be performed only in birds that are producing an increased quantity of urine, because normal birds do not have liquid urine because of the presence of large amounts of urate crystals.

Microorganisms in urine sediments usually originate in the intestinal tract or cloaca, and they represent contamination of the sample. Large numbers of bacteria, however, may be indicative of renal infection, especially when casts are present. Because bacteria frequently contaminate avian urine samples and multiply during storage, resulting in artificially high bacterial numbers, fresh samples should be examined.

ELECTROLYTES AND ACID-BASE BALANCE

Water consumption in birds is influenced by species, age, size, environmental temperatures, and both the type and amount of food that is consumed. Water intake often relates inversely to body size and ranges between 5% and 30% of body weight per day. Young birds tend to consume more water than adults. Carnivorous birds as well as those that have evolved in arid environments normally drink little water.

Water deprivation, hemorrhage, or administration of hypertonic saline produces thirst in birds, which is caused by the release of angiotensin II. Angiotensin II induces the release of arginine vasotocin (i.e., antidiuretic hormone [ADH]), aldosterone, and corticosterone. Arginine vasotocin increases the reabsorption of water in the renal tubules and collecting ducts; other neurohormonal factors also play a role in the hypothalamic regulation of water intake. Disorders of the hypothalamus and deficiency of ADH from the posterior pituitary result in diabetes insipidus, thereby causing polydipsia and polyuria. These conditions have been reported in chickens and a few other species. A water-deprivation test or administration of exogenous ADH can be performed to differentiate polyuric disorders of birds. In chickens, water deprivation increases the plasma osmolality from 315 to 325 mOsm/L after 24 hours and to 340 mOsm/L after 72 hours. During

dehydration and 24-hour water deprivation, the urine osmolality of normal birds is greater than 450 mOsm/L.

The ability of the avian kidney to conserve and excrete water has a wider range than that of mammals. The fractional excretion of water in birds can be as high as 33% during hydration and as low as 1% during dehydration. Cessation of renal water loss during dehydration results partially from shutdown of the cortical nephrons; it is not strictly a function of the tubular resorption of water.

Sodium

Sodium is the primary osmotically active electrolyte in the plasma and urine of birds. Dietary sodium is absorbed in the intestines and carried to the kidneys, where it is excreted by glomerular filtration. Depending on the need for sodium by the bird, sodium may be resorbed into the plasma or secreted by the renal tubules and then excreted.

Birds with salt (i.e., nasal) glands can excrete 60% to 88% of the sodium by an extrarenal route. The paired salt glands are located just above the orbits in most marine birds. Ducts from these glands deliver secretions into the nasal cavity, which flow through the nares and drip off the tip of the rhinotheca (i.e., beak). Nasal secretion of sodium occurs not only in marine species but also in some desert species, such as desert partridges (*Ammoperdix beji*) and ostriches (*Struthio camelus*), in response to high temperatures. Salt glands also are found in ducks and geese. The typical concentration of sodium in the salt-gland secretions of most species that have been studied ranges between 450 and 1000 mEq/L. The rate of sodium secretion by the salt glands varies among species, however, as do the degrees of hydration and salt loading. The primary stimulus for salt-gland secretion is plasma osmolality, but hormonal influences also affect nasal secretion, which is increased by adrenal corticosteroids and aldosterone.

Hyponatremia in most species occurs when the plasma sodium concentration is less than 130 mEq/L. Diseases affecting the kidneys, gastrointestinal tract, or perhaps, the salt gland can be associated with excessive sodium loss. Excessive hydration because of polydipsia or iatrogenic delivery of low-sodium intravenous fluids (e.g., 5% dextrose in water) also can result in hyponatremia. Hyponatremia can be corrected by addressing the cause of the sodium loss, control of overhydration, or use of fluid therapy with an appropriate electrolyte balance.

Hypernatremia occurs when the plasma sodium concentration exceeds 160 mEq/L and with excessive dietary salt intake, decreased water intake, or increased water loss. After salt loading, hypernatremia occurs more rapidly in birds without functional salt glands. Marine birds that are given freshwater over a period of time exhibit atrophy of the salt glands, thereby resulting in hypernatremia after the ingestion of salt water. Hyper-natremia associated with salt loading can be associated with excessive dietary sodium or via intravenous fluids containing excessive sodium. Hypernatremia associated with excessive free-water loss occurs with diarrhea, renal failure, or rarely, diabetes insipidus.

Chloride

Chloride is the anion of highest concentration in the extracellular fluid. Chloride and sodium represent the primary osmotically active component of plasma. For most species, hypochloridemia is indicated by a plasma chloride concentration of less than 100 mEq/L, whereas hyperchloridemia is indicated by a plasma chloride concentration greater than 120 mEq/L. These conditions rarely are reported in birds. Hyperchloridemia can be associated with dehydration and salt loading.

Potassium

Potassium is the major intracellular cation. Therefore, a factitious increase in the serum or plasma potassium concentration occurs with hemolysis or delayed separation of the cells in the sample. True hyperkalemia in most species is indicated by a plasma potassium concentration of greater than 4.0 mEq/L. Hyperkalemia results from renal failure with decreased secretion of potassium, acidosis, and severe tissue necrosis. Hypokalemia in most species of birds is indicated by a plasma potassium concentration of less than 2.0 mEq/L. Hypokalemia can be associated with chronic diarrhea, prolonged anorexia, and alkalosis. Use of potassium-poor fluids during fluid therapy in chronically anorectic birds may dilute the plasma potassium to a hypokalemic level; this also may enhance the renal loss of potassium. Diuretic therapy rarely is used in birds, but it may enhance renal potassium loss as well. Imbalances of plasma potassium may result in muscle weakness, serious cardiac disturbances (e.g., sinus bradycardia and arrest) or both. Hypokalemia can be corrected with the addition of potassium to supportive fluids.

Calcium

Control of calcium metabolism is mediated by parathormone (PTH), calcitonin, and vitamin D_3 (i.e., 1,25-dihydrocholecalciferol, calciferol). Other hormones, such as estrogens, corticosteroids, thyroxine (T_4), and glucagon, also influence calcium metabolism. The primary function of PTH is to maintain normal plasma calcium concentrations by its action on bone, kidney, and intestinal mucosa. When plasma concentrations of ionized calcium decrease, the parathyroid glands are stimulated to

release PTH. The primary effect of this is to mobilize calcium from bone; however, increased calcium absorption by intestinal mucosa and calcium reabsorption by renal tubules also aid in the restoration of normal plasma ionized calcium concentration. Parathormone also enhances the renal excretion of phosphorus to maintain a normal calcium:phosphorus ratio.

Calcitonin is produced by the ultimobranchial glands of birds. Avian C cells, which are the calcitonin-secreting cells, migrate from the sixth pharyngeal pouch during embryonic development to form the ultimobranchial gland. In some species of birds, C cells also can be found in parathyroid or thyroid tissue. Calcitonin has the opposite action from that of PTH. Therefore, as the plasma calcium concentration increases, calcitonin is released to prevent excessive calcium reabsorption from bones.

Calciferol, which stimulates calcium and phosphorus absorption by the intestinal mucosa, increases the sensitivity of bone to the effects of PTH and is important for bone mineralization. The kidney is involved with the conversion of vitamin D_3 to its hormonally active state, 1,25-dihydroxycholecalciferol (calciferol). Renal synthesis of 1,25 dihydroxycholecalciferol is regulated, at least partially, by PTH.

Birds differ from mammals by the increased development of medullary bone in the long bones (of hens) before egg laying, hypercalcemia in response to estrogen (and reproductive activity) in females, and the ability of hens to use 10% of their total body calcium stores for egg production on a daily basis for extended periods without detrimental physiologic consequences. Calcium deposition occurs in the medullary spaces of the femur, tibiotarsus, and other nonpneumatic long bones in female birds during the first 10 days before egg laying. This is referred to as medullary bone formation, and it is under the influence of the ovarian hormones, estrogen and testosterone. Medullary bone formation occurs 1 to 2 weeks before the increase in total plasma calcium concentration and renal hydroxylase activity that increases formation of the hormonally active vitamin D_3. During the ovulation-oviposition cycle, periods of medullary bone formation alternate with periods of medullary bone depletion.

Prolactin and sex hormones influence the 1-hydroxylation of 25-hydroxyvitamin D_3 in the kidney, which in turn plays an important role in calcium metabolism. This activity increases just before egg laying and corresponds to the increase in total blood calcium concentration. Therefore, the renal vitamin D endocrine system is involved in the increased intestinal calcium absorption during the ovulation-oviposition cycle of laying hens.

The total blood calcium concentration of a laying hen ranges from 20 to 30 mg/dL. Blood calcium occurs as ionized calcium, which is the biologically active form, or as un-ionized calcium, which is the protein-bound form.

Estrogen stimulates the production of calcium-binding proteins such as vitellogenin and albumin; therefore, the total plasma calcium concentration increases because of an increase in protein-bound calcium. This occurs several weeks before egg laying in chickens. The ionized calcium level remains unchanged.

Calcium for egg formation is derived from intestinal absorption and bone mobilization. If the dietary calcium is adequate, then most of the eggshell calcium is derived from intestinal absorption. Bone is an important source of eggshell calcium during the night, when food is not being consumed, or if the dietary calcium intake is inadequate.

The normal plasma concentration of calcium in most nonlaying birds ranges from 8.0 to 11.0 mg/dL. Approximately one-third to one-half of the plasma calcium is bound to albumin. Therefore, the total plasma calcium concentration is affected by the plasma albumin concentration; however, only the portion bound to albumin is affected. The total plasma calcium concentration usually decreases with hypoalbuminemia and increases with hyperalbuminemia. A significant correlation between total calcium and albumin or total protein occurs in birds. Correction formulas have been developed for African Grey parrots (*Psittacus erithacus*):

$$\text{Adjusted Ca (mmol/L)} = \text{Ca (mmol/L)} \\ - 0.015 \text{ Albumin (g/L)} + 0.4$$

and Peregrine falcons (*Hierofalco peregrinus*):

$$\text{Adjusted Ca (mmol/L)} = \text{Ca (mmol/L)} \\ - 0.02 \text{ Total protein (g/L)} + 0.67$$

with significantly low or high total protein values.

The proportion of ionized calcium is affected by the acid-base balance. The ionized calcium level increases during metabolic acidosis and decreases during metabolic alkalosis.

Most species of birds are considered to be hypocalcemic when the plasma calcium concentration is less than 8.0 mg/dL, and hypocalcemia has been associated with dietary calcium and vitamin D_3 deficiency, excessive dietary phosphorus, alkalosis, and hypoalbuminemia. African Grey parrots often exhibit a hypocalcemic syndrome with a plasma calcium concentration of less than 6.0 mg/dL that results in seizure disorders. The pathophysiology of this condition is unknown, but it has been considered to be a form of nutritional hypoparathyroidism or, possibly, a result of hypovitaminosis D_3. Secondary nutritional hyperparathyroidism commonly is observed in birds that are fed calcium-poor diets (e.g., all-seed or all-meat diets). Affected birds have a decreased plasma calcium concentration, normal plasma phosphorus concentration, and increased plasma alkaline phosphatase (AP) activity.

Hypercalcemia in most species of birds is indicated by a plasma calcium concentration of greater than 11 mg/dL. Hypercalcemia has been associated with hypervitaminosis D_3, osteolytic bone lesions secondary to neoplasms, and hyperalbuminemia. Causes of hypercalcemia in mammals, such as primary and pseudohyperparathyroidism, certain plant toxicities, and hypoadrenocorticism, have not been documented in birds.

Phosphorus

Plasma phosphorus is primarily regulated via renal excretion stimulated by PTH. Young, growing birds tend to have higher plasma phosphorus concentrations compared with adult birds.

Hypophosphatemia in birds is indicated by plasma phosphorus concentrations of less than 5 mg/dL. This may occur with hypovitaminosis D_3 (hypocalcemia also occurs), malabsorption, or starvation. Long-term corticosteroid therapy also may result in hypophosphatemia in birds; other disorders in mammals that result in hypophosphatemia have not been reported in birds.

Hyperphosphatemia in birds is indicated by plasma phosphorus concentrations of greater than 7.0 mg/dL, and it may occur with severe renal disease because of reduced glomerular filtration, hypervitaminosis D_3 resulting in increased intestinal phosphorus absorption, and excessive dietary phosphorus. Hypoparathyroidism also may be considered in some cases of hyperphosphatemia in birds. Improper sample handling often is the cause of factitious avian hyperphosphatemia. Hemolysis produces a false increase in phosphorus concentrations, and plasma that is held in contact with erythrocytes and other cells for too long results in leakage of intracellular phosphorus.

Acid-Base Balance

The normal pH of birds is maintained between 7.33 and 7.45, and the buffering systems that regulate blood pH in mammals appear to be present in birds. The bicarbonate/carbonic acid buffer system is the most important because of the rapid rate of CO_2 elimination by the lungs after conversion from H_2CO_3. Therefore, alterations in plasma bicarbonate and CO_2 content are useful in the detection of acid-base disturbances in birds. Because most CO_2 in plasma is derived from bicarbonate, the clinical interpretation of the total CO_2 concentration is the same as that of the bicarbonate concentration. The total CO_2 concentration rarely is reported, but concentrations between 20 and 30 mmol/L are considered to be normal for most species. Increases in the total CO_2 concentration are suggestive of a metabolic alkalosis or a compensation for a respiratory acidosis, whereas decreases are suggestive of a metabolic acidosis or a respiratory alkalosis, as occurs with excessive ventilation. During active shell formation in laying hens, the plasma bicarbonate concentration decreases, thereby resulting in a metabolic acidosis.

Blood gases rarely are determined in birds. Avian erythrocytes continue to be metabolically active after blood collection, and alterations in blood gas values in vitro can occur quickly. These alterations are influenced by temperature; therefore, blood gas analysis should be performed as quickly as possible after sample collection. Portable blood gas analyzers that are designed for bedside monitoring of human patients may provide a quick, reliable method for monitoring blood gases in birds.

LABORATORY EVALUATION OF THE AVIAN LIVER

Plasma Enzymes

Interpretation of liver enzyme activity, as commonly used in mammalian medicine, has been applied to birds. Experimental studies involving the sensitivity and specificity of these enzymes, however, have been limited to only a few avian species. Because the specificity and sensitivity of these enzymes may vary with the species and the type of hepatic disease, only generalized statements regarding alterations in enzyme activity can be made. Plasma enzyme activity used to detect hepatic disease in birds can reflect either hepatocellular injury or increased enzyme production.

Aspartate Aminotransferase

High aspartate aminotransferase (AST) activity has been reported in the liver of birds. High AST activity also has been found in the skeletal muscle, heart muscle, brain, and kidney. The distribution of AST among tissues varies with the species, thereby making interpretation of increased plasma AST activity challenging. In general, increases of plasma AST activity in birds are suggested when such activity is greater than 275 IU/L. Increases result from either hepatic or muscle injury. Plasma AST activity is considered to be markedly increased when the activity is greater than 800 IU/L. Activity of this magnitude is suggestive of severe hepatic insult, especially in the presence of biliverdinuria or biliverdinemia.

Alanine Aminotransferase

Plasma alanine aminotransferase (ALT) activity is neither a specific nor a sensitive test for hepatocellular disease in birds. Plasma ALT activity in most species of normal birds ranges from 19 to 50 IU/L and may be more useful for the detection of hepatic disease in carnivorous birds. Because increased plasma ALT activity is not specific for hepatic

disease, such increases also may occur with injury to the skeletal muscle. Plasma ALT activity increases with significant liver or muscle injury in birds (especially carnivores) and has no advantage compared with AST as a test for hepatocellular disease.

Lactate Dehydrogenase

Plasma lactate dehydrogenase (LD) activity is nonspecific for hepatocellular disease in birds. Plasma LD activity is less than 1000 IU/L in normal birds, and increased activity often is associated with hepatocellular disease or muscle damage. Compared with plasma AST and ALT activity, plasma LD activity increases and declines more rapidly after injury to the liver or muscle. Determination of the plasma LD activity has no diagnostic advantage compared with plasma AST activity, especially because the former typically has a wide normal reference range in birds. The LD isoenzymes could be helpful in determining the source of the elevated plasma LD activity; however, verification studies involving LD isoenzymes in various avian tissues would be required for a large number of avian species. Because avian erythrocytes have high LD activity, hemolysis results in increased plasma LD activity.

Glutamate Dehydrogenase

Although not commonly offered by most veterinary laboratories, plasma glutamate dehydrogenase (GLDH) activity appears to be a sensitive test for hepatocellular disease in birds. Because GLDH is a mitochondria-bound enzyme, it is released when severe cell injury has occurred. Significant GLDH activity has been found in the liver, kidney, and brain of pigeons, chickens, ducks, turkeys, and budgerigars. In general, plasma GLDH activity of greater than 10 IU/L is considered to be increased and indicative of hepatic necrosis. The degree of increase in the plasma GLDH activity reflects the severity of the hepatocellular injury. Plasma GLDH activity does not appear to increase with muscle injury, as do the activities of AST, ALT, and LD, thereby making GLDH the most liver-specific plasma enzyme among those species of birds that have been evaluated. Plasma GLDH appears to have a shorter half-life than AST and ALT, and it can be used to evaluate not only the severity of the hepatocellular injury but also the duration (if the insult is not ongoing).

Sorbitol Dehydrogenase

Sorbitol dehydrogenase (SD) appears to be a liver-specific cytosolic enzyme, and it may be useful in establishing the diagnosis of hepatocellular injury in birds. Plasma SD has a short half-life, and its activity may remain increased for shorter periods of time than those of AST and other enzymes. Plasma SD assays usually are unavailable at most veterinary laboratories. Plasma SD appears to have no diagnostic advantage compared with plasma GLDH.

Alkaline Phosphatase

Plasma AP activity in birds primarily results from osteoblastic activity. Therefore, increases in the plasma AP activity are suggestive of skeletal growth, nutritional secondary hyperparathyroidism, healing fractures, and the preovulation condition in hens. Plasma AP activity is not useful in the detection of hepatobiliary disease in birds. Aflatoxin B_1-induced liver necrosis and bile duct hyperplasia have not significantly increased the serum AP activity in the pigeon, cockatiel (*Nymphicus hollandicus*), great horned owl (*Bubo virginianus*), and red-tailed hawk (*Buteo jamaicensis*).

γ-Glutamyltransferase

Plasma γ-glutamyltransferase (GGT) activity does not predictably increase in birds with hepatobiliary disease. Measurable GGT activity occurs in the kidney, brain, and intestines of birds; however, disorders of these tissues do not increase the plasma GGT activity. The highest GGT activity is found in the kidney of birds. The plasma activity does not increase with renal disease, however, because the enzyme is excreted in the urine. The serum GGT activity has not significantly increased in pigeons, cockatiels, great horned owls, and red-tailed hawks with aflatoxin B_1-induced hepatic necrosis and cholestasis. The plasma GGT concentration, however, has increased in pigeons with hepatic disease, which is suggestive that the plasma GGT activity may increase in some species of birds depending on the nature of the hepatic insult.

Biliverdin and Bilirubin

Because the avian liver generally lacks the enzyme biliverdin reductase, which is required to convert biliverdin to bilirubin, the primary bile pigment in birds is biliverdin, which is a green pigment. Clinical icterus with an increased plasma bilirubin concentration has been reported in ducks and macaws (*Ara* sp.). Presumably, some biliverdin may be reduced to bilirubin by nonspecific extrahepatic enzymes or bacteria; however, bilirubin is considered to be a poor indicator for hepatobiliary disease in most birds. The healthy avian kidney is efficient in clearing bile pigments from the blood; therefore, green-colored urine and urates are suggestive of biliverdinuria and significant liver disease in birds. The presence of biliverdinemia is indicated by green sera or plasma, which reflects severe hepatobiliary disease in birds, and is associated with a poor prognosis for survival. Most veterinary laboratories do not offer biliverdin testing. Biliverdin is an unstable bile pigment that is sensitive to light degrada-

tion. The yellow color of the plasma in many avian species may be associated with carotenoid pigments from the diet and should not be misinterpreted as bilirubinemia.

Bile Acids

Because plasma enzymes are neither sensitive nor specific for the detection of liver disease in birds and also do not reflect the degree of liver disease, other blood biochemical tests are necessary to evaluate avian liver metabolism and excretion. Moreover, biliverdin and bilirubin concentrations in the blood are either not available or applicable to the detection of liver disease. Bile acid determination, however, is a sensitive test for liver function in some species of birds. Bile acids are produced in the liver, excreted in the bile, reabsorbed by the intestines into the portal circulation, and removed from the blood by the hepatocytes. This process is referred to as the enterohepatic circulation. Bile acids normally occur in very small amounts in the peripheral blood of healthy birds. Deoxycholic acid, which is a common bile acid in mammals, is not found in the bile of chickens and, possibly, other species of birds. The primary bile acids in birds are chenodeoxycholic acid, cholic acid, and allocholic acid, with the latter two being prominent in the bile of carnivorous birds. Fasting plasma bile acid concentrations are lower than postprandial concentrations, and postprandial plasma bile acid concentrations do not significantly vary between birds with or without a gallbladder.

Increases in fasting plasma bile acid concentrations are suggestive of abnormal hepatic uptake, bile acid storage, excretion, or hepatic perfusion. When measuring the bile acid concentration, a 12-hour fast is recommended because of the digestive physiology of birds. The emptying time of the ingluvies or crop varies both with diet and among species of birds; thus, the timing of postprandial sampling for bile acid testing is difficult. Moreover, ill birds often have a slow gastrointestinal transit time—or even stasis. Conversely, increased gastrointestinal motility may interfere with bile acid release from the liver and absorption from the intestines. A 24-hour fast is recommended in carnivorous birds for bile acid testing. The enzymatic method for determination of bile acids is preferred and has been validated in a few species. Bile acids are stable in plasma for as long as 48 hours at room temperature, but lipemia and hemolysis interfere with bile acid testing.

Reference ranges for fasting plasma bile acid concentrations have not been determined for many species of birds. The plasma bile acid concentration of normal birds is greater than that of mammals. The reference range for African Grey parrots, cockatoos (*Cacatua* sp.), pigeons, and macaws is 18 to 71 μmol/L. Amazon parrots (*Amazona* sp.) have normal fasting bile acid concentrations of between 19 and 144 μmol/L.

Cholesterol

Cholesterol is eliminated in the form of bile acids; therefore, increases in the plasma cholesterol concentration may be associated with extrahepatic biliary obstruction, hepatic fibrosis, and bile duct hyperplasia. Hypercholesterolemia also can be associated with conditions other than liver disease, such as hypothyroidism, high-fat diets, and lipemia. Postprandial increases in cholesterol may occur as well. The normal plasma cholesterol concentrations of most species range between 100 and 250 mg/dL. Hypocholesterolemia may occur with end-stage liver disease, maldigestion or malabsorption, and starvation.

Other Tests

Other abnormalities that may be suggestive of hepatic insufficiency in birds include hypoalbuminemia, hypoglycemia, hyperammonemia, and decreased levels of coagulation factors. Hypoglycemia and hypoalbuminemia could result from chronic liver disease in birds but rarely are reported. An increased plasma ammonia concentration with hepatic encephalopathy resulting from severe hepatic disease has not been documented in birds. Coagulation studies are performed only rarely in birds but could be used to help establish the diagnosis of hepatic insufficiency.

LABORATORY EVALUATION OF PLASMA AND SERUM PROTEINS

The normal plasma protein concentration in birds is less than that in mammals, and it generally ranges from 2.5 to 4.5 g/dL. Albumin, which represents 40% to 50% of the total plasma protein in birds, is produced in the liver. Other plasma proteins also produced in the liver include transport proteins, proteins of coagulation, fibrinogen, enzymes, and hormones. Immunoglobulins produced by B lymphocytes and plasma cells represent a significant component of the total plasma protein concentration. The normal plasma protein concentration is essential to the maintenance of the normal colloidal osmotic pressure, which preserves normal blood volume and pH. Hens demonstrate a marked increase in plasma total protein concentration just before egg production. This estrogen-induced hyperproteinemia is associated with an increase in vitellogenin and lipoproteins, which are necessary for yolk production. These proteins are produced in the liver, transported in the blood, and incorporated into the oocytes of the ovary.

The biuret method is the method of choice for determining plasma or serum total protein concentration in birds. This method provides accurate and repeatable results when the total protein concentrations fall between 1 and 10 g/dL. Because proteins in the serum are primarily responsible for changes in the refractive index, a refractometer commonly is used to obtain a total plasma or serum protein concentration in birds. Temperature-compensated refractometers, as well as those that are not temperature compensated, tend to overestimate the total protein concentration. Lipemia and hemolysis affect the accuracy of the refractometric method, which frequently is used for a rapid estimate of the plasma protein concentration. The biuret method, however, is more accurate.

The plasma albumin concentrations that are obtained range from 0.8 to 2.0 g/dL in normal birds. These values may not be accurate, however, because most analyzers require serum samples. Protein electrophoresis provides a more accurate measure of the albumin concentration as well as those of other plasma proteins. The total protein concentration as obtained by the biuret method combined with electrophoretic separation of plasma proteins represents an accurate absolute concentration of the plasma proteins. The primary plasma protein fractions include albumin, alpha globulins (alpha-1 and alpha-2), beta globulins (beta-1 and beta-2), and gamma globulin. A prealbumin fraction may be present in some species (e.g., psittacines). Normal concentrations for albumin, alpha globulin, beta globulin, and gamma globulin as obtained by protein electrophoresis from psittacine birds range from 1.5 to 3.0 g/dL, 0.1 to 0.5 g/dL, 0.2 to 0.6 g/dL, and 0.2 to 0.7 g/dL, respectively. The normal albumin:globulin (A:G) ratio for most psittacine birds is between 1.5 and 3.5. Acute-phase proteins in cases of inflammation typically result in increases of the alpha and globulin fractions of the electrophoretic tracing. Chronic inflammatory disorders such as active hepatitis also may increase the alpha and beta globulin fractions. Some of the immunoglobulins (e.g., IgM and IgA) may migrate into the beta globulin fraction. The gamma globulin fraction is composed of immunoglobulins such as IgA, IgM, IgG, and IgE. A polygammopathy is indicative of active chronic inflammatory diseases, especially those associated with infectious agents such as *Chlamydia*, *Aspergillus*, and *Mycobacterium* sp. Decreased gamma globulin fractions may be indicative of immunodeficiency.

Hyperproteinemia in most birds is indicated by plasma total protein concentrations of greater than 4.5 g/dL. Hyperproteinemia usually is the result of dehydration, acute or chronic inflammation, or a preovulatory condition in hens. Increased albumin and globulin concentrations with a normal A:G ratio commonly are associated with dehydration. Hyperproteinemia associated with hypoalbuminemia and hyperglobulinemia results in a decreased A:G ratio and frequently is associated with chronic inflammatory diseases in birds. Such diseases include chlamydiosis, aspergillosis, tuberculosis, and egg-related peritonitis. A decreased A:G ratio associated with a normal total plasma protein concentration often is caused by a decreased level of albumin and increased levels of globulins, especially gamma globulins, during these chronic disorders. Hyperproteinemia associated with normal albumin and elevated globulin concentrations is suggestive of acute inflammatory diseases or preovulatory conditions in egg-laying hens. Usually the electrophoretic patterns demonstrate elevations in alpha and beta globulins; however, increases in gamma globulins also may be observed in birds with these conditions. Hyperproteinemia associated with hyperalbuminemia and hypoglobulinemia results in an increased A:G ratio and suggests dehydration in birds with low plasma globulin concentrations. Dehydrated birds subjected to chronic stress or other immunosuppressive conditions may demonstrate this type of plasma protein profile.

Hypoproteinemia in birds frequently is associated with hypoalbuminemia and a decreased A:G ratio. Hypoalbuminemia occurs with poor nutrition or severe liver disorders that result in decreased production of albumin. Intestinal malabsorption and maldigestion also may cause hypoalbuminemia in birds. In addition, hypoproteinemia may result from severe protein loss, such as occurs with marked external hemorrhage, renal disease with chronic proteinuria, or protein-losing enteropathies (e.g., intestinal parasitism and bacterial enteritis). Overhydration during fluid therapy may result in an apparent hypoproteinemia as well.

LABORATORY EVALUATION OF GLUCOSE METABOLISM

The blood glucose concentration in normal birds ranges from 200 to 500 mg/dL. The plasma glucose concentration varies according to a circadian rhythm; however, this variation is clinically insignificant in healthy birds. The normal blood glucose concentration is maintained by hepatic glycogenolysis during short-term fasting. Specifically, short-term fasting (e.g., 1–8 days) in birds does not decrease glucose utilization per unit body weight, as it does in fasted mammals. During fasting, the greatest energy loss is associated with fat depletion and protein mobilization, thereby resulting in the loss of body weight in birds, which is seen as a reduction in the pectoral muscle mass. The blood glucose concentration remains remarkably stable during short-term fasting in birds, and it is more stable in carnivorous birds during prolonged periods of fasting compared with granivorous birds.

Whereas insulin plays a key role in mammalian glucose homeostasis, glucagon plays a major role in the maintenance of normal avian blood glucose concentrations. This idea is supported by the relative abundance of alpha cells in the pancreas of granivorous birds and a lower insulin:glucagon ratio compared with that of mammals. The distribution of the pancreatic islet cells of carnivorous birds resembles that of mammals; therefore, their glucose metabolism may differ from granivorous birds. Glucagon is produced by pancreatic alpha cells that maintain normal plasma concentrations of 1 to 4 ng/mL, which is 10- to 50-fold greater than the normal mammalian concentrations. The blood glucagon concentration increases by 100% to 200% in birds during a 24- to 48-hour fast. The blood glucagon concentration is increased with an increase in free fatty acids, insulin, and cholecystokinin. Glucose decreases the release of pancreatic glucagon. Significant increases in glucose and hyperaminoacidemia stimulate the release of insulin from pancreatic beta cells.

Hypoglycemia in birds is indicated by blood glucose concentrations of less than 200 mg/dL and results from prolonged starvation, severe liver disease (e.g., Pacheco disease), septicemia, enterotoxemia, or endocrine disorders (e.g., hypothyroidism). Delayed separation of serum or plasma from avian blood cells does not significantly decrease the glucose level in the sample, as it does in mammalian blood, because avian erythrocytes use fatty acids rather than glucose for energy.

Hyperglycemia in birds is indicated by blood glucose concentrations of greater than 500 mg/dL. Hyperglycemia occurs with diabetes mellitus, catecholamine release, and glucocorticosteroid excess such as occurs with stress or administration of corticosteroids. Excess glucocorticosteroids result in a mild to moderate increase in the blood glucose concentration (≤600 mg/dL) in birds. Exertion, excitement, and extreme temperatures stimulate the release of catecholamines, which also result in a mild to moderate increase in the blood glucose concentration. Concentrations of greater than 700 mg/dL are suggestive of diabetes mellitus in birds. The pathophysiology of diabetes mellitus in birds is variable, however, and appears to be associated with excess glucagon in the presence of hyperglycemia. Birds suffering from diabetes mellitus demonstrate polyuria and urinary glucose concentrations exceeding 1 mg/dL. Pancreatic islet cell tumors and pancreatitis have been suggested as being causes of diabetes mellitus in psittacine birds. In some species (e.g., toucans [Ramphastidae]), diabetes mellitus occurs commonly and appears to be related to a fruit diet.

LABORATORY DETECTION OF MUSCLE INJURY

Creatine kinase is a muscle-specific enzyme in birds that can be used to detect muscle cell damage. The normal plasma CK activity in most species ranges from 100 to 500 IU/L. Increased plasma CK activity can result from muscle cell injury or marked exertion and frequently is observed in birds that are struggling from restraint during blood collection or suffering from seizure disorders. Muscle tissue damage can occur with traumatic injury, intramuscular injections of irritating fluids, or systemic infections that affect the skeletal or cardiac muscle.

Skeletal muscle injury also should be considered when plasma AST activity is increased. Measurement of plasma CK activity can be useful for determining if muscle injury versus hepatocellular injury is the cause of increased plasma AST activity. Thus, an increased plasma AST activity without an increased plasma CK activity is suggestive of hepatocellular disease in birds. Severe skeletal muscle injury often results in marked increases of the plasma CK activity and moderate increases of the plasma AST activity. Plasma AST appears to have a longer half-life than CK, and after a single insult to muscle, as may occur with an intramuscular injection of an irritating drug, the CK activity may return to normal before the AST activity. Regarding situations in which the plasma CK activity has returned to normal after muscle injury but the plasma AST activity remains increased, an erroneous diagnosis of hepatobiliary disease may be made. Unlike plasma CK activity, plasma AST activity normally does not increase significantly with capture and restraint of struggling birds, but under these conditions, a bird with a preexisting hepatocellular injury may have increases in both the AST and the CK activity.

Increased plasma ALT activity may occur with muscle injury. Plasma ALT appears to have a longer half-life compared with plasma CK; therefore, it remains increased longer than CK after muscle injury.

Plasma LD activity also increases with muscle injury. Because the plasma half-life of LD is shorter than that of CK, the two enzymes can be evaluated concurrently to differentiate hepatocellular damage from muscle injury. In most birds, increased plasma LD activity with normal CK activity is suggestive of hepatocellular disease without muscle involvement. Validation and evaluation of LD isoenzymes may be helpful in differentiating hepatic versus muscle disorders; however, most veterinary laboratories do not routinely offer LD isoenzyme determination.

LABORATORY EVALUATION OF ENDOCRINE DISORDERS

Thyroid

Both T_4 and triiodothyronine (T_3) have been isolated from birds. Most of the secreted hormone is T_4, whereas T_3 is formed peripherally by diodination of T_4. Circulating T_4 and T_3 are bound to protein. A T_4-binding globulin is absent in birds; therefore, most of the thyroid hormones are bound to albumin. These hormones also are bound sec-

ondarily to other proteins (e.g., prealbumin and alpha globulin). The binding of thyroid hormones to albumin and other blood proteins is weak, however, thereby resulting in higher free-T_4 percentages in the blood of birds compared with those in mammals. Compared with T_4, T_3 is more metabolically active at the cellular level. The ratio of T_4 to T_3 varies with the species, however. Thyroid hormones are excreted primarily in the bile and urine. In birds, T_3 and T_4 have relatively short half-lives compared with those in mammals, and a significant diurnal rhythm is more easily demonstrated in birds compared with mammals. In chickens, plasma T_4 concentrations decrease during the light phase and increase during the dark phase of the light cycle. Plasma T_3 concentrations behave in the opposite manner. The pattern of food intake may influence this rhythm.

Competitive protein binding and radioimmunoassay are sensitive methods used to measure the plasma or serum T_4 and T_3 concentrations in birds. Protein-bound iodine determination is not a sensitive test for iodine-containing hormones in birds, primarily because avian blood contains a large amount of nonhormonal iodoproteins compared with mammalian blood.

Secretion of thyroid hormones by the thyroid gland is governed by the concentration of circulating thyroid hormones. A decrease in the circulating concentration of thyroid hormones stimulates the pituitary gland to release thyrotropin-releasing hormone, which stimulates the release of thyrotropin (TSH, thyroid-stimulating hormone) via neuroendocrine-controlled mechanisms. In turn, the release of TSH stimulates the secretion of thyroid hormones.

A TSH-stimulation test has been used to evaluate thyroid function in a variety of birds. In general, a prestimulation plasma T_4 concentration is obtained to compare with a poststimulation sample, which is obtained 4 to 6 hours after the intramuscular administration of TSH. A dosage of 1 IU of TSH per bird, regardless of the body weight, typically is used. A normal response is indicated by a 2.5-fold or greater increase in the T_4 level after TSH stimulation. Responses of lesser magnitude are suggestive of hypothyroidism. Measurements of T_3 concentrations appear to be inconsistent and unreliable. Low baseline total T_4 concentrations are poor indicators of hypothyroidism in birds, because many healthy birds normally have low T_4 concentrations compared with those in mammals. This may, however, reflect diurnal variation. Also, other conditions (e.g., stress and systemic disease) can decrease plasma T_4 concentrations. Therefore, TSH-stimulation testing provides a more reliable method for detecting hypothyroidism in birds.

Other blood biochemical abnormalities often associated with hypothyroidism in birds include increases in cholesterol, triglycerides, uric acid, AST, and LD. Hypothyroidism in birds also may result in a mild normocytic, normochromic nonregenerative anemia.

Hyperthyroidism is rare in birds. An increased plasma concentration of T_4 and T_3 is suggestive of hyperthyroidism.

Parathyroid

The primary function of PTH is maintenance of the normal plasma calcium concentration by its action on bone, kidney, and intestinal mucosa. Unfortunately, plasma PTH analysis in birds is commercially unavailable. Therefore, detection of disorders associated with blood PTH concentrations (e.g., hyper- and hypoparathyroidism) depends on the evaluation of blood calcium and phosphorus concentrations in birds. Hypoparathyroidism has not been reported in birds.

Adrenal

Corticosterone is the primary glucocorticoid that is produced by the avian adrenal gland. Corticosterone secretion in birds is regulated by adrenocorticotropic hormone (ACTH), which is released from the pituitary gland in response to corticotropin-releasing factor. The plasma corticosterone concentration increases during times of stress. Corticosterone also has mineralocorticoid activity. Plasma corticosterone concentrations exhibit a diurnal rhythm as well, with maximum concentrations occurring at the beginning of the day. Plasma corticosterone concentrations also are influenced by other physiologic factors, such as the ovulatory cycle of hens and changes in the seasons.

Plasma corticosterone concentrations in birds can be determined by radioimmunoassay. Single baseline corticosterone determinations may have little value in establishing the diagnosis of hyperadrenocorticism in birds. An ACTH-stimulation test may be more valuable, however, when pre- and 60- to 90-minute post–ACTH stimulation corticosterone concentrations are compared. Normal birds should demonstrate a greater than 10-fold increase in post–ACTH stimulation plasma corticosterone concentration compared with pre–ACTH stimulation concentration. Stimulation dosages of 50 and 125 µg of ACTH have been used in birds for this test.

Hyperadrenocorticism in birds usually is caused by excessive administration of exogenous glucocorticosteroid; excess endogenous corticosterone is rare. The effects are variable as well as dependent on both dose and duration. Hematologic changes include lymphopenia, leukocytosis, and heterophilia. Blood biochemical changes include hypercholesterolemia and mild hyperglycemia, with blood glucose concentrations ranging between 500 and 600 mg/dL. Glucosuria also should be expected.

Adrenal insufficiency (i.e., Addison disease) also is rare in birds. The decreased production of corticosterone or aldosterone (or both) in this condition results in a decreased plasma sodium:potassium (Na : K) ratio. An Na : K ratio of less than 27, hypoglycemia, hypercalcemia, and low urine specific gravity are suggestive of adrenal insufficiency. Because hyperkalemia from other causes (e.g., delayed separation of plasma from cells, acidosis, hemolysis, and renal disease) results in a decreased Na : K ratio, an ACTH-stimulation test may be helpful in confirming the presence of adrenal insufficiency.

SUGGESTED READINGS

Alberts H, Halsema WB, de Bruijne JJ, et al. A water deprivation test for the differentiation of polyuric disorders in birds. Avian Pathol 1988;17:385–389.

Anderson CB. Determination of chicken and turkey plasma and serum protein concentrations using refractometry and the biuret method. Avian Dis 1989;33:93–96.

Battison AL, Buczkowski S, Archer FJ. The potential use of plasma glutamate dehydrogenase activity for the evaluation of hepatic disease in the cockatiel (*Nymphicus hollandicus*). Vet Clin Pathol 1996;25:43–47.

Bollinger T, Wobeser G, Clark RG. Concentration of creatine kinase and aspartate aminotransferase in the blood of wild mallards following capture by three methods for banding. J Wildl Dis 1989;25:225–231.

Bromidge ES, Wells JW, Wight PAL. Elevated bile acids in the plasma of laying hens fed rapeseed meal. Res Vet Sci 1985;39:378–382.

Clarkson MJ, Richards TG. The liver with special reference to bile acid formation. In: Bell DJ, Freeman BM, eds. Physiology and biochemistry of the domestic fowl. New York: Academic Press, 1971:1085–1114.

Clubb SL, Schubot RM, Joyner K. Hematologic and serum biochemical reference intervals in juvenile cockatoos. J Assoc Avian Vet 1991;5:16–26.

Clubb SL, Schubot RM, Joyner K. Hematologic and serum biochemical reference intervals in juvenile eclectus parrots (*Eclectus roratus*). J Assoc Avian Vet 1990;4:218–225.

Clubb SL, Schubot RM, Joyner K. Hematologic and serum biochemical reference intervals in juvenile macaws (*Ara* sp.). J Assoc Avian Vet 1991;5:154–162.

Clyde VL, Orosz SE, Munson L. Severe hepatic fibrosis and bile duct hyperplasia in four Amazon parrots. J Avian Med Surg 1996;10:252–257.

Cray C, Bossart G, Harris D. Plasma protein electrophoresis: principles and diagnosis of infectious disease. Proc Annu Conf Assoc Avian Vet 1995:55–59.

Duke GE. Alimentary canal: secretion and digestion, special digestive functions, and absorption. In: Sturkie PD, ed. Avian physiology. 4th ed. New York: Springer-Verlag, 1986:289–302.

Griminger P, Scanes CG. Protein metabolism. In: Sturkie PD, ed. Avian physiology. 4th ed. New York: Springer-Verlag, 1986:326–344.

Harms CA, Hoskinson JJ, Bruyette DS, et al. Development of an experimental model of hypothyroidism in cockatiels (*Nymphicus hollandicus*). Am J Vet Res 1994;55:399–404.

Harvey S, Scanes CG, Brown KI. Adrenals. In: Sturkie PD, ed. Avian physiology. 4th ed. New York: Springer-Verlag, 1986:479–493.

Hazelwood RL. Carbohydrate metabolism. In: Sturkie PD, ed. Avian physiology. New York: Springer-Verlag, 1986:303–325.

Hochleithner M. Biochemistries. In: Ritchie BW, Harrison GJ, Harrison LR, eds. Avian medicine: principles and application. Lake Worth, FL: Wingers Publishing, 1994:223–245.

Hochleithner M. Reference values for selected psittacine species using a dry chemistry system. J Assoc Avian Vet 1989;3:207–209.

Hoefer HL. Bile acid testing in psittacine birds. Semin Avian Exotic Pet Med 1994;3:33–37.

Johnson AL. Reproduction in the female. In: Stukie PD, ed. Avian physiology. New York: Springer-Verlag, 1986:403–431.

Lewandowski AH, Campbell TW, Harrison GJ. Clinical chemistries. In: Harrison GJ, Harrison LR, eds. Avian medicine and surgery. Philadelphia: WB Saunders, 1986:192–200.

Lothrop C, Harrison GJ, Schultz D, et al. Miscellaneous diseases. In: Harrison GJ, Harrison LR, eds. Avian medicine and surgery. Philadelphia: WB Saunders, 1989:525–527.

Lothrop CD Jr. Diseases of the endocrine system. In: Rosskopf WJ, Woerpel RW, eds. Diseases of cage and aviary birds. 3rd ed. Baltimore: Williams & Wilkins, 1996:368–379.

Lothrop CD Jr, Loomis MR, Olsen JH. Thyrotropin stimulation test for evaluation of thyroid function in psittacine birds. J Am Vet Med Assoc 1985;186:47–48.

Lumeij JT. A contribution to clinical investigative methods for birds, with special reference to the racing pigeon (*Columbia livia domestica*) [thesis]. Utrecht, Proefschrift, 1987.

Lumeij JT. Avian clinical enzymology. Semin Avian Exotic Pet Med 1994;3:14–24.

Lumeij JT. Fasting and postprandial bile acid concentrations in racing pigeons (*Columbia livia domestica*) and mallards (*Anas platyrhynchus*). J Assoc Avian Vet 1991;5:197–200.

Lumeij JT. Hepatology. In: Ritchie BW, Harrison GJ, Harrison LR, eds. Avian medicine: principles and application. Lake Worth, FL: Wingers Publishing, 1994:522–537.

Lumeij JT, de Bruijne JJ, Slob A. Enzyme activities in tissues and elimination half-lives of homologous muscle and liver enzymes in the racing pigeon (*Columbia livia domestica*). Avian Pathol 1998;17:851–864.

Lumeij JT, Meidam M, Wolfswinkel J. Changes in plasma chemistry after drug induced liver disease or muscle necrosis in racing pigeons (*Columbia livia domestica*). Avian Pathol 1988;17:865–874.

Lumeij JT, Overduin LM. Plasma chemistry reference values in Psittaciformes. Avian Pathol 1990;19:235–244.

Lumeij JT, Remple JD. Plasma bile acid concentrations in response to feeding in peregrine falcons (*Falco peregrinus*). Avian Dis 1992;36:1060–1062.

Lumeij JT, Wolfswinkel J. Blood chemistry reference values for use in Columbine hepatology. Avian Pathol 1988;17:515–517.

Sopano JJ, Whitesides JF, Pedersoli WM, et al. Comparative albumin determination in ducks, chickens, and turkeys by electrophoretic and dye-binding methods. Am J Vet Res 1988;49:325–326.

Sturkie PD. Kidneys, extrarenal salt excretion, and urine. In: Sturkie PD, ed. Avian physiology. 4th ed. New York: Springer-Verlag, 1986:359–382.

Wentworth BC, Ringer RK. Thyroids. In: Sturkie PD, ed. Avian physiology. 4th ed. New York: Springer-Verlag, 1986:452–465.

CHAPTER

33

CLINICAL CHEMISTRY

OF REPTILES

Blood biochemistry profiles frequently are used to assess the health of reptilian patients; however, controlled studies designed to clarify the meaning of changes in the blood chemistries of reptiles compared with those of domestic mammals generally are lacking. Therefore, reptilian clinical chemistry has not achieved the same critical evaluation as that in domestic mammalian medicine. In general, interpretations of reptilian blood biochemistries are considered to be the same as those for domestic mammals, with the consideration that external factors (e.g., environmental conditions) have greater influence on the normal physiology and health of ectothermic vertebrates compared with endotherms. Reptilian blood biochemistries are influenced by species, age, gender, nutritional status, season, and physiologic status, thereby making the interpretation of results challenging.

Normal reference values for specific blood biochemical tests in a few reptilian species have been reported. Environmental conditions and physiologic parameters such as nutritional status, gender, and age often have not been considered when establishing reference intervals, however, thereby making those intervals less meaningful. Methods of sample collection, handling, and biochemical analysis are additional sources of variation in the published reference values. Therefore, published references generally are used as a broad guide to the interpretation of blood biochemical results in reptiles. Because of the difficulty in

obtaining meaningful reference intervals for each reptilian species seen in clinical practice, most clinicians use decision levels when assessing such patients. As discussed with the interpretation of avian blood biochemical results (see Chapter 32), decision levels may vary among clinicians dealing with reptiles, depending on laboratory results and experience. The values suggested in this text are general guidelines that can be used as decision levels when evaluating each analyte in the reptilian blood biochemical profile. As suggested with valued avian patients, the process of evaluating the blood chemistries of reptilian patients can be refined by obtaining a set of normal values from that patient when housed under a given set of environmental and nutritional parameters. Therefore, when that patient becomes ill, a more meaningful set of reference values, which are specific for that individual patient, can be used to evaluate the chemistry results.

SAMPLE COLLECTION AND HANDLING

Blood samples for biochemical studies can be collected from reptiles using a variety of methods; the choice depends on the species, volume needed, size of the reptile, physiologic condition of the patient, and preference of the collector (see Chapter 18). Depending on the collection site, blood samples from reptiles often are contaminated with lymphatic fluid. Most of the analytes in lymph, such as glucose, calcium, phosphorus, sodium, urea, and enzymes, are comparable with those of plasma or serum in reptiles; however, total protein and potassium have a significantly lower concentration in lymph compared with blood. Therefore, the amount of lymph contamination in the blood sample should be considered when interpreting the blood biochemical parameters of reptiles. Many clinicians prefer to collect blood using an anticoagulant (e.g., lithium heparin) for blood biochemical testing of reptiles, primarily because a greater sample volume can be achieved for plasma compared with serum. Collection of blood into lithium heparin also allows for evaluation of both the hemogram and blood biochemistries using one sample. Plasma is preferred over serum, because clot formation in reptilian blood is unpredictable and often prolonged, thereby producing significant changes in some of the chemistries (e.g., serum electrolytes). Reptilian blood clots slowly because of a low intrinsic thromboplastin activity and a strong natural, circulating antithrombin factor, which compensates for the sluggish flow of blood.

Often, the sample collected from small reptiles is of sufficient size only for a few tests, not for a complete panel. Therefore, the clinician must decide which tests are most beneficial in the evaluation of the reptilian patient. Blood biochemical tests that appear to be most useful include total protein, glucose, uric acid, aspartate aminotransferase (AST), creatine kinase (CK), calcium, and phosphorus. Other tests that also may be helpful include creatine, lactate dehydrogenase (LD), sodium, potassium, chloride, total CO_2, and protein electrophoresis. Many modern blood chemistry analyzers require a small sample size (10–30 μL) to perform many of these tests. Commercial veterinary laboratories often offer chemistry profiles that require a minimal amount of serum or plasma (0.5 mL). Blood chemistry analyzers that use dry reagents and reflectance photometry for "in-house" testing may be used for reptilian samples as well.

The plasma of most reptiles is colorless; however, it may be orange to yellow because of carotenoid pigments in the diets of herbivores such as the green iguana (*Iguana iguana*). The plasma of some snakes such as pythons may be a greenish yellow because of carotenoids and riboflavin. Some lizards normally have a green plasma because of high concentrations of biliverdin.

LABORATORY EVALUATION OF REPTILIAN KIDNEYS

The paired kidneys of many reptilian species are located within the pelvic canal. The elongated kidneys of snakes are located in the dorsal caudal part of the coelomic cavity, with the right kidney being cranial to the left. The ureters of snakes empty into the urodeum of the cloaca, as they do in birds. Most species of lizards and chelonians (i.e., turtles, tortoises, and terrapins) have a urinary bladder. Terrestrial chelonians and, possibly, lizards use the urinary bladder to store water.

The reptilian renal cortex contains only simple nephrons (i.e., cortical nephrons) with a tubular system devoid of loops of Henle. Therefore, reptiles cannot concentrate their urine. Nitrogenous wastes excreted by the reptilian kidney include variable amounts of uric acid, urea, and ammonia, depending on the animal's natural environment. Freshwater turtles that spend much of their lives in water excrete equal amounts of ammonia and urea, whereas those with amphibious habits excrete more urea. Sea turtles excrete uric acid, ammonia, and urea. Alligators excrete ammonia and uric acid. Terrestrial reptiles such as tortoises must conserve water, and ammonia, urea, and other soluble urinary nitrogenous wastes require large amounts of water for excretion. Therefore, to conserve water, terrestrial reptiles produce more insoluble nitrogenous waste in the form of uric acid and urate salts, which are eliminated in a semisolid state.

Blood biochemical detection of renal disease in reptiles is more difficult than in mammals because of the physiologic differences in their kidneys. Blood urea nitrogen (BUN) and creatinine concentrations generally are poor indicators of renal disease in reptiles; however, plasma urea nitrogen concentrations may be more useful in the evaluation of renal disease among aquatic reptiles that primarily excrete urea. Because terrestrial reptiles primarily are uricotelic, the normal urea nitrogen concentration in these species is less than 15 mg/dL, with the exception of terrestrial chelonians (especially desert species), which typically have plasma urea nitrogen concentrations that normally vary from 30 to 100 mg/dL. This is considered to be a mechanism to elevate the plasma osmolarity to reduce water loss from the body. The plasma osmolarity of freshwater turtles and crocodilians is approximately the same as that of common domestic mammals, but it is higher in terrestrial reptiles. An increase in plasma urea nitrogen concentration in reptiles may be suggestive of severe renal disease, prerenal azotemia, or a high dietary urea intake. The BUN, however, does not reliably increase under these conditions in reptiles.

Creatinine is a normal constituent of mammalian urine, but the amount formed in most reptiles is negligible (< 1mg/dL). The blood creatinine concentration generally is considered to be of poor diagnostic value in the detection of renal disease in reptiles. The blood creatine concentration may, in fact, have diagnostic value in the detection of renal disease in some reptilian species, but the test is unavailable from most veterinary laboratories.

Uric acid is the primary catabolic end product of protein, nonprotein nitrogen, and purines in terrestrial reptiles, and it represents 80% to 90% of the total nitrogen excreted by the kidneys. The normal blood uric acid concentration in most reptiles is less than 10 mg/dL.

Hyperuricemia is indicated by uric acid values of greater than 15 mg/dL, and it usually is associated with renal disease. Renal diseases that are associated with hyperuricemia include severe bacteremia, septicemia, nephrocalcinosis, and nephrotoxicity. Plasma uric acid is neither a sensitive nor a specific indicator for renal disease in reptiles. Hyperuricemia associated with renal disease most likely reflects the loss of two-thirds (or more) of the functional renal mass. Hyperuricemia in reptiles also can be associated with gout or recent ingestion of a high-protein diet. Carnivorous reptiles tend to have higher blood uric acid concentrations than herbivorous reptiles, and their plasma uric acid concentrations generally peak the day after a meal, thereby resulting in a 1.5- to 2.0-fold increase in uric acid. Gout can result from an overproduction of uric acid (i.e., primary gout) or from an acquired disease that interferes with the normal production and excretion of uric acid (i.e., secondary gout). Conditions that result in secondary gout among reptiles include starvation, renal disease (especially tubular damage), severe and prolonged dehydration, and excessive dietary purines (i.e., herbivorous reptiles fed diets rich in animal proteins). Hyperuricemia associated with renal disease and gout often result in greater than twofold increases in uric acid concentrations.

The reptilian kidney has high alanine aminotransferase (ALT) and alkaline phosphatase activity. Significant increases in the plasma activities of these enzymes, however, do not occur with renal disease, because most of the enzymes released from damaged renal cells are released in urine, not in plasma.

Reptiles rarely exhibit polyuria with renal disease. Therefore, urinalysis rarely is performed to assess renal disease.

ELECTROLYTES AND ACID BASE

Water Balance

Species, diet, and environmental conditions such as temperature and humidity influence the water consumption of reptiles. Desert species require less water than temperate and tropical species. Some reptiles have developed methods for conserving water. For example, tortoises and some lizards store water in the urinary bladder. Many reptiles can achieve water uptake through the cloaca by soaking. Water also is conserved in reptiles by the elimination of nitrogenous waste in the form of uric acid and urate salts, which are excreted in a semisolid state.

Sodium and Chloride

Dietary sodium is absorbed in the intestines and transported to the kidneys, where it then is excreted or resorbed, depending on the reptile's need for sodium. Some reptiles have nasal salt glands that participate in the regulation of sodium, potassium, and chloride in the blood. Therefore, disorders of the salt gland may affect the electrolyte balance.

The normal serum or plasma sodium concentration ranges between 120 and 170 mEq/L. The normal plasma sodium concentrations of tortoises and freshwater turtles range between 120 and 150 mEq/L. Sea turtles tend to have higher normal sodium plasma concentrations, which range between 150 and 170 mEq/L. The normal plasma sodium concentrations of lizards range between 140 and 170 mEq/L, and those of snakes, such as boas and pythons, range between 130 and 160 mEq/L. Hyponatremia can result from excessive loss of sodium associated with disorders of the gastrointestinal tract (i.e., diarrhea), kidneys, or possibly, the salt gland. Iatrogenic hyponatremia can occur with overhydration of the reptilian patient with intravenous or intracoelomic fluids that are low in sodium. Hypernatremia results from dehydration, either from excessive water loss or inadequate water intake, and from excessive dietary salt intake.

Chloride is the principle anion in the blood, and along with sodium, it represents the primary osmotically active component of plasma in most reptiles. The normal serum or plasma chloride concentration of reptiles varies among species but generally ranges between 100 and 130 mEq/L. Plasma chloride concentrations of turtles tend to range between 100 and 110 mEq/L, whereas those of most lizards and snakes range between 100 and 130 mEq/L. The blood chloride concentration provides the least clinically useful information regarding the electrolytes. Hypochloremia in reptiles is rare and, when present, is suggestive of the excessive loss of chloride ions or of overhydration with fluids that are low in chloride ions. Hyperchloremia is associated with dehydration and, possibly, renal tubular disease or disorders of the salt glands.

Potassium

Normal serum or plasma potassium concentrations also vary among reptilian species, but they generally range between 2 and 6 mEq/L. The normal plasma potassium concentrations of most turtles, lizards, and snakes range between 2 and 6, 3 and 5, and 3 and 6 mEq/l, respectively. Common imbalances of serum or plasma potassium include inadequate dietary potassium intake or excessive gastrointestinal potassium loss (i.e., hypokalemia) or decreased renal secretion of potassium (i.e., hyperkalemia). Hypokalemia also can be associated with severe alkalosis.

Hyperkalemia can result from excessive dietary potassium intake or severe acidosis as well.

Acid/Base

The normal blood pH of turtles and most other reptiles ranges between 7.5 and 7.7 at 23° to 25°C. The normal blood pH of some snakes and lizards may fall below 7.4. The blood pH of reptiles is labile, however, and it changes with fluctuations in temperature. An increase in temperature or excitement may cause the blood pH to decrease. The blood pH may increase during anesthesia, from a normal value of 7.5 to 7.6 to a new value of 7.7 to 7.8. As in mammals, the oxygen dissociation curve for reptilian hemoglobin shifts to the left as the pH increases, thereby producing an increased affinity of hemoglobin for oxygen but a decreased release to tissues. The buffering systems that regulate blood pH in mammals most likely are the same in reptiles, with the bicarbonate/carbonic acid buffer system being the most important because of the rapid rate of CO_2 elimination via the lungs after conversion from H_2CO_3. Total plasma CO_2 or bicarbonate concentrations rarely are reported in reptiles; however, normal total CO_2 values for most reptiles are expected to range between 20 and 30 mmol/L. A marked fasting physiologic metabolic alkalosis occurs in postprandial alligators because of an anion shift, with bicarbonate replacing chloride in the blood as chloride is lost (as HCl) via gastric secretions. Therefore, a postprandial decrease of chloride and increase of bicarbonate concentrations are seen in alligators.

Calcium and Phosphorus

Both blood calcium metabolism and the amount of ionized calcium in reptilian plasma are mediated by parathormone (PTH), calcitonin, and activated vitamin D_3 (1,25-dihydrocholecalciferol). Other hormones, such as estrogen, thyroxin, and glucagon, also may influence calcium metabolism in reptiles. The primary function of PTH is to maintain normal blood calcium levels by its action on bone, kidneys, and intestinal mucosa. Low blood levels of ionized calcium stimulate the release of PTH, which results in calcium mobilization from bone, increased calcium absorption from the intestines, and increased calcium reabsorption from the kidneys.

The exact role of calcitonin in reptiles is unknown, but it most likely has a physiologic role opposite that of PTH. Increases in the blood calcium level stimulate the release of calcitonin from the ultimobranchial gland, which inhibits calcium reabsorption from bone.

The active form of vitamin D_3 stimulates the absorption of calcium and phosphorus by the intestinal mucosa. Photochemical production of the active form of vitamin D_3 by exposure to ultraviolet radiation (wavelength, 290–320 nm) is believed to be essential for normal calcium metabolism in reptiles, especially basking species.

Female reptiles exhibit features of calcium metabolism similar to those of birds during egg production. During egg development, female reptiles exhibit hypercalcemia in response to estrogen and reproductive activity. The increase in total plasma calcium is associated with an increase in protein-bound calcium during follicular development before ovulation, and the total plasma calcium level may increase by two- to fourfold.

The normal plasma calcium concentration for most reptiles ranges between 8 and 11 mg/dL, and it varies both with the species and the physiologic status of the reptile. For example, some species of tortoises have low blood calcium concentrations (<8 mg/dL).

Hypocalcemia in most reptiles occurs when the plasma calcium concentration is less than 8 mg/dL. Hypocalcemia can occur with dietary calcium and vitamin D_3 deficiencies, excessive dietary phosphorus, alkalosis, hypoalbuminemia, or hypoparathyroidism. Secondary nutritional hyperparathyroidism is a common disorder of herbivorous reptiles such as green iguanas. Herbivorous diets often are deficient in calcium and contain excessive amounts of phosphorus. In addition, dietary deficiency in vitamin D_3 or lack of proper exposure to ultraviolet light predisposes reptiles to hypocalcemia. Juvenile reptiles (especially green iguanas) with secondary nutritional hyperparathyroidism commonly develop metabolic bone disease with fibrous osteodystrophy and bone fractures. Adult reptiles often develop muscle tremors, paresis, and seizures with hypocalcemia. Carnivorous reptiles that are fed all-meat, calcium-deficient diets also develop hypocalcemia associated with nutritional imbalances in calcium and phosphorus. Secondary renal hyperparathyroidism may result in hypocalcemia as well.

Hypercalcemia in reptiles is indicated by a plasma calcium concentration of greater than 20 mg/dL, which occurs with excessive dietary or parenteral vitamin D_3 and calcium levels. Typically, this is an iatrogenic condition that is associated with oversupplementation of calcium and vitamin D_3. Other differentials for hypercalcemia include primary hyperparathyroidism, pseudohyperparathyroidism, and osteolytic bone disease; however, these disorders rarely are reported in reptiles.

The normal plasma phosphorus concentration for most reptiles ranges between 1 and 5 mg/dL. Hypophosphatemia may result from starvation or a nutritional deficiency of phosphorus. Hyperphosphatemia is indicated by a plasma phosphorus concentration of greater than 5 mg/dL. Disorders resulting in hyperphosphatemia include excessive dietary phosphorus, hypervitaminosis D_3, and renal disease. Rare causes of hyperphosphatemia include severe tissue trauma and osteolytic bone disease.

A factitious hyperphosphatemia can occur when serum or plasma is not promptly separated from the clot, thereby allowing phosphorus to be released from erythrocytes.

LABORATORY EVALUATION OF THE REPTILIAN LIVER

Liver enzymes in reptiles appear to be similar to those in birds and mammals. The LD and AST activities are high in reptilian liver tissue, and although few critical studies have examined the biochemical testing of reptilian blood to evaluate hepatic disease, increases in the plasma activities of these enzymes may suggest hepatocellular disease. The plasma AST activity is not considered to be organ specific, because activity for this enzyme can be found in many tissues. In general, normal plasma AST activity for reptiles is less than 250 IU/L. Increased plasma AST activity suggests hepatic or muscle injury. Generalized diseases such as septicemia or toxemia, however, may damage these tissues, thereby producing increased plasma AST activity.

The plasma LD activity also is considered to have a wide tissue distribution in reptiles. Therefore, increases in the plasma LD (activity, >1000 IU/L) may be associated with damage to the liver, skeletal muscle, or cardiac muscle. Hemolysis also may result in increased plasma LD activity.

Like AST, plasma ALT is not considered to be organ specific in reptiles. The normal plasma ALT activity for reptiles usually is less than 20 IU/L. Although ALT activity occurs in the reptilian liver, increases in the plasma ALT activity may not be as reliable in the detection of hepatocellular disease compared with increases in the plasma AST or LD activity.

Alkaline phosphatase also is widely distributed in the reptilian body, and the plasma activity of this enzyme is not considered to be organ specific. Little information is available concerning the interpretation of increased plasma alkaline phosphatase activity in reptiles; however, increased activity may reflect increased osteoblastic activity.

Biliverdin, a green bile pigment, generally is considered to be the primary end product of hemoglobin catabolism in reptiles. Green plasma results from the accumulation of biliverdin in reptilian blood, and it usually is a pathologic finding that suggests hepatobiliary disease in these animals. A nonpathologic accumulation of biliverdin in the blood of some reptilian species, however, which are rarely presented for clinical evaluation, also can occur. The physiologic advantage of this is not known. Biliverdin appears to be less toxic to tissues compared with bilirubin, and the normal biliverdin concentration in the plasma of some species of lizards (i.e., *Prasino haema*) can be greater than 1000 μmol/L.

LABORATORY EVALUATION OF PLASMA AND SERUM PROTEINS

The plasma total protein concentration of normal reptiles generally ranges between 3 and 7 g/dL. Female reptiles demonstrate marked increases in their plasma total protein concentration during active folliculogenesis. This estrogen-induced hyperproteinemia is associated with increased levels of the proteins (primarily globulins) necessary for yolk production. The plasma total protein concentration returns to normal after ovulation.

The biuret method is the most accurate for determining the plasma or serum total protein concentration. The refractometer method, however, commonly is used to rapidly estimate the plasma protein concentration in reptilian blood.

Protein electrophoresis provides an accurate assessment of the serum or plasma albumin concentration in reptilian blood. Absolute concentrations of the various plasma proteins are obtained by determining the total protein concentration using the biuret method in conjunction with electrophoretic separation of the proteins.

Hyperproteinemia is indicated by total protein values of greater than 7 g/dL in most reptiles, and it occurs with dehydration or hyperglobulinemia associated with chronic inflammatory diseases. The alpha, beta, and gamma globulins may increase with infectious diseases.

Hypoproteinemia, as indicated by a total protein value of less than 3 g/dL, commonly is associated with chronic malnutrition in reptiles. Other causes, however, such as malabsorption, maldigestion, protein-losing enteropathies, severe blood loss, and chronic hepatic or renal disease, also should be considered.

LABORATORY EVALUATION OF GLUCOSE METABOLISM

The normal blood glucose concentration of most reptiles ranges between 60 and 100 mg/dL, but this is subject to marked physiologic variation. The blood glucose concentration of normal reptiles varies with species, nutritional status, and environmental conditions. For example, an increase in temperature produces hypoglycemia in turtles but hyperglycemia in alligators. In aquatic reptiles, hypoxia associated with diving results in a physiologic hyperglycemia because of anaerobic glycolysis. Normal oral glucose tolerance curves in reptiles differ both among species and with temperature.

Common causes of hypoglycemia in reptiles include starvation and malnutrition, severe hepatobiliary disease, and septicemia. Clinical signs associated with hypoglycemia in reptiles include tremors, loss of righting reflex, torpor, and dilated, nonresponsive pupils.

Hyperglycemia in reptiles often results from the iatrogenic delivery of excessive glucose. A persistent, marked hyperglycemia and glucosuria are suggestive of diabetes mellitus, which is a rarely reported disorder of reptiles. Hyperglycemia also may occur with glucocorticosteroid excess.

LABORATORY DETECTION OF MUSCLE INJURY

Creatinine kinase is considered to be a muscle-specific enzyme and is used to test for muscle cell damage. Increases in the plasma CK activity can result from muscle cell injury or exertion. Elevations in plasma CK frequently are observed in reptiles that are struggling to resist restraint during blood collection or exhibiting seizure activity. Increased plasma CK activity resulting from muscle cell damage occurs with traumatic injury, intramuscular injections of irritating drugs or fluids, and systemic infections that affect skeletal or cardiac muscle. Brain tissue generally has high CK activity; however, whether brain lesions contribute significantly to plasma CK is not known.

Muscle injury also results in mild to moderate increases in plasma AST and LD activities. These enzymes are not organ specific for muscle, however, and their activities could increase with hepatobiliary disease. When plasma CK activity is not increased during increased AST and LD activity, hepatobiliary disease should be suspected. Damage to both liver and skeletal muscle can occur simultaneously, such as occurs with trauma and septicemia, which would result in elevated plasma AST, LD, and CK activities.

LABORATORY EVALUATION OF ENDOCRINE DISORDERS

Laboratory evaluation of reptilian thyroid and adrenal function is uncommon. Because of the ectothermic nature of reptiles, their physiologic status, which includes endocrine physiology, is highly dependent on the external environment. Therefore, correction of environmental and nutritional deficits usually results in restoration of normal physiologic health.

SUGGESTED READINGS

Austin CC, Jessing KW. Green-blood pigmentation in lizards. Comp Biochem Physiol 1994;109A:619–626.

Bissell DM. Heme catabolism and bilirubin formation. In: Ostrow JD, ed. Bile pigments and jaundice: molecular, metabolic, and medical aspects. New York: Marcel Dekker, 1986:133–156.

Boyd JW. Serum enzymes in the diagnosis of diseases in man and animals. J Comp Pathol 1988;98:381–404.

Boyer TH. Metabolic bone disease. In: Mader DR, ed. Reptile medicine and surgery. Philadelphia: WB Saunders, 1996:385–392.

Campbell TW. Clinical pathology. In: Mader DR, ed. Reptile medicine and surgery. Philadelphia: WB Saunders, 1996:248–257.

Coulson RA, Hernandez T. Reptiles as research models for comparative biochemistry and endocrinology. J Am Vet Med Assoc 1971;159:1672–1677.

Crawshaw GJ, Holz P. Comparison of plasma biochemical values in blood and blood-lymph mixtures from red-eared sliders, *Trachemys scripta elegans*. Bull Assoc Rept Amphib Vet 1996;6:7–9.

Davies PMC. Anatomy and physiology. In: Cooper JE, Jackson OF, eds. Diseases of the reptilia. San Diego: Academic Press, 1981;I:9.

Dessauer HC. Blood chemistry of reptiles: physiological and evolutionary aspects. In: Gans C, Parsons TC, eds. Biology of the reptilia. New York: Academic Press, 1970;3C:1–72.

Donoghue S, Langenberg J. Nutrition. In: Mader DR, ed. Reptile medicine and surgery. Philadelphia: WB Saunders, 1996:148–174.

Frye FL. Biomedical and surgical aspects of captive reptile husbandry. 2nd ed. Melbourne, FL: Krieger Publishing, 1991;209–277.

Frye FL, Centofanti BV. Successful treatment of iatrogenic (diet-related) hypervitaminosis D and hypercalcemia in an iguana (*Iguana iguana*). In: Proceedings of the Fourth International Colloquium on the Pathology and Therapeutics of Reptiles and Amphibians, Bad Nauheim, Germany, 1991:244–250.

Holz P, Holz RM. Evaluation of ketamine, ketamine/xylazine, and ketamine/medazolam anesthesia in red-eared sliders (*Trachemys scripta elegans*). J Zool Wildl Med 1994;25:531–537.

Jacobson ER. Blood collection techniques in reptiles: laboratory investigations. In: Fowler ME, ed. Zoo and wild animal medicine: current therapy. 3rd ed. Philadelphia: WB Saunders, 1993:144–152.

Jacobson ER, Gaskin, JM, Brown MB, et al. Chronic upper respiratory tract disease of free-ranging desert tortoises, *Xerobates agassizii*. J Wildl Dis 1990;27:296–316.

Marcus LC. Veterinary biology and medicine of captive amphibians and reptiles. Philadelphia: Lea & Febiger, 1981:1–53.

Ramsay EC, Dotson TK. Tissue and serum enzyme activities in the yellow rat snake (*Elaphe obsoleta quadrivitatta*). Am J Vet Res 1995;56:423–428.

Reeves RB. The interaction of body temperature and acid-base balance in ectothermic vertebrates. Annu Rev Physiol 1977;39:559–586.

Stein G. Hematologic and blood chemistry values in reptiles. In: Mader DR, ed. Reptile medicine and surgery. Philadelphia: WB Saunders, 1996:473–483.

34

CLINICAL CHEMISTRY
OF FISH AND AMPHIBIANS

FISH

Blood biochemical evaluation is not routinely part of the clinical assessment of piscine patients. Like fish hematologic studies, much of the blood biochemical studies have focused on economically important species, such as salmonids (salmon and trout), catfish, and cyprinids (carp, goldfish, and Koi). Routine assay methods for the biochemical evaluation of mammalian blood appear to be useful for fish blood; however, interpretation of the results is difficult.

SAMPLE COLLECTION AND HANDLING

Blood samples for biochemical studies of fish are collected in the same manner as that described for hematologic studies (see Chapter 19). When collecting blood, emersion and handling of fish for as little as 30 seconds can elicit changes in plasma biochemical analytes such as electrolytes and ammonia. Changes in plasma electrolyte concentrations resulting from transmembrane shifts of H^+, Na^+, Cl^-, and H_2O also may continue until the erythrocytes and plasma are separated. The magnitude of these changes varies directly with the handling time and with

the time that elapses between blood collection and analysis. In vitro changes after blood collection can be minimized by separating plasma from the erythrocytes as soon as possible after the specimen is obtained.

Blood may be collected into an anticoagulant such as lithium heparin to harvest a plasma sample. Plasma is preferred over serum. The long time required for piscine clot formation may produce significant changes in some of the blood biochemical values. Furthermore, a larger sample volume can usually be obtained when using an anticoagulant. Collection of blood into lithium heparin also allows for evaluation of the hemogram and plasma chemistry parameters with use of only a single sample.

The sample size is often small, especially when blood is collected from small fish. Therefore, the clinician must decide which tests would be most beneficial in the evaluation of piscine patients. Blood biochemical tests that may be useful include those for total protein, glucose, aspartate aminotransferase (AST), ammonia, creatinine, calcium, sodium, chloride, potassium, and bicarbonate.

LABORATORY EVALUATION OF THE PISCINE KIDNEY

Both grossly and histologically, the anatomy of the piscine kidney varies among species. Freshwater species have larger and more numerous glomeruli compared with those of marine species, some of which have aglomerular kidneys. When present, fish glomeruli resemble those of mammals. Fish kidneys lack a loop of Henle, and collecting ducts occur only in freshwater species. Fish also lack a true urinary bladder, although an enlargement of the distal ureter, which is of mesothelial rather than endothelial origin, resembles a bladder in some species. The primary urinary function occurs in the caudal kidney.

Normal Renal Physiology of Freshwater Fish

The kidney of freshwater teleosts (i.e., bony fish) have well-developed glomeruli, proximal and distal tubules, and collecting ducts. The proximal tubule has two subunits. The first (segment I) is homologous to the proximal tubule of tetrapod vertebrates, and the second (segment II) is found only in fish. Freshwater bony fish faced with a water volume load and salt loss maintain a high glomerular filtration rate (GFR) and urine production rate to counteract the marked osmotic uptake of water, whereas they conserve sodium chloride (NaCl) by reabsorption in the renal tubules and collecting ducts. The final processing of urine occurs in the water-impermeable "urinary bladder," where ion reabsorption is substantial.

Normal Renal Physiology of Saltwater Fish

The kidneys of marine teleosts have fewer and smaller glomeruli compared to those of freshwater species, and the distal tubule is usually missing. Glomeruli and proximal tubules also are missing in some marine species. Marine teleosts face water volume depletion and salt loading. In these fish, some reabsorption of urine occurs in the tubules and the "urinary bladder," which is permeable to water.

Normal Renal Physiology of Sharks and Rays

The kidneys of elasmobranchs (i.e., cartilaginous fish such as sharks, skates, and rays) are extremely complex and composed of glomeruli, proximal tubules and distal tubules that are divided into segments, and collecting tubules and ducts. The GFR of marine elasmobranchs approaches that of freshwater teleosts to balance the osmotic influx of water across the gill. The proximal tubules of these fish can secrete NaCl, and both fluid and salt are reabsorbed in the distal tubule to establish an osmotic gradient, thereby facilitating a tubular countercurrent system to promote the passive reabsorption of urea. The high urea concentration of marine elasmobranchs causes the plasma to be slightly hyperosmotic to the surrounding seawater. Thus, marine elasmobranchs face a net osmotic influx of water, because their gill epithelium is permeable to water but not to NaCl. The high plasma urea concentration of these

fish would be fatal without the presence of trimethylamine oxide (TMAO), which, when present at 50% of the urea concentration, counteracts the toxic effects of urea. Both plasma urea and TMAO are derived from hepatic biosynthesis, and the concentrations are maintained by low branchial (i.e., gill) permeability and renal tubular reabsorption.

Plasma Urea, Uric Acid, Creatine, and Creatinine

Piscine kidneys primarily are involved in ion excretion and osmoregulation. Because these kidneys contribute little to the excretion of nitrogenous wastes, interpretation of the plasma concentrations of urea nitrogen, uric acid, and creatinine may not be useful in the evaluation of renal disease in fish. Most fish produce small amounts of urea, but urea is the major end product of nitrogen metabolism only in marine elasmobranchs, a few teleosts inhabiting areas of extreme conditions, and coelacanths. Little is known concerning factors that regulate urea metabolism in teleosts. The gills, however, appear to predominate over the kidneys as the major organ of urea excretion in most fish (even marine elasmobranchs). Therefore, increases in the plasma urea concentration may be more indicative of branchial epithelial disease than of renal disease in fish. Freshwater teleosts living in alkaline lakes with high pH have high plasma urea concentrations because of a possible interaction of acid-base with urea production. Plasma urea concentrations increase in species such as the lungfish (*Protopterus* sp.), which can survive out of water (i.e., estivation) for extended periods. These fish primarily are ammoniotelic when living in water, but during estivation, the plasma ammonia concentration decreases to negligible levels and the urea concentration increases to avoid ammonia toxicity. The plasma urea concentration also increases in cyprinids (carp, goldfish, and Koi) exposed to high environmental levels of ammonia.

The normal plasma urea concentration of freshwater and marine teleosts is less than 10 mg/dL and 5 mg/dL, respectively. Marine elasmobranchs (sharks and rays) have a normal mean plasma urea concentration that ranges between 350 and 1000 mg/dL. Decreases in the plasma urea concentration, especially in marine elasmobranchs, suggest hepatic disease or starvation. Renal disease in marine elasmobranchs also may produce a decreased plasma urea concentration.

Fish produce small amounts of uric acid, creatine, and creatinine, but little is known regarding their physiologic role. Creatine represents more than 50% of the nitrogenous waste that is excreted through the kidney. Therefore, the plasma creatine concentration may be valuable in the assessment of renal disease among fish. Unfortunately, studies have not been performed to evaluate the use of creatine as an indicator of such renal disease, and most veterinary laboratories do not offer creatine assays.

Creatinine is formed from creatine, and it also is secreted by piscine kidneys. The normal plasma creatinine concentration of teleosts ranges between 0.5 and 2.0 mg/dL. In the English sole (*Parophrys vetulus*), increases in the plasma creatinine concentration have been associated with renal disease, although the urea concentrations remain normal.

Divalent Ions

Excess divalent and monovalent ions are excreted in marine teleosts by different routes after the oral ingestion of seawater. The kidneys excrete divalent ions such as magnesium and sulfate, and increases in the plasma concentrations of these ions may indicate renal disease in these fish.

LABORATORY EVALUATION OF ELECTROLYTES AND ACID-BASE BALANCE

Osmoregulation

Teleost (i.e., bony fish) plasma is hyperosmotic to freshwater but hypo-osmotic to seawater. Freshwater teleosts are hyperregulators, and they face hyperhydration and ion losses by diffusion. They maintain osmotic and ionic homeostasis by active uptake of ions across the intestinal and branchial epithelium. Marine teleosts are hyporegulators and maintain plasma osmolality at approximately one-third that of seawater and slightly greater than that of freshwater teleosts. The resulting osmotic water loss is compensated for by drinking seawater. A Na$^+$/K$^+$/Cl$^-$ cotransporter drives the water uptake in the intestinal epithelium, and the high uptake of monovalent ions is compensated for by excretion of these ions via the gills. Therefore, marine teleosts ingest saltwater to balance the osmotic loss of water across the gills, and freshwater teleosts excrete large volumes of dilute urine to balance the osmotic uptake of water. Plasma urea, TMAO, and NaCl concentrations in marine elasmobranchs (sharks and rays) raise the osmotic pressure to slightly greater than that of the ambient seawater. Therefore, marine elasmobranchs, unlike marine teleosts, do not lose water across the gills; rather, they gain small amounts that allow for urine formation. Thus, marine elasmobranchs do not drink seawater. A decrease in plasma urea concentration and osmolality occurs in marine elasmobranchs during fasting because of a decrease in urea biosynthesis. These decreases also occur when marine elasmobranchs move to environments with lower salinity because of increases in renal urea clearance.

Sodium Chloride

Marine teleosts display a higher branchial permeability to salt; therefore, the unidirectional Na and Cl fluxes are 10- to 50-fold greater than those of freshwater teleosts. Ionic gradients across the gill epithelium are of the same magnitude as those of freshwater fish, but they are reversed in direction. Because the kidney of marine teleosts cannot produce urine, which is hyperosmolar relative to plasma, extrarenal salt secretion must occur. The mitochondria-rich chloride cells of the gills are most likely the sites of ionic and/or acid-base regulation involving Na/H[NH$_4$] and Cl/HCO$_3$ exchanges in fish.

The rectal gland is the site of extrarenal salt secretion in marine sharks and rays. This gland produces a solution that is iso-osmotic to the plasma but that contains more NaCl than seawater (in a manner similar to the NaCl transport system in the thick, ascending limb of the loop of Henle in mammals). An increase in plasma volume, rather than in NaCl concentration, appears to stimulate rectal gland secretions in marine elasmobranchs.

Fish have adapted to marine or freshwater environments by using osmotic and ionic regulating mechanisms allowing them to maintain a relatively constant plasma and intracellular salt concentration as well as cellular volume. Whereas the kidney is the primary osmoregulatory organ of terrestrial vertebrates, fish use organs such as the gills, intestines, rectal glands, and to a lesser extent, the kidneys to regulate fluid volume and salt concentration.

The normal plasma sodium and chloride concentrations of freshwater teleosts are approximately 150 mEq/L and 130 mEq/L, respectively. Hyponatremia and hypochloremia in freshwater fish can be associated with gill and renal disease or with acidic or soft-water environments.

Potassium

The normal plasma potassium concentration of freshwater fish is approximately 3 mEq/L. Greater than 95% of the potassium ingested by marine fish is absorbed in the intestines, and the excess is excreted extrarenally as part of the slime coat. Hypokalemia may be associated with alkalosis, gastrointestinal or cutaneous potassium loss, or nitrite toxicity. Hyperkalemia may be associated with acidosis and decreased renal secretion of potassium in freshwater teleosts.

Calcium

The normal plasma calcium concentration of freshwater and marine teleosts is approximately 5 mEq/L and 6.5 mEq/L, respectively. Because water is a readily available source of calcium, the plasma calcium concentration is influenced by the environmental calcium concentration. Fish have access to a continuous supply of calcium, so they must limit their calcium intake (unless the environmental calcium levels are low). In freshwater teleosts, calcium is transported by the chloride cells in the gills to the blood. Calcium ions enter these cells passively along the electrochemical gradient via calcium channels in the apical cell membrane. Stanniocalcin is a hormone that is unique to certain fish (e.g., teleosts) and that acts as a calcium-channel blocker to prevent the development of hypercalcemia. Fish do not have parathyroid glands or a parathormone-like hormone. How fish that do not produce stanniocalcin regulate their blood calcium concentrations is not yet known.

Acid-Base Balance

Acid-base regulation in fish is more challenging compared with that of terrestrial animals, because the composition of water varies to a greater degree than that of air. Large and rapid changes in oxygen and carbon dioxide (CO_2) levels, electrolyte concentrations, and temperature are significant challenges to acid-base regulation. The branchial epithelium is the site of gas exchange and principal ion regulation in fish; ions readily transfer across the gill surface. Therefore, changes in the water ionic composition affect the ionic transfer process across the branchial epithelium, which in turn affects osmotic and acid-base regulation.

Fish have a low blood CO_2 concentration compared with that of terrestrial animals. This results from the high rate of gill ventilation and the much larger capacity of water for carbon monoxide (CO) dissolution. The small environmental CO_2 and arterial CO_2 differences limit the ability of fish to compensate for changes in arterial CO_2 by hyper- or hypoventilation. Therefore, changes in CO_2 are too small to contribute significantly to the acid-base balance in fish. However, even though respiratory regulation contributes little to acid-base balance, fish have a larger epithelial ionic transfer capacity than that of air-breathing mammals, and they also have the capacity for a net gain of bicarbonate from the environment to facilitate normalization of the acid-base status. This epithelial ionic transfer is a function of the chloride cells located in juxtaposition to the secondary circulatory system of the central venous gill sinus. Ionic transfer for acid-base regulation also occurs, although to a lesser extent, across the skin and kidney of fish.

LABORATORY EVALUATION OF BRANCHIAL EPITHELIUM

Because the gills of fish are important organs for osmotic, ionic, and acid-base regulation as well as for removal of nitrogenous waste, changes in the blood biochemistry may

reflect damage to the branchial epithelium. Injury to gill tissue may result in thickening of the branchial epithelium and an increased distance for diffusion from blood to water. In turn, this may lead to an increased plasma concentration of analytes normally excreted by the branchial epithelium. Therefore, acid-base disturbances, electrolyte imbalances, and increases in the blood ammonia and urea concentrations may occur with damage to the branchial epithelium of fish.

Ammonia

Ammonia is the major end product of nitrogen metabolism in most fish except marine elasmobranchs. Ammonia is the most reduced and energy-efficient nitrogenous waste product of the biologic oxidation of dietary or structural proteins. The primary mechanism of ammonia excretion in freshwater teleosts is branchial excretion. The skin also contributes to ammonia excretion, especially in marine teleosts. The kidneys excrete less than 15% of ammonia.

The mechanism of branchial ammonia excretion primarily involves diffusion along a concentration gradient from blood to water and an electroneutral Na^+/NH_4^+ exchange located on the apical membranes of the branchial epithelial cells. Electroneutral H^+/NH_4^+ exchange also may occur in the gill membranes of fish. Marine teleosts excrete ammonia by NH_4^+ diffusion along an electrochemical gradient from blood to water.

The inflammation, swelling, and mucinification that occur with gill damage result in an increased diffusion distance between blood and water, thereby creating an increased blood ammonia concentration. Environmental toxins, changes in the environmental pH and ammonia concentrations, or infections can damage the gills of fish, thus resulting in increased blood ammonia concentrations. Increases in the environmental pH and ammonia concentration also can increase the blood ammonia concentration by the inhibition of ammonia diffusion, thereby reversing the blood-to-water gradient.

Both the site of blood collection and the duration of restraint affect the blood ammonia concentration in fish. Venous blood contains 50% to 600% more ammonia than arterial blood. During restraint, the release of ammonia from hypoxic muscles and the interference with branchial excretion also can increase the blood ammonia concentration in fish.

LABORATORY EVALUATION OF THE PISCINE LIVER

Little information is available regarding laboratory evaluation of the liver in fish. The liver tissue of teleosts may contain significant concentrations of AST and alanine aminotransferase. The plasma activity of these enzymes may elevate with severe hepatocellular disease in some piscine species.

Bile pigments in most fish include both bilirubin and biliverdin; however, the percentages of these pigments vary between species. The serum usually is a light yellow color because of the presence of bilirubin. Hepatic disease in fish may not reliably cause an increased plasma bilirubin concentration. The serum from some fish (e.g., certain eels) is bluish green because of the presence of biliverdin.

LABORATORY EVALUATION OF ENDOCRINE DISORDERS

The neuroendocrine system of fish is similar to those of other vertebrates. Because fish have a very close interaction with the ambient aquatic environment, their endocrine system may differ functionally from those of terrestrial animals. For example, hormones such as prolactin, growth hormone, cortisol, glucagon, and somatostatin have important ionic regulating functions in fish that are not observed in terrestrial vertebrates. Fish also have unique hormones, including somatolactin, melanophore-concentrating hormone, urotensin, and stanniocalcin. Parathormone and aldosterone are not found in fish, however, and this implies the absence of a requirement for these hormones because of their close association with their aquatic environment.

Thyroid

Fish thyroid tissue appears to behave similarly to that of terrestrial mammals. It is stimulated by a thyroid-stimulating hormone to release thyroxine (T_4), which is de-iodinated to triiodothyronine (T_3) in target organs such as the gills and liver. Increases in plasma T_3 and T_4 concentrations are associated with significant physiologic functions in fish, such as the adaptation of salmonids to seawater.

Adrenal (Interrenal Tissue)

The interrenal tissue of fish is homologous to the adrenal tissues of higher vertebrates. The major corticosteroid produced by this tissue in most jawed fish is cortisol. The major corticosteroid in elasmobranchs is 1α-hydroxycorticosterone. Cortisol is involved in energy metabolism, ion regulation, and response to stress. Cortisol secretion is stimulated by the stress response and results in hyperglycemia.

AMPHIBIANS

Blood biochemical evaluation is not routinely part of the clinical assessment of amphibian patients. Routine assay methods for the biochemical evaluation of mammalian blood appear to be useful for amphibians. Interpretation of the results is difficult, however, because little information is available regarding plasma or serum chemistry values. *Table 34.1* demonstrates the expected normal serum biochemical values in bullfrogs (*Rana catesbeiana*). Extrinsic factors such as environmental temperature and humidity, photoperiod, season, water-quality parameters, diet, and population density likely affect the normal plasma biochemistries. Intrinsic factors such as gender and age also likely influence the variation in plasma biochemistry values. As an example, female bullfrogs have higher plasma total protein, calcium, and sodium concentrations than male bullfrogs.

Because adult newts and salamanders and gilled aquatic amphibian larvae are more fish-like than adult toads and frogs, the interpretation of changes in their plasma biochemistry profiles may be more like those in fish. The plasma biochemical changes in adult toads and frogs may be more like those of reptiles.

> ### TABLE 34.1 NORMAL SERUM BIOCHEMISTRY REFERENCE VALUES FOR AMERICAN BULLFROGS (*RANA CATESBEIANA*) KEPT AT 20°C TO 25°C

Urea (mg/dL)	3.00 ± 1.00[a]
Creatinine (mg/dL)	0.99 ± 0.20
Uric acid (mg/dL)	0.06 ± 0.05
Total plasma protein (g/dL)	4.40 ± 0.30 (females)
	3.70 ± 0.80 (males)
Albumin (g/dL)	1.60 ± 0.30
Aspartate aminotransferase (IU/L)	45 ± 21
Lactate dehydrogenase (IU/L)	33 ± 20
Calcium (mg/dL)	8.7 ± 0.6 (females)
	7.4 ± 0.6 (males)
Phosphorus (mg/dL)	3.3 ± 0.7
Sodium (mEq/L)	111 ± 3.0 (females)
	105 ± 4.0 (males)
Potassium (mEq/L)	2.7 ± 0.4
Chloride (mEq/L)	77 ± 6.0
Total carbon dioxide (mmol/L)	25 ± 4.5
Anion gap (calculated)	9.9 ± 6.5

Modified from Cathers T, Lewbart GA, Correa M, et al. Serum chemistry and hematology values for anesthetized American bullfrogs (*Rana catesbeiana*). J Zool Wildl Med 1997;28:171–174.
[a] All values represent mean ± standard deviation.

Blood samples for use in biochemical studies of amphibians are collected in the same manner as that described for hematologic studies (see Chapter 20). Blood to be evaluated for hematology and plasma biochemistry generally is collected into an anticoagulant (e.g., lithium heparin). Plasma is preferred to serum, because a larger sample volume usually can be obtained when collecting plasma.

SUGGESTED READINGS

Fish

Butler PJ, Metcalfe JD. Physiology of elasmobranch fishes. Berlin: Springer-Verlag, 1988.

Casillas E, Myers MS, Rhodes LD, et al. Serum chemistry of diseased English sole, *Parophyrs vetulus* Girard, from polluted areas of Puget Sound, Washington. J Fish Dis 1986;8:437–449.

Cornelius CE. Bile pigments in fishes: a review. Vet Clin Pathol **19???**; 20:106–115.

Evans DH: Osmotic and ionic regulation. In: Evans DH, ed. The physiology of fishes. Boca Raton, FL: CRC Press, 1993:315–341.

Heisler N. Acid-base regulation. In: Evans DH, ed, The physiology of fishes. Boca Raton, FL: CRC Press, 1993:343–378.

Heming TA. Clinical studies of fish blood: importance of sample collection and measurement techniques. Am J Vet Res 1989;50:93–97.

Hille S. A literature review of the blood chemistry of rainbow trout *Salmo gairdneri*. J Fish Biol 1982;20:535–569.

Hoar WS, Randall DJ, eds. Fish physiology. Orlando, FL: Academic Press, 1984.

Perry SF, McDonald G. Gas exchange. In: Evans DH, ed. The physiology of fishes. Boca Raton, FL: CRC Press, 1993:251–278.

Railo E, Nikinmaa M, Soivio A. Effects of sampling on blood parameters in the rainbow trout, *Salmo gairdneri* Richardson. J Fish Biol 1985;26:725–732.

Stoskopf MK, ed. Fish medicine. Philadelphia: WB Saunders, 1993.

Wood CM. Ammonia and urea metabolism and excretion. In: Evans DH, ed. The physiology of fishes. Boca Raton, FL: CRC Press, 1993: 329–425.

Amphibians

Cathers T, Lewbart GA, Correa M, et al. Serum chemistry and hematology values for anesthetized American bullfrogs (*Rana catesbeiana*). J Zool Wildl Med 1997;28:171–174.

Duellman WE, Trueb L. Biology of amphibians. Baltimore: The John Hopkins University Press, 1994.

Mitruka BM, Rawnsley HM. Clinical biochemical and hematological reference values in normal experimental animals. 2nd ed. New York: Masson Publishing USA, 1981:89–145.

Wright KM. Amphibian husbandry and medicine. In: Mader DR, ed, Reptile medicine and surgery. Philadelphia: WB Saunders, 1996: 436–458.